A Functional Approach to
NEUROANATOMY

EARL LAWRENCE HOUSE, Ph.D.

Professor of Anatomy
New York Medical College
Flower and Fifth Avenue Hospitals
New York City

BEN PANSKY, Ph.D.

Research Associate
New York Medical College
Flower and Fifth Avenue Hospitals
New York City

Illustrations by Ben Pansky, Ph.D.

Second Edition

The Blakiston Division
McGRAW-HILL BOOK COMPANY, INC.
New York Toronto Sydney London

To Grace and Julie,
our devoted wives,
whose patience, understanding, and encouragement
made this book possible

A Functional Approach to NEUROANATOMY

 Library of Congress Catalog Card Number: 67-13902

30467

1234567890 QB 732106987

PREFACE

This book was written primarily with the medical student in mind; it is designed to meet the needs of basic courses in neuroanatomy at a time when time itself has become a great factor in medical education. So overwhelming is the material confronting the medical student that a clear, concise textbook, systematically organized, is almost a necessity if he is to achieve any semblance of comprehension and understanding in the limited time afforded each subject he undertakes.

Our approach is functional, to be sure, but above all it is systematic, strictly adhering to the systems once the basic fundamental considerations of evolution, development, and anatomy have been covered. The early chapters dealing with the basic fundamentals of the nervous system are comprehensive and thoroughly illustrated, nonetheless, since we have always felt that a solid, basic comprehension of the fundamentals of embryology and anatomy is an essential prerequisite for an understanding of the intricacies of both the normal and the abnormal functions of the nervous system. To us, a basic foundation and systematic method seem to be the most logical, the most interesting, and at the same time, the most utilitarian approach to a subject whose name itself somehow seems to imply complexity.

It might be argued that too great stress is placed on reflex activity and the descriptions of the reflex pathways in each of the system chapters. However, one must admit that though the conscious pathways are those most likely to be presented and described in many courses or discussions of human neuroanatomy, it is the reflex mechanisms which are the foundation upon which the more complex nervous system is built. Since the reflexes represent the first order of nervous activity in the body, they are placed first in the discussion. Furthermore, since reflexes play such an essential part in our every movement and reaction, we feel justified in our elaboration and complete discussion of their activity.

To further our aim, the illustrations are presented not only to clarify but to amplify the text. They have been simplified into concise black and white line drawings with a minimum of labeling. In many instances numerous small illustrations are used in lieu of one or two large overwhelming drawings in order to eliminate some of the involved complications which often defeat the purpose of illustrations. It is our hope that the student will be able to direct his efforts to learning from the illustrations rather than to deciphering them.

In common with other teachers in all fields, it has been our observation that repetition is an essential of the learning process. Thus, every chapter is followed by a summary which should enable, perhaps even encourage, the student to work frequent reviews into an already overcrowded schedule.

Considerable emphasis is placed on clinical considerations. This, we feel, is important, since it strengthens motivation not only by demonstrating a reason for learning the material as it is presented, but it also assuages the appetite of the neophyte doctor for all things directly pertaining to the practice of medicine. This is a spark lodged in the hearts of all beginners which should be fanned, not dampened, at the outset of their young careers.

It should be obvious that a book of this kind could not be written without the published findings of many individuals and teams of investigators from all over the world. However, the list of contributors is now becoming so vast that to be completely impartial a distractingly large, overwhelming list of references would be a necessity. We have, therefore, omitted from the text proper all specific bibliographic references, not because the authors have failed to appreciate the importance of the contributors in this field, but for the sake of smoother reading. Thus, at the risk of offending countless men whose works are worthy of note we thought it preferable to place a modest, general bibliography at the end of the book.

We are indebted to McGraw-Hill Book Company, W. B. Saunders Company, J. B. Lippincott Company, Williams & Wilkins Company, and Little, Brown and Company, for permission to use or modify illustrations from several of their publications which in each case have been duly accredited.

We are grateful to J. Harold Walton, M.D., editor of Ciba Clinical Symposium, for permission to modify figures 21-2 and 21-10 through 21-18, inclusive, based upon original paintings of Dr. Frank Netter from the article, "The Hypothalamus," Ciba Clinical Symposia, Vol. 8, No. 4, by W. R. Ingram, Ph.D.; Mr. Joseph Kerrigan, General Publicity and Projects Supervisor of the Schering Corporation, for permission to use or modify material from certain of their publications; Drs. Alfred Ebel, Nicholas Panin, Milton Holtzman, Jose Cibeira, and Andor Weiss for the use of their outline on Common Vascular Brain Syndromes; Drs. Frank Borrelli, Chairman, and Rita Girolamo, Professor, Department of Radiology, New York Medical College, for making the X-rays, arteriograms, and brain scans available to us.

The authors also wish to express their appreciation to the Research Committee of the New York Medical College for their support of the project, and to our students, especially Drs. Gustave Mork, Charles Burton, and Harvey Cooper for reading and making suggestions concerning the manuscript. Particular thanks go to Dr. Iris F. Norstrand of King's County Hospital and Dr. William K. Jordan of the University of Arkansas for their careful review of clinical aspects, especially the material on clinical neurologic testing techniques.

We also deeply appreciate the guidance, advice, and generosity of the publisher, McGraw-Hill Book Company of New York, without which the book could not have been prepared.

E. Lawrence House
Ben Pansky

CONTENTS

1 TRENDS IN EVOLUTION

It it beyond the scope of this chapter to cover exhaustively the evolution of the central nervous system. All that can be accomplished is to give some insight into the origins of certain portions of the system and indicate how these portions are related to the human brain. Little stress has been put upon the specific time or place in phylogeny where certain parts came into being, for to the authors, the "why" seemed more important than the "how" or "when."

There are basic properties in all protoplasm that set it apart from the inorganic. Among these properties is the ability to transmit an impulse. This is known as *conductivity*. Another characteristic is *contractility*. Fundamentally, this is the shortening of the cell along a given axis.

In order to survive, a cell must maintain an intimate relationship with its surroundings, the *environment*. This is true in two senses: the organism must make adjustments to changing conditions in the environment; and through the environment come nutritive substances essential for the life of the organism. For example, the single-celled amoeba, exposed to excessive warmth on one side, reacts to the temperature change by alternately pushing out and drawing in its pseudopodia. In order to accomplish this, information concerning the change must be conducted from the affected side across the cell to initiate the movement that occurs there. Similarly, food particles produce a local change, initiating the development of a current within the cell, which responds by sending out processes to engulf the particle.

With the evolution of the multicellular animal (Metazoa) new problems arise. Where once the entire cell surface of the amoeba was in contact with the surroundings, in the Metazoa there are many cells located some distance from the exterior. Thus, the deep cells require a different type of adjustment than those located superficially. Hence, the Metazoa must localize a certain amount of protoplasmic specialization. On this account, the property of conduction becomes concentrated in some cells while that of contractility is concentrated in others. Thus, *nervous* and *muscular* tissue develop.

If muscular activity is to be translated into purposeful movement, it first does so in response to environmental changes. Hence, it is essential that a mechanism be developed which will carry information concerning surface changes to the deeper-lying tissue. Responding to this need, cells, originally located at the surface, become elongated, one end remaining exposed to the exterior while the other extends inward to the muscle (Fig. 1-1). In this manner, the unit of structure of the nervous system, the *neuron,* evolved.

With an ever-increasing number of cells associated with an increase in activities, environmental changes assume greater significance. Therefore, specialized endings, the *receptors,* arise. The receptors transform various kinds of physical or chemical changes into nerve impulses which can then be transmitted to the muscle, the *effector*. Since primitive receptors are situated at the surface, they are classified as *exteroceptors* or *contact exteroceptors.*

To a certain point in phylogeny (i.e., the coelenterates—jellyfish, corals, and hydroids) it is possible to carry on activities with a diffuse arrangement of neurons (Fig. 1-2). However, in

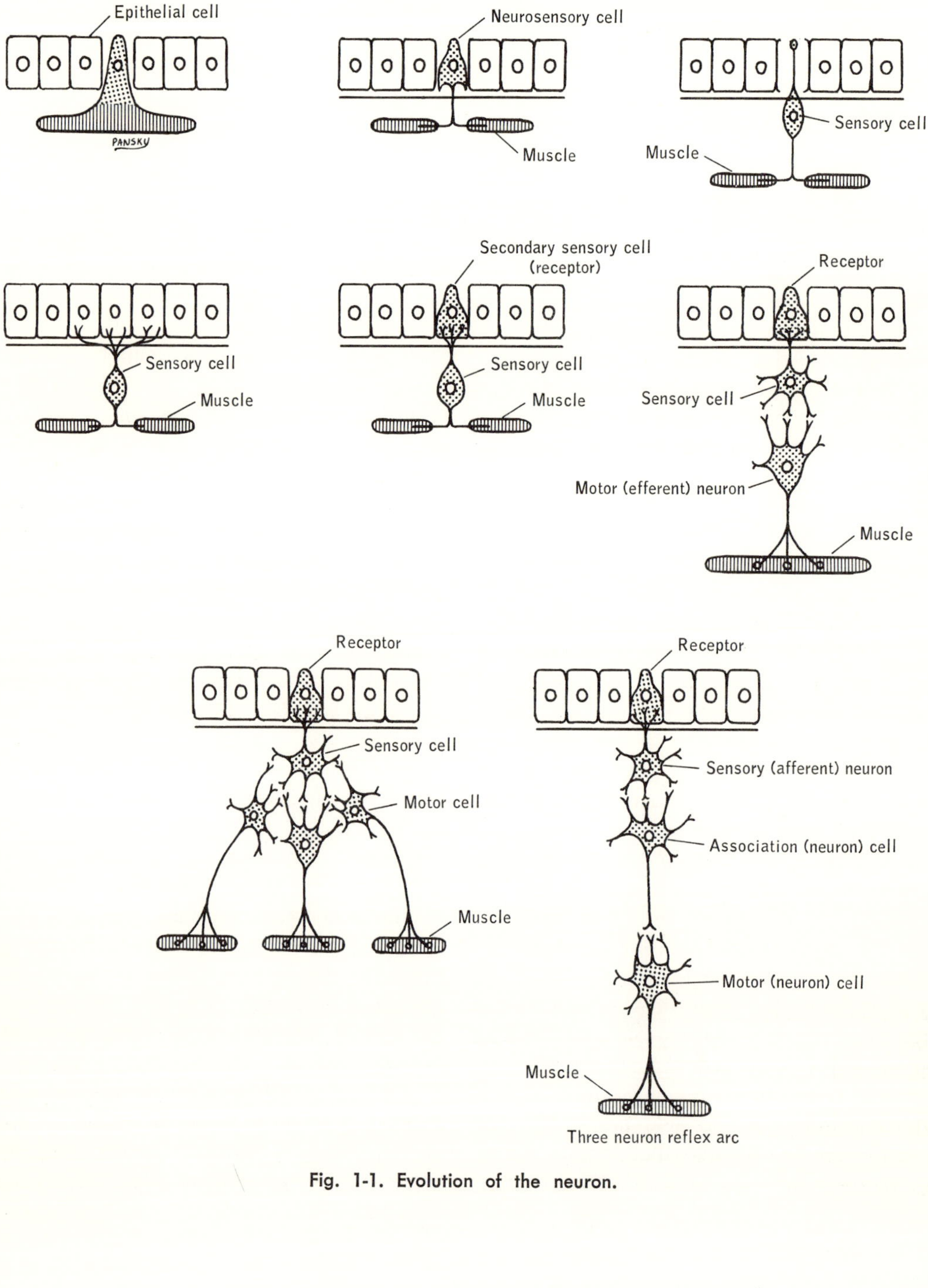

Fig. 1-1. Evolution of the neuron.

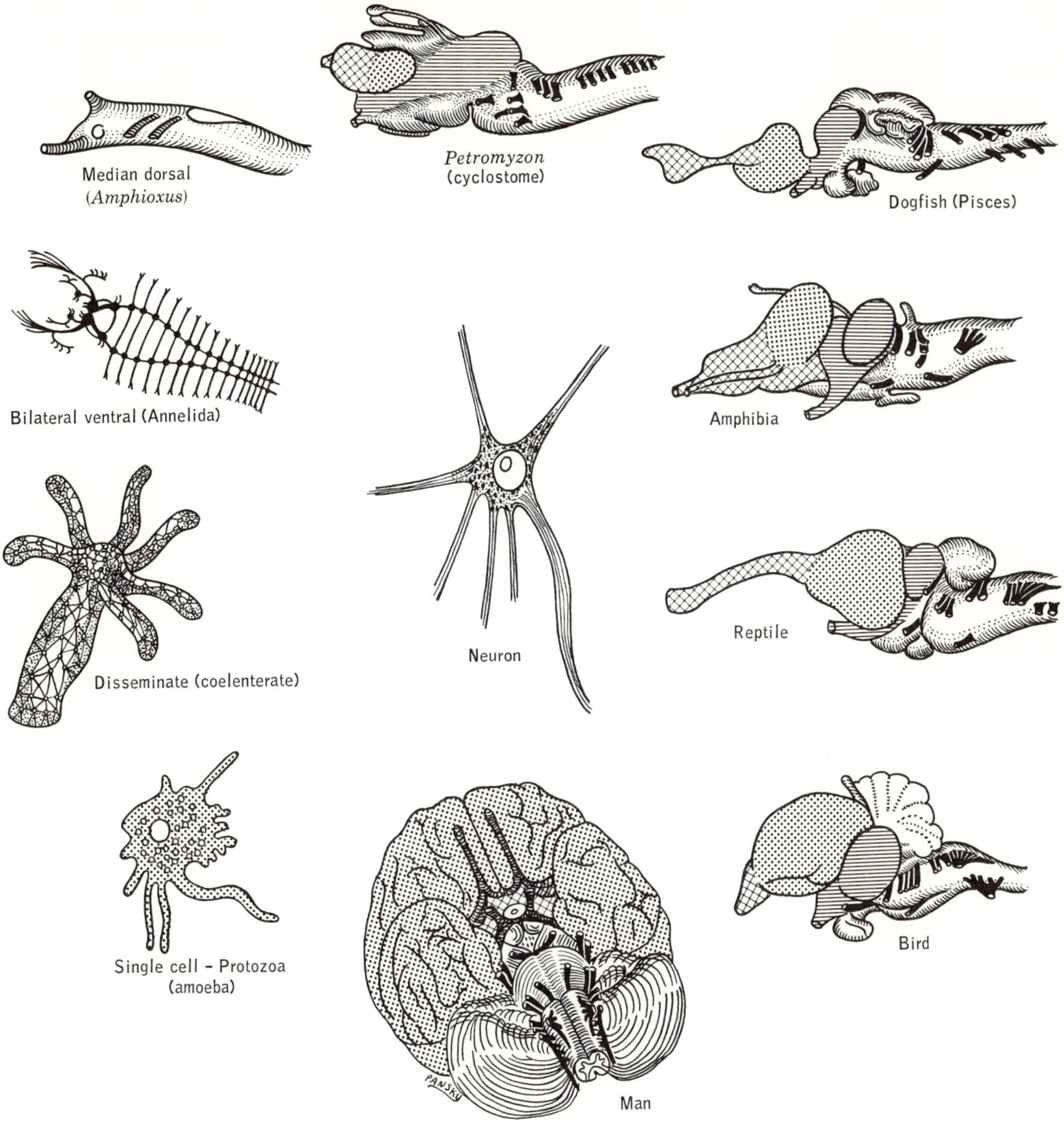

Fig. 1-2. Evolution of the central nervous system.

more complex forms, such a plan would be too cumbersome. For this reason, the establishment of the central nervous system becomes a necessity.

With the appearance of a center, the neuron now carries an impulse from the receptor to the center rather than to the effector, directly. Since this impulse is directed toward the center, such a neuron is classified as *afferent* (*sensory*). To produce activity of the muscle, another neuron, beginning in the central nervous system, carries impulses away from the latter toward the effector. This is the *efferent* (*motor*) neuron (Fig. 1-1). The afferent and efferent neurons are not in physical continuity, the fine terminals of the former merely making contact with the latter. This contact zone, where an impulse must be transferred from one fiber to another, is called the *synapse*. In this way is established the simplest form of *reflex arc,* composed of an afferent neuron with its receptor, a center where the synapse occurs, and the efferent neuron with its effector (Fig. 1-1). Primitive circuits of this type are not uncommon among cyclostomes (lampreys and hagfish, Fig. 1-2).

Certain features of this primordial system remain basically unchanged regardless of subsequent complexities. First, the cell bodies of afferent neurons remain outside the central nervous system, usually grouped together in structures known as *ganglia*. The actual collection of all sensory cells in ganglia, however, is not seen in animals below plagiostomes (sharks and dogfish). Second, the transfer of an impulse from the afferent neuron occurs in the center. Third, the cell bodies of efferent neurons lie in the central nervous system.

As animal complexity progresses, a picture of ever-increasing body length is apparent. This leads to the development of new areas of muscle essential to the over-all movement of the body, e.g., when some environmental change occurs at the caudal end of the animal, it is necessary for muscles at the anterior end to contract. In response to such demands, several changes occur. First, the primitive nervous system elongates.[1] Second, the afferent neuron, upon entry into the center, bifurcates into ascending and descending branches. In this way, contacts with efferent neurons at other levels are made possible. This phenomenon can be demonstrated in *Amphioxus*. Third, a new neuron appears, interposed between the afferent and efferent fiber. Such an arrangement is of particular significance since it increases the number of synapses enormously. This new fiber is referred to as the *association neuron,* present in cyclostomes. With the coming of this fiber, the *three-neuron reflex arc* is formed (Fig. 1-1). The establishment of long bundles of association neurons makes possible the activation of the entire effector apparatus.

As soon as one cell layer is superimposed upon another, an internal environment is created. This is further complicated by the development of internal organs (viscera), each specialized for the performance of a specific function. However, if these organs are to take their place in the total body economy, it is necessary for them also to respond to change. Therefore, a portion of the nervous system evolves for the purpose of controlling the viscera. This is the *autonomic (visceral) system.* Even in plagiostomes (Fig. 1-1), the basis for such a mechanism has been laid down, but in a very diffuse arrangement. Birds, however, are the first to display all the parts seen in man.

With each upward step in evolution, other problems appear. One of the earliest of these is the maintenance of *equilibrium.* Another arises with the budding of limbs and the development of articulations. It is easily understood that the movement of the appendages can be achieved only through the alternating contractions of opposing sets of muscles. It should also be clear that the simple contraction of a muscle is not enough to produce the desired effect but that varying degrees of contraction are also essential. To meet these conditions, additional neural elements must be added. First, information about the extent of muscle contraction must reach the center, together with impulses arising at or near articulations. Hence, special receptors appear, in muscles, tendons, and joints, associated with a new set of afferent neurons. Thus, the *proprioceptive system* originates. In order to accommodate such new mechanisms, the central nervous system expands, an enlargement appearing at the rostral end of the cord. This is the *hindbrain,* or *rhombencephalon,* a structure already established in *Amphioxus.* Next, to satisfy the demands of equilibrium, there develops a fluid-filled, tubulosaccular structure equipped with hair cell receptors. The latter are related to

[1] The definitive phylogenetic link between the diffuse system of lower forms and the true cord of vertebrates is in dispute. A well-defined cord is already present in *Amphioxus* (Fig. 1-2).

afferent neurons which terminate in the hindbrain—*the vestibular system.* This system is enhanced, particularly in fish and aquatic Amphibia, by the lateral line apparatus. Through such circuits, the reflex control of the body musculature necessary in maintaining the animal in natural balance is made possible. A third change is concerned with the coordination of reflexes initiated through both the proprioceptive and vestibular systems. This requires the development of a special coordination center, conveniently located with respect to both systems. Hence, a small outgrowth from the dorsal side of the hindbrain, near its rostral end, occurs. This is the *cerebellum.* Although there is evidence that this region is present in cyclostomes, it becomes grossly discernible for the first time in plagiostomes.

The head, possessing such new features as the mouth and its associated structures, particularly the branchial apparatus (gill arches), is in the process of developing.[2] Since the portion of the brain lying nearest to these parts is the hindbrain, the efferent neurons regulating their movement originate at that brain level.

A greater awareness of environmental changes at some distance from the body not only enhances the chances for survival but also facilitates the finding of food and the location of a mate. This leads to the formation of a special set of receptors, the *teloreceptors* (distance receptors).

Probably the first to appear among the special senses is *gustation* (taste), the receptors for which doubtless represent a further specialization of the more primitive chemoreceptors of the skin. Taste buds have been demonstrated both externally and internally, on the gills and in the pharynx, in cyclostomes. The concentration of these receptors on the tongue is seen for the first time in land Amphibia.

About the same time, the *olfactory* apparatus appears. Like the gustatory receptors, olfactory cells develop from tissue originally lying on the body surface. Early in phylogenesis such chemoreceptors become concentrated near the rostral end of the primitive head. Since smell plays such a vital role in locating food, the olfactory organ becomes closely related to the mouth. Later, the nose assumes importance in both the detection of natural enemies and the recognition of the opposite sex. Furthermore, this system plays a part in the preparation of certain viscera for the ingestion of food.

With the increasing importance of the olfactory system, large brain centers, where associations may be made to activate both muscles and viscera, are necessary. Consequently, in a region adjacent to the olfactory receptors but well rostral to the hindbrain, a new part develops. Because of its anterior location, it is known as the *forebrain,* or *prosencephalon.* From its inception, this new portion shows a tendency toward bilaterality, the more lateral outgrowths representing simple *cerebral hemispheres,* while the medial portion, between the former, is the *diencephalon.* On a very primitive scale, these parts may be seen in cyclostomes (Fig. 1-2).

The *auditory system* appears as a modification of an outgrowth from the vestibular mechanism. A tubular prolongation, extending from one of the vestibular sacs, coils upon itself several times, while new hair cells project into the lumen. This is the *cochlear duct,* the hair cells of which are adapted to the selection of the atmospheric waves known as sound. The afferent neurons associated with these receptors terminate in the hindbrain.

The retina, or light-sensitive portion of the eye, containing the receptors for the visual system, is a modification of primitive photoreceptors originally located in the skin of lower animals. As in the cochlea, its structure is too complex to describe here.

For anyone who has watched animals or who has thought about his own purely reflex reactions to sight or sound, it is easy to understand the need for brain centers where impulses carried by these new systems can be dispersed to the entire body musculature. Therefore, an enlargement occurs in the region between the hindbrain and forebrain. This is the *midbrain,* or

[2] Branchiomeric nuclei are becoming distinct in *Petromyzon* (lamprey).

mesencephalon. The first animals to show visual reflex centers, the *corpora bigemina,* in the mesencephalon are the plagiostomes.

At this point, it might be advantageous to study the gross aspects of the central nervous system of an animal which has evolved many of the parts previously mentioned and whose nervous system, therefore, with certain functional modifications, represents the human brain stem. For this purpose, the dogfish is an excellent subject (Figs. 1-3, 1-4).

Animals whose nervous systems have attained even the relatively simple state seen in the dogfish require a center for better integration and coordination of afferent impulses. The diencephalon, up to this stage, represents the highest level of the sensory mechanism. At the same time, bundles of secondary neurons arise in synaptic relation with the terminations of afferent neurons. These secondary neurons carry sensory impulses rostrally into the diencephalon, especially into that portion of it known as the *thalamus.* Each of the sensory modalities, whether pain, temperature, touch, proprioception, sight, or sound, has such secondary connections. The *hypothalamus,* the most ventral part

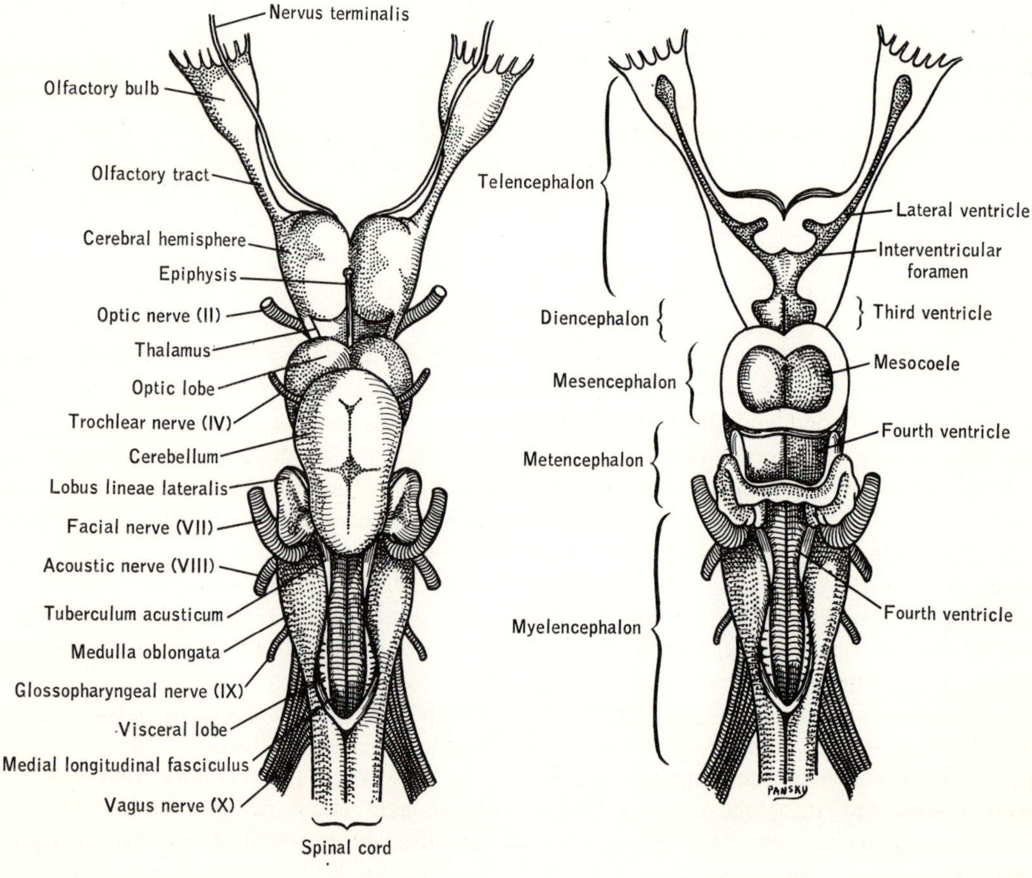

Fig. 1-3. *A.* Dorsal view of the brain of the dogfish. *B.* Dorsal view of the brain of the dogfish with the ventricles open. (*Adapted from Ranson and Clark, The Anatomy of the Nervous System, 10th ed., W. B. Saunders Company, Philadelphia, 1959*).

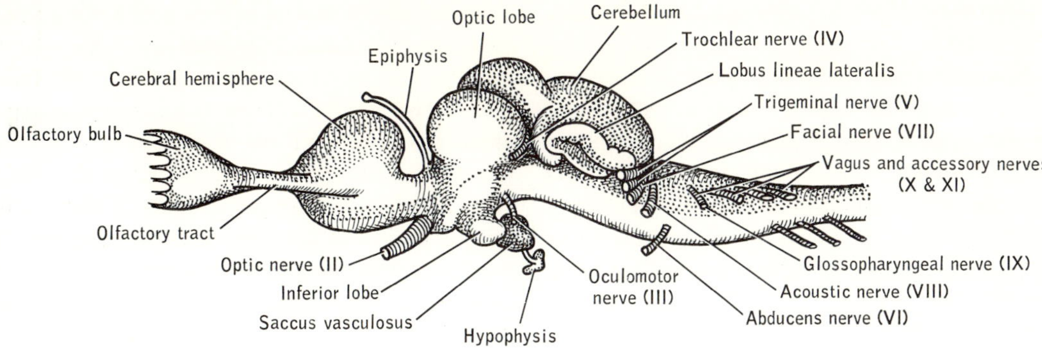

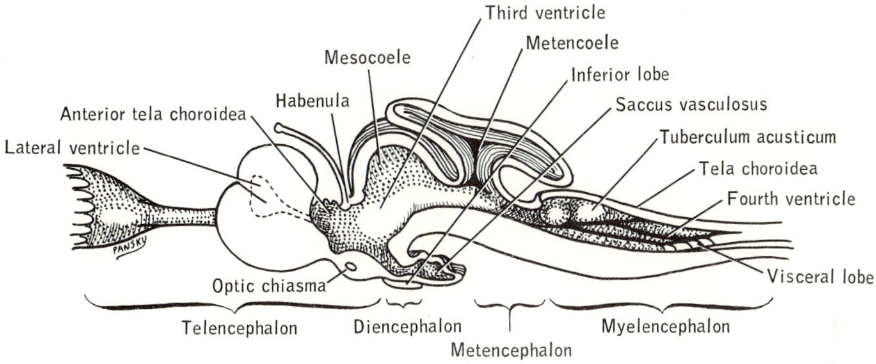

Fig. 1-4. *Above,* lateral view of the brain of the dogfish. *Below,* midsagittal section of the brain of the dogfish. (*Adapted from Ranson and Clark, The Anatomy of the Nervous System, 10th ed., W. B. Saunders Company, Philadelphia, 1959.*)

of the diencephalon, becomes particularly important as a higher control center for visceral activity.

The first impression of the human brain, when comparing it with that of the dogfish, is that everything has changed. However, one should constantly keep in mind that with each step upward in the evolutionary series, new parts are merely added to the old; sometimes they are modified and often almost obscured, but nothing is thrown away. Furthermore, some parts tend to grow enormously, while others remain relatively underdeveloped.

The most striking difference noticed in the brain of man is the tremendous growth of the cerebral hemispheres (Fig. 1-2). This growth is primarily because of the stablishment of a *reception center* for afferent impulses where they can be *perceived* and *interpreted* as pain, touch, sound, etc.; a place for the storage of sensory information in the *learning* process; and a place for the retention of sensation-action patterns, which is *memory*. Finally, such areas as these must be connected with the newly acquired *motor regions* of the hemisphere in order to initiate voluntary action.

Another obvious change in the human brain occurs in order to increase the area of the hemisphere without enlarging the brain, as a whole, to a disproportionate size. Hence, the superficial, cellular covering of the hemispheres, called the *cortex,* is thrown into prominent folds, or *gyri,* separated by grooves, the *sulci.*

One of the structures which has become completely buried by the growth of the hemispheres is the diencephalon. In man, sensory systems still send their fibers here. However, the thalamus now serves, among other things, as a kind of substation where incoming afferent impulses are sorted and directed to the cerebral cortex.

In the light of the increase in higher motor control over muscular activity, the ventral surface of the midbrain in man becomes relatively much larger than in lower forms, in order to accommodate masses of fibers descending from cerebral motor centers. These fiber bundles are known as *cerebral peduncles.*

The dorsal aspect of the midbrain, likewise obscured by the hemispheres, shows four swellings instead of the two seen in the dogfish. The more recently evolved caudal pair, associated with the auditory system, shows some differentiation in land Amphibia but is not easily seen until the reptilian stage is attained (Fig. 1-2).

Another outstanding feature of the human brain is the largeness of the cerebellum. This is due to two major factors: the assumption of an erect position; and the fine, learned activities made possible by the evolution of the hands. Associated with the enlargement of this portion of the brain, major fiber bundles appear. The *pons,* located on the ventral side of the hindbrain, and the *brachium pontis,* which carries fibers from the pons to the cerebellum, are a part of this mechanism.

Having observed some of the underlying processes which lead to the emergence of the central nervous system, it is now appropriate to take up a detailed study of its gross anatomy.

2 ANATOMY OF THE BRAIN

TELENCEPHALON

General Topography of the Cerebral Hemispheres

The cerebral hemisphere consists of three parts: the pallium, or cortex, the rhinencephalon, and the basal nuclei. Each hemisphere has three poles: frontal, occipital, and temporal; four lobes: frontal, occipital, parietal, and temporal; and three surfaces: dorsolateral, medial, and basal. To the lobes should be added the insula (island of Reil, Fig. 2-3) which lies at the bottom of the lateral fissure, obscured by overlying parts of the frontal and temporal lobes.

Pallium, or Cortex

Dorsolateral Surface. (Figs. 2-1, 2-2.) Each hemisphere is divided into lobes by distinct fissures, or sulci, and by arbitrary lines. The central sulcus, the lateral fissure, the preoccipital notch, and the parieto-occipital fissure serve as landmarks by which the frontal, parietal, occipital, and temporal lobes are set apart.

Frontal Lobe. This is bounded posteriorly by the central sulcus (fissure of Rolando) and inferiorly by the lateral cerebral fissure (fissure of Sylvius). The lateral cerebral fissure consists of two portions: a short stem which divides into two rami—the anterior horizontal and the anterior ascending—and a long posterior ramus. The central sulcus is situated about the middle of the lateral surface of the hemisphere. Running parallel to the central sulcus is the precentral, usually divided into an upper and lower part. From the precentral sulcus, the superior and inferior frontal sulci run rostrally. These sulci divide the frontal lobe into the following gyri: precentral and superior, middle, and inferior frontal, the latter being further subdivided into the orbital, triangular, and opercular (Broca's area) portions.

Temporal Lobe. The temporal lobe is separated superiorly from the frontal by the lateral cerebral fissure and from the parietal lobe by an arbitrary line drawn between the angle of the posterior ramus of the lateral fissure and the occipital pole; posteriorly, it is separated from the occipital lobe by a line connecting the superior end of the parieto-occipital fissure and the preoccipital notch. The superior temporal sulcus begins near the temporal pole and runs parallel to the lateral fissure. Ventral to it is a less distinct and disconnected sulcus, the middle temporal, most of which lies on the basal surface of the hemisphere. These sulci limit the superior and middle temporal gyri. On the dorsal surface of the superior temporal gyrus, lying in the lateral fissure, are the transverse temporal gyri.

Parietal Lobe. This lobe lies posterior to the central sulcus which separates it from the frontal lobe. It is separated inferiorly from the temporal lobe by the lateral fissure and a line extending from the angle of the posterior ramus of the

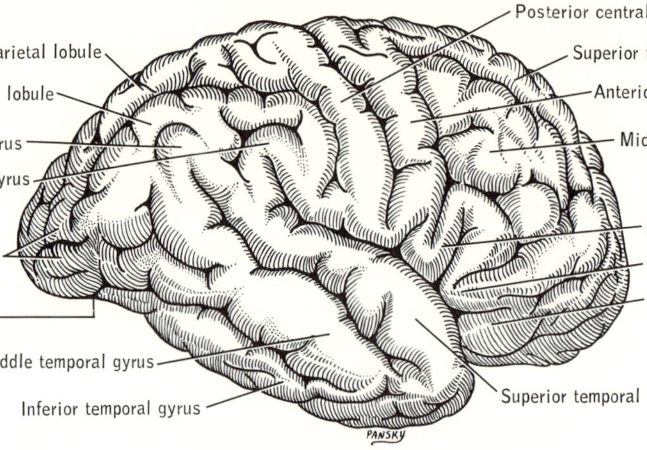

Fig. 2-1. Lateral view of the human cerebral hemispheres illustrating the principal gyri.

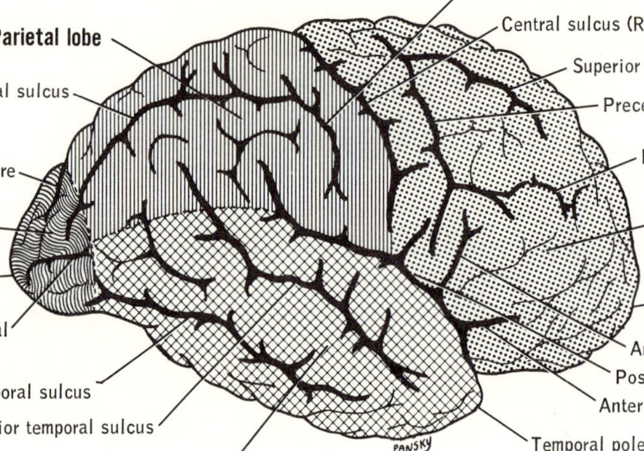

Fig. 2-2. Lateral view of the human cerebral hemispheres illustrating the principal sulci and lobes.

lateral fissure to the occipital pole. Parallel to the central sulcus is the postcentral sulcus, which may consist of two disconnected parts—a superior and an inferior. The intraparietal sulcus, extending dorsocaudally from the postcentral, runs in a course roughly paralleling the dorsal border of the hemisphere but some distance ventral to it. Between the central and postcentral sulci lies the postcentral gyrus. The cortical area dorsal to the intraparietal sulcus is referred to as the superior parietal lobule; that portion ventral to it is the inferior parietal lobule.

Related to extensions of the lateral cerebral fissure and the superior temporal sulcus, but lying in the inferior parietal lobule, are the supramarginal and angular gyri, respectively.

Occipital Lobe. Only a small portion of this lobe is seen from the lateral side. It is separated anteriorly from the parietal and temporal lobes by a line extending from the superior end of the parieto-occipital fissure to the preoccipital notch.

The Insula (Island of Reil). (Fig. 2-3.) After removing the overhanging operculum and parts of the frontal, parietal, and temporal lobes, the insula is seen to be somewhat conical in shape, surrounded at its base by the circular sulcus. The apex of the cone is directed rostrocaudally. Extending medially from the apex to the basal surface of the hemisphere is the limen insulae. On its lateral aspect a fairly prominent sulcus, the central sulcus of the insula, can be seen. Caudal to the central sulcus is the long gyrus; rostral to it are several "short gyri" of the insula.

Medial Surface. (Figs. 2-4 to 2-6.) Since the medial surface merges gradually with the basal, it is almost impossible to describe either without overlap. Further, portions of the lobes described with the dorsolateral surface are also represented here.

Among the most obvious features seen on the medial aspect of the brain is the corpus callosum, which consists of the rostrum, genu, body, and splenium. The corpus callosum is separated from the adjoining cortex by the sulcus of the corpus callosum, which begins just ventral to the rostrum and curves dorsally and posteriorly around the corpus, becoming confluent with the hippocampal fissure along the basomedial surface. The cortex which parallels the corpus callosum and its sulcus is the gyrus cinguli. Along the outer periphery of this gyrus is the sulcus cinguli (callosomarginal fissure). This begins a short distance ventral to the rostrum of the corpus callosum and runs dorsally around the gyrus cinguli, terminating in the formation of two branches. The longer branch appears to be a posterior continuation of the sulcus, ending just behind the splenium of the corpus callosum. This branch is the subparietal sulcus. The shorter branch, known as the marginal ramus, curves superiorly to reach the border of the hemisphere. A very short continuation of the central sulcus can be traced from the dorsolateral surface to the medial surface. A short ascending branch from the sulcus cinguli, lying anterior to the central sulcus, extends almost to the superior border of the hemisphere. This is the paracentral sulcus. An arbitrary line drawn from the central sulcus to the sulcus cinguli serves as a boundary line between the frontal and parietal lobes on the medial surface.

There are several other important fissures. The calcarine fissure consists of two parts. The rostral, deeper portion begins behind the splenium of the corpus callosum and extends to the parieto-occipital fissure. The second part continues from this point posteriorly to the dorsal surface of the hemisphere just above the oc-

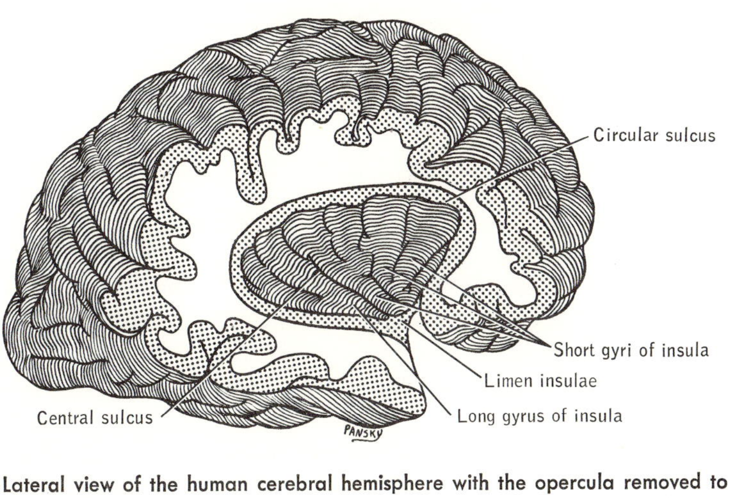

Fig. 2-3. Lateral view of the human cerebral hemisphere with the opercula removed to expose the insula (island of Reil).

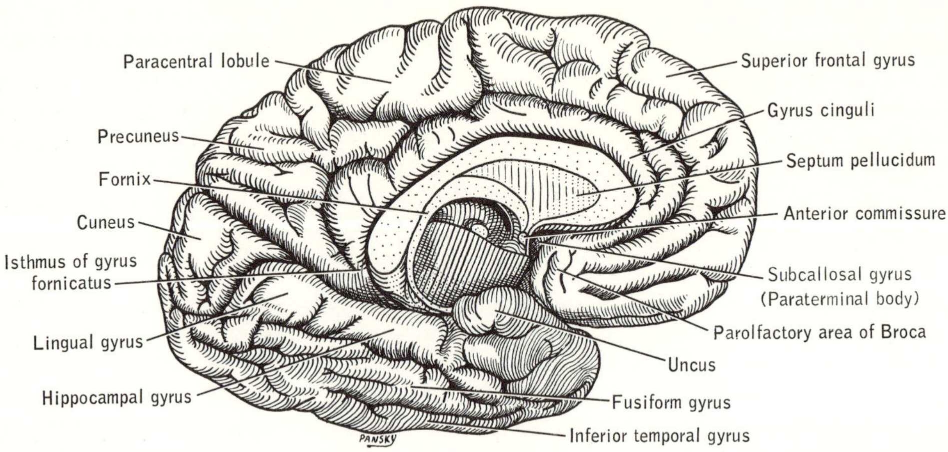

Fig. 2-4. Human cerebral hemisphere as seen from the medial side, showing the principal gyri.

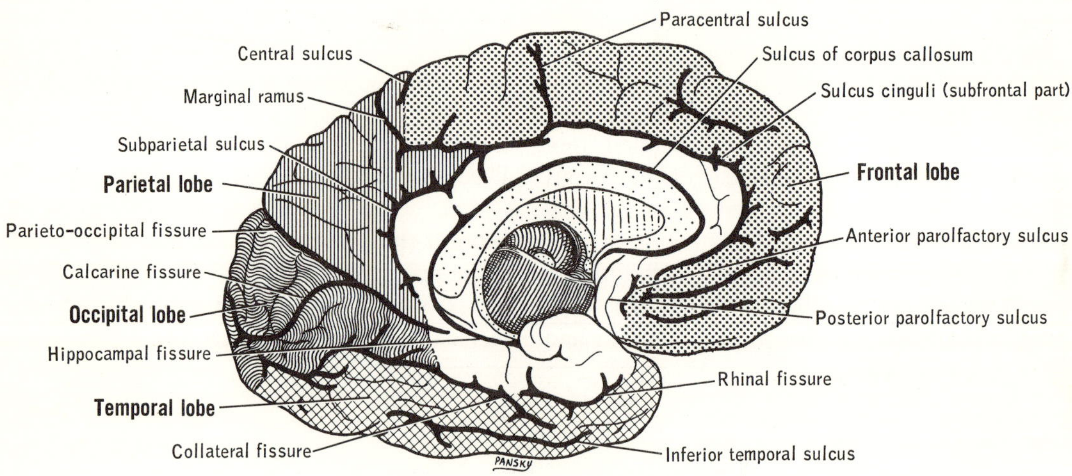

Fig. 2-5. Human cerebral hemisphere as viewed from the medial side, showing the lobes together with the principal sulci.

cipital pole. The parieto-occipital fissure angles dorsally from the high point of the arch of the calcarine fissure to the dorsal border of the hemisphere. The hippocampal fissure is a continuation of the sulcus of the corpus callosum. It curves around inferior to the splenium of the corpus callosum and continues anteriorly toward, but not to, the temporal pole. The collateral fissure begins near the occipital pole and runs rostrally, parallel to the inferior temporal sulcus and separated from the latter by the fusiform gyrus. Occasionally, in its rostral course, the collateral fissure passes without interruption into the rhinal fissure. An arbitrary line drawn downward from the rostral end of the calcarine fissure to the collateral fissure serves as the anterior boundary of the occipital lobe.

Frontal Lobe. The chief representation of this lobe on the medial surface is the superior frontal gyrus which continues over the border of the hemisphere from the dorsolateral surface. Its inferior border is the cingular sulcus. Its posterior boundary is a line drawn from the central sulcus to the cingular sulcus.

Parietal Lobe. This is represented by a continuation, over the dorsal border of the hemisphere, of the superior parietal lobule. It is limited inferiorly by the subparietal sulcus. That portion of the parietal lobe lying between the marginal ramus of the sulcus cinguli and the parieto-occipital fissure is the precuneus.

Paracentral Lobule. This is the term applied to the cortex surrounding the dorsomedial end of the central sulcus, bounded rostrally by the paracentral sulcus and posteriorly by the marginal ramus of the sulcus cinguli.

Occipital Lobe. This consists of two portions, the cuneus and a part of the lingual gyrus. The former is a wedge-shaped area lying between the parieto-occipital fissure superiorly and the calcarine fissure inferiorly. That part of the lingual gyrus which contributes to the occipital lobe lies posterior to an arbitrary line drawn vertically downward from the inferior end of the subparietal sulcus to the collateral fissure. It may be seen bulging superiorly within the arch of the posterior part of the calcarine fissure.

Basal Surface. (Figs. 2-7, 2-8.) This consists of the territory lying in a horizonal plane rostral to the temporal poles.

A distinct groove that begins near the frontal pole, lateral to the longitudinal fissure and diverging slightly from the midline in its posterior course, is the olfactory sulcus, occupied by the olfactory bulb and tract. Between this sulcus and the longitudinal fissure is the gyrus rectus. Lateral to the olfactory sulcus is a variable number of irregular orbital sulci and gyri.

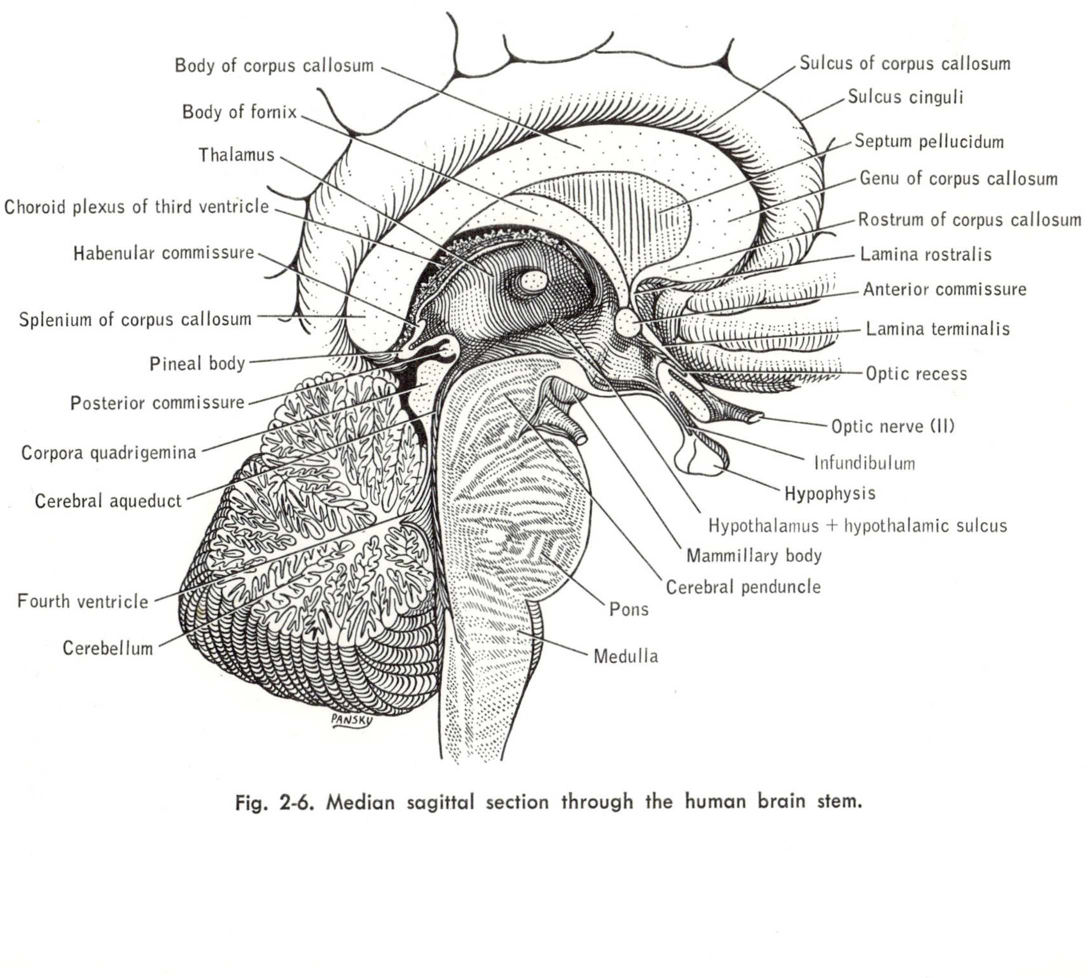

Fig. 2-6. Median sagittal section through the human brain stem.

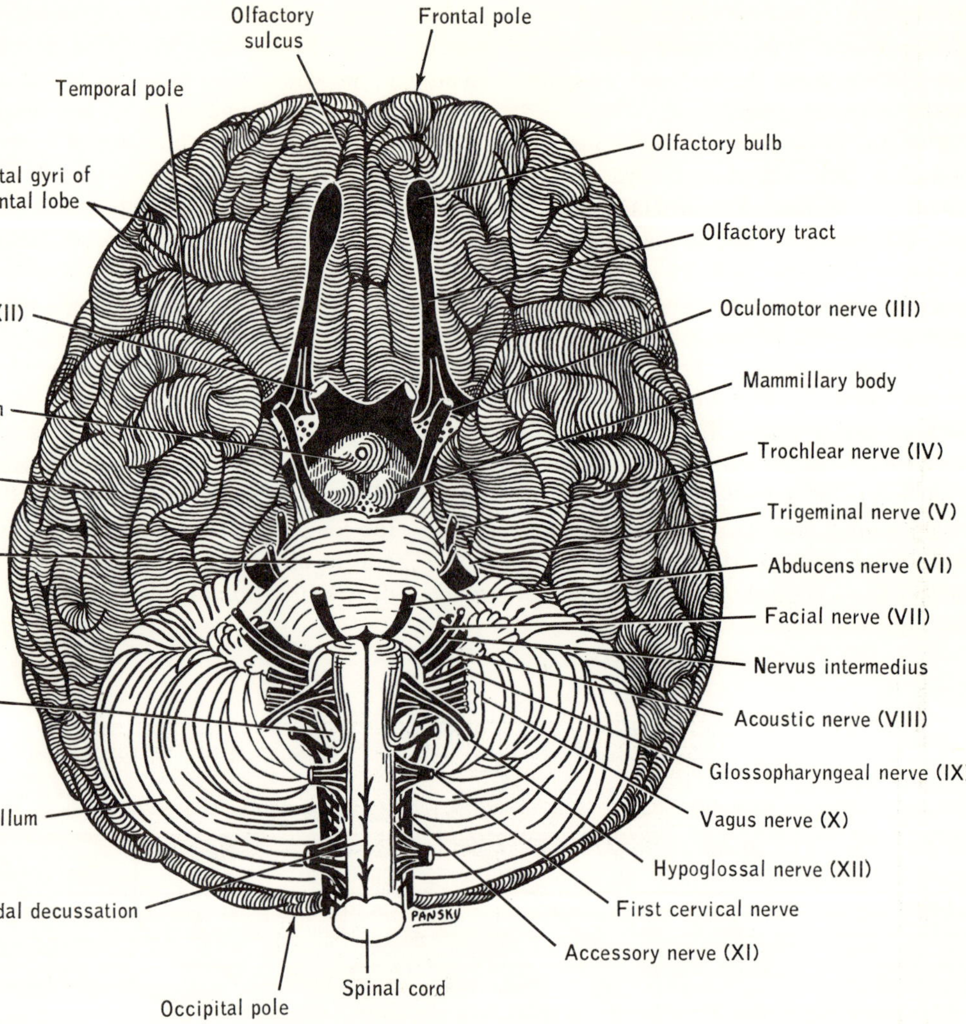

Fig. 2-7. Basal aspect of the human brain.

Rhinencephalon

This is the most ancient portion of the hemisphere and has no representation on the dorsolateral surface, being predominantly situated on the basal and medial surfaces.

The olfactory bulb and tract occupy the olfactory sulcus on the basal surface of the frontal lobe. The olfactory tract runs posteriorly into the olfactory trigone. From the trigone, diverging toward the medial side of the hemisphere, is the *medial olfactory stria.* Also from the trigone, the *lateral olfactory striae* course laterally and posteriorly, becoming continuous with the hippocampal gyrus. The anterior part of the hippocampal gyrus plus the lateral olfactory stria are often referred to collectively as the pyriform lobe (area). Behind the olfactory trigone, bounded posteriorly by the optic tract, is the *anterior perforated substance.* The posterior part of the anterior perforated substance is known as the *diagonal gyrus* (diagonal band of Broca), which can be traced to the medial side of the hemispheres just ventral to the rostrum of the corpus callosum. This area is called the *paraterminal body* (subcallosal gyrus). In front of the paraterminal body, a very narrow band, the *hippocampal rudiment,* extends from the rostrum of the corpus callosum toward the medial olfactory stria and then continues completely around the outer surface of the corpus callosum. In some brains a swelling occurs in the anterior perforated substance. This is the *olfactory tubercle* (tuberculum olfactorum).

The position of the gyrus cinguli has already been noted. Posteriorly, this gyrus is continuous with a narrow cortical band which runs ventral to the splenium of the corpus callosum. This band is the *isthmus* (Fig. 2-4). It extends rostrally to merge with the hippocampal gyrus, which is a thick convolution lying between the hippocampal fissure dorsally and the collateral and rhinal fissures ventrally. The hippocampal gyrus bends sharply around the rostral end of the hippocampal fissure to form the *uncus* (Fig. 2-4). In the older terminology, the gyrus cinguli, isthmus, hippocampal gyrus, and uncus are grouped together as the *gyrus fornicatus,* or *limbic lobe* (Fig. 2-4). This designation was based upon the belief that the limbic lobe belongs exclusively to the rhinencephalon. More recent evidence indicates that it might be preferable to consider the hippocampal gyrus and uncus as a part of the temporal lobe rather than part of the rhinencephalon. Similarly, that part of the gyrus cinguli which lies rostral to the line of division between the frontal and parietal lobes may be said to belong to the frontal lobe, while that portion posterior to it, including the isthmus, belongs to the parietal lobe.

Basal Ganglia (Figs. 2-9 to 2-17.)

Four nuclear masses comprise the basal ganglia (nuclei): the caudate, lenticular (lentiform), amygdaloid, and claustrum. When the

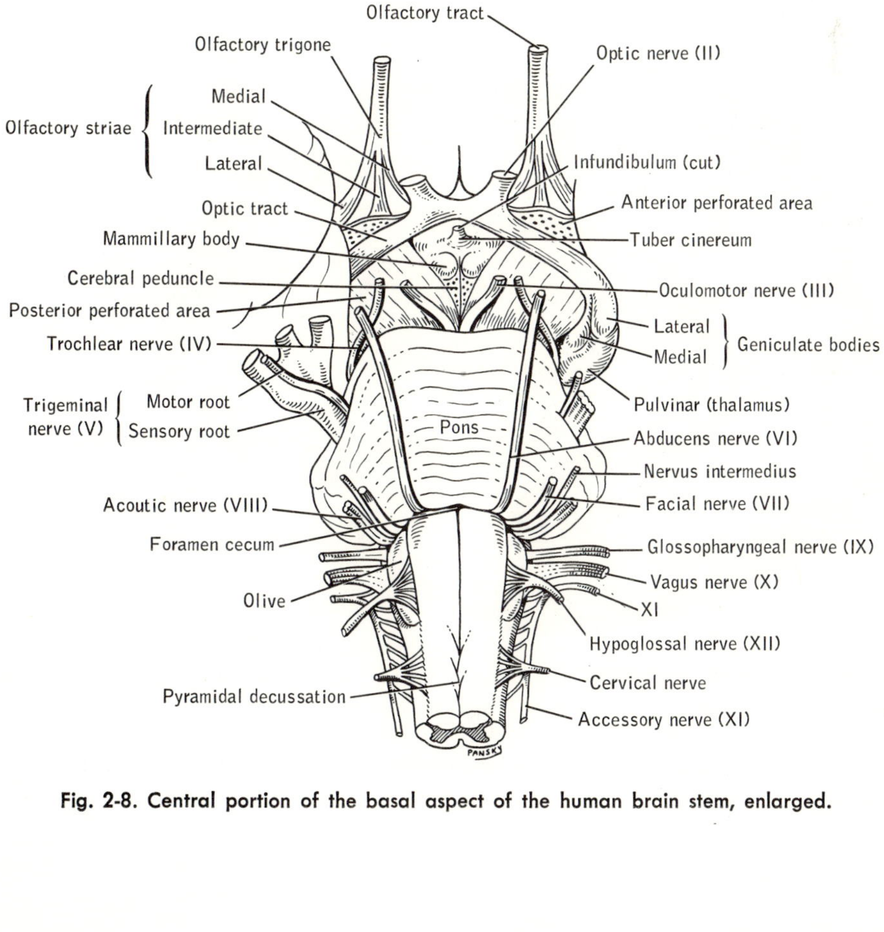

Fig. 2-8. Central portion of the basal aspect of the human brain stem, enlarged.

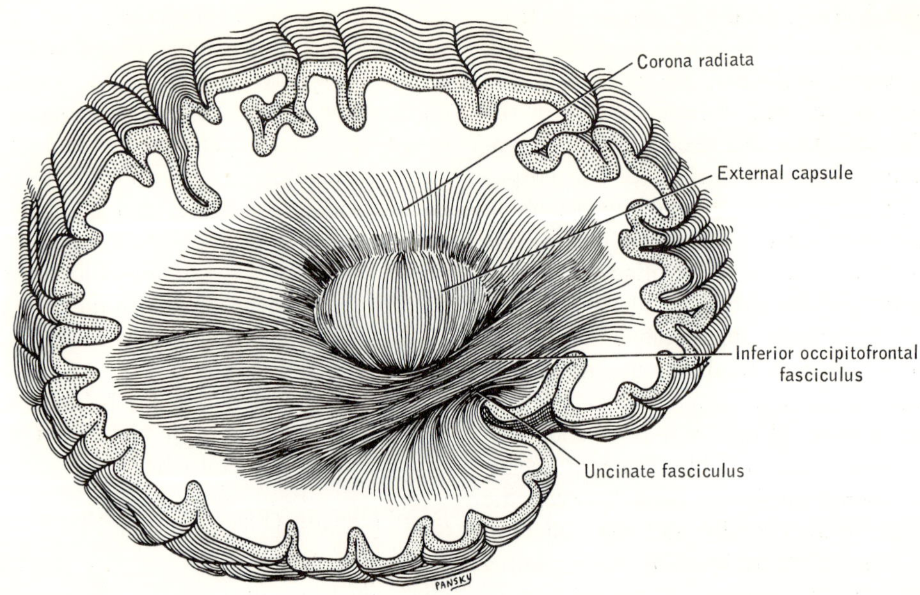

Fig. 2-9. Lateral aspect of a dissection of a human cerebral hemisphere after both opercula and insula have been removed. (*Adapted from Ranson and Clark, The Anatomy of the Nervous System, 10th ed., W. B. Saunders Company, Philadelphia, 1959.*)

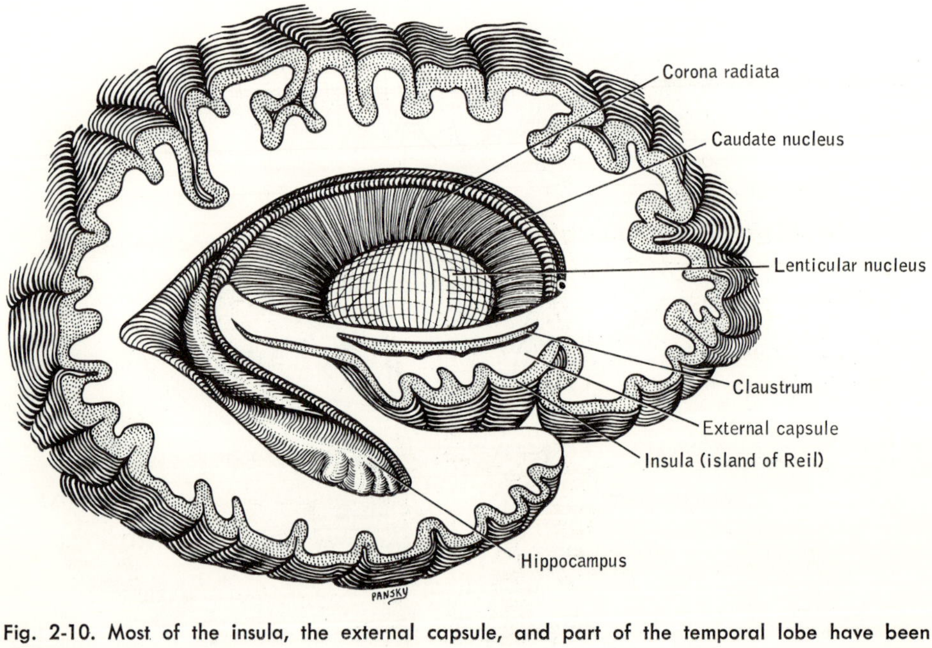

Fig. 2-10. Most of the insula, the external capsule, and part of the temporal lobe have been removed.

Figs. 2-10 to 2-13. Lateral views of a series of dissections of the human cerebral hemisphere. (*Adapted, in part, from Ranson and Clark, The Anatomy of the Nervous System, 10th ed., W. B. Saunders Company, Philadelphia, 1959.*)

internal capsule and the adjacent caudate and lenticular nuclei are considered together, the term *corpus striatum* is applied.

Caudate Nucleus. (Figs. 2-10 to 2-17.) The pear-shaped head of this nucleus is large, and its rostral extremity lies just dorsal to the anterior perforated substance. As the nucleus curves posteriorly, it tapers down into a slender tail, which extends almost to the temporal pole, ending at the amygdaloid nucleus. Anteriorly,

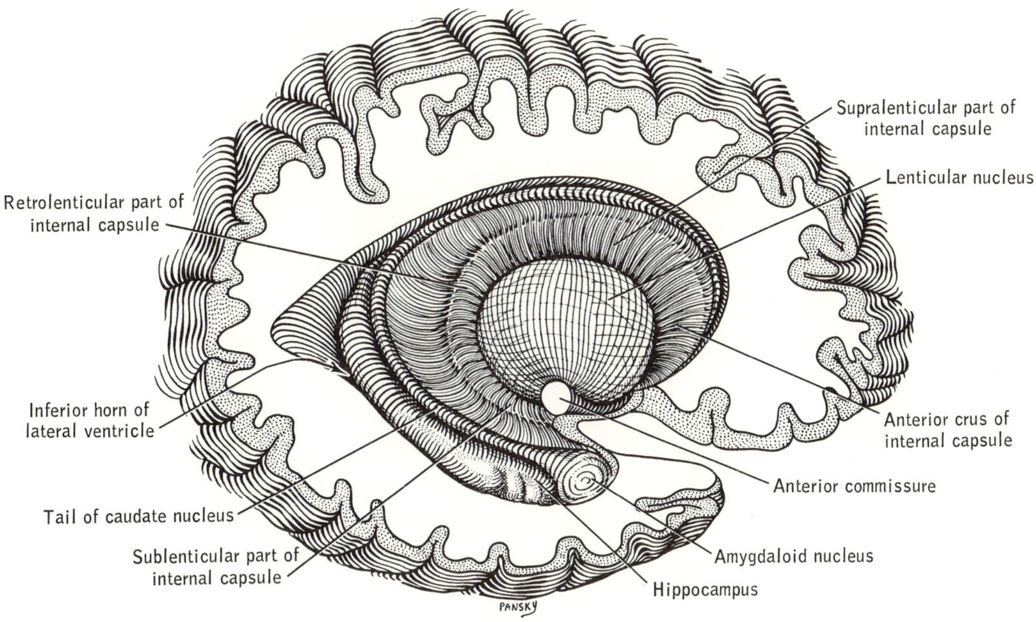

Fig. 2-11. All of the insula has been removed, together with a larger portion of the temporal lobe.

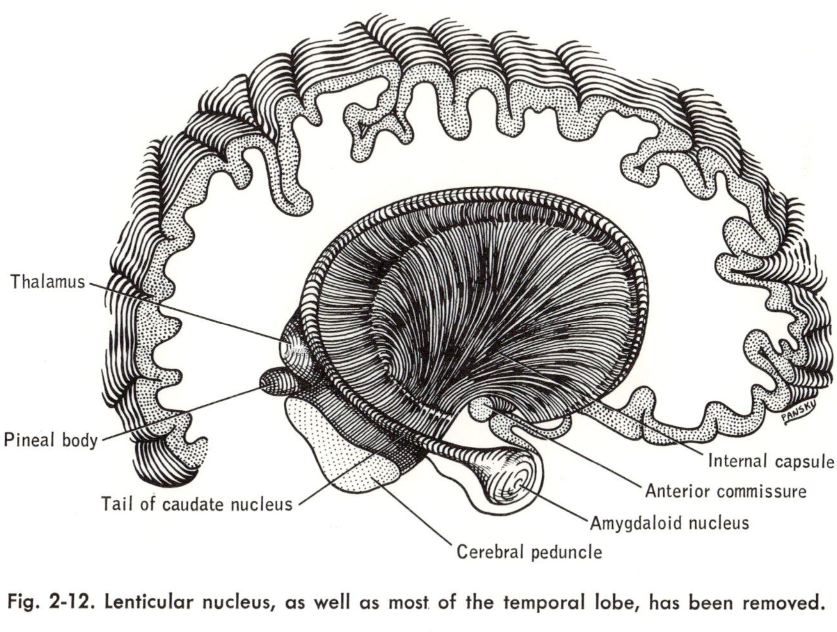

Fig. 2-12. Lenticular nucleus, as well as most of the temporal lobe, has been removed.

rostral to the internal capsule, the head of the caudate is fused with the lenticular nucleus.

Lenticular Nucleus. (Figs. 2-10, 2-11, 2-14 to 2-17.) This gray mass is buried deeply in the white core of the hemisphere. It is shaped somewhat like a biconvex lens, the convexity of which is directed laterally. Where it is fused with the caudate nucleus, it lies just above the anterior perforated substance. The ventral surface is closely related to the roof of the inferior horn of the lateral ventricle. The lateral surface underlies the insula, from which it is separated by the

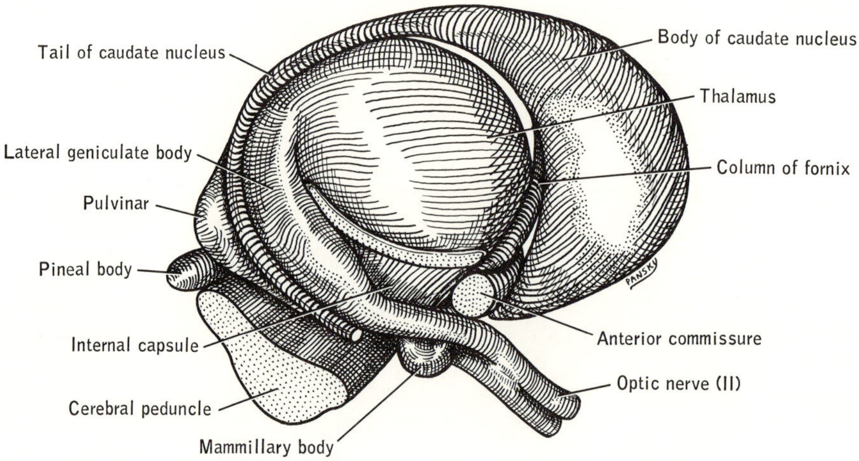

Fig. 2-13. Cortical parts, as well as internal capsule, have been removed.

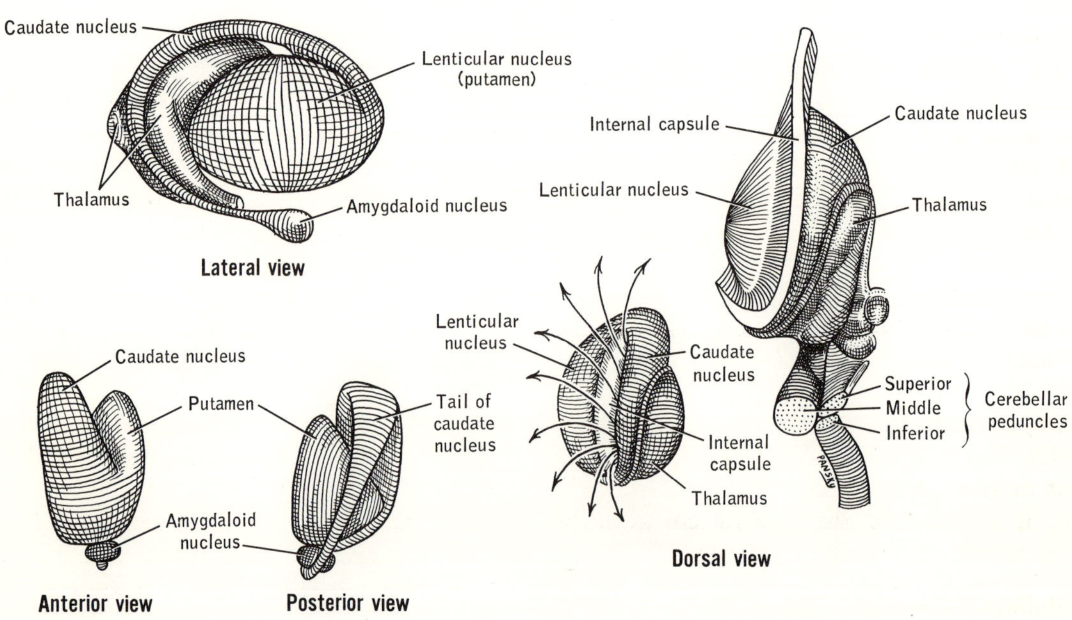

Fig. 2-14. Diagrammatic representation of the basal ganglia as seen from various aspects. ***(Adapted from Krieg, Functional Neuroanatomy, 2d ed., McGraw-Hill Book Company, Inc., Blakiston Division, New York, 1953.)***

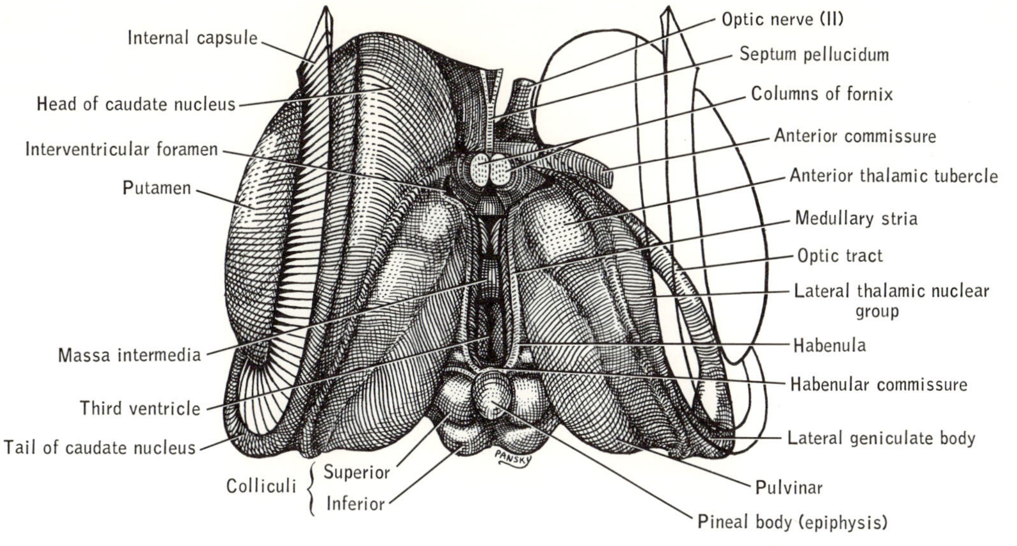

Fig. 2-15. Basal ganglia, diencephalon, and a portion of the mesencephalon as seen from the dorsal side.

external capsule and claustrum. The medial surface lies against the internal capsule. This nucleus appears to be subdivided by two thin fibrous layers. The most lateral, the *external medullary lamina,* divides the nucleus into a lateral, cell-rich zone known as the *putamen.* Medial to this lamina lies the *globus pallidus.* The latter is further divided into an internal and external zone by the *internal medullary lamina.*

Claustrum. This is a thin gray mass embedded in the white substance of the hemisphere between the lateral side of the lenticular nucleus and the insula. It is separated from the lenticular nucleus by a thin white lamina of nerve fibers, the external capsule. (Figs. 2-10, 2-17.)

Amygdaloid Nucleus. (Figs. 2-11, 2-12, 2-14.) This is a small, round aggregate of nuclear masses lying far forward in the temporal lobe. It merges with the cerebral cortex lateral to the anterior perforated substance.

Medullary Substance of the Cerebral Hemispheres

The medullary substance underlies the cortex. It varies greatly in thickness in different areas and consists of myelinated fibers. Generally, these fibers are classified as *projection, association,* and *commissural.*

Projection Fibers

These are two types: afferent (corticipetal) or efferent (corticifugal), depending upon the direction of the impulse toward or away from the cortex, respectively. Many of the projection fibers are grouped together in named bundles: the internal capsule and the fornix.

Internal Capsule. (Figs. 2-11, 2-12, 2-14 to 2-18.) This is the great fiber mass containing both afferent and efferent fibers of the neopallium. In a horizontal section, it has the form of an obtuse angle with its apex pointing medially. The fact that it more nearly resembles a fan can be appreciated only in a gross dissection. That portion of the capsule which lies between the head of the caudate and the rostral end of the lenticular nucleus is called the *anterior limb.* The fibers here tend to be directed rostrally and dorsally. The region of the angle is known as the *genu.* The remainder is called the *posterior limb.* The latter part is applied to the medial surface of the lenticular nucleus, wrapping

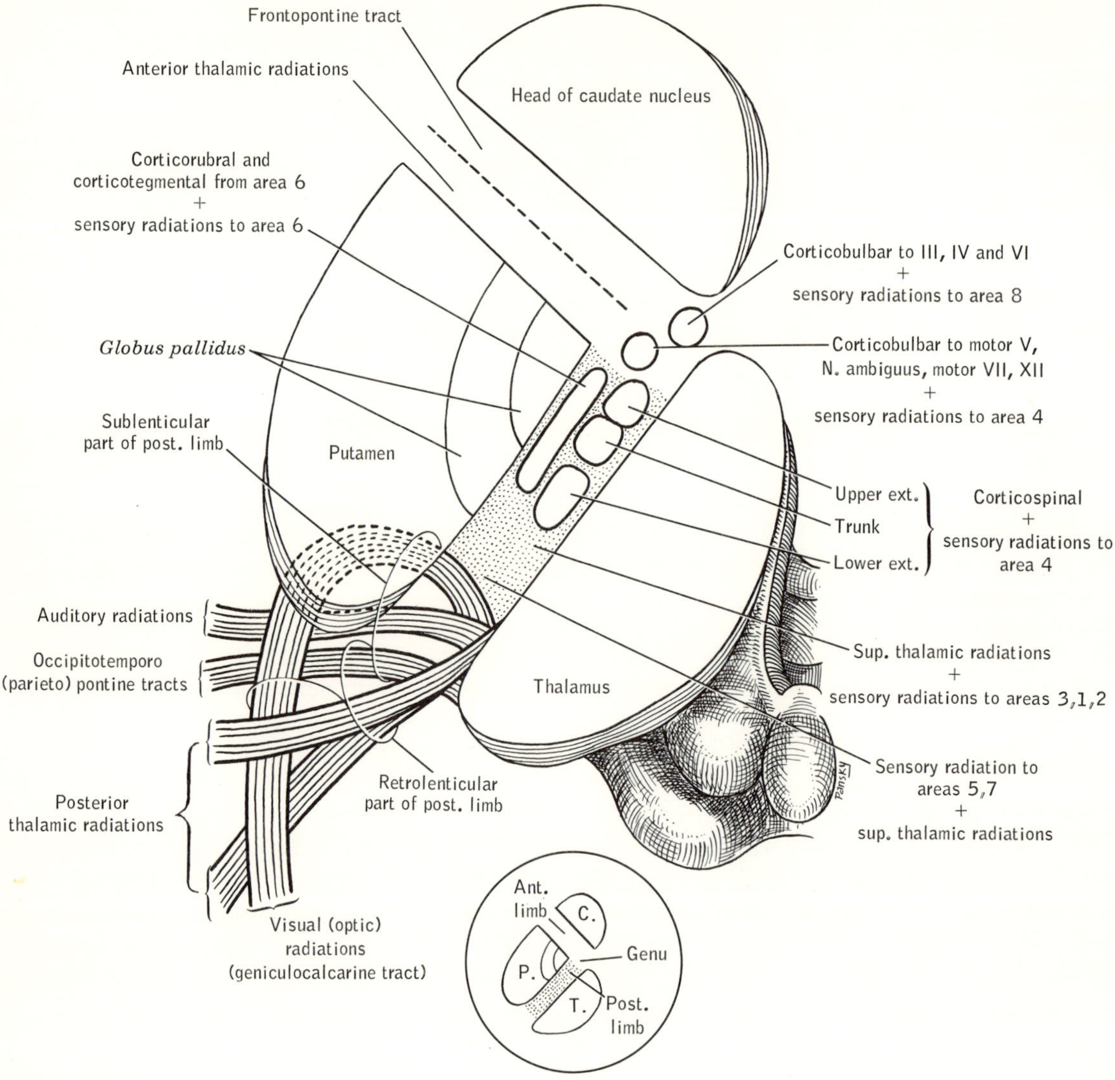

Fig. 2-16. Diagrammatic representation of the left internal capsule showing its relations and major components.

around its posterior aspect as well as its posteroventral surface. The posterior limb consists of three parts: the *lenticulothalamic,* between the thalamus and the lenticular nucleus, in which the fibers are directed approximately vertically; the *retrolenticular* portion, behind the lenticular nucleus, in which the fibers run posteriorly; and the *sublenticular,* beneath the posterior half of the lenticular nucleus, in which the fibers are directed laterally. The efferent fibers of the capsule converge inferiorly into the *cerebral peduncles* of the mesencephalon. Dorsal to the lenticular nucleus the fibers of the capsule spread out to form the *corona radiata.*

Fornix. (Fig. 2-19.) These are projection fibers of the archipallium. They originate in the hippocampus, which they leave via the *fimbria*. The fibers curving upward from each fimbria comprise the *crus* of the fornix. The crura pass medially and dorsally, approaching each other beneath the splenium of the corpus callosum. Here the fibers run rostrally, directly beneath the corpus callosum, as the *bodies of the fornix*. Anteriorly, the fibers arch to form the *columns of the fornix,* which terminate in the mammillary bodies and other parts of the hypothalamus.

Association Fibers (Figs. 2-9, 2-20 to 2-23.)

These are also divided into two groups. The first are short, running in the deeper parts of the cortex, interconnecting closely adjoining areas (intracortical); or they may run just below the cortex (subcortical), uniting neighboring gyri. Many of the subcortical fibers appear U-shaped and are designated as arcuate. The second type are long, running deep in the medullary centers and uniting widely separated cortical regions in the same hemisphere. Most of the convolutions contain numerous intracortical and subcortical fibers which are not specifically named. There are, however, some fairly distinct sets belonging to the long type.

Cingulum. (Figs. 2-20, 2-23.) These fibers lie in the white substance of the gyrus cinguli, close to the corpus callosum. They begin in the parolfactory area of the cortex, caudal to the rostrum of the corpus callosum. They swing dorstally, following the gyrus until they reach the level of the splenium, at which point they curve

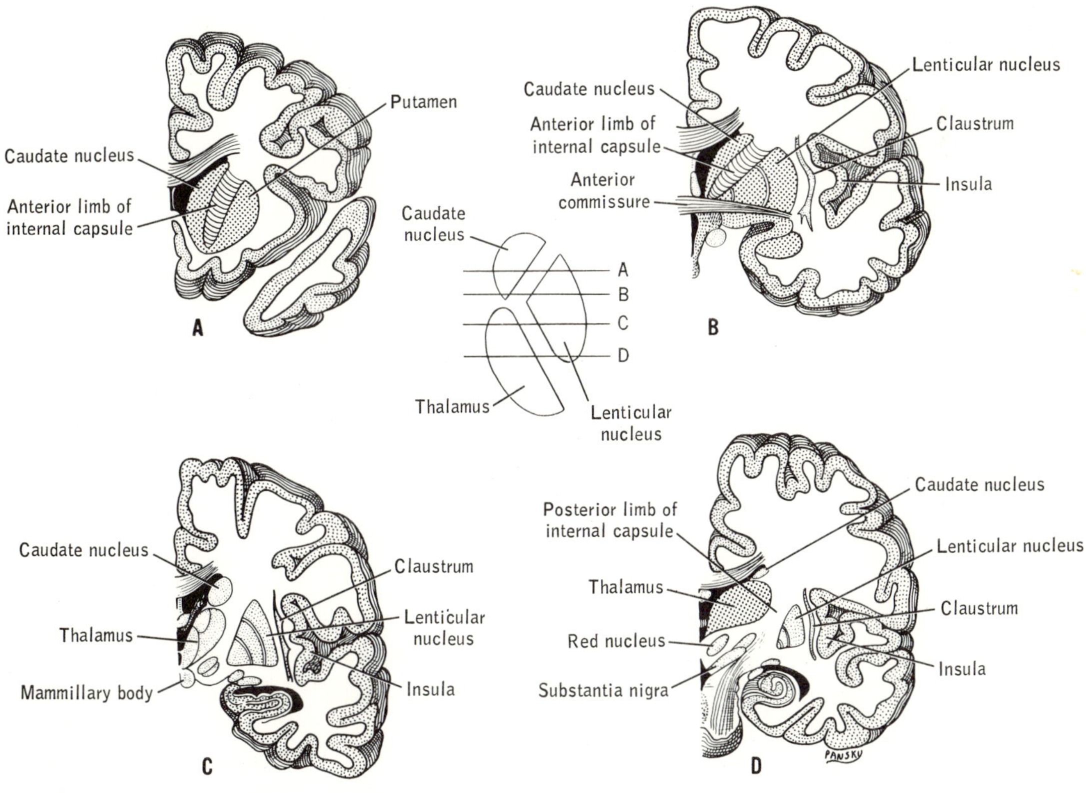

Fig. 2-17. Series of vertical sections through several levels of the basal ganglia and internal capsule, arranged in a rostral-caudal sequence.

caudally, then rostrally, into the hippocampus and uncus.

This bundle helps interconnect parts of the frontal, parietal, and temporal lobes.

Superior Longitudinal Fasciculus. (Figs. 2-20, 2-21.) This begins in the frontal lobe and passes through the frontal and parietal opercula, with some fibers terminating posteriorly in the occipital lobe and others ventrally in the temporal lobe.

Superior Occipitofrontal Fasciculus. (Figs. 2-20, 2-22.) This bundle passes posteriorly from the frontal lobe along the dorsal border of the caudate nucleus and beneath the corpus callosum. In many places, it parallels the superior longitudinal fasciculus, but it is separated from the latter by the corona radiata.

Inferior Occipitofrontal Fasciculus. (Figs. 2-9, 2-20, 2-21.) These fibers extend from frontal to occipital lobes but are in a more ventral plane than the superior occipitofrontal fasciculus. They run along the ventrolateral edge of the lenticular nucleus. In the frontal lobe, they adjoin the uncinate fasciculus.

Uncinate Fasciculus. (Figs. 2-9, 2-20, 2-22.) These fibers begin in the orbital gyri of the frontal lobe, arch over the lateral fissure, and end in the rostral part of the temporal lobe.

Inferior Longitudinal Fasciculus. (Figs. 2-20, 2-23.) These fibers extend from the temporal

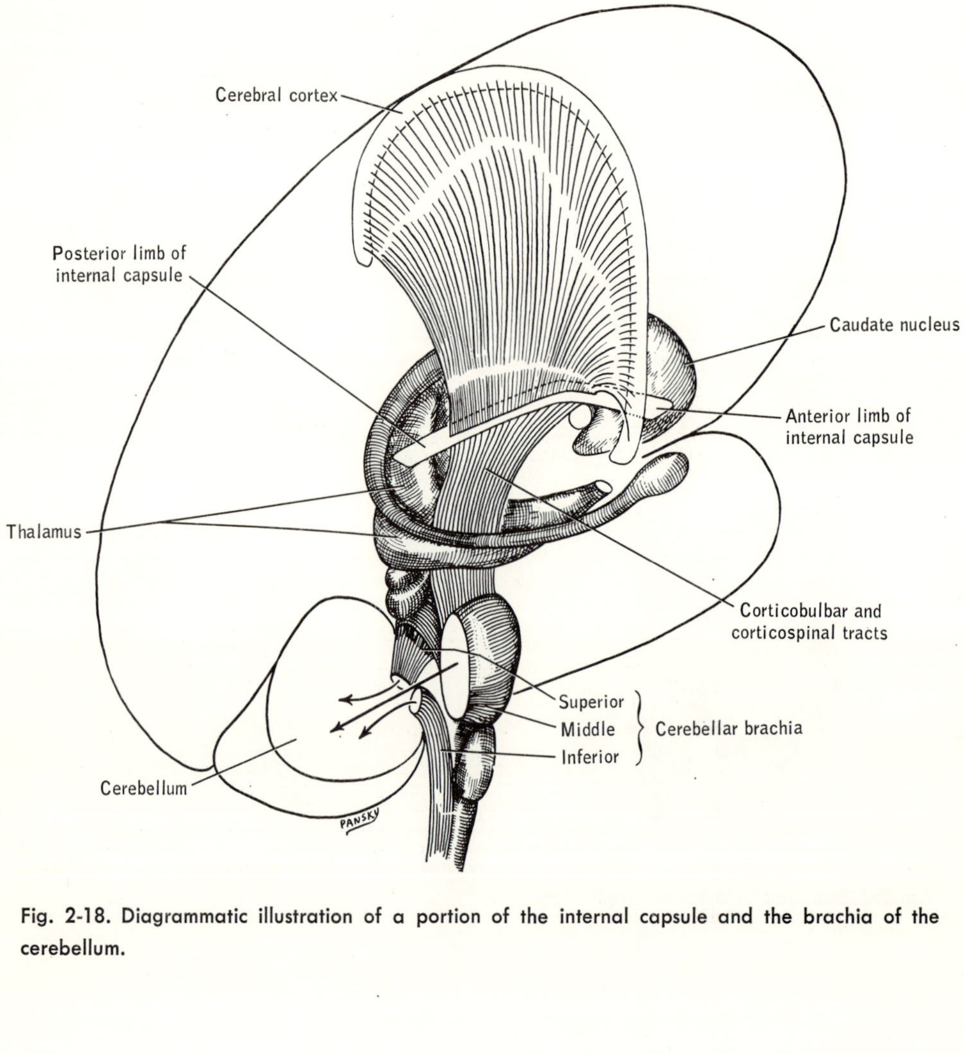

Fig. 2-18. Diagrammatic illustration of a portion of the internal capsule and the brachia of the cerebellum.

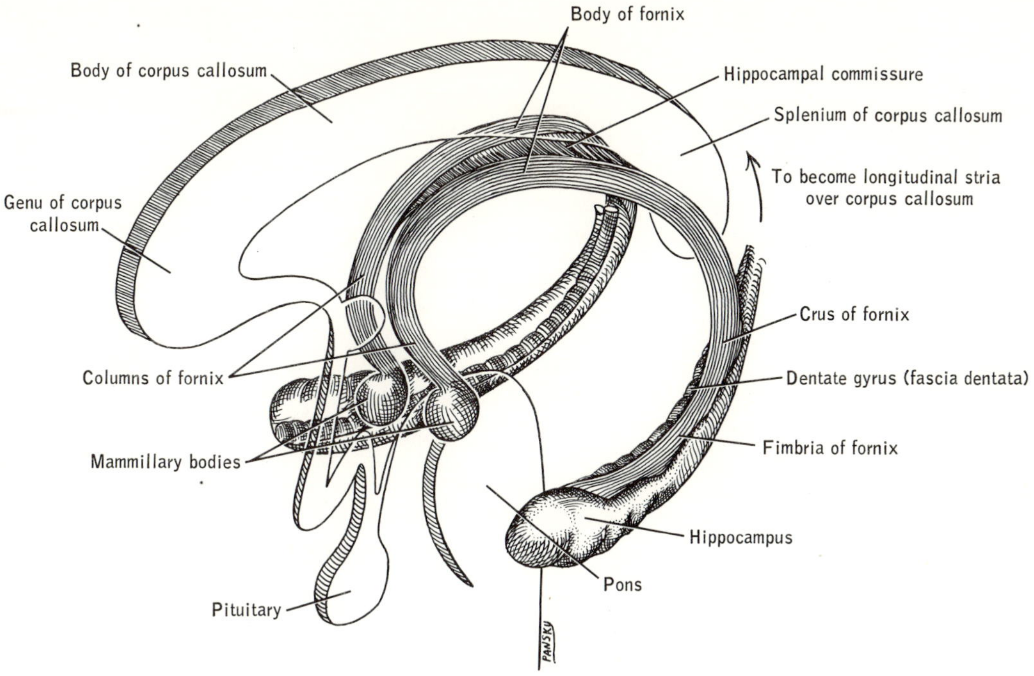

Fig. 2-19. Diagrammatic representation of a reconstruction of the fornix.

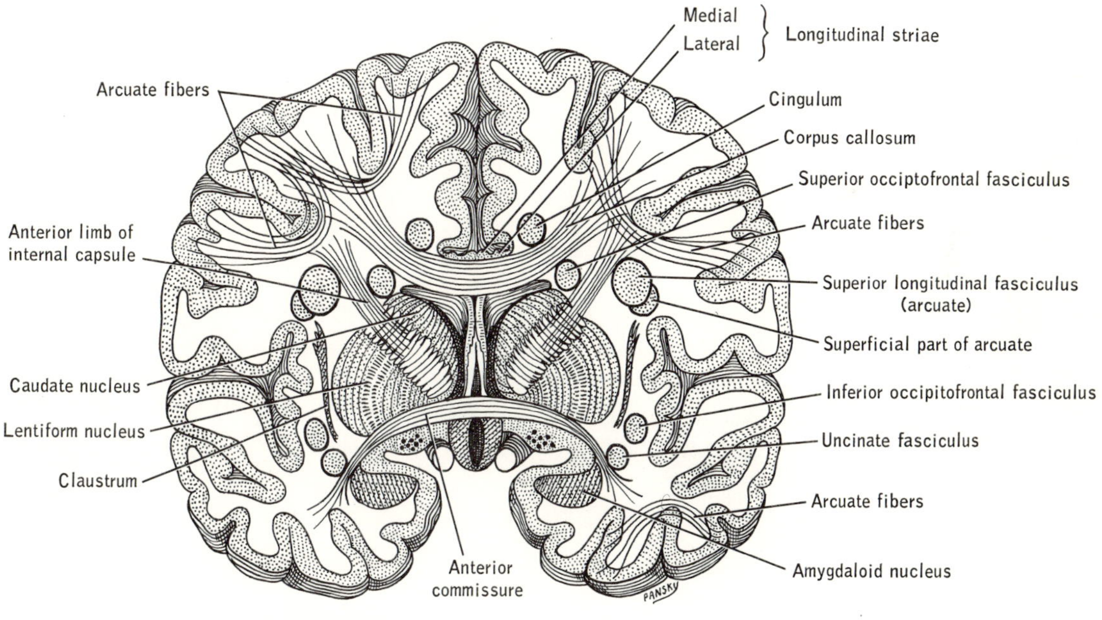

Fig. 2-20. Vertical section of the cerebral hemispheres at the level of the anterior commissure, showing the locations of the association bundles.

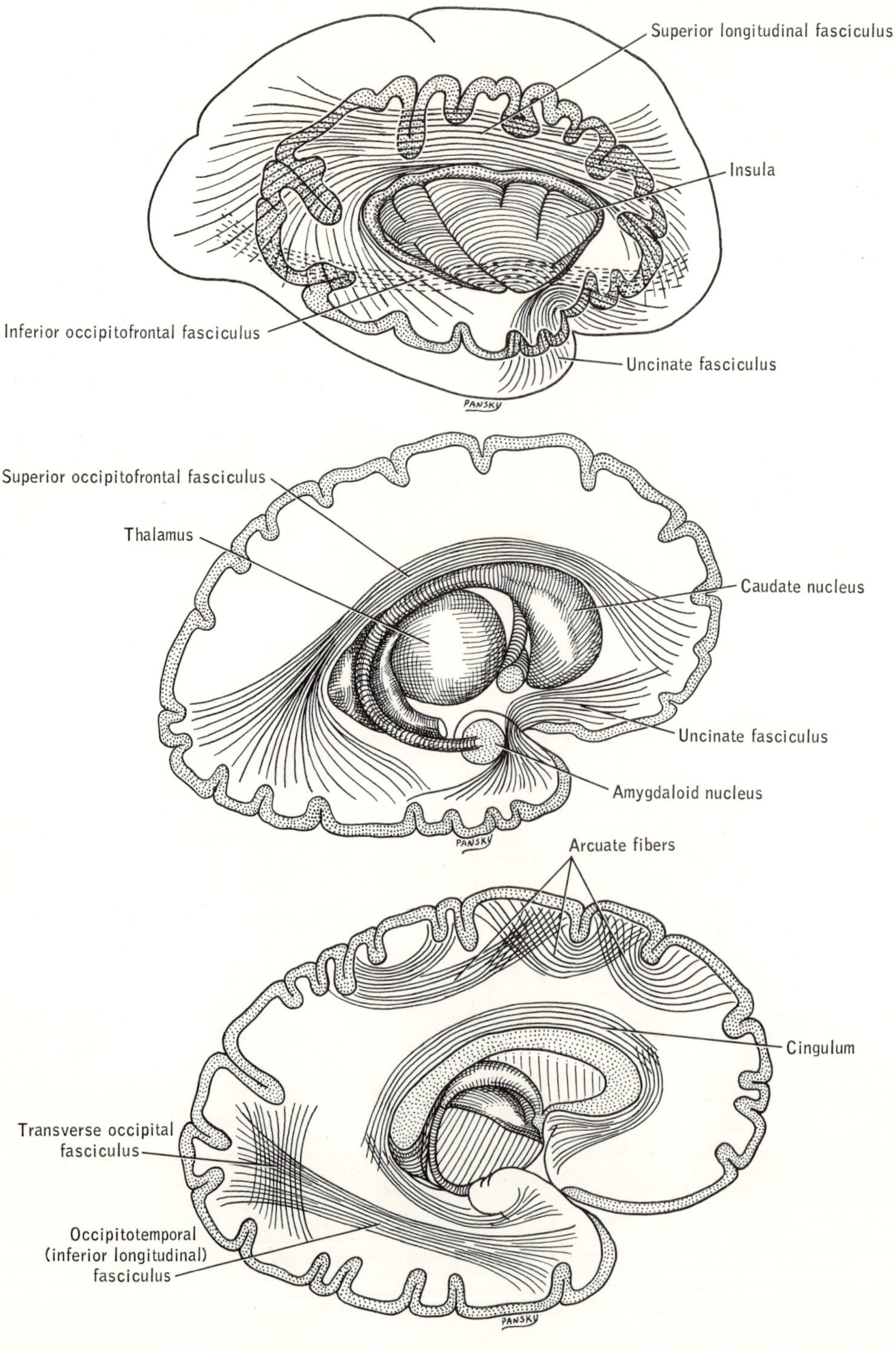

Figs. 2-21 to 2-23. Some of the long and short association bundles as seen from sagittal dissections through the cerebral hemisphere.

pole, pass through the length of the temporal lobe, and terminate in the occipital lobe.

Commissural Fibers (Figs. 2-6, 2-19, 2-20.)

These are fibers from an area of the cortex of one hemisphere which cross the midline to areas of the opposite hemisphere. The hemispheres are joined by three such fiber groups: the corpus callosum and the anterior and hippocampal commissures.

Corpus Callosum. (Figs. 2-6, 2-24, 2-25.) This massive accumulation of fibers is one of the most obvious structures on the medial surface of the hemisphere. Most of the fibers connect corresponding areas of cortex of the neopallial portions of the two hemispheres. Fibers of the corpus callosum intermingle with those of the corona radiata of the internal capsule as the latter fan out toward the cortex. The fibers which pass by way of the genu of the corpus callosum to the frontal lobes form the so-called forceps anterior (forceps minor) while those traversing the splenium of the corpus callosum to the occipital lobes form the forceps posterior (forceps major). The tapetum of the corpus callosum is composed of fibers passing through the body of that structure.

Anterior Commissure. This is a bundle of fibers which crosses through the lamina terminalis. The majority of fibers interconnect portions of the rhinencephalon (archipallium). The anterior fibers of the commissure unite the olfactory tubercle, anterior olfactory nucleus, and olfactory bulb. The posterior fibers terminate in the middle temporal gyrus. (Fig. 2-20.)

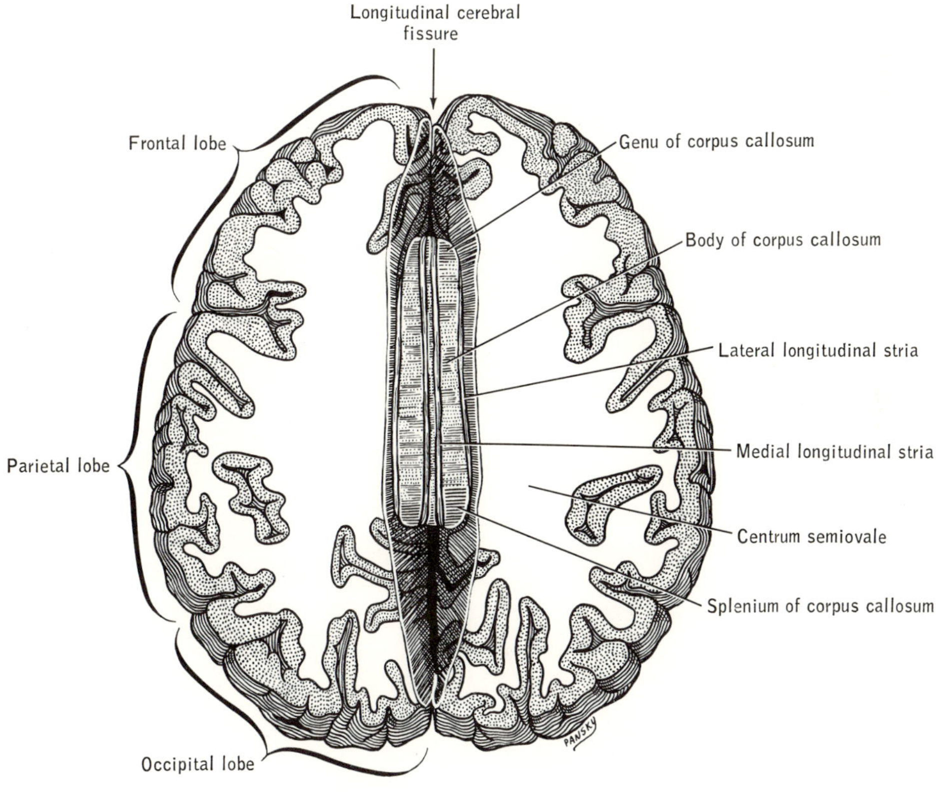

Fig. 2-24. Horizontal section of the human telencephalon taken just above the dorsal surface of the corpus callosum.

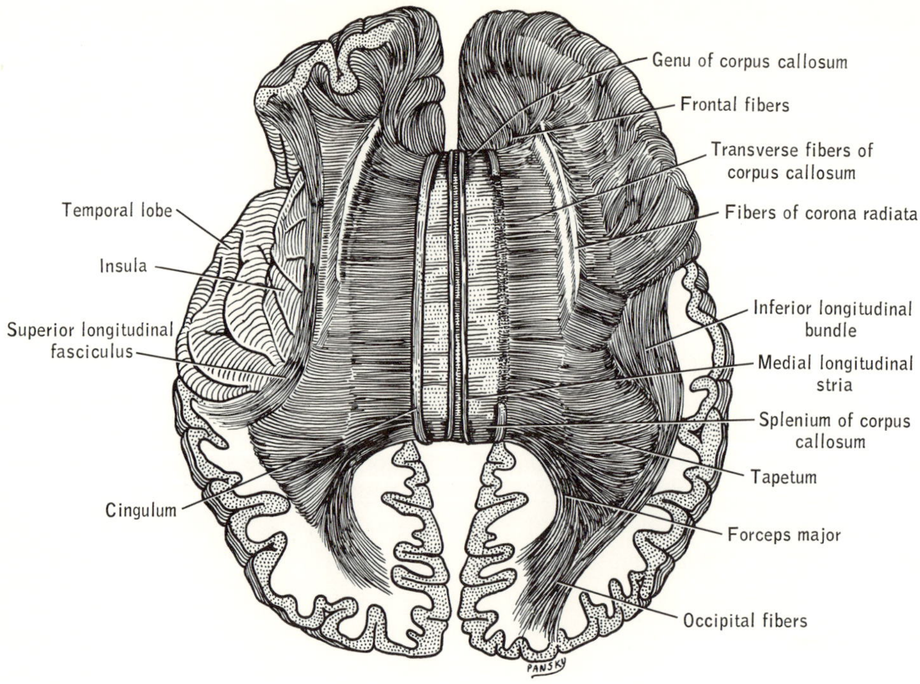

Fig. 2-25. Dissection of the human telencephalon showing the radiations of the corpus callosum as seen from the dorsal aspect.

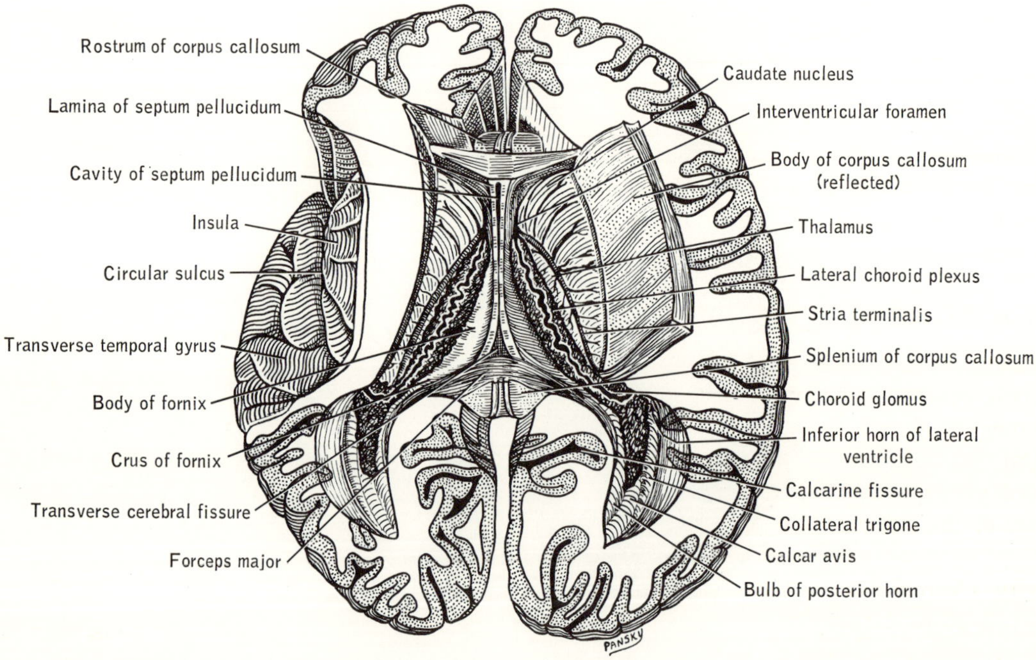

Fig. 2-26. Dissection of the human telencephalon, viewed from the dorsal side, with the corpus callosum reflected on the right side and removed on the left to illustrate the lateral ventricles.

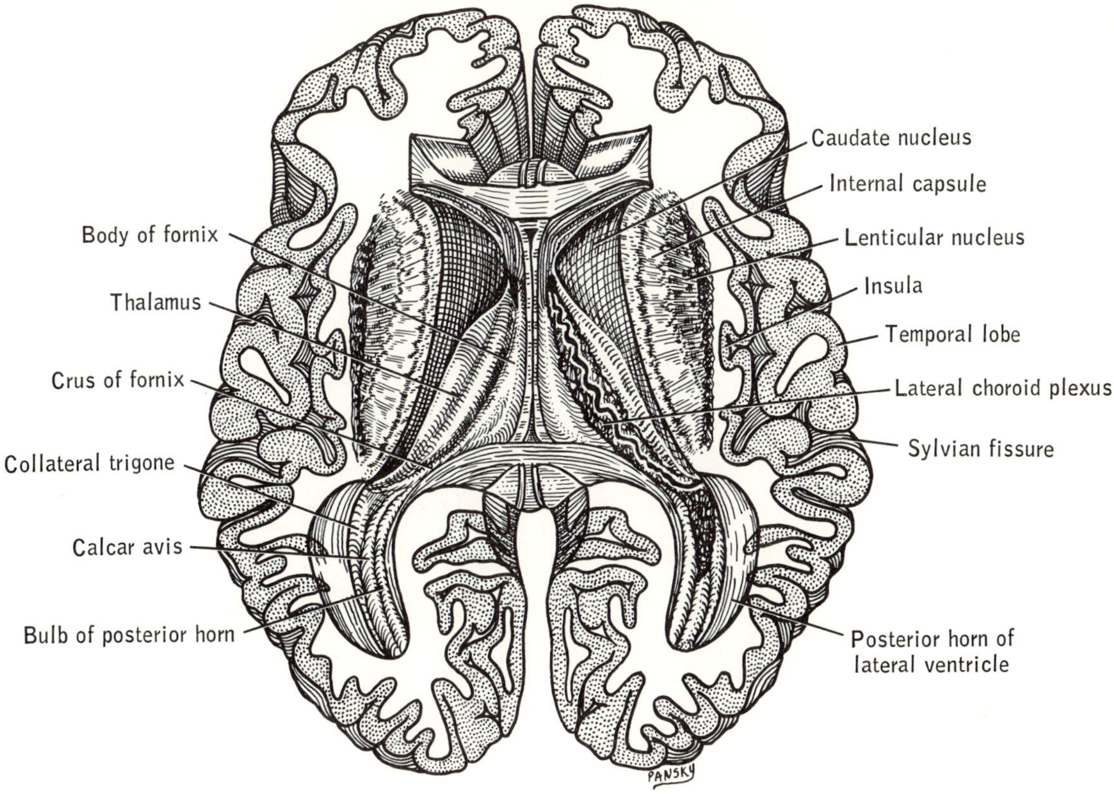

Fig. 2-27. Dissection of the human telencephalon, as seen from above, with the temporal lobe partially removed to illustrate the relationship of the basal ganglia to the lateral ventricle.

Hippocampal Commissure. (Fig. 2-19.) These fibers, which unite the two hippocampi, cross through the bodies of the fornices, where the fornices diverge from the midline.

Septum Pellucidum (Figs. 2-6, 2-26 to 2-28.)

This is a thin-walled septum which fills the interval between the corpus callosum and the columns of the fornix and separates the two lateral ventricles. It consists of two vertically placed sheets, separated by a narrow cleft, the cavity of the septum.

Cavity (Ventricle) of the Telencephalon (Figs. 2-26 to 2-36.)

Within each hemisphere is an ependymal-lined cavity called the *lateral ventricle,* consisting of several parts: anterior horn, body, collateral trigone, posterior horn, and inferior horn.

Anterior Horn

This is the portion extending rostrally from the interventricular foramen. It is triangular in outline, the sloping floor also serving as the lateral side. Medially, the wall is vertical and is composed of the septum pellucidum. The head of the caudate nucleus forms the floor and lateral wall. The roof and rostral end are formed by the fibers of the corpus callosum.

Body

This extends posteriorly from the interventricular foramen to the splenium of the corpus callosum. The medial wall is again vertical and

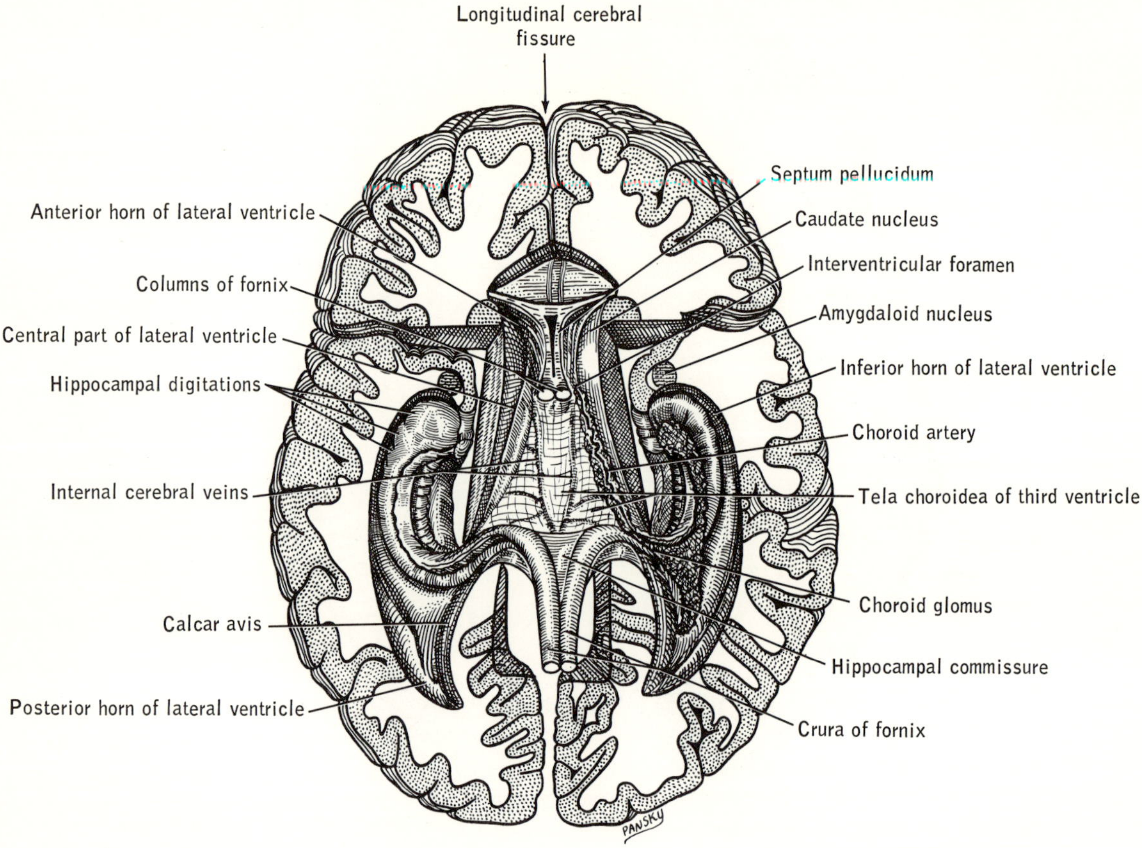

Fig. 2-28. Dissection of the human telencephalon, as seen from above, with the fornix reflected to expose both the tela choroidea of the third ventricle and the hippocampal commissure.

composed of the septum pellucidum. The roof is formed by the corpus callosum. The lateral wall, which slopes gradually to meet the roof at an acute angle, is formed from below upward, by the fornix, the choroid plexus, dorsal surface of the thalamus, stria, and vena terminalis, and the caudate nucleus.

Collateral Trigone

This is a region at the posterior end of the body, from which the posterior and inferior horns diverge.

Posterior Horn

This portion extends into the occipital lobe. Here, the roof and lateral wall form an arch composed chiefly of the tapetum of the corpus callosum. On the medial wall, two swellings are evident. The more dorsal is called the bulb of the posterior horn, caused by the occipital portion of the radiations of the corpus callosum. The larger, more ventral one, known as the calcar avis, is caused by the deep indentation of the calcarine fissure.

Inferior Horn

This curves ventrally and then rostrally from the collateral trigone. It extends through the medial part of the temporal lobe almost to the temporal pole. The roof is composed chiefly of the white substance of the lobe, the stria terminalis, and tail of the caudate nucleus. Rostral

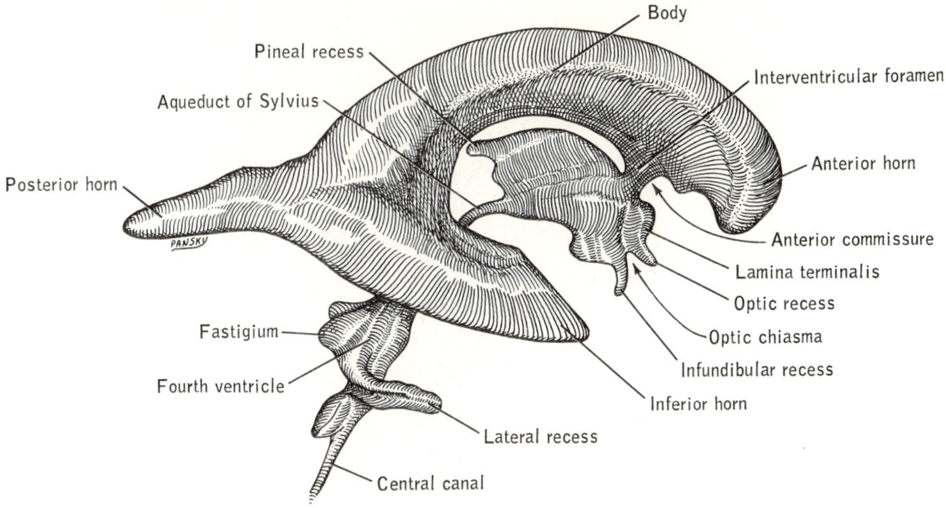

Fig. 2-29. Cast of the ventricular system of the brain, viewed from the right. (*Adapted from Woerdeman, Atlas of Human Anatomy, McGraw-Hill Book Company, Inc., Blakiston Division, New York, 1950.*)

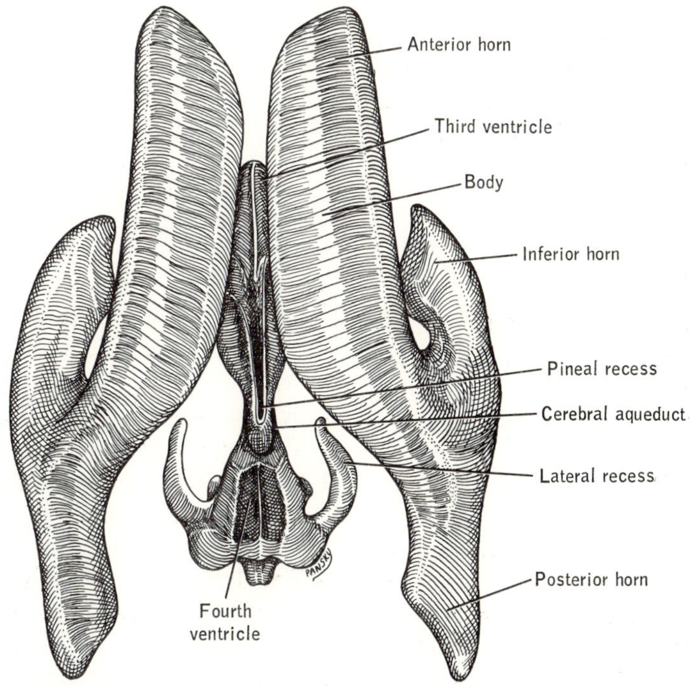

Fig. 2-30. Cast of the ventricular system of the brain, viewed from above. (*Adapted from Woerdeman, Atlas of Human Anatomy, McGraw-Hill Book Company, Inc., Blakiston Division, New York, 1950.*)

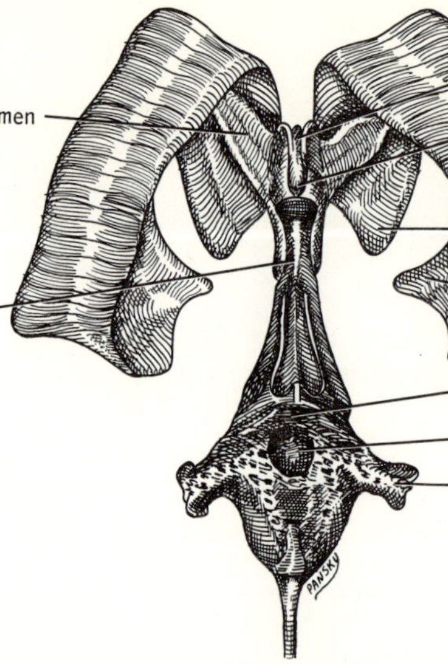

Fig. 2-31. Cast of the ventricular system of the brain, seen from the posterior side. (*Adapted from Woerdeman, Atlas of Human Anatomy, McGraw-Hill Book Company, Inc., Blakiston Division, New York, 1950.*)

to the end of the caudate nucleus lies the amygdaloid nucleus, which bulges into the end of the ventricle. The medial wall and floor, in order from medial to lateral, are formed by the fimbria, choroid plexus, hippocampus, and collateral eminence.

DIENCEPHALON

The diencephalon (Figs. 2-6, 2-34) is almost completely hidden when the hemispheres are in place. Several parts are described, namely: epithalamus, thalamus, subthalamus, and hypothalamus.

Epithalamus (Figs. 2-6, 2-34.)

This consists of the *pineal body* (epiphysis), *habenular trigone, stria medullaris,* and *habenular commissure.* The last lies just rostral to the pineal body and serves to connect the nuclei in the habenular trigone. The posterior commissure, which lies just behind the attachment of the pineal body, is sometimes described as part of this region.

Thalamus

External Morphology

This is the largest portion of the diencephalon. It is bounded ventrally by the hypothalamic sulcus, its caudal limit is at the level of the posterior commissure and cerebral aqueduct, its rostral limit is at the interventricular foramen, and dorsally it is related to the stria medullaris and the roof of the third ventricle. The two halves of the thalamus are frequently joined across the midline by a bridge of gray substance known as the *massa intermedia.*

The *lateral surface* (Figs. 2-13, 2-14, 2-15, 2-16) is intimately applied to the posterior limb of the internal capsule.

The *dorsal surface* (Figs. 2-15, 2-34) is free and slightly convex. The thalamus appears as two obliquely placed oval masses, the long axis of each extending from the anterior tubercle caudally through the pulvinar. This posterior part of the thalamus overlaps the rostral mesencephalon. The stria and vena terminalis lie in a groove which separates the lateral edge of the dorsal surface from the caudate nucleus. Medially, the dorsal surface is separated from the medial surface by the *taenia thalami,* the edge of the ependymal roof of the third ventricle. This dividing line is usually made more prominent by the stria medullaris thalami. The dorsal surface is further divided into a lateral and medial portion by a slight, oblique groove, the choroid sulcus. The area lateral to this groove is covered by the *lamina affixa,* the ependyma lying in the floor of the lateral ventricle which became secondarily fused to the thalamus during development. The area medial to the groove is covered by the pia in the floor of the transverse fissure of the cerebrum.

The *ventral surface* (Figs. 2-6, 2-34) adjoins the subthalamus. Caudally it is continuous with the tegmental region of the mesencephalon, through which most ascending fibers enter the thalamus. The caudal region (Fig. 2-39), sometimes called the *metathalamus,* contains two swellings, the *medial* and *lateral geniculate bodies.*

Internal Morphology (Figs. 2-33, 2-34.)

The thalamus is a large mass of gray matter divided into a number of nuclear groups. No attempt will be made here to describe each of these nuclei (Chap. 22). However, some of the more gross aspects will be considered.

The dorsal surface of the thalamus has a thin covering of fibers called the *stratum zonale.* Along the lateral surface is the external medullary lamina. Medially, beneath the ependymal

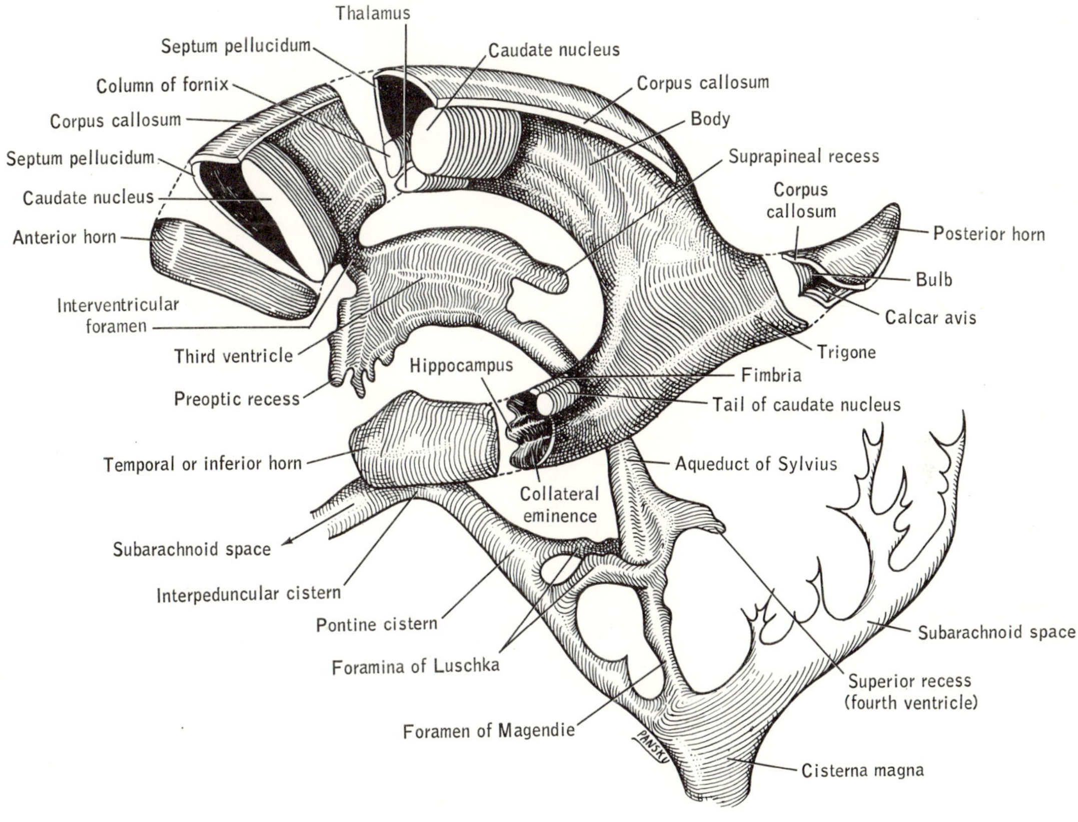

Fig. 2-32. Diagrammatic representation of the ventricular system of the human brain, showing the relations of various structures to the walls of the ventricles.

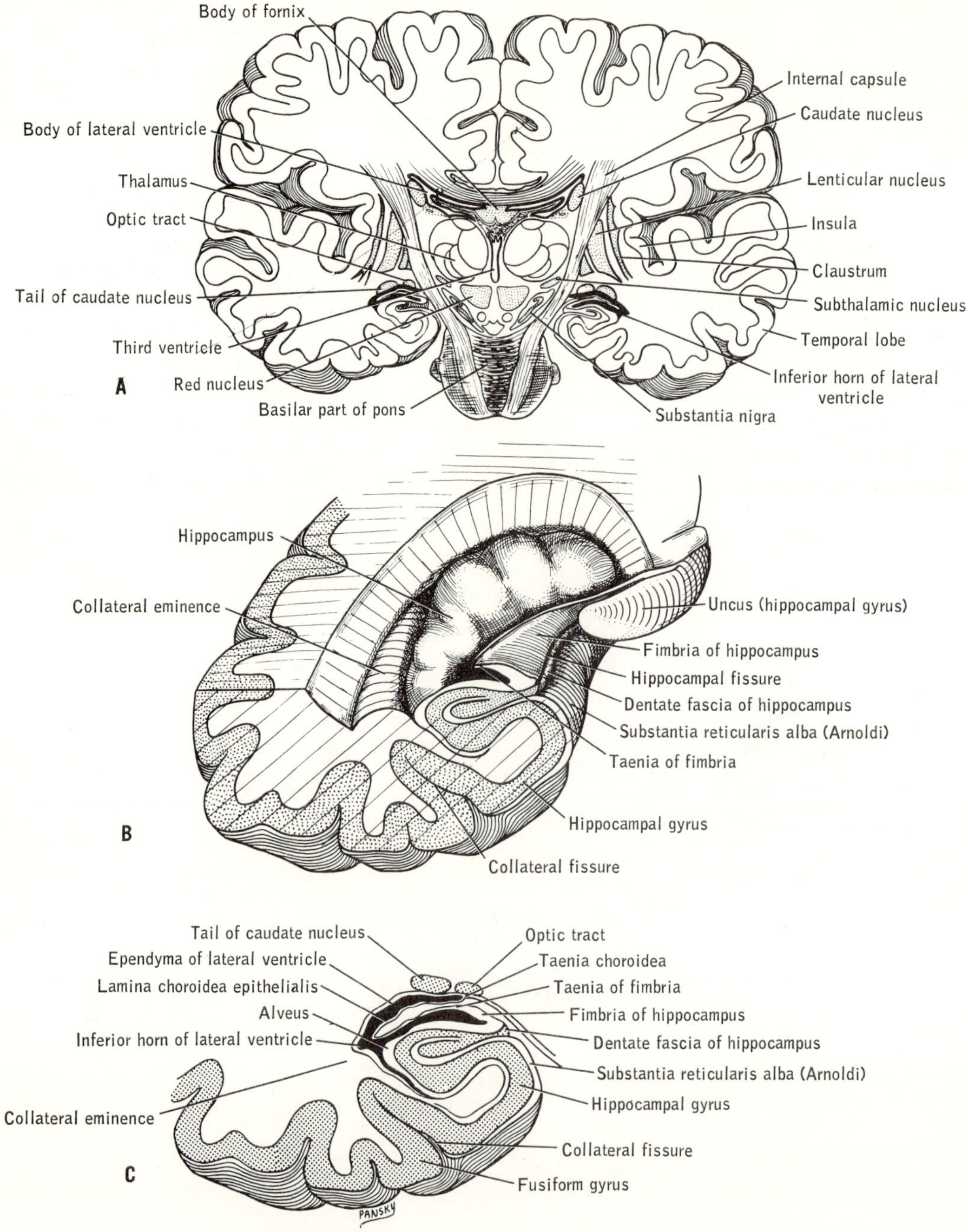

Fig. 2-33. *A.* Vertical section through the human brain at the level of the third ventricle. (*Adapted from Woerdeman, Atlas of Human Anatomy, McGraw-Hill Book Company, Inc., Blakiston Division, New York, 1950.*) *B.* Dissection of the inferior horn of the lateral ventricle. C. Enlargement of a part of *A* to show the hippocampus, the choroid plexus, and inferior horn of the lateral ventricle.

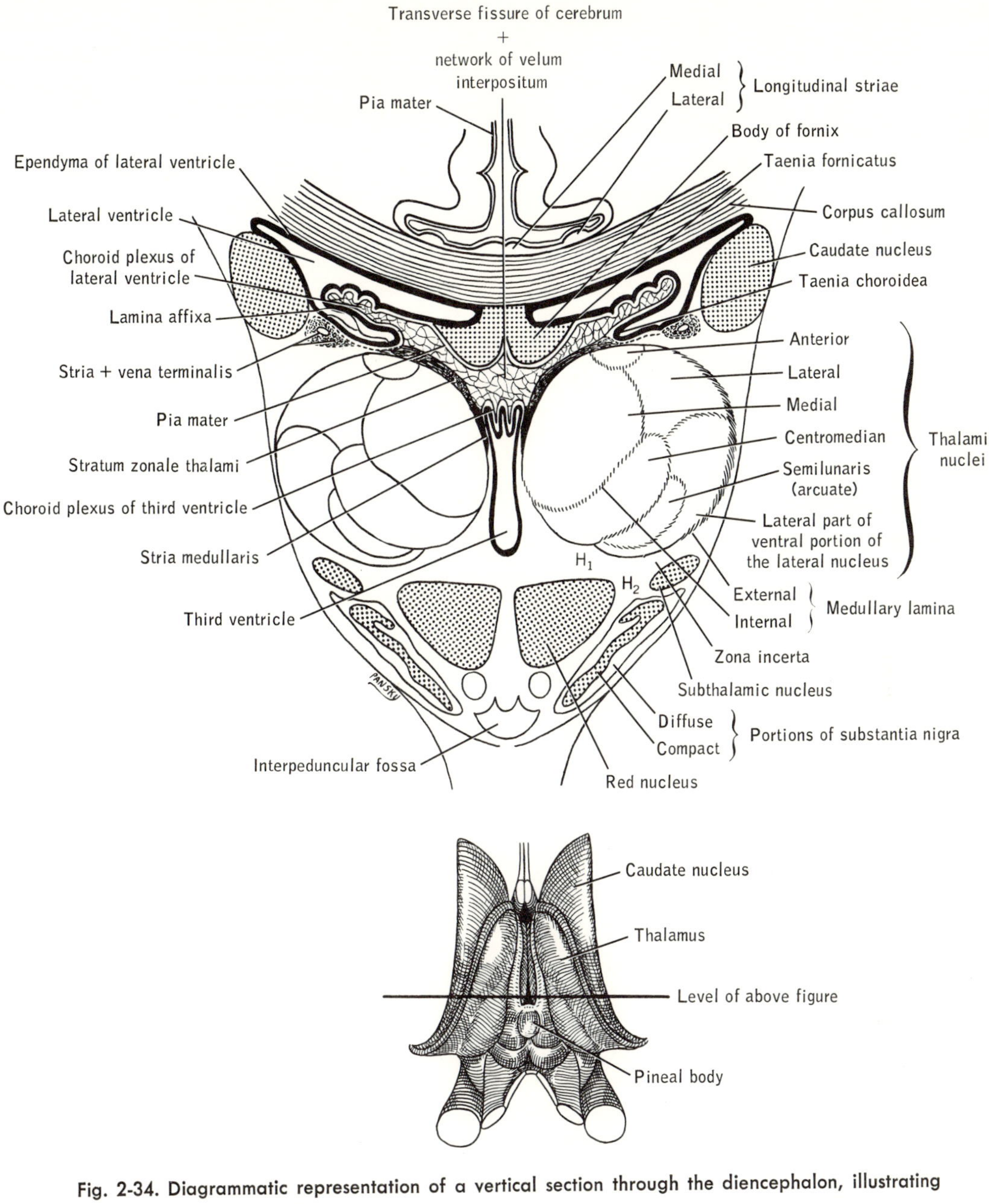

Fig. 2-34. Diagrammatic representation of a vertical section through the diencephalon, illustrating the thalamus and its adjoining structures.

lining of the third ventricle, lies a homogeneous zone of gray substance called the *central gray* (matter). This area is lacking in myelinated fibers and is occupied by several nuclear groups. The stratum zonale sends fibers ventrally into the substance of the thalamus, forming the *internal medullary lamina.* This divides the thalamus into a medial and a lateral portion. Rostrally, in the region of the anterior tubercle, the internal lamina splits, partially separating the anterior thalamus from the medial and lateral.

The Subthalamus (Figs. 2-33, 2-34.)

This is a transition zone between the thalamus and tegmental portion of the mesencephalon. Both the *red nucleus* and the *substantia nigra* of the mesencephalon protrude into the caudal portion of the subthalamus. Lateral to it is the region where the internal capsule joins the cerebral peduncles. The hypothalamus lies medially and rostrally.

Hypothalamus

External Morphology (Figs. 2-6 to 2-8.)

This region lies ventral to the hypothalamic sulcus. It consists of several parts, including the lamina terminalis, optic recess, optic chiasma, infundibulum, tuber cinereum, and mammillary bodies. The optic chiasma, infundibulum, tuber cinereum, posterior perforated substance, and mammillary bodies lie between the cerebral peduncles in the interpeduncular fossa. The enlarged upper end of the infundibulum is called the *median eminence* and is part of the tuber cinereum. Its inferior end is the posterior lobe (neural lobe) of the hypophysis.

Internal Morphology

The medial portion of the hypothalamus is predominantly cellular, containing many nuclear groups (Chap. 21). The lateral portion of the hypothalamus contains scattered nerve cells and many longitudinally running myelinated fibers. The hypothalamus may also be subdivided transversely into a supraoptic area, overlying the chiasma; a tuberal or central portion, containing the median eminence and the infundibulum; and the posterior, mammillary region, containing the mammillary bodies.

Cavity of the Diencephalon
(Figs. 2-29 to 2-34.)

This is a narrow, perpendicular cavity called the third ventricle. Its lateral walls are formed by the thalamus dorsally and the hypothalamus ventrally. On the lateral wall, the hypothalamic sulcus extends from the cerebral aqueduct caudally to the interventricular foramen (of Monro). In most cases, the third ventricle is traversed by a bridge of gray substance, the *massa intermedia*.

At the anterior end of the ventricle, the lamina terminalis extends upwards from the region of the optic chiasma to the anterior commissure. Between the chiasma and the ventral edge of the lamina lies the optic recess.

In the floor of the ventricle are the optic chiasma, the infundibulum, tuber cinereum, mammillary bodies, and subthalamus.

The roof is narrow, a thin lamina of ependyma stretching between the medullary striae. To this is added the vascular pia, forming the choroid tela, the folds of which invaginate into the ventricle as the choroid plexus.

Three foramina are associated with the ventricle: one for each of the lateral ventricles (interventricular foramina, or foramina of Monro) and an opening for the cerebral aqueduct.

MESENCEPHALON

External Structure (Figs. 2-15, 2-34 to 2-36.)

Dorsal Surface

When cerebrum and cerebellum have been removed, it is seen that the dorsal surface of the mesencephalon consists of four rounded swellings, the *quadrigeminal bodies, or colliculi.* Two furrows, in the form of a cross (cruciate sulcus) divide the four into paired superior and inferior colliculi. The pineal body overlaps the rostral end of the longitudinal groove. From the caudal end of this same groove is a band of fibers, the *frenulum veli,* which ends in the anterior medullary velum of the metencephalon (cerebellum). The rootlets of the fourth nerve (IV) emerge from the brain on either side of the midline just caudal to the inferior colliculus.

Lateral Surface

Laterally (Figs. 2-35, 2-36), two fiber bands, associated with each colliculus, are represented

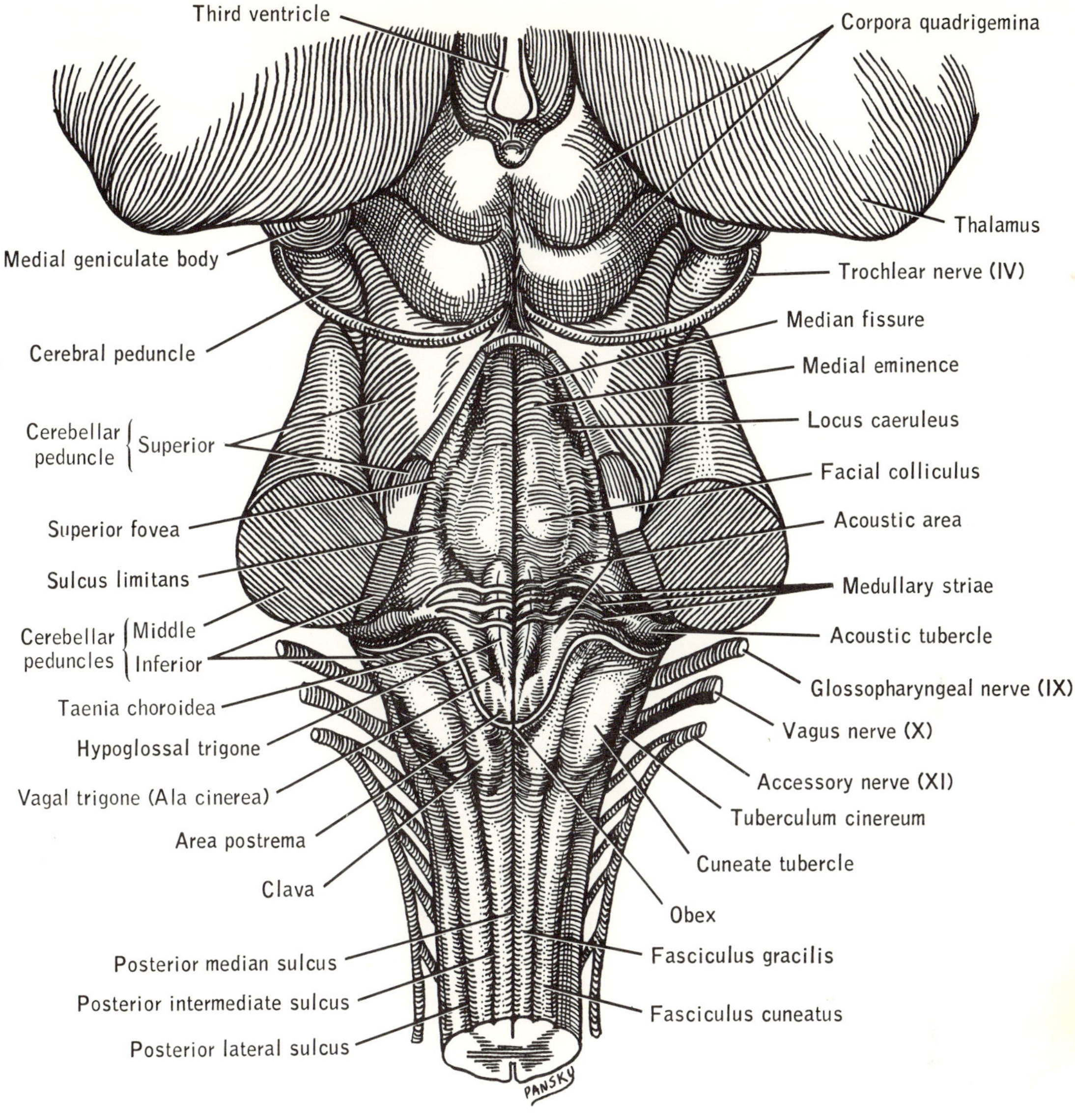

Fig. 2-35. Dorsal view of the human brain stem with the cerebellum removed to expose the rhomboid fossa.

by elevations. One band, the brachium of the inferior colliculus, joins the inferior colliculus to the medial geniculate body of the thalamus. The other, the brachium of the superior colliculus connects the superior colliculus to the lateral geniculate body of the thalamus.

Basal Surface

On this side (Figs. 2-7, 2-8), the cerebral peduncles diverge laterally from the rostral edge of the pons, leaving a triangular depression, the *interpeduncular fossa,* between them. Within the fossa, there is a groove on the medial side of

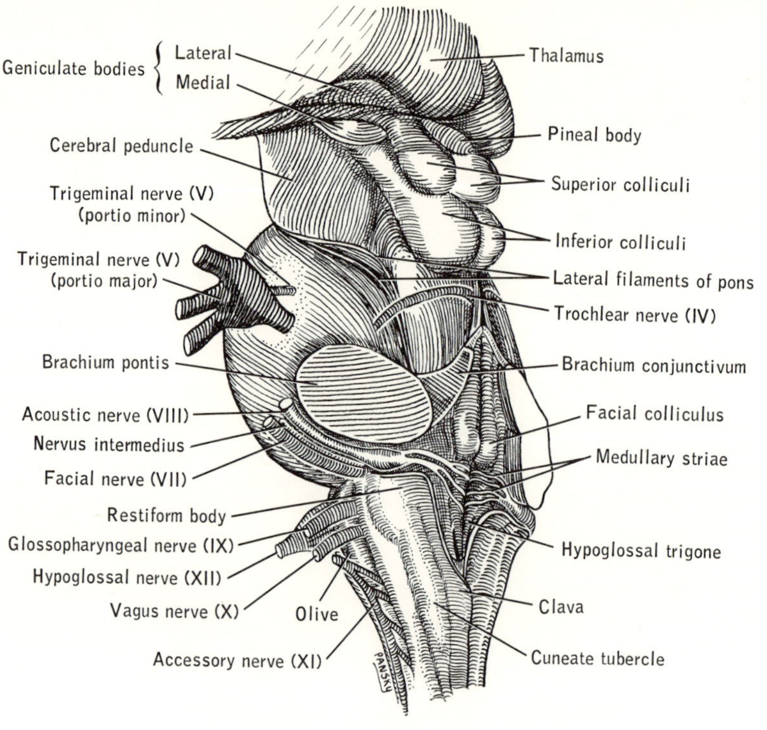

Fig. 2-36. Human brain stem viewed from the side.

each peduncle, the sulcus of the oculomotor nerve (III), through which the rootlets of that nerve emerge from the brain. On the lateral aspect of the peduncle, there is also a longitudinal groove, called the lateral sulcus of the mesencephalon. Just above this sulcus is a faint indication of fibers curving dorsally toward the inferior colliculus. These represent the *lateral lemniscus*.

Cavity of the Mesencephalon
(Figs. 2-6, 2-29 to 2-32.)

The cavity of the mesencephalon, the *cerebral aqueduct* (of Sylvius), is a small canal usually triangular in shape with the apex directed ventrally. It is surrounded by a thick zone of gray matter, the central gray stratum, which is continuous with a similar zone along the third ventricle of the diencephalon.

Internal Structure (Figs. 2-37, 2-38, 2-39.)

Dorsal to the aqueduct is the tectum, or lamina quadrigemina, made up of both white and gray substance. Ventral to the aqueduct, the mesencephalon can be divided into two parts: the basis pedunculi and the tegmentum. The former is the most ventral part and consists of a large area of longitudinally running fibers. The tegmentum is an area of reticular formation composed of both nuclear gray masses and fibers continuous with the tegmentum of the pons. A large area of pigmented nerve cells, the *substantia nigra* lies between the tegmentum and the peduncle. Among the fiber groups located in the tegmentum are the lemniscus system, the dorsal and medial longitudinal fasciculi, the brachium conjunctivum and its decussation, the brachium of the inferior colliculus, and fibers of the third and fourth cranial nerves. The dorsal and ventral tegmental decussations are associated with the tectospinal and rubrospinal tracts. Certain cell groups are also located here: the dorsal and ventral tegmental nuclei, the interpeduncular nucleus, the red nucleus, the nuclei of the third and fourth cranial nerves, and the mesencephalic nucleus of the fifth cranial nerve.

METENCEPHALON

This consists of two parts, the cerebellum and pons.

Cerebellum

External Morphology (Figs. 2-6, 2-41 to 2-44.)

The surface of the cerebellum, the cortex, is thrown into folds, called folia, the long axis of which runs transversely across the cerebellum. This portion of the brain consists of three parts: a single central portion, the *vermis;* and two *hemispheres* located on either side. Dorsally, the vermis forms a median elevation not clearly separated from the hemispheres. This is the superior vermis. Ventrally, the vermis lies at the bottom of a deep fissure (cerebellar notch) and is here referred to as the inferior vermis.

A deep groove, the *primary fissure,* divides the cerebellum into lobes—*anterior* and *posterior*. The anterior lobe is the area rostral to the fissure and includes a major portion of the superior vermis and a portion of the hemispheres. From front to back the vermis consists of the *lingula,* the *central lobule,* and the *culmen mon-*

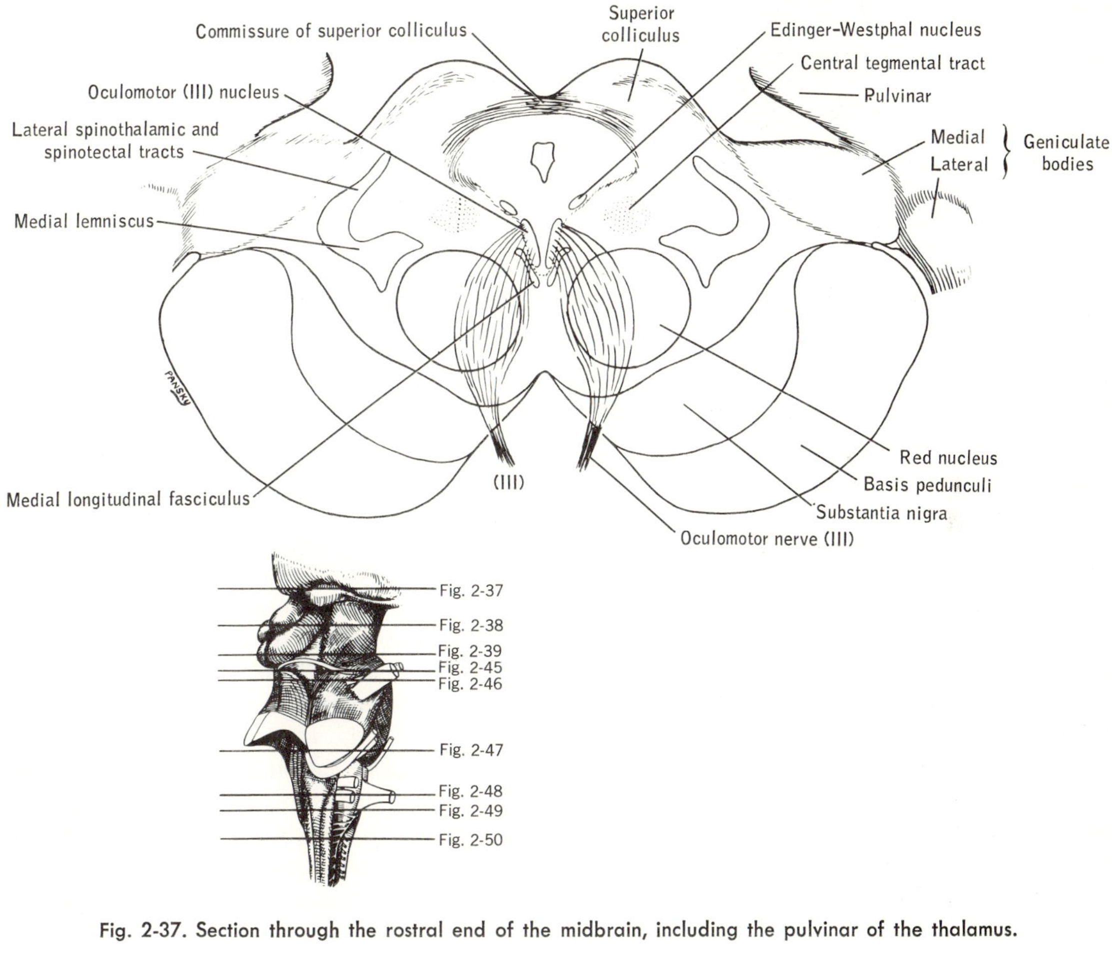

Fig. 2-37. Section through the rostral end of the midbrain, including the pulvinar of the thalamus.

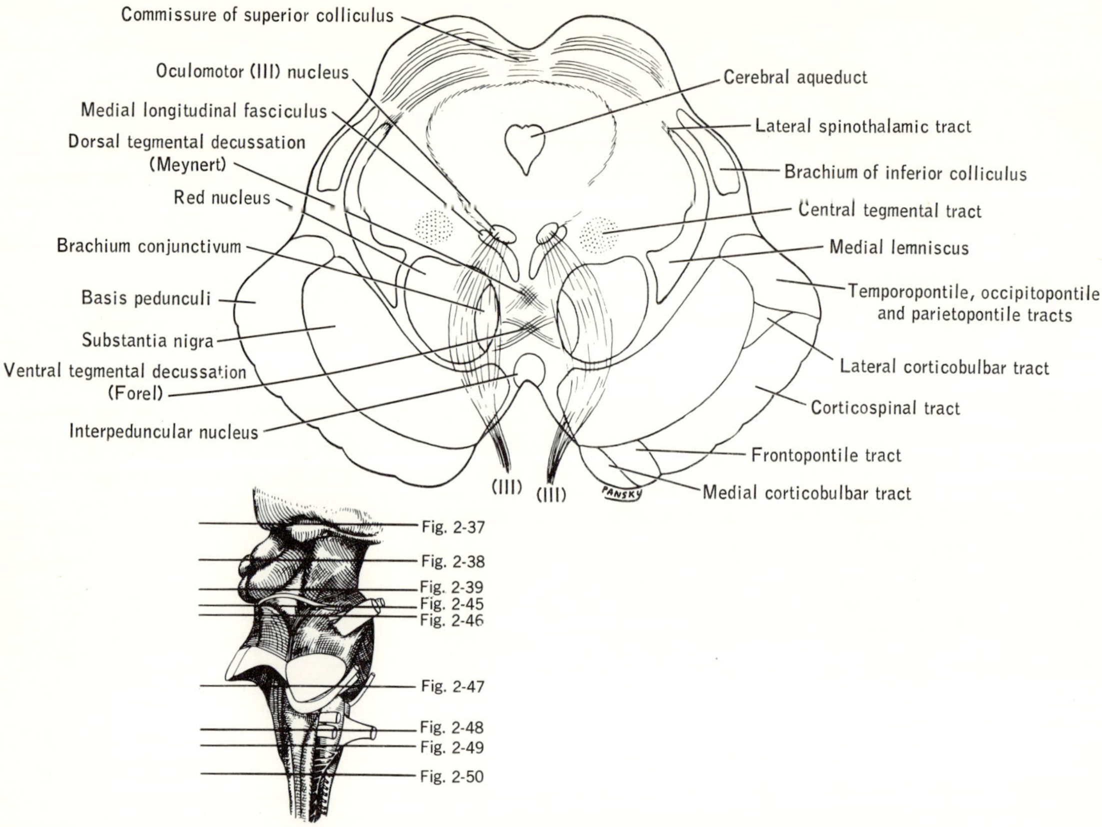

Fig. 2-38. Section of the midbrain at the caudal level of the superior colliculus.

ticuli. The regions of the hemispheres included in the anterior lobe are called the ala centralis and the anterior quadrangular lobule.

The posterior lobe lies behind the primary fissure and includes the caudal portion of the superior vermis, all of the inferior vermis, and the major portion of the hemispheres. That portion of the superior vermis included in the posterior lobe is the *declive* (of Monticulus). From front to back, the inferior vermis consists of *the folium, tuber, pyramis,* and *uvula.* The most rostral part of the hemisphere found in the posterior lobe is the posterior quadrangular (simple) lobule. It is bounded posteriorly by the *postclival sulcus.* Behind this sulcus lies the *ansiform lobule,* sometimes divided by the *horizontal cerebellar sulcus* into the *superior* and *inferior similunar lobule* which sometimes shows a partial division in its caudal portion. This is the gracile lobule (Chap. 18). A small lateral projection between the tonsil and the flocculus, the paraflocculus, is also described (Chap. 18). On the ventral surface of the posterior lobe, the ansiform lobule is not sharply delimited from the more anterior, *biventer lobule;* by many neuroanatomists, the biventer lobule is considered to be a part of the ansiform lobule. Two small rounded areas, lying on either side of the vermis, are called the *paramedian lobules* (tonsils).

Along the most caudal border of the ansiform or biventral, lobule, lies the *posterolateral fissure,* which separates this lobule from the small, almost vestigial *flocculonodular* lobe. The latter includes the most inferior portion of the vermis, the *nodulus,* and two small portions on either side

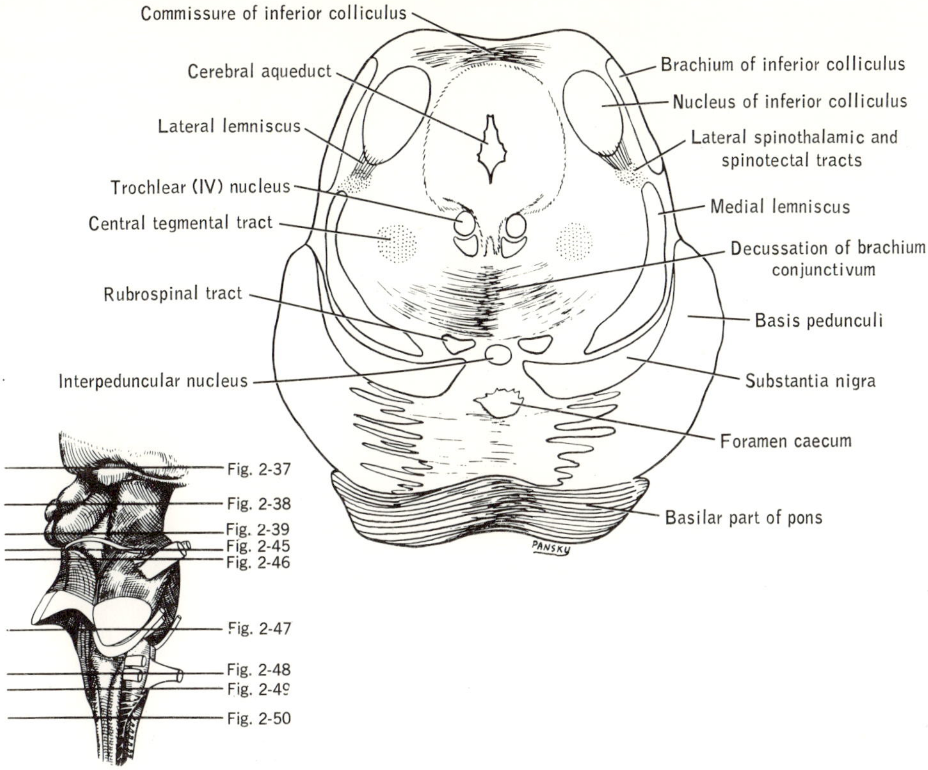

Fig. 2-39. Section of the midbrain at the level of the inferior colliculus.

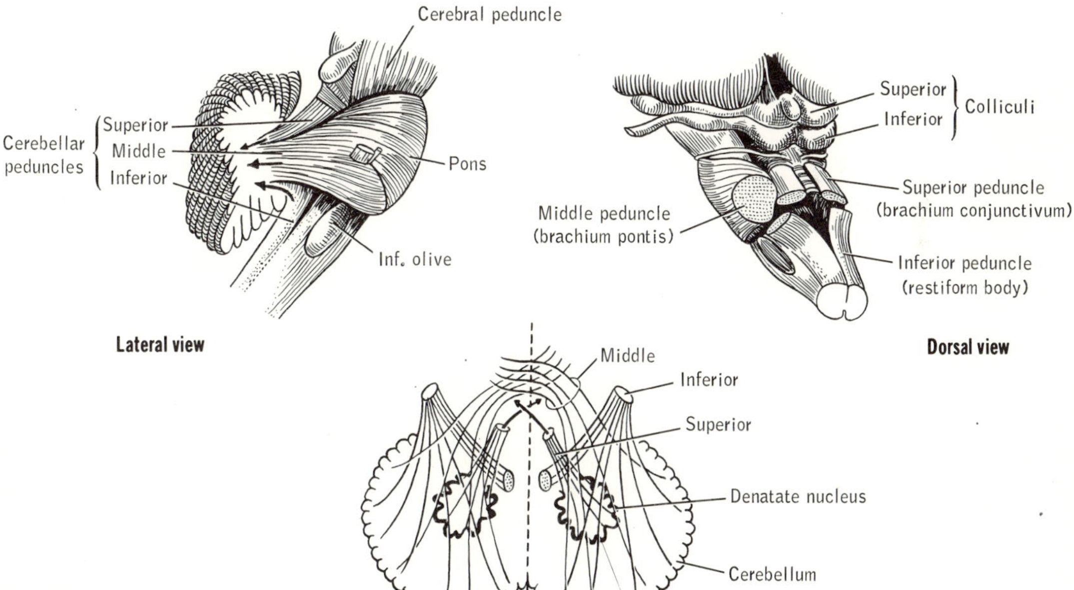

Fig. 2-40. Diagrams of the brain stem to show the three cerebellar peduncles.

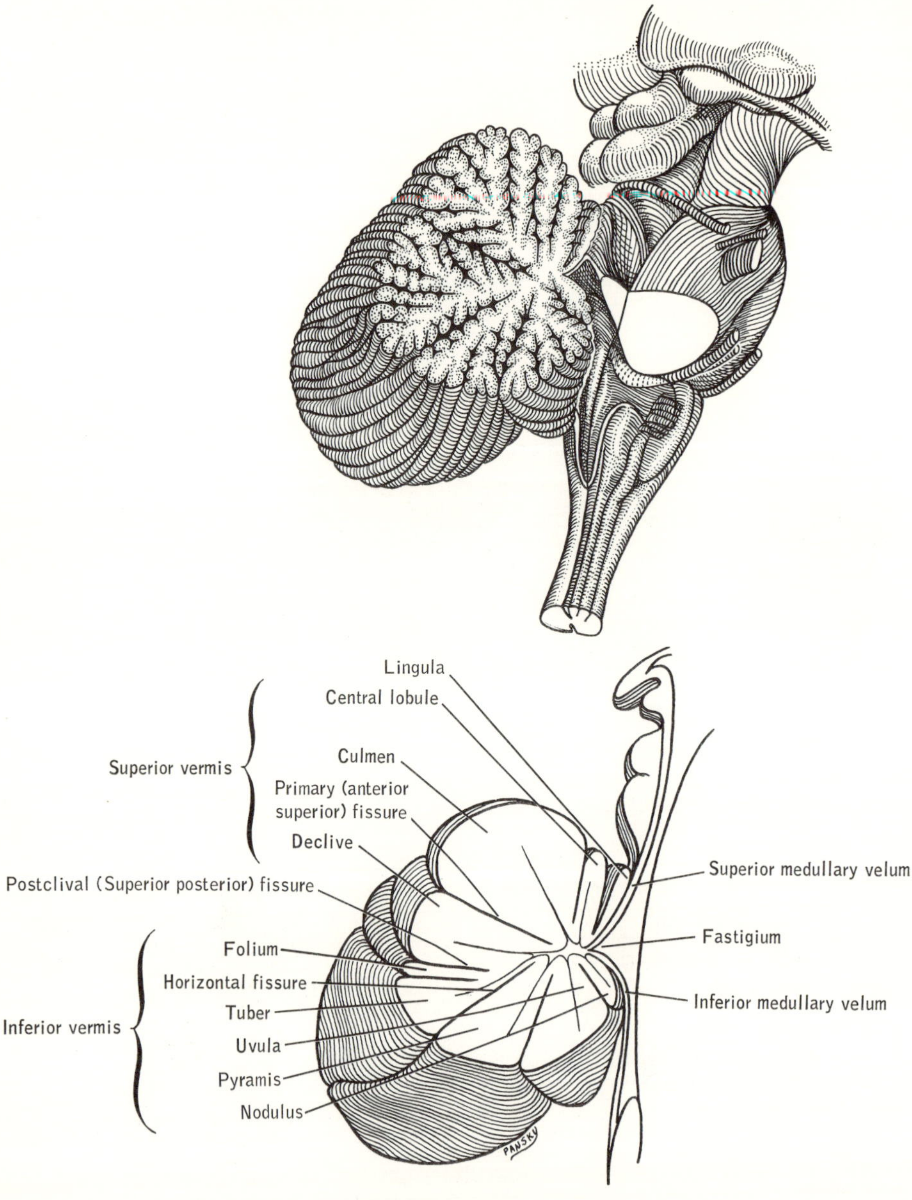

Fig. 2-41. Midsagittal section through the cerebellum.

associated with the hemispheres, the *flocculus* and a connecting band, the *peduncle of the flocculus*.

Internal Structure (Figs. 2-40, 2-44.)

The details of cortical structure will be given elsewhere (Chap. 18). Long, narrow folds of cortex, called folia, cover a central core of white substance which is continuous from one hemisphere to the other through the vermis. Embedded in the medullary core are groups of gray substance, the cerebellar nuclei. The largest and most lateral is an irregular lamina of gray substance which resembles a crumpled sac with an open mouth, the hilus, directed medially. This is the *dentate nucleus*. Close to the hilus lies a narrow, vertical plate of cells called the *emboliform nucleus*. Medial to the inferior portion of the latter lie one or more rounded gray areas called the *globose nuclei*. Closely adjoining the midline, in the core of the vermis, are the *fastigial nuclei*.

Cerebellar Connections (Figs. 2-14, 2-18, 2-35, 2-40.)

The cerebellum is connected with the brain stem by large fiber bundles called the cerebellar peduncles or cerebellar brachii. The lowest, or *inferior peduncle* (*restiform body*), runs rostrally along the lateral wall of the fourth ventricle, bending sharply to enter the cerebellum.

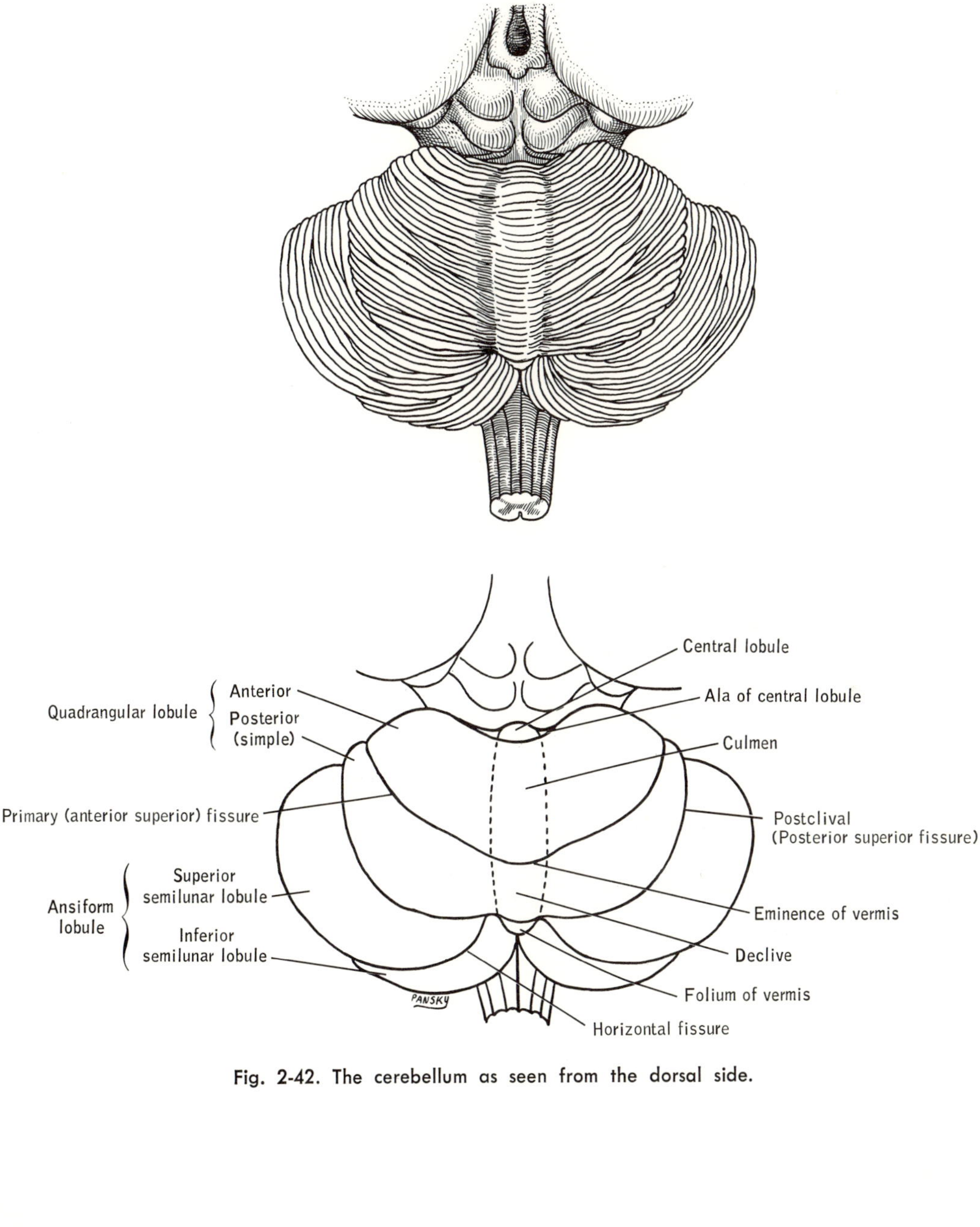

Fig. 2-42. The cerebellum as seen from the dorsal side.

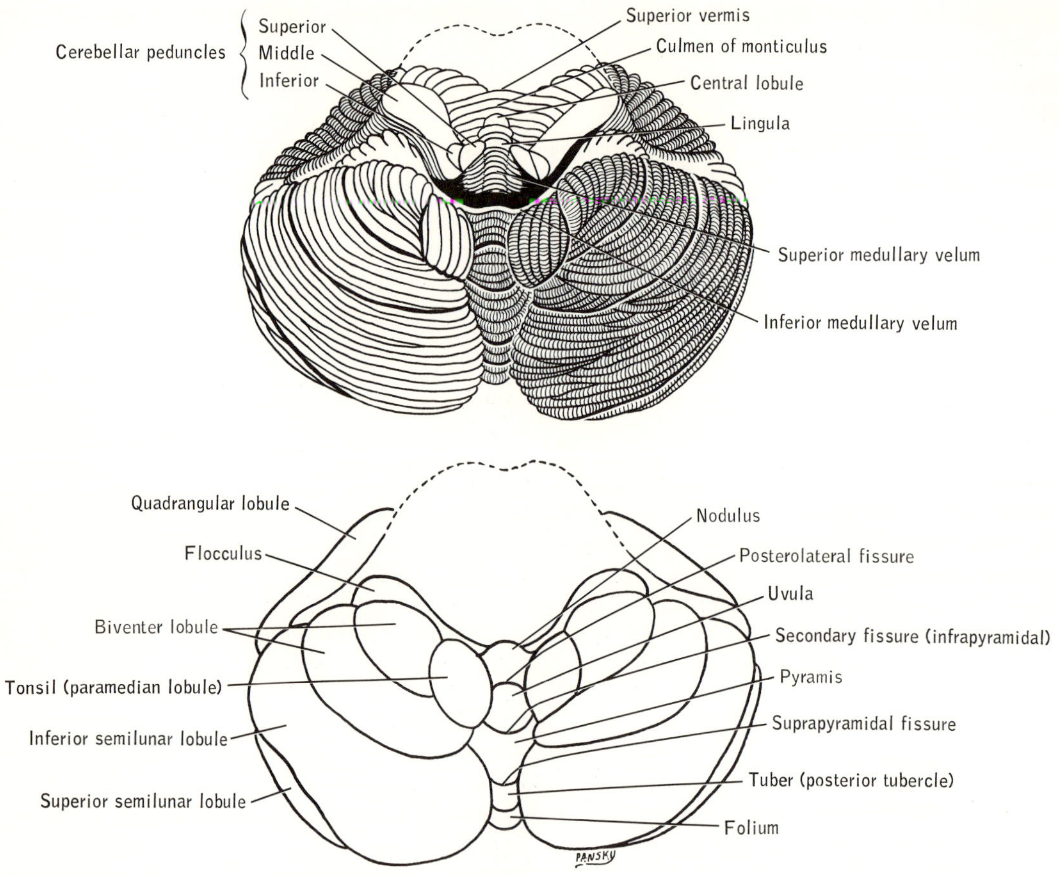

Fig. 2-43. The cerebellum as seen from below.

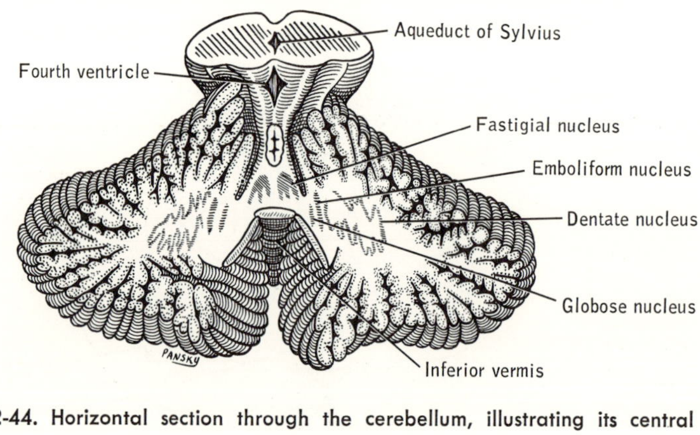

Fig. 2-44. Horizontal section through the cerebellum, illustrating its central nuclei.

The largest and most lateral of the brachii is the *middle peduncle* (*brachium pontis*), the fibers of which ascend dorsally from the lateral aspect of the pons. The *superior peduncle* (*brachium conjunctivum*), runs ventrally and rostrally along the lateral wall of the superior part of the fourth ventricle.

Pons

External Structure (Figs. 2-6 to 2-8.)

The dorsal surface of the pons is completely obscured by the cerebellum, where it forms the floor of the fourth ventricle. The ventral surface is convex, both longitudinally and transversely. A median groove, called the basilar sulcus, extends the full length of the ventral surface of the pons. The trigeminal nerve roots emerge from the ventrolateral aspect of the pons near the point where pons and brachium pontis become confluent.

Internal Structure (Figs. 2-45 to 2-47.)

The pons is composed of two parts which are structurally different: the *dorsal,* or *tegmental, region,* which is similar to and continuous with the medulla; and the *ventral,* or *basal,* portion.

The basilar portion of the pons is the largest. It is composed of scattered, longitudinally running fiber bundles, irregular in size and shape. There are also groups of fibers passing laterally from the pons to the brachium pontis. Interspersed among all the bundles are gray masses, the *nuclei pontis.*

The smaller tegmental portion contains several gray masses, among which are the dorsal and ventral cochlear nuclei; certain of the vestibular

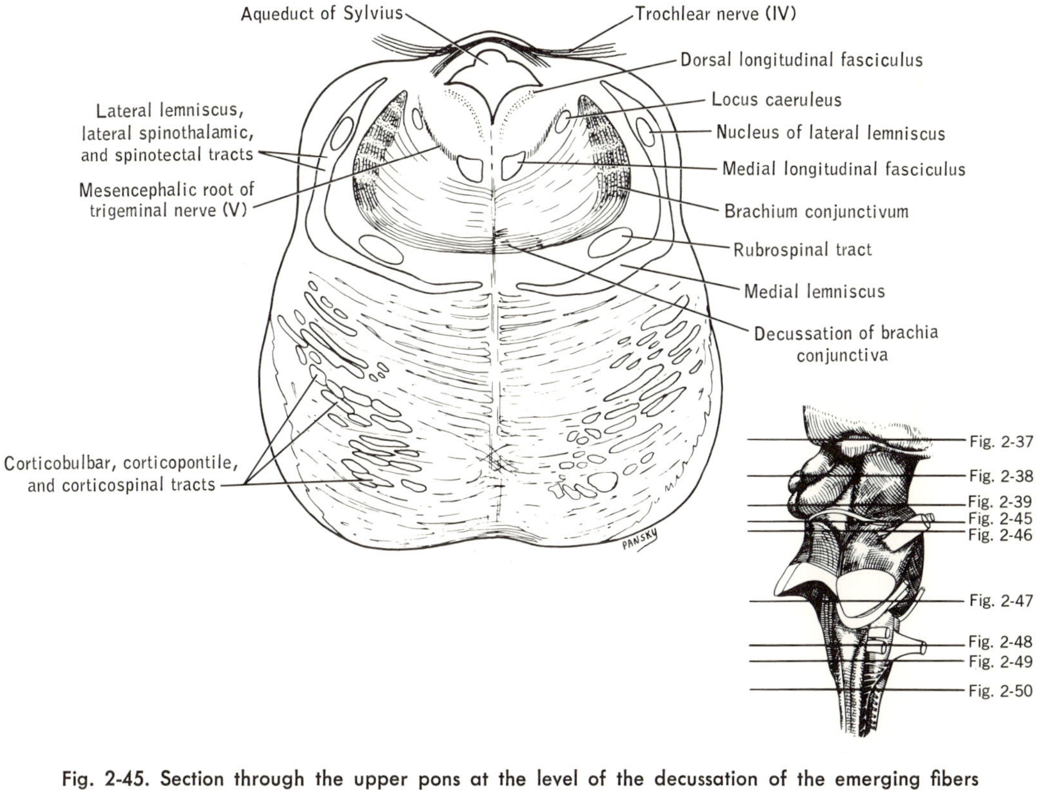

Fig. 2-45. Section through the upper pons at the level of the decussation of the emerging fibers of the trochlear nerve (IV).

nuclei; the superior olivary nucleus; the nuclei of the abducens (VI) and facial (VII) cranial nerves; and the spinal, main sensory, and motor nuclei of the trigeminal (V) cranial nerve. There are also important fiber groups here: trapezoid body; fibers of the abducens, facial, and trigeminal nerves, including the mesencephalic root of the latter; the medial longitudinal fasciculus; the medial lemniscus; the inferior, middle, and superior cerebellar peduncles.

MYELENCEPHALON

Medulla Oblongata

External Structure (Figs. 2-6 to 2-8, 2-38, 2-39.)

A line just rostral to the highest rootlet of the first cervical nerve represents the caudal boundary of the medulla. It is separated from the pons by a transverse sulcus. In shape, it resembles a truncated cone with apex pointed toward the spinal cord.

The surface of the medulla is traversed by several longitudinal fissures and sulci, which serve to divide it into several areas. On the dorsal surface of the caudal part of the medulla is the *dorsal* (posterior) *median fissure,* which is continued caudally onto the spinal cord. Lateral to this is the *dorsal lateral sulcus,* made outstanding by rootlets of the glossopharyngeal (IX), vagus (X), and accessory (XI) cranial nerves. Between the dorsal median and dorsal lateral fissures lies the *dorsal intermediate sulcus.* On the ventral midline is the *ventral* (anterior) *median fissure,* which continues downward onto the cord and ends rostrally at the

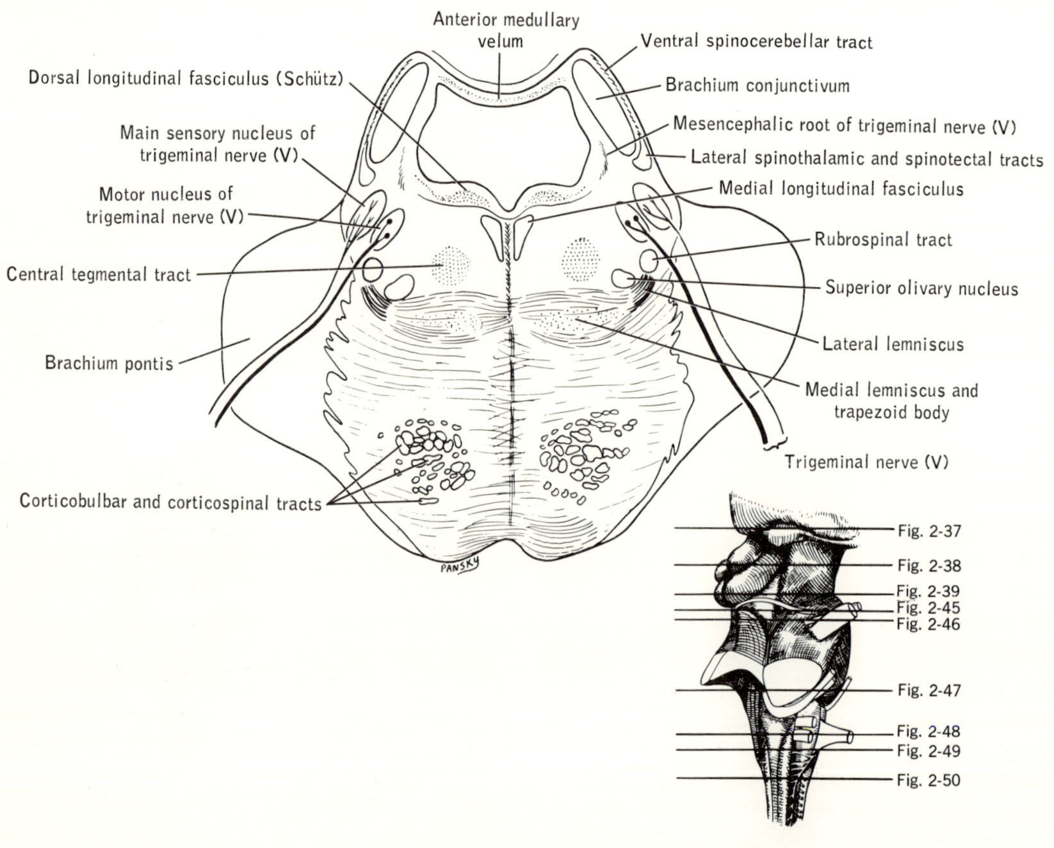

Fig. 2-46. Section through the mid-pons at the level of the trigeminal nerve (V).

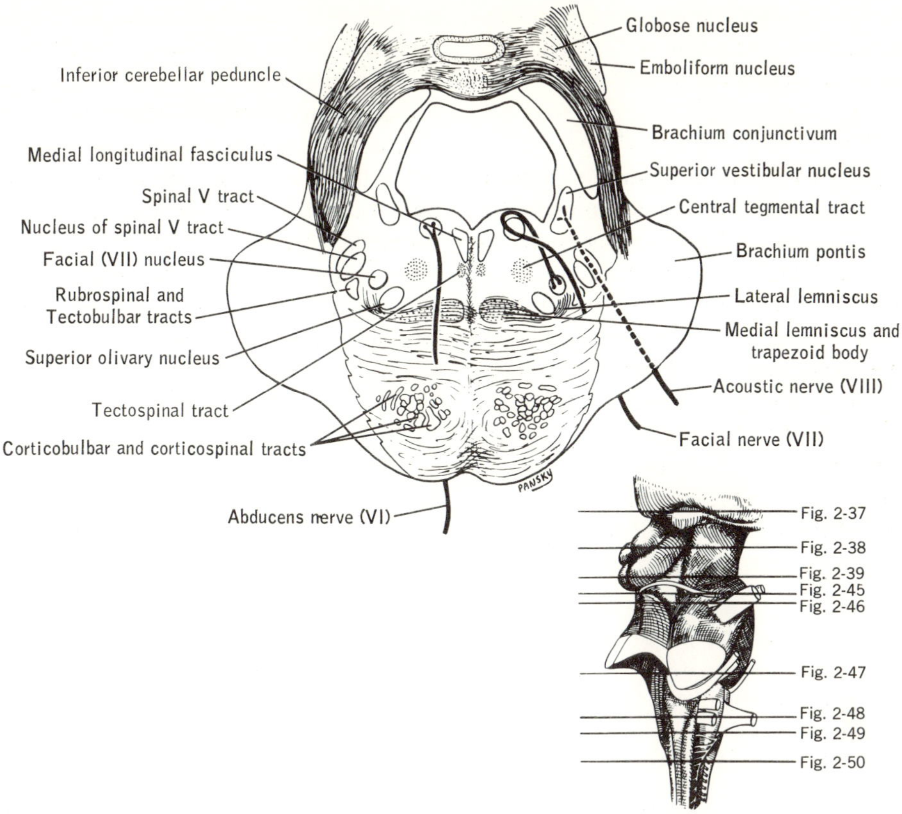

Fig. 2-47. Section through the lower pons at the level of the nuclei of nerves (VI) and (VII).

caudal border of the pons as the *foramen cecum*. Lateral to the ventral median fissure is a less distinct groove called the *ventral lateral sulcus*. Along this line emerge fibers of the hypoglossal (XII) nerve. This groove also continues onto the cord.

Between the dorsal median fissure and the dorsal intermediate sulcus is the *fasciculus gracilis,* the direct continuation of the same bundle from the cord. Lateral to the dorsal intermediate sulcus is the *fasciculus cuneatus*. Rostrally these fasciculi end in swellings because of the presence of their nuclei of termination. The nucleus gracilis lies in the region called the *clava,* while the nucleus cuneatus lies in the *cuneate tubercle*. Just above the middle of the medulla, the clava and cuneate tubercle are shifted far laterally and are replaced by the inferior cerebellar peduncle. Running parallel to the cuneate fasciculus, between the latter and the roots of the ninth, tenth, and eleventh cranial nerves, is another longitudinal ridge called the *tuberculum cinereum*.

The lateral area of the medulla, between the dorsal lateral and ventral lateral sulci, is a continuation of the corresponding lateral funiculus of the cord. However, in the rostral end of this funiculus is a prominent oval swelling, the *olive*. Fibers running dorsally either from the ventral median fissure or from the groove between the pyramid and olive are called the *ventral external arcuate fibers*. They join the restiform body.

The ventral area, betwen the ventral median fissure and the ventral lateral sulcus, consists mainly of an elongated swelling, the *pyramid*. Each tapers toward the spinal cord, and at the caudal end of the medulla, the pyramids undergo nearly complete decussation, in which region the median fissure is almost obliterated.

Internal Structure (Figs. 2-48 to 2-50.)

It is a mixture of gray and white substance. Among the tracts and fiber bundles are the following: the pyramids and their decussation; the fasciculus gracilis and cuneatus; the medial longitudinal fasciculus (MLF); the spinal tract of the trigeminal nerve; the internal arcuate fibers; the restiform body; tractus solitarius; the spinal vestibular tract; and the medial lemniscus. Emerging fibers of the hypoglossal, vagus, acoustic, and abducens nerves are also seen. The nuclei located here are nucleus gracilis and cuneatus; nucleus of the spinal tract of the trigeminal nerve; spinal vestibular nucleus; dorsal motor nucleus of the vagus; nucleus of the hypoglossal; nucleus ambiguus; the inferior olivary nucleus; the dorsal and ventral cochlear nuclei; the accessory cuneate and accessory olivary nuclei. In addition to these special circumscribed fiber bundles and nuclei, there are the dorsal and ventral spinocerebellar fibers; the tectospinal tract; and the olivocerebellar fibers. Also scattered among the fibers in the region dorsal to the olive are nests of cells, the *reticular nuclei.*

Cavity of the Hindbrain
(Figs. 2-29 to 2-32, 2-35.)

The cavity of the hindbrain is the *fourth ventricle.* It lies between the cerebellum dorsally and the tegmentum of the pons and medulla ven-

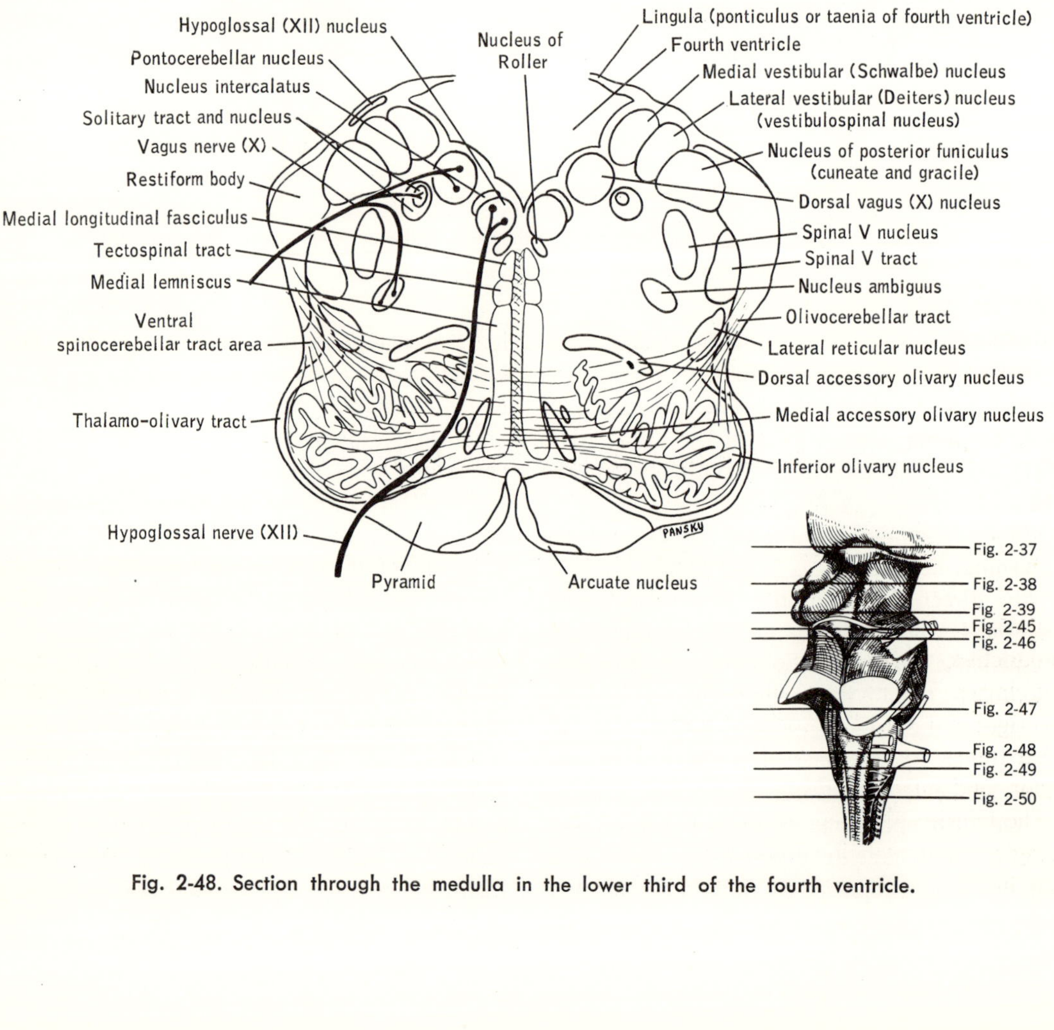

Fig. 2-48. Section through the medulla in the lower third of the fourth ventricle.

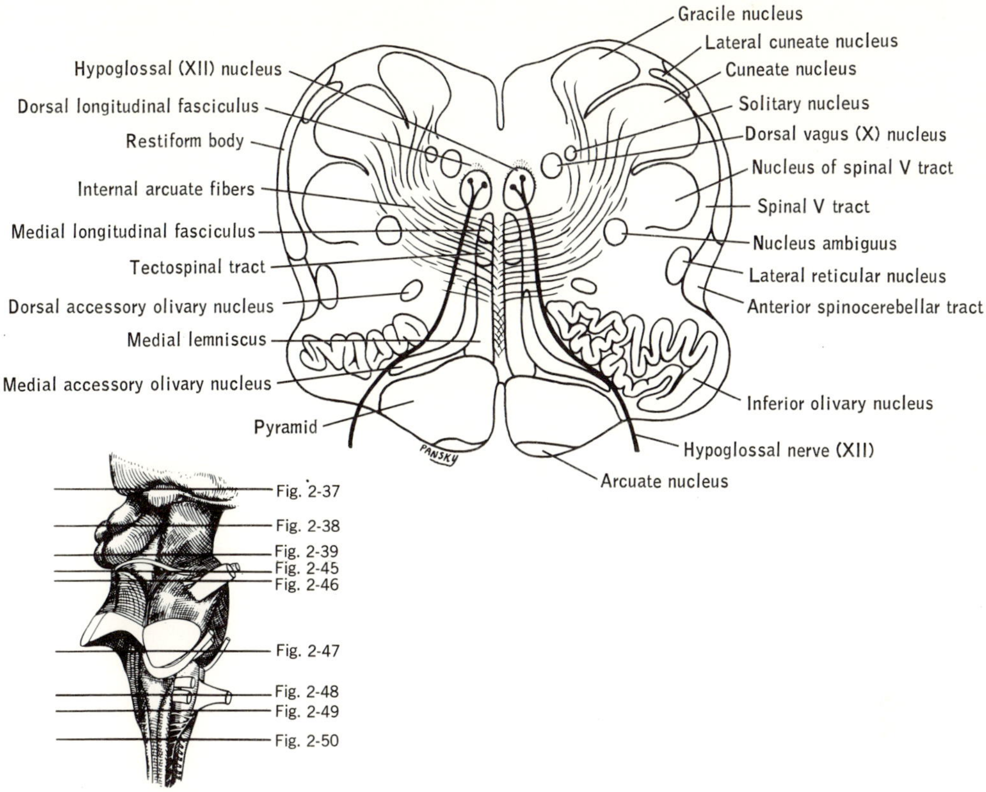

Fig. 2-49. Section through the medulla at the level of the sensory decussation.

trally. Rostrally, it is continuous with the cerebral aqueduct, while caudally, through the canal of the closed portion of the medulla, it is confluent with the central canal of the spinal cord. In the broadest portion of the ventricle, the *lateral recess* extends to the surface of the restiform body. Each recess opens laterally into the subarachnoid space through a foramen of Luschka.

Because of its shape, the floor of the ventricle (Fig. 2-35) is called the *rhomboid fossa.* The boundaries, from rostral to caudal, are brachia conjunctiva, restiform bodies, cuneate tubercles, and clavae. The median sulcus divides the fossa into right and left halves. The fossa is usually divided transversely into three parts: inferior, superior, and intermediate.

The inferior part has the shape of an inverted triangle, the base being represented by an arbitrary line joining the horizontal part of the *taenia* on either side. The taenia is a band through which the ependymal roof is attached to the boundary of the ventricle. The apex, the *calamus scriptorius,* is directed caudally. Lateral and parallel to the median sulcus is the *sulcus limitans.* In the latter is a small depression, the *inferior fovea.* From the fovea, a groove extends caudally and medially to form the inferolateral boundary of the *hypoglossal trigone.* Caudal to the hypoglossal trigone is another triangular area, the *ala cinerea,* separated from the former by an obliquely placed band of thickened ependyma called the *funiculus separans.* The elevated zone lying between the sulcus limitans and the median sulcus is the *median eminence,* found throughout the length of the rhomboid fossa.

The superior part is also triangular in shape, with the apex directed rostrally. Its base is formed by a line drawn transversely through the upper

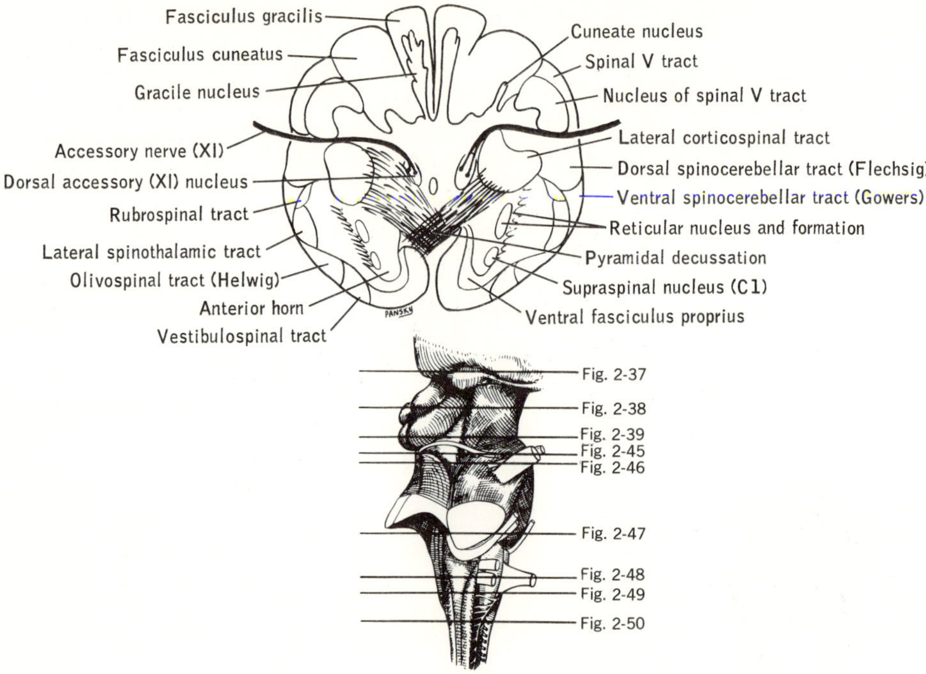

Fig. 2-50. Section through the lower medulla at the level of the pyramidal decussation.

ends of the *superior fovea.* The superior fovea are depressions in the sulcus limitans lying rostral to the inferior fovea. Medial to the superior fovea, the median eminence enlarges to become the *facial colliculus.* The region lateral to the sulcus limitans in the superior part of the rhomboid fossa is the *locus caeruleus.*

The intermediate part is that portion of the fossa which lies between the parallel bases of the superior and inferior zones. Horizontal ridges, the *medullary striae,* cross this region.

In addition to the three zones just mentioned, the *area acoustica* is also described. It includes a portion of the superior, intermediate, and inferior parts of the fossa. It is triangular in outline, the base being the sulcus limitans while its laterally directed apex points toward the end of the lateral recess of the fourth ventricle.

The roof of the fourth ventricle (Figs. 2-41, 2-46) is formed by three structures: the anterior medullary velum; the white substance of the cerebellum; and the choroid tela. Rostrally, the white substance of the cerebellum is stretched thin between the dorsal borders of the brachii conjunctiva as far as the caudal border of the tectum of the mesencephalon. This thin area is the *anterior medullary velum.* Near the midline, the lingula of the cerebellar vermis adheres to it. In a narrow zone near the middle of the ventricle, the roof is formed by the white core of the cerebellum. Caudal to the latter lies the choroid tela, composed of ependyma to which the vascular pia has been fused. The vessels of the tela invaginate into the fourth ventricle along two lines, one vertical, the other horizontal. This is the choroid plexus of the fourth ventricle. There is a median opening in the roof into the subarachnoid space, called the foramen of Magendie.

CLINICAL CONSIDERATIONS

Craniocerebral Topography (Figs. 2-51–2-53.)

It is essential for the clinical neurologist interested in the localization of cerebral lesions, and

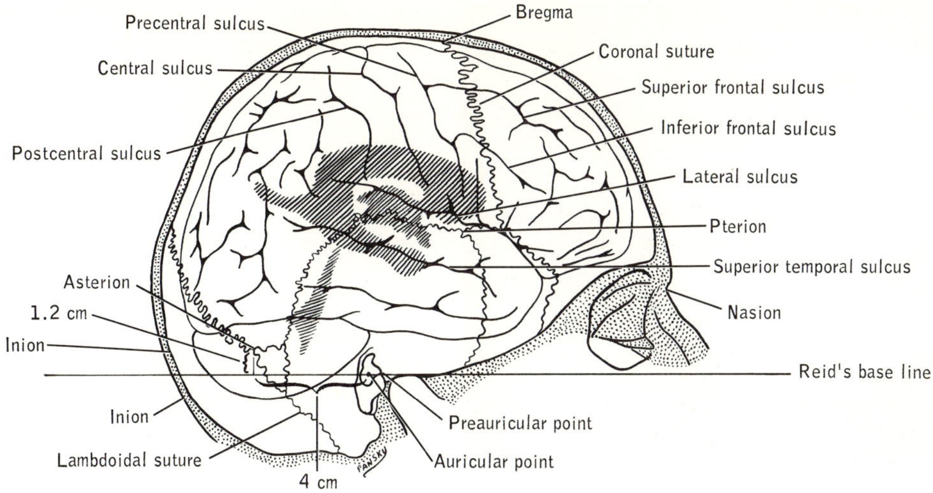

Fig. 2-51. Craniocerebral topography.

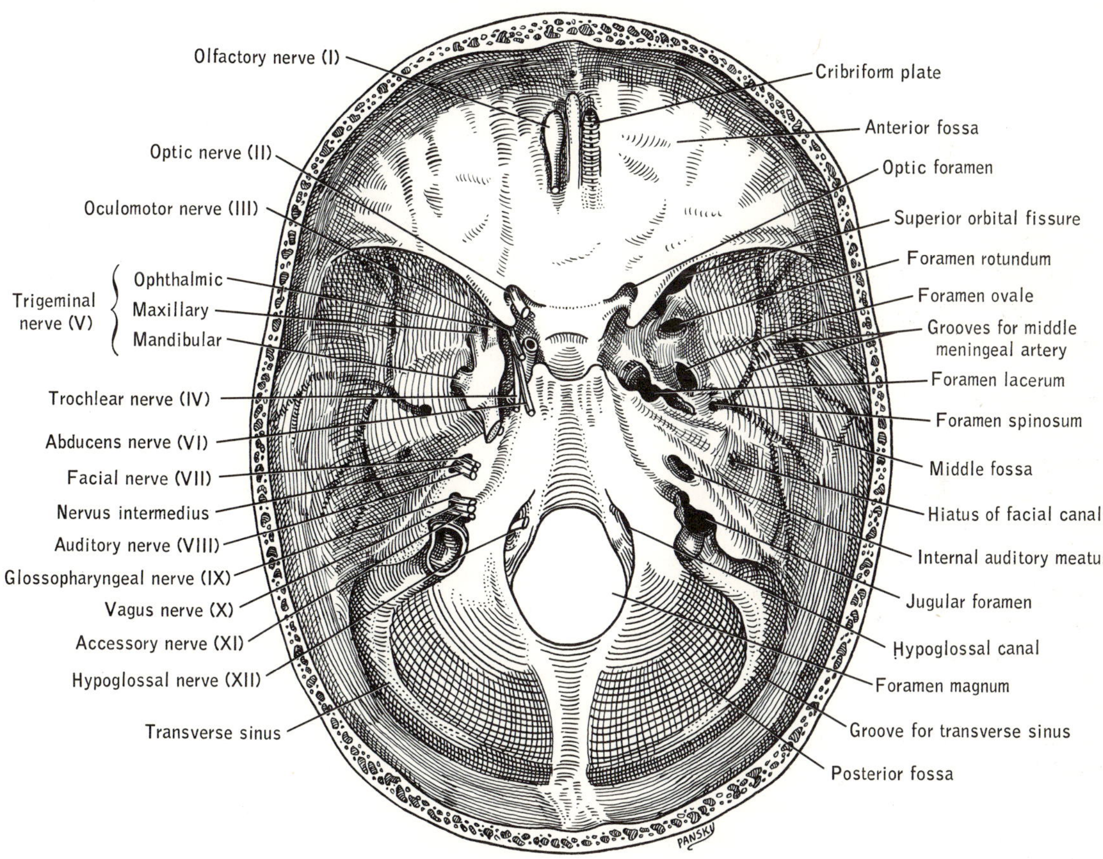

Fig. 2-52. Basal portion of the skull seen from above: cranial fossae, foramina, and grooves on the right; nerves on the left.

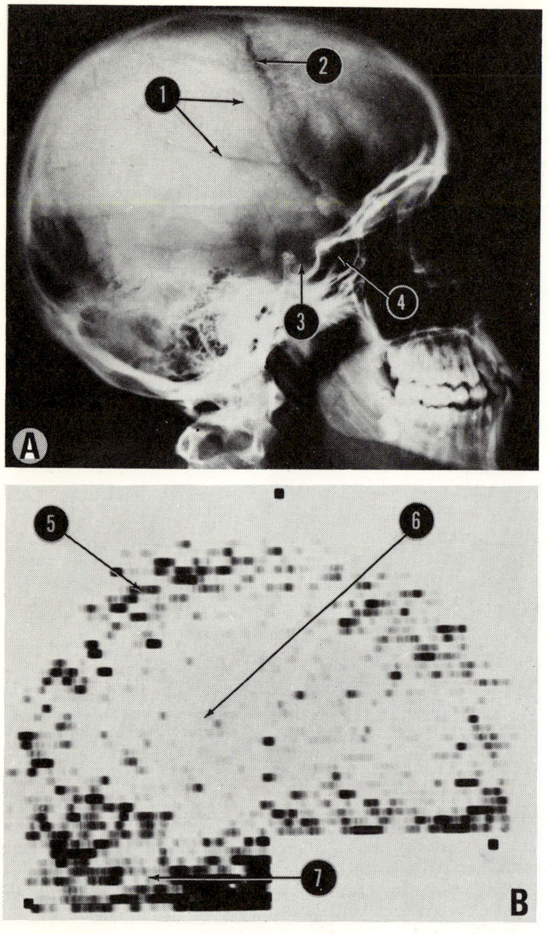

Fig. 2-53. *A.* X-ray of the normal skull viewed from the right side: (1) grooves for the branches of the middle meningeal artery; (2) coronal suture; (3) sella turcica; (4) sphenoidal sinus. *B.* Normal cranial scan after isotope injection: (5) soft tissue of the scalp; (6) background of normal brain tissue; (7) temporal and occipital muscles. (*Courtesy of Drs. Frank Borrelli and Rita Girolamo of the Department of Radiology, New York Medical College.*)

for the neurosurgeon who may be called upon to investigate such pathologic change, to have an understanding of the relationships between the bones of the skull and the brain. A general review of the **skull** will be of considerable assistance in fully appreciating this relationship.

The position of the cerebral landmarks varies within normal limits, and it is therefore possible to locate them in a general way only.

Dorsolateral Surface Relations (Fig. 2-51.)

Base of Cerebrum. This is indicated by a line (Reid's line) drawn from the inferior margin of the orbit through the upper margin of the external auditory meatus.

Longitudinal Fissure. This corresponds to the midline or sagittal line of the scalp between the external occipital protuberance (inion) and the midpoint of the frontonasal suture (nasion).

Lateral Cerebral Fissure (Sylvian). The pterion (sylvian point), 3.5 cm behind and 1.2 cm above the frontozygomatic suture, corresponds to the point where the lateral cerebral fissure divides into its ascending and posterior rami. A line drawn from the pterion to a point 2 cm below the parietal eminence overlies the posterior ramus. Another 2-cm line, perpendicular to the previous line, also originating from the pterion, overlies the ascending ramus. A third line, drawn 2 cm rostrally from the pterion, corresponds to the anterior horizontal ramus of the fissure.

Central Sulcus. This is determined by a line joining two points: the superior, 1.25 cm behind the center of the sagittal line; the inferior, determined by the intersection of a line perpendicular to Reid's base line, originating at the preauricular point, and the line outlined for the posterior ramus of the sylvian fissure.

Pre- and Postcentral Sulci. These are parallel to the line of the central sulcus, lying 1.5 cm in front of or behind it, respectively.

Superior Frontal Sulcus. This is indicated by a line drawn rostrally, parallel to the longitudinal fissure and about 3 cm lateral to it.

Parieto-occipital Fissure. This is a posterior continuation of the line drawn from the posterior ramus of the sylvian fissure to the sagittal line. The last 2.5 cm of this continuation overlie the fissure.

Interparietal Sulcus. This can be best represented by a curved line running from a point on the central sulcus, 3 cm above the sylvian point. It parallels the longitudinal fissure located halfway between the latter and the parietal eminence.

It then turns downward, ending about midway between the lambda and the parietal eminence.

Basal Surface Relations (Fig. 2-52.)

This aspect of the brain is related to the anterior, middle, and posterior cranial fossae located in the floor of the cranial cavity.

Anterior. The basal surface of the frontal lobe occupies this fossa, resting upon the orbital plates of the frontal bone. The olfactory bulb and tracts lie in the olfactory grooves of the ethmoid bone, with the olfactory nerve fibers entering the skull through the cribriform plates.

Middle. This is occupied predominantly by the temporal lobe laterally and the hypothalamus medially. Associated with the latter, are the optic chiasma, resting in the chiasmatic groove, and the pituitary gland, lying in the sella turcica of the sphenoid bone. Certain of the cranial nerves exit from the skull through this fossa: the optic through the optic foramen; oculomotor, trochlear, and abducens, plus the ophthalmic division of the trigeminal, through the superior orbital fissure; the maxillary division of the trigeminal through the foramen rotundum; and the mandibular division of the trigeminal through the foramen ovale. A small branch, the great superficial petrosal of the seventh cranial nerve, enters the fossa through the hiatus of the facial canal. The carotid artery lies in the carotid groove, entering the fossa through the foramen lacerum, while the middle meningeal artery enters through the foramen spinosum, occupying grooves in the lateral aspect of the fossa. Medially, above the carotid groove on the petrous temporal bone, lies the shallow trigeminal impression. Still other small vessels and nerves associated with this fossa are too numerous to mention here.

Posterior Fossa. This houses the cerebellum, pons, and medulla oblongata. The pons and the medulla rest upon the dorsum sellae and basilar portion of the occipital bone. The junction between the cord and medulla lies in the foramen magnum, through which also pass the vertebral arteries and the spinal portion of the accessory nerve. The remainder of the cranial nerves leave the skull through the foramina of this fossa: the facial and acoustic, through the internal auditory meatus; the glossopharyngeal, vagus, and accessory, through the jugular foramen; and the hypoglossal, through the hypoglossal canal (anterior condyloid foramen).

SUMMARY

- Telencephalon
  - Pallium (hemispheres)
    - Lobes
      - Frontal
      - Parietal
      - Occipital
      - Temporal
      - Insula
    - Fibers
      - Projection
        - Internal capsule
        - External capsule
        - Extreme capsule (fornix)
      - Association
        - Long
          - Cingulum
          - Superior longitudinal fasciculus
          - Superior occipitofrontal fasciculus
          - Inferior occipitofrontal fasciculus
          - Uncinate fasciculus
        - Short
          - Arcuate
          - Intracortical
      - Commissures
        - Corpus callosum
          - Rostrum
          - Genu
          - Body
          - Splenium
        - Anterior
    - Lateral ventricle
      - Anterior horn
      - Body
      - Collateral trigone
      - Posterior horn
      - Inferior horn
  - Basal nuclei (ganglia)
    - Caudate
    - Lenticular
      - Putamen
      - Globus pallidus
    - Claustrum
    - Amygdaloid
  - Rhinencephalon
    - Olfactory bulb
    - Olfactory tract
    - Olfactory trigone
    - Olfactory striae
      - Medial
      - Intermediate
      - Lateral
    - Dentate gyrus
    - Hippocampus
    - Diagonal band of Broca
    - Fibers
      - Projection
        - Medial forebrain bundle
        - Fornix
          - Fimbria
          - Crus
          - Body
          - Column
        - Stria medularis
        - Stria terminalis
      - Commissural
        - Hippocampal
        - Stria terminalis
        - Anterior
      - Association
        - Longitudinal striae

- Diencephalon
  - Epithalamus
    - Habenula
    - Habenular commissure
    - Medullary striae
    - Epiphysis (pineal body)
    - (Posterior commissure)
  - Thalamus (Chap.22)
    - Nuclei
      - Anterior nucleus
      - Medial division
      - Lateral division
      - Caudal (metathalamus)
        - Lateral geniculate body
        - Medial geniculate body
    - Fibers
      - Optic tract
      - Brachium of inferior colliculus
  - Subthalamus (Chap.19)
    - Nuclei
      - Red
      - Substantia nigra
      - Subthalamic
    - Fibers
      - Brachium conjunctivum
  - Hypothalamus (Chap.21)
    - Mammillary bodies
    - Tuber cinereum
    - Infundibulum
    - Neurohypophysis
    - Optic chiasma
    - Fornix
  - Third ventricle

- Mesencephalon
  - Corpora quadrigemina
    - Superior colliculus and brachium
    - Inferior colliculus and brachium
    - Root of trochlear nerve
  - Tegmentum
    - Nuclei
      - Oculomotor
      - Trochlear
      - Mesencephalic of trigeminal
      - Red
      - Interpeduncular
      - Tegmental
    - Fibers
      - Brachium conjunctivum
      - Medial lemniscus
      - Lateral lemniscus
      - Mesencephalic of trigeminal
      - Ventral tegmental decussation
      - Dorsal tegmental decussation
      - Medial longitudinal fasciculus
  - Cerebral peduncle
    - Basis pedunculi
      - Interpeduncular fossa
      - Oculomotor nerve
    - Substantia nigra
  - Cerebral aqueduct

- Metencephalon
  - Cerebellum (Chap. 18)
    - Peduncles
      - Superior (brachium conjunctivum)
      - Middle (brachium pontis)
      - Inferior (restiform body)
    - Nuclei
      - Fastigial
      - Globose
      - Emboliform
      - Dentate
    - Vermis
      - Superior
      - Inferior
    - Hemispheres
      - Superior
      - Inferior
      - Flocculus
  - Pons
    - Basal pons
      - Brachium pontis
      - Trigeminal nerve root
      - Nuclei of basal pons
      - Pyramidal system
      - Pontocerebellar system
    - Tegmentum
      - Fibers
        - Brachium conjunctivum
        - Trapezoid body
        - Lateral lemniscus
        - Medial lemniscus
        - Spinal of trigeminal
        - Mesencephalic of trigeminal
        - Vestibulospinal tract
        - Medial longitudinal fasciculus
      - Nuclei
        - Vestibular
        - Facial
        - Superior salivatory
        - Abducens
        - Motor of trigeminal
        - Spinal of trigeminal
        - Chief sensory of trigeminal
        - Mesencephalic of trigeminal
        - Ventral cochlear
        - Dorsal cochlear
        - Superior olive
        - Nucleus of trapezoid body
        - Nucleus of lateral lemniscus
    - Fourth ventricle
      - Roof
        - Brachium conjunctivum
        - Anterior medullary velum
      - Floor
        - Medial eminence
        - Facial colliculus
        - Superior fovea
        - Medullary striae
        - Acoustic trigone
        - Locus caeruleus

- Myelencephalon
  - External structures
    - Pyramid
    - Decussation of pyramids
    - Ventral and dorsal external arcuate fibers
    - Inferior olive
    - Abducens nerve root
    - Facial nerve root
    - Acoustic nerve root
    - Glossopharyngeal nerve root
    - Vagus nerve root
    - Accessory nerve root
    - Hypoglossal nerve root
    - Fasciculus cuneatus and tubercle (clava)
    - Fasciculus gracilis and tubercle
    - Tuberculum cinereum
    - Restiform body (inferior brachium)
  - Internal structures
    - Gracile nucleus
    - Cuneate nucleus
    - Spinal V nucleus and tract
    - Inferior olive
    - Olivocerebellar fibers
    - Vestibular nuclei
    - Cochlear nuclei
    - Accessory nuclei
    - Hypoglossal nucleus
    - Nucleus ambiguus
    - Dorsal motor nucleus of vagus
    - Superior salivatory nucleus
    - Inferior salivatory nucleus
    - Tractus and nucleus solitarius
    - Restiform body (inferior brachium)
    - Internal arcuate fibers
    - Medial lemniscus
    - Medial longitudinal fasciculus
    - Vestibulospinal tract
    - Reticular formation
    - Pyramid
  - Fourth ventricle
    - Roof
      - Choroid tela and plexus
      - Posterior medullary velum
      - Restiform body
    - Floor
      - Acoustic area
      - Medullary striae
      - Vagal triangle
      - Hypoglossal triangle
      - Inferior fovea
      - Superior fovea
      - Facial colliculus

3 ANATOMY OF THE SPINAL CORD

EXTERNAL STRUCTURE (Figs. 3-1, 3-2.)

The spinal cord averages 16 to 18 in. (40 to 45 cm) in length. It is nearly oval in cross section, with the longer diameter in the transverse plane. The diameter is not uniform throughout its length. There are cervical and lumbar enlargements to accommodate the nerve supply to the upper and lower extremities. Caudal to the lumbar enlargement, the cord diminishes rapidly, having a cone-shaped termination called the *conus medullaris,* from the apex of which extends the *filum terminale internum,* which descends to be attached to the coccyx.

The cord is divided into areas by several longitudinal grooves (Fig. 3-2). In the midventral line is the deep *ventral median fissure,* which indents the cord to at least one-third of its dorsoventral diameter. Opposite this, on the dorsal surface, is the shallow *dorsal median sulcus.* A median septum extends inward from this sulcus, helping to divide the cord into symmetric halves. Lateral to the ventral median fissure are the *ventral lateral sulci.* Along these grooves emerge the ventral rootlets of the 31 pairs of spinal nerves. Parallel, but some distance lateral to the dorsal median sulcus, are the *dorsal lateral sulci,* along which the dorsal rootlets of the spinal nerves enter the cord. Beginning in the upper thoracic region and becoming quite definite on the cervical cord is another sulcus, lying between the dorsal median and dorsal lateral sulci. This is the *dorsal intermediate sulcus.*

Each half of the cord is divided into columns called funiculi. The *anterior funiculus* is found between the ventral median and ventral lateral sulci; the *lateral funiculus* lies between the ventral lateral and dorsal lateral sulci; the *posterior funiculus* is situated between the dorsal median and dorsal lateral sulci. In the cervical region, the posterior funiculus is subdivided by the dorsal intermediate sulcus into a medial *fasciculus gracilis* and a lateral *fasciculus cuneatus.* In the region of the upper five or six cervical nerves, rootlets of the accessory nerve (XI) emerge from the lateral funiculus.

The cord is a segmented structure, and it gives rise to 31 pairs of nerves. Arbitrary lines drawn through the most rostral root filaments of each pair serve as demarcation between the segments. The highest of these lines is the boundary between the cervical cord and the medulla.

INTERNAL STRUCTURE (Fig. 3-3.)

The cord is composed of two fundamentally different materials. In fresh specimens the more peripheral part appears glistening white, because of the fatty myelin sheaths covering the longitudinally-running fibers contained in the area. This region is called the *white matter.* Internal to the white substance lies an H-shaped mass which appears less white, since it contains fine, nonmyelinated fibers together with all the neuron cell bodies of the spinal cord. This is the *gray*

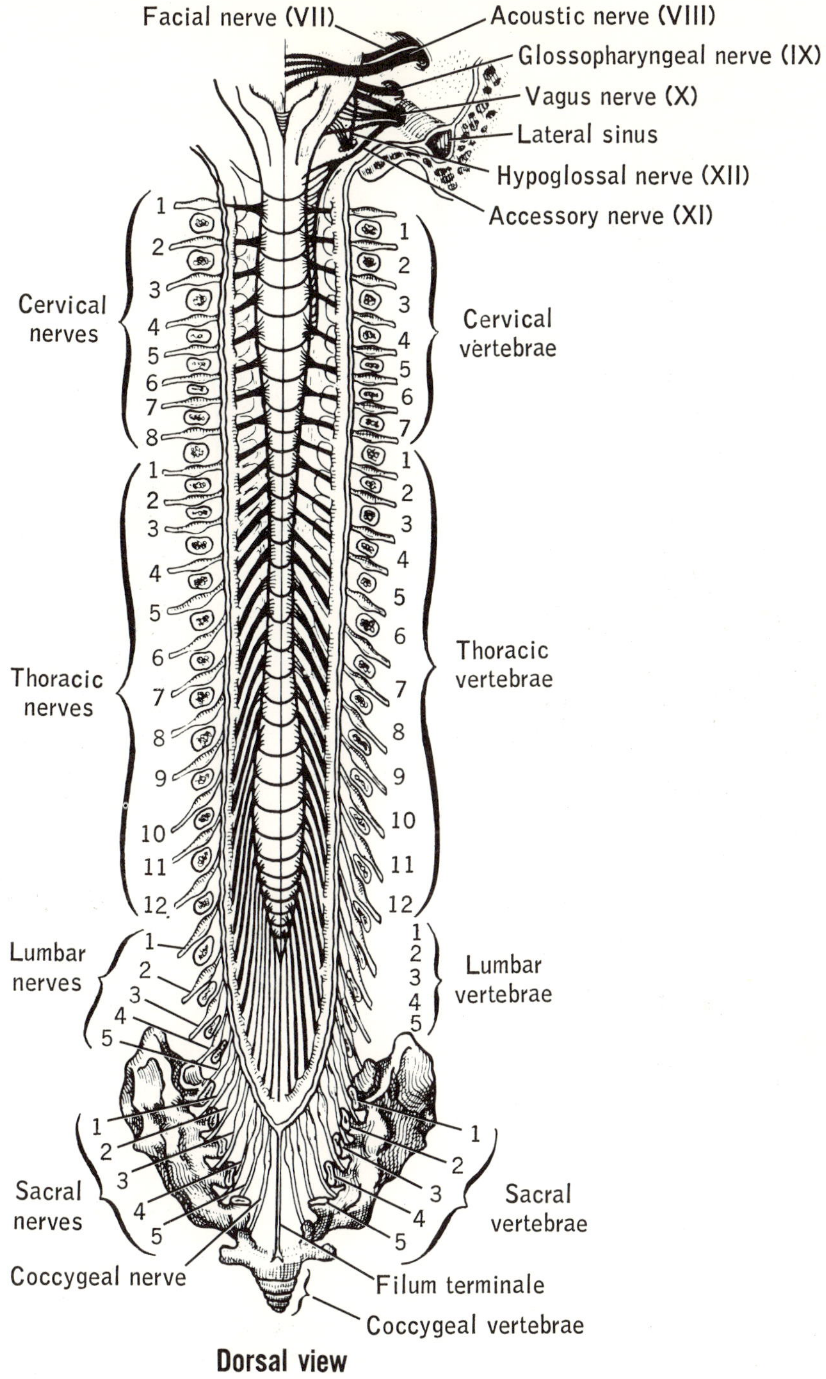

Fig. 3-1. Gross aspects of the spinal cord and lower brain stem viewed from the dorsal side with bone and meninges removed.

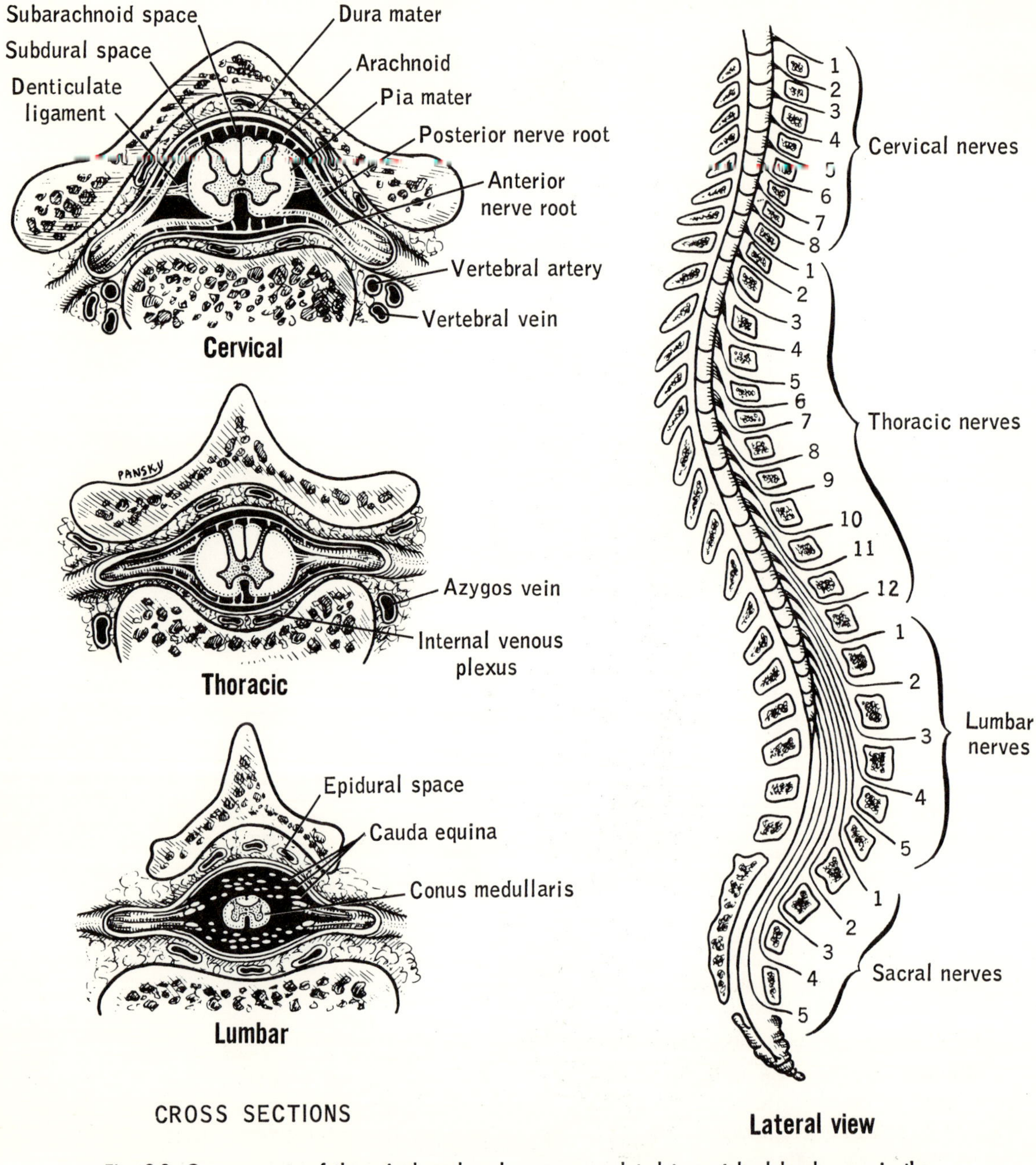

Fig. 3-2. Gross aspects of the spinal cord and nerves as related to vertebral levels seen in the sagittal plane. The relations of the cord and nerves to the meninges together with variations in size and shape of the cord at different levels is shown in a series of three cross sections.

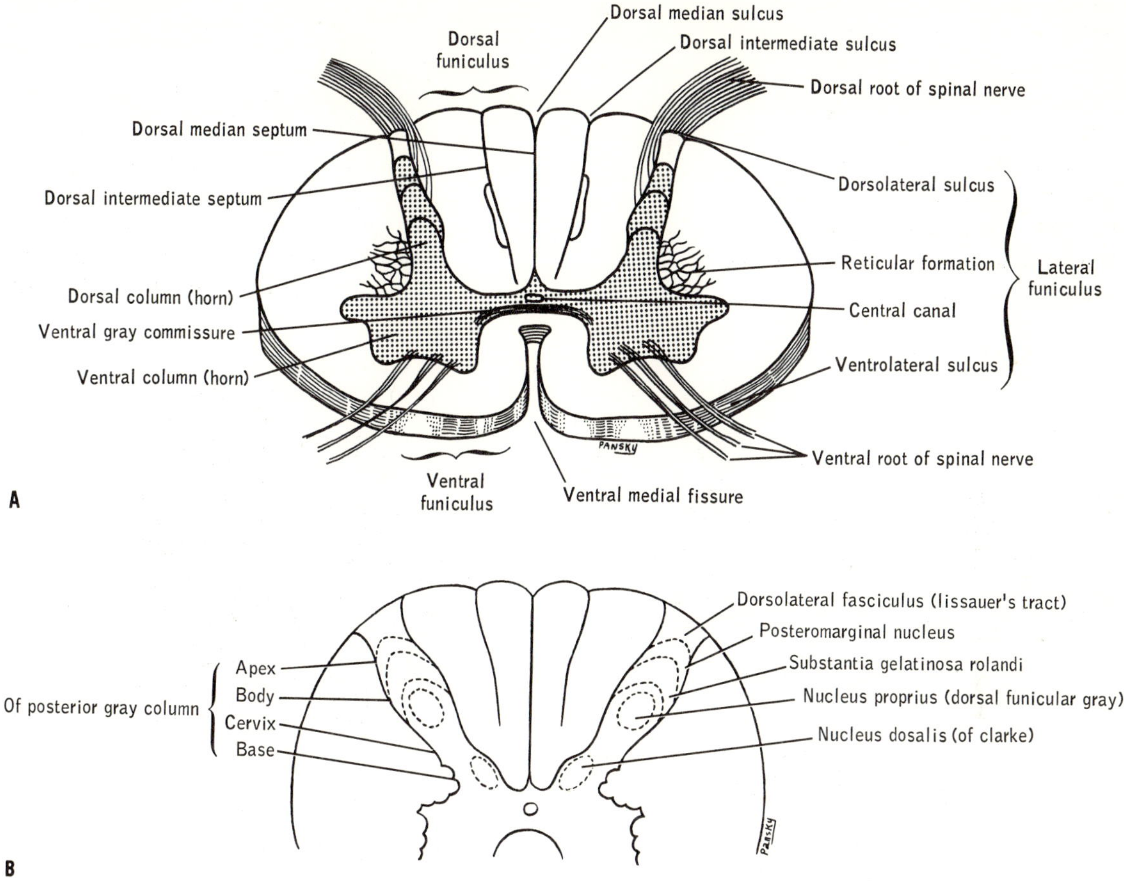

Fig. 3-3. *A.* Transverse section of the spinal cord at the level of C-5 to indicate the general arrangements of its parts. *B.* Diagram of the dorsal gray columns of the spinal cord showing the divisions and principal nuclei.

matter, which, like the white, extends through the length of the cord as columns.

Gray Substance (Figs. 3-3 to 3-5.)

Although the shape of the gray mass varies from level to level, the *posterior gray column* tends to be relatively narrow and in some places nearly reaches the bottom of the dorsal lateral sulcus. The posterior gray column consists of three parts, namely: apex, caput, and cervix. At the apex, the gray matter is of a consistency different from that found in other parts of the column and is known as the *substantia gelatinosa* (Rolandi).

Just lateral to the cervix of the posterior column is an area of mixed white and gray. This is the *reticular substance* of the cord and is most prominent in the cervical region.

The *anterior columns* are shorter and broader than the posterior, directed toward but not approaching the ventral lateral sulcus.

In the thoracic and upper lumbar levels, a lateral protrusion of gray matter appears. This is the *lateral* or *intermediolateral column.*

The strip of gray matter connecting the limbs of the "H" is the *gray commissure,* near the middle of which lies the *central canal.* The position of this canal divides the commissure into an *an-*

terior and *posterior* gray commissure. Ventral to the former is a narrow band of myelinated fibers referred to as the *anterior white commissure*.

The gray substance contains all the nerve cell bodies of the cord as well as many glial supporting elements. In the posterior columns, afferent neurons terminate, while association neurons of the reflex arcs and secondary neurons to higher levels arise. In the intermediolateral columns, present throughout thoracic and upper lumbar cord segments, are found the cell bodies of the preganglionic neurons of the autonomic system. The ventral columns contain cells of neurons supplying skeletal muscle. (Fig. 3-6.)

Within the gray substance, the neuron cell bodies tend to be assembled in groups. In the posterior gray columns, the aggregation of cells at the apex is known as the *posteromarginal nucleus,* ventral to which lies a much larger cell mass, the *substantia gelatinosa* (Rolandi). At

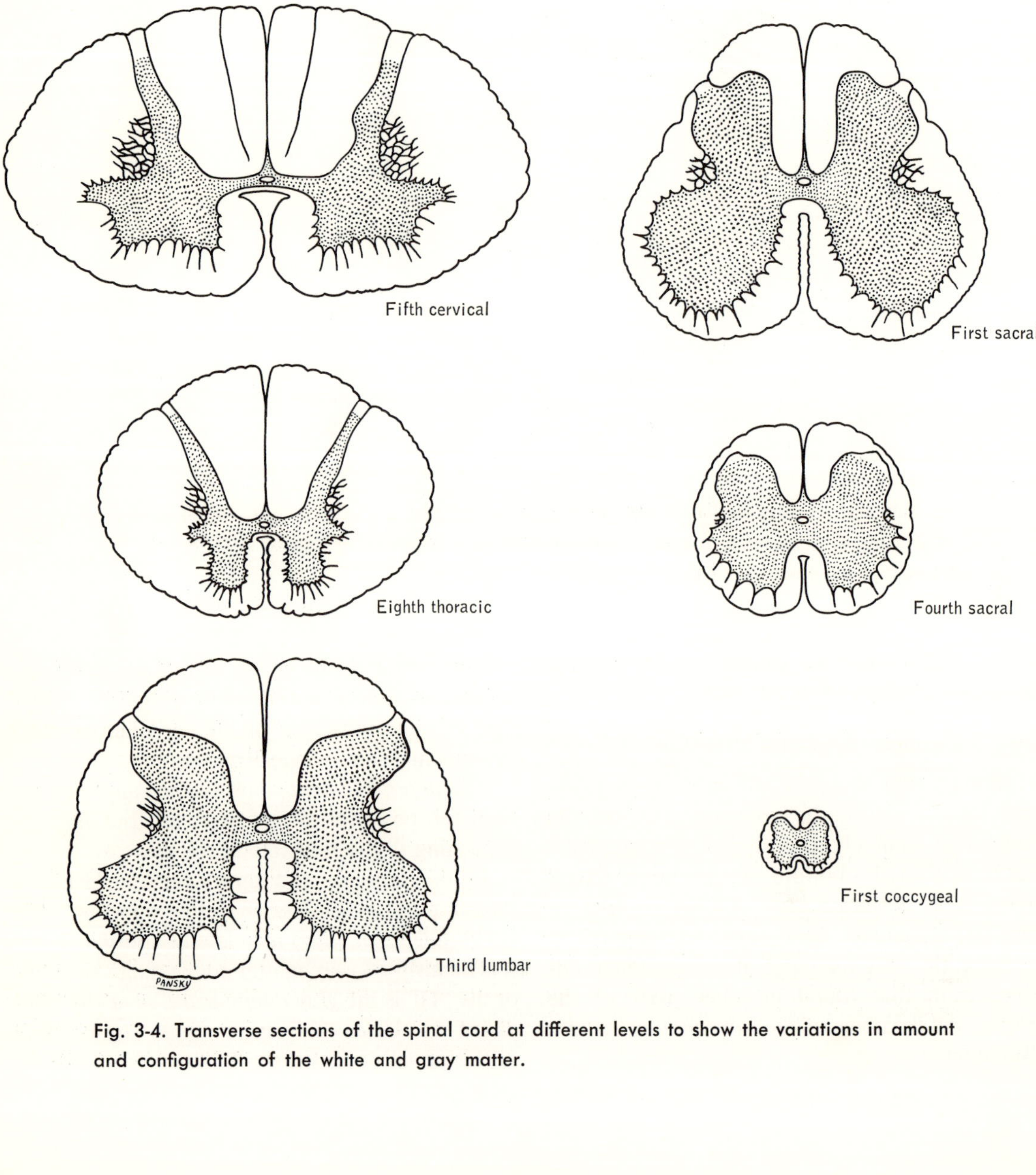

Fig. 3-4. Transverse sections of the spinal cord at different levels to show the variations in amount and configuration of the white and gray matter.

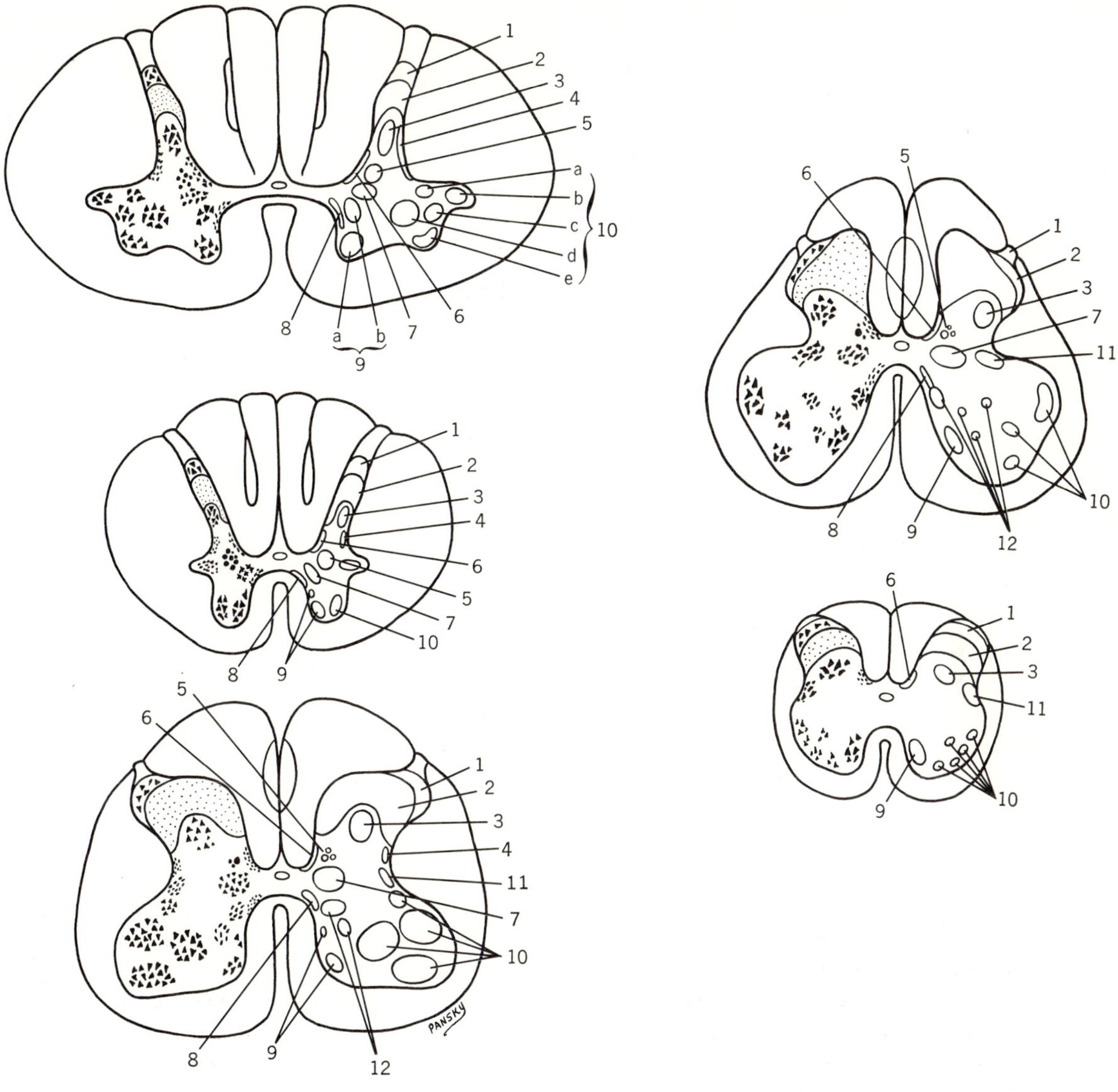

Fig. 3-5. Transverse sections of the spinal cord with the nuclear subdivisions of the gray matter indicated. (1) Posteromarginal cells (n. magnocellularis pericornualis); (2) substantia gelatinosa of Rolando (n. sensibilis proprius); (3) nucleus proprius cornu dorsalis (n. magnocellularis centralis; n. spinothalamicus; n. centrodorsalis); (4) nucleus reticularis; (5) Clarke's column (n. dorsalis; n. magnocellularis basalis; n. spinocerebellaris); (6) nucleus commissuralis posterior (dorsomedial diffuse cell group of Jacobsohn); (7) nucleus intermediomedialis; (8) nucleus commissuralis anterior (ventromedial diffuse cell group of Jacobsohn); (9) nucleus medialis: (*a*) anteromedial, (*b*) posteromedial (medial motor); (10) nucleus lateralis: (*a*) posterolateral, (*b*) mediolateral, (*c*) anterolateral, (*d*) central, (*e*) anterior; (11) intermediolateral column (n. sympatheticus lateralis); (12) nucleus myoleioticus (n. sympatheticus medialis).

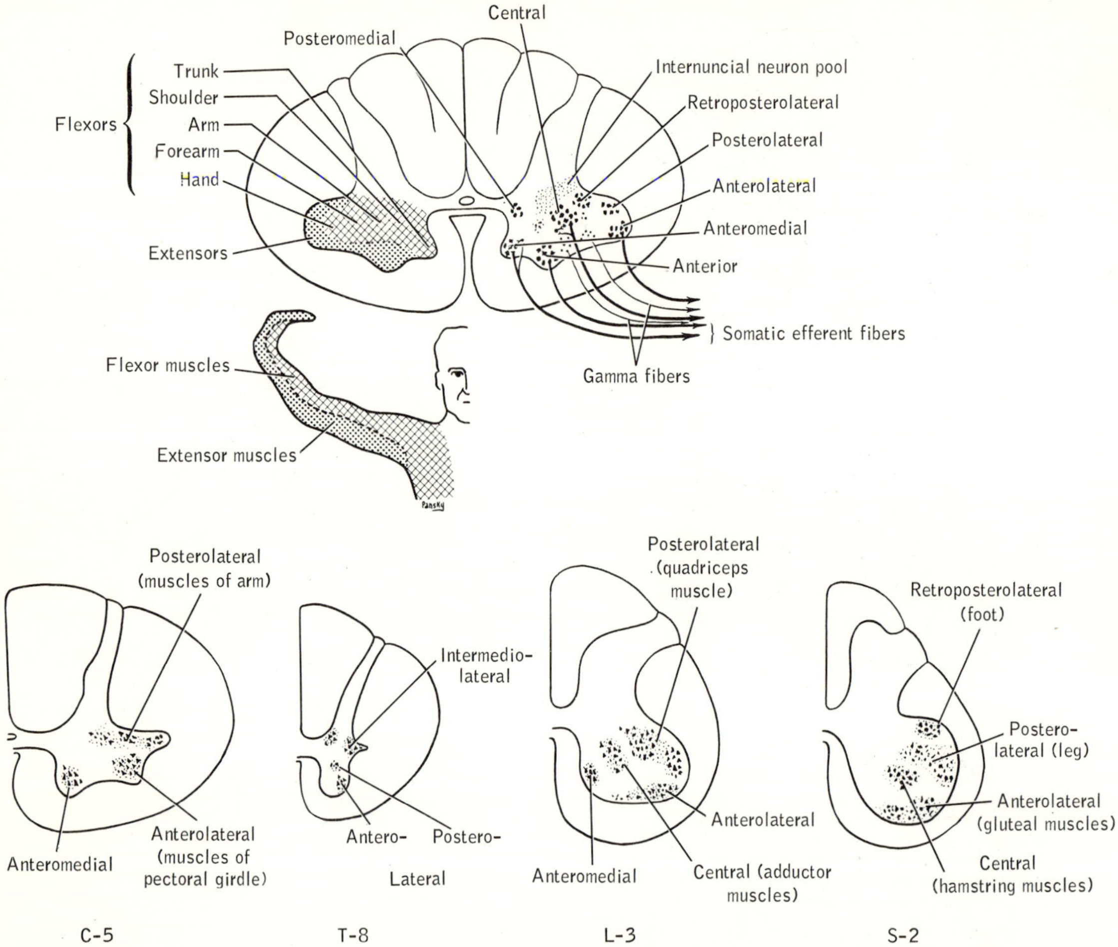

Fig. 3-6. *Upper figure.* Diagram of the motor nuclei in the anterior gray column of a lower cervical cord segment. On the left the relations of the motor neurons to the muscle groups innervated are shown. Note that more distal muscles are supplied by neurons in the dorsolateral position and the flexors are innervated by more deeply placed neurons than are the extensors. Axon collaterals from efferent neurons are shown "recurring" to synapse with Renshaw cells. *Lower figure.* Diagram of motor nuclei and the muscle groups innervated. (*Modified after Crosby, Humphrey, and Lauer,* 1962.)

thoracic levels, a group of cells collected on the medial side of the base of the dorsal column forms the nucleus dorsalis (Clarke's column). In the ventral column, the cells are generally divided into lateral and medial groups, each of which is again subdivided (Fig. 3-4). In the midcervical region, a central group is also found. Generally, it is believed that the cells in the medial group give rise to axons destined for the axial musculature, while the lateral, which are more marked in the cervical and lumbar enlargement, are concerned with the muscles of the girdles and extremities.

White Substance (Figs. 3-3, 3-7.)

The ratio of white substance to gray varies from level to level in the cord, the actual amount of white being greatest in the cervical region.

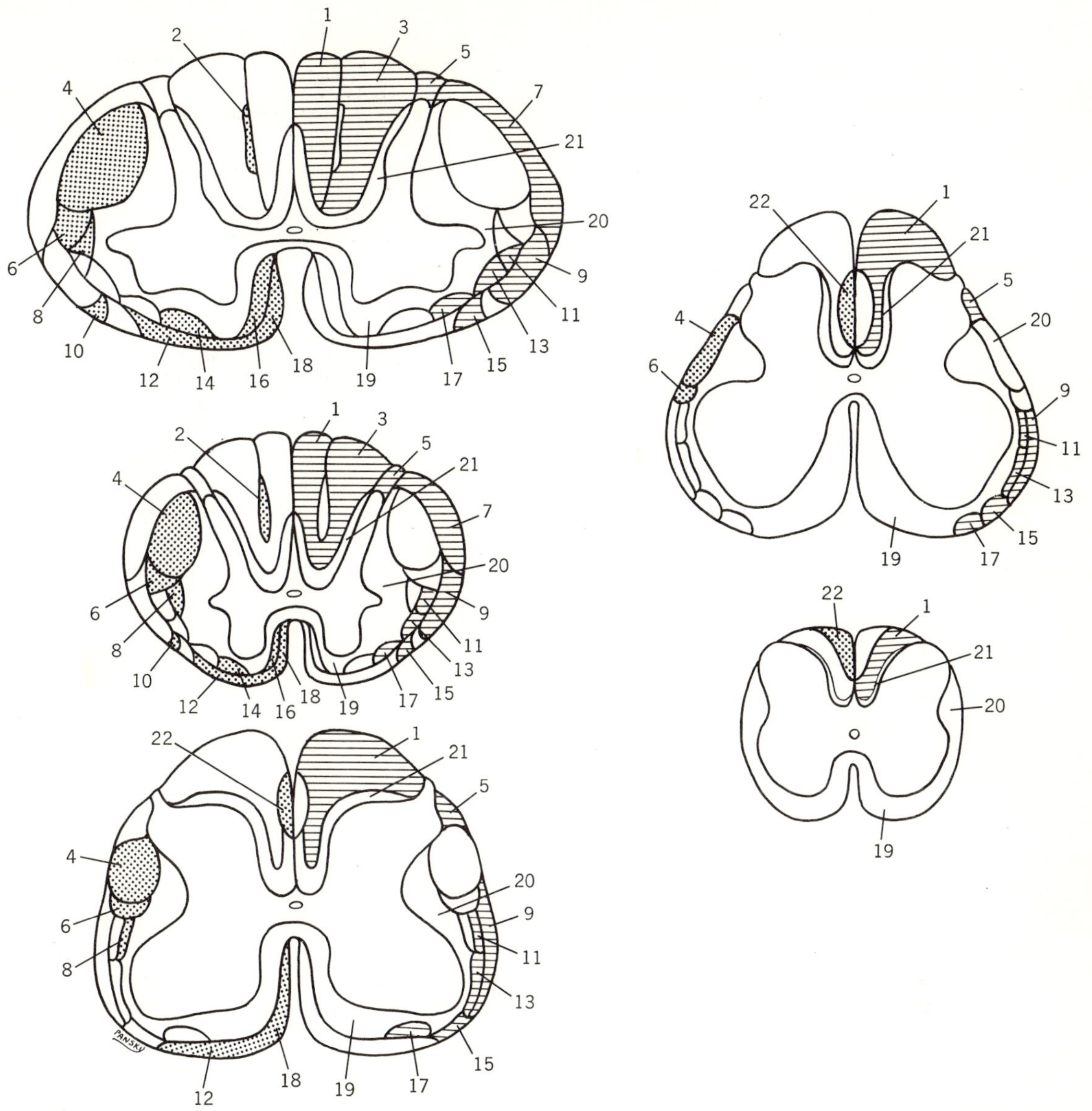

Fig. 3-7. Transverse sections of the spinal cord: ascending tracts in the white matter on the right, descending on the left. The tracts indicated by numbers 19, 20, and 21 are mixed. (1) Fasciculus gracilis, (2) comma tract (interfascicular fasciculus), (3) fasciculus cuneatus, (4) lateral corticospinal tract, (5) dorsal lateral tract, (6) rubrospinal tract, (7) dorsal spinocerebellar tract, (8) vestibulospinal tract (lateral), (9) ventral spinocerebellar tract, (10) olivospinal tract (tract of Helwig), (11) lateral spinothalamic tract, (12) anterior vestibulospinal tract, (13) spinotectal tract, (14) tectospinal tract (colliculospinal tract), (15) spino-olivary tract, (16) ventral corticospinal tract, (17) ventral spinothalamic tract, (18) sulcomarginal tract, (19) fasciculus proprius anterior (ground bundle), (20) fasciculus proprius lateralis (ground bundle), (21) fasciculus proprius posterior (ground bundle), (22) septomarginal tract.

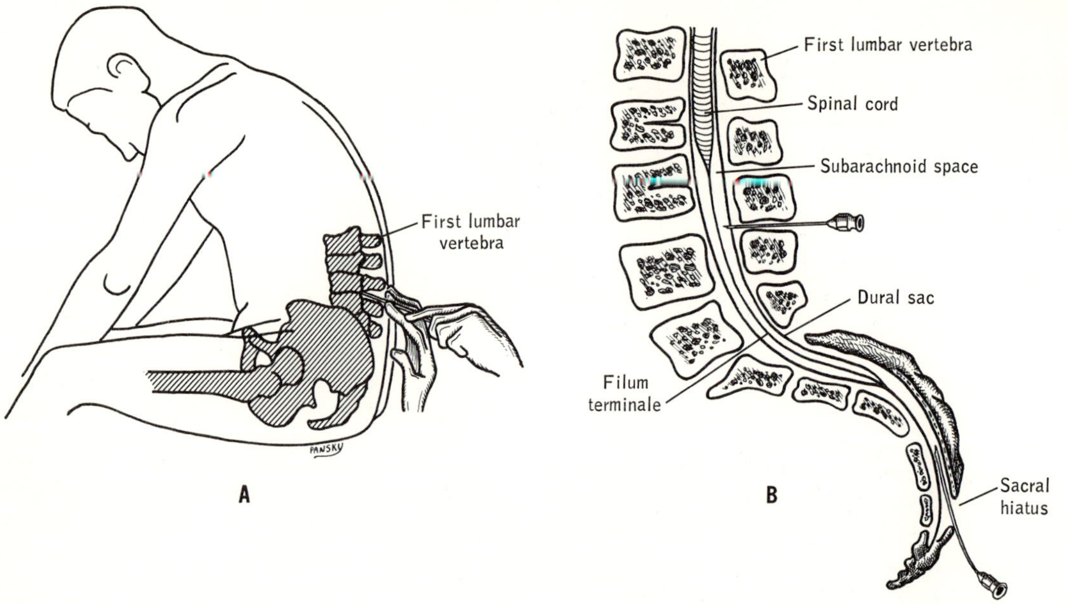

Fig. 3-8. *A.* Lumbar (spinal) anesthesia. *B.* Spinal and caudal anesthesia.

Although most of the bundles of fibers in the white matter are not clearly defined, the area overlying the apex of the dorsal gray column is pale by comparison with other white areas. This is called the *dorsal lateral fasciculus* (Lissauer's tract).

The white matter, like the gray, is supported and held together by numerous glial elements.

CLINICAL CONSIDERATIONS

An understanding of the relationships between the spinal cord, the vertebral column, and the body surface is important not only to the neurosurgeon but to the diagnostician and anesthetist as well.

Spinovertebral Topography
(Figs. 3-8, 3-9.)

Fourth Lumbar Interspace

This is used both for spinal anesthesia and for withdrawal of cerebrospinal fluid. It may be located by a line drawn across the dorsum at the level of the iliac crests.

Sacral Hiatus

This is important in sacral block. The articulation between sacrum and coccyx must be located by palpation. The needle is inserted into the gap between the bones and then directed upward along the axis of the sacrum for a distance of 2.5 to 4.0 cm.

Posterior Sacral Foramina

These may be used for transsacral anesthesia.

First Foramen. This lies about opposite the tip of the transverse process of the fifth lumbar vertebra.

Second Foramen. This lies about 1 cm medial and slightly below the posterior superior iliac spine.

Third, Fourth, and Fifth Foramina. These are approximately in a line drawn caudally from the point of the second foramen, separated from each other by a distance of about 2.5 cm.

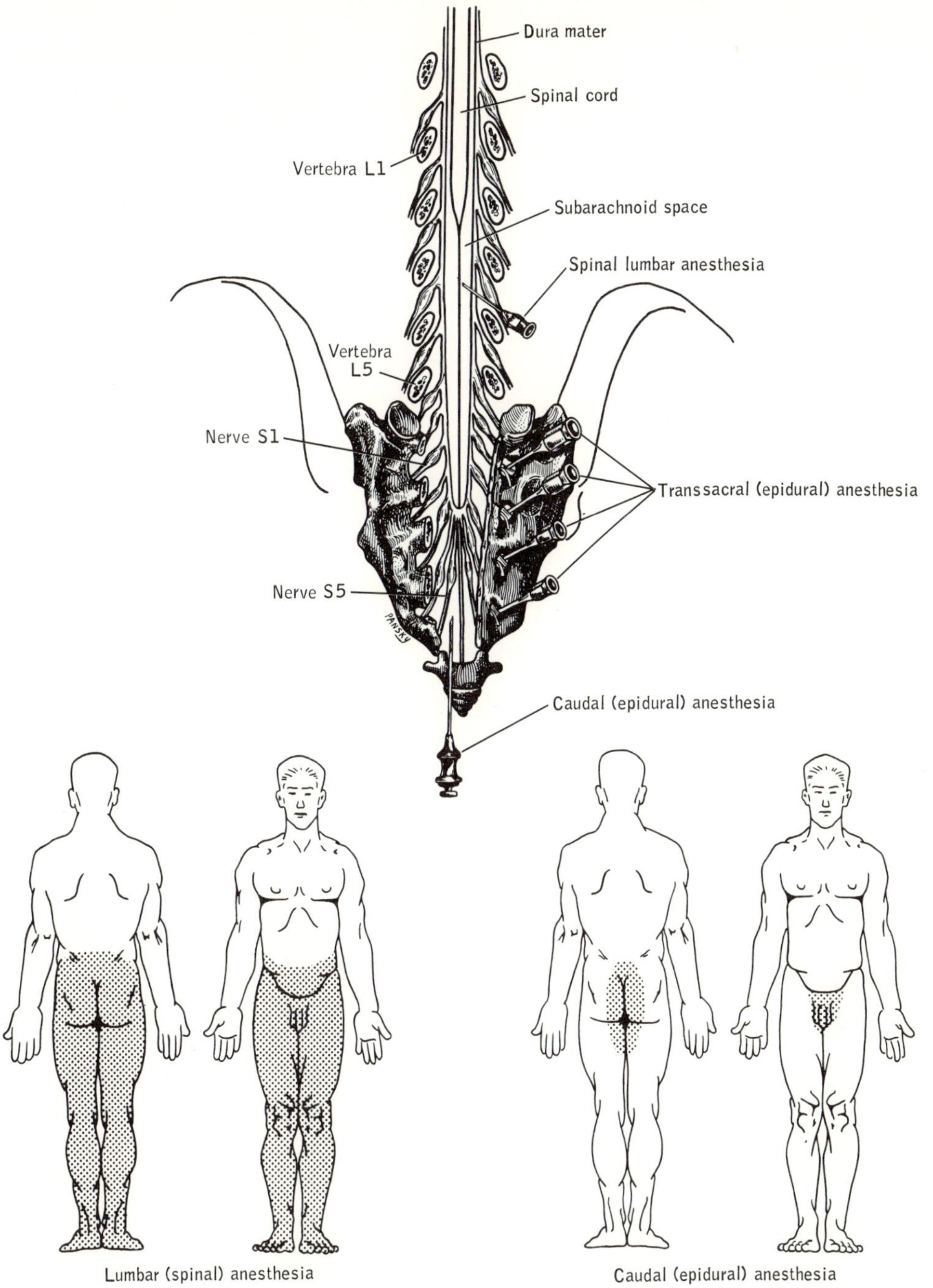

Fig. 3-9. Spinal, caudal, and transsacral anesthesia. Areas of anesthesia are also indicated.

SUMMARY

- Spinal cord
  - Gray
    - Columns
      - Dorsal
        - Apex – Posteromarginal nucleus
        - Body – Substantia gelatinosa rolandi
        - Cervix – Nucleus proprius
        - Base – Nucleus dorsalis (of Clarke)
      - Intermediolateral (T1-L3; S2-S4)
      - Ventral
        - Medial
          - Dorsal
          - Ventral
        - Central
        - Lateral
          - Retrodorsal
          - Dorsal
          - Ventral
    - Commissures
      - Anterior
      - Posterior
  - White
    - Funiculi
      - Dorsal
        - Fasciculus gracilis
        - Fasciculus cuneatus
      - Intermediodorsal
      - Lateral
        - Ascending
          - Dorsal spinocerebellar
          - Ventral spinocerebellar
          - Lateral spinothalamic
          - Spinotectal
          - Spino-olivary
        - Descending
          - Lateral corticospinal
          - Lateral reticulospinal
          - Rubrospinal
      - Ventral
        - Ascending
          - Ventral spinothalamic
        - Descending
          - Ventral corticospinal
          - Medial tectospinal
          - Medial reticulospinal
          - Vestibulospinal
    - Commissures
      - Anterior
      - Posterior

4 COVERINGS AND VASCULARIZATION OF THE CENTRAL NERVOUS SYSTEM

MENINGES

The fibrous coverings of the central nervous system are of great importance in support, protection, and nourishment. They consist of three major layers, from without inward: the dura mater, the arachnoid, and the pia mater. Associated with these layers are three spaces: a potential epidural space, external to the dura; a subdural space, between the dura and the arachnoid; and a subarachnoid space, between the arachnoid and the pia.

Coverings of the Brain

Dura Mater (Figs. 4-1 to 4-3.)

This is the outermost covering. It is a thick, tough membrane which serves as both the internal periosteum for the cranial bones and a support for the brain. It consists, therefore, of two layers, an external, endosteal layer, and an inner, meningeal layer. The former is intimately attached to the bones and is closely applied to the meningeal layer except in the areas of the venous sinuses. The meningeal layer is smooth and is lined, on its inner surface, by mesothelium. At the foramina in the base of the skull, the dura joins the epineurium of the exiting cranial nerves and also becomes continuous with the external periosteum (pericranium). At the foramen magnum it joins the spinal dura. The meningeal layer also sends four major processes deep into the cranium, forming compartments for portions of the brain. These are the falx cerebri; the tentorium cerebelli; the falx cerebelli; and the diaphragma sellae.

Falx Cerebri. This descends into the longitudinal fissure between the cerebral hemispheres. Anteriorly, it is attached to the crista galli of the ethmoid. Posteriorly, it becomes continuous with the tentorium cerebelli. Its superior convex border is attached to the skull on either side of the midline as far posteriorly as the internal occipital protuberance. The *superior sagittal sinus* is lodged in it. The inferior margin is concave and free and contains the *inferior sagittal sinus.*

Tentorium Cerebelli. This forms a tentlike roof for the posterior cranial fossa, sloping downward from its median attachment to the falx cerebri toward its lateral attachments on the petrous temporal bone. It separates the occipital lobes of the cerebral hemispheres and the superior surface of the cerebellum. Its rostral border is free and bounds the incisure (opening) of the tentorium. The cerebral peduncles descend through this gap. The tentorium is attached to the ridges of the occipital bone posteriorly. The *transverse sinuses* are enclosed along this attachment. Laterally and rostrally, the edges are attached along a groove on the superior angle of the petrous temporal bone. The *superior petrosal sinus* runs along this attached border. Anteriorly, the tentorium continues to the clinoid processes of the sphenoid bone. In the midline, along its attachment to the falx cerebri, is the *straight sinus*.

Falx Cerebelli. This is a small triangular projection which dips into the posterior cerebellar notch. Above, it is attached to the most posterior part of the inferior surface of the tentorium and posteriorly to the internal occipital crest.

Diaphragma Sellae. This is a small sheet which overlies the sella turcica, forming a covering for the hypophysis. In its center is a small opening for the pituitary stalk (infundibular stem).

Arachnoid (Figs. 4-5 to 4-7.)

This is a delicate membrane lying internal to the dura mater. It surrounds the brain rather

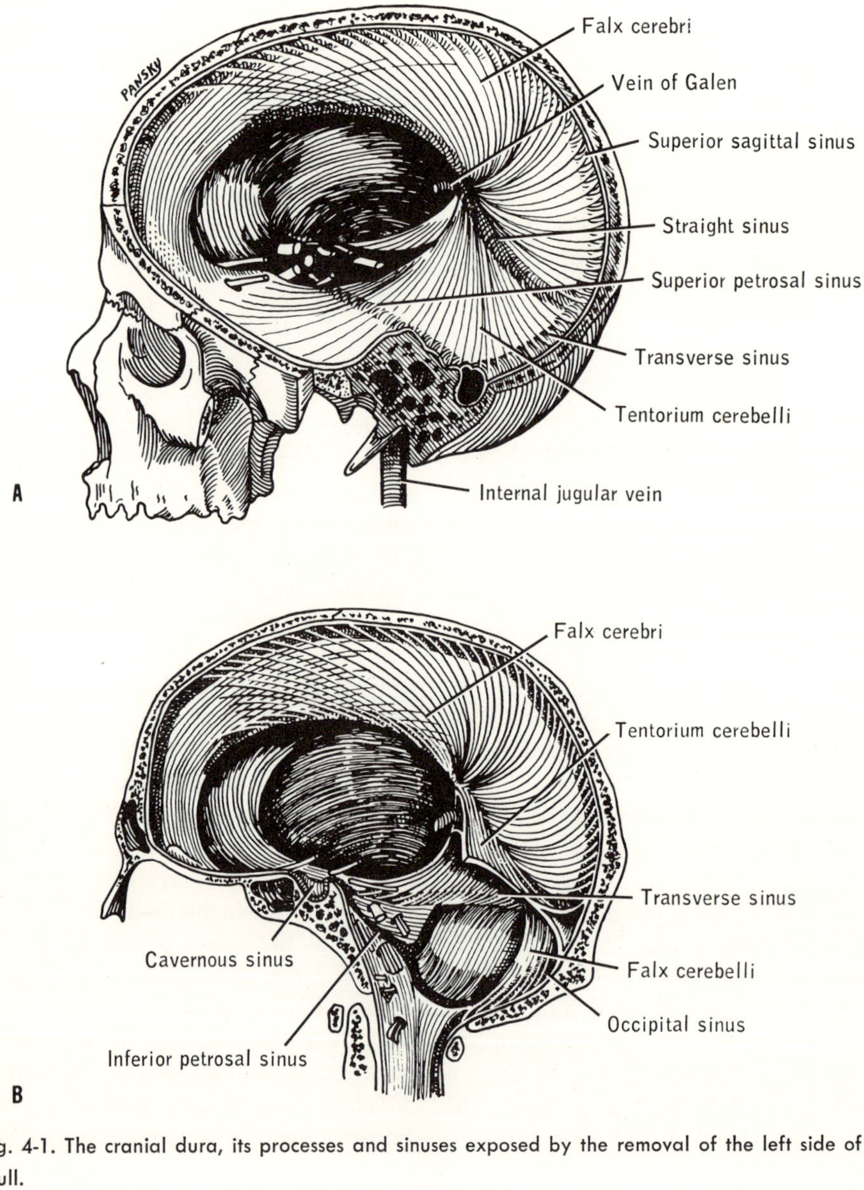

Fig. 4-1. The cranial dura, its processes and sinuses exposed by the removal of the left side of the skull.

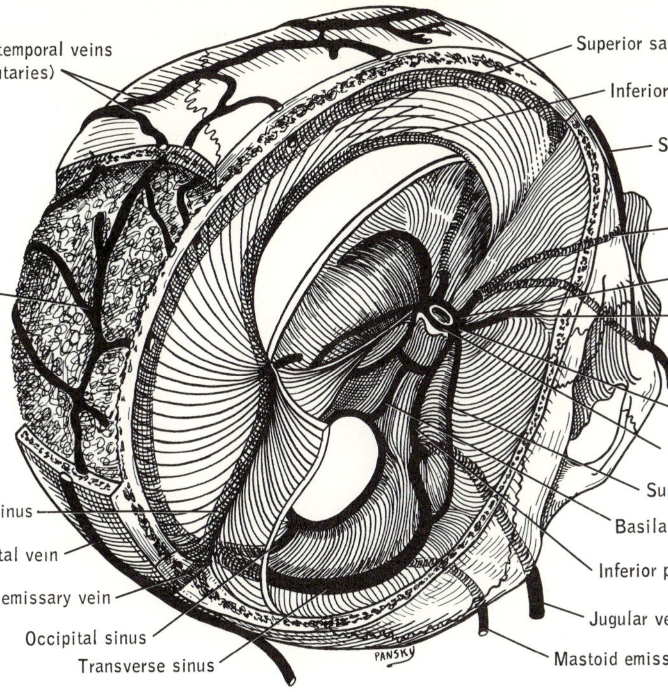

Fig. 4-2. The cranial dural sinuses exposed by the removal of the right side of the skull. The emissary, diploic, and superficial veins of the cranium are also shown.

loosely and does not dip into the sulci or fissures, except the longitudinal fissure. Projections of arachnoid invaginate the overlying dura, particularly in the region of the superior sagittal sinus and the *venous lacunae,* which adjoin the sinus. These are the *arachnoid villi* (granulations, Pacchionian bodies). Where the arachnoid lies close to the brain, delicate trabeculae of connective tissue traverse the subarachnoid space to join the pia mater. In certain regions around the base of the brain, the arachnoid and the pia are separated by considerable intervals, called cisterns. The major cisterns are the *cerebellomedullaris,* (*cisterna magna*); the *interpeduncular;* the *pontine;* and the *chiasmatic.*

Cisterna Cerebellomedullaris (Magna). This is a region where the arachnoid is reflected from the inferior surface of the cerebellar hemispheres and the dorsum of the medulla. It is continuous with the subarachnoid space of the vertebral column through the foramen magnum.

Cisterna Interpeduncularis. This is the space where the arachnoid crosses between the two temporal lobes, enclosing the cerebral peduncles and the interpeduncular fossa. It is continuous rostrally with the chiasmatic cistern and caudally with the pontine cisterna.

Three other cisterns are also recognized: the bilateral *cisterna fossae cerebri lateralis,* where the arachnoid bridges the lateral fissures; and the *cisterna venae magnae cerebri,* a single space lying between the splenium of the corpus callosum and the superior surface of the cerebellum.

Pia Mater (Figs. 4-4, 4-5, 4-7.)

This layer, deep to the arachnoid, is a vascular membrane composed of very small plexuses of blood vessels held together by delicate connective tissue fibers and covered externally by mesothelial cells. The pia, especially the mesothelial component, dips into the substance of the brain along the penetrating blood vessels, forming a lining for the perivascular spaces. Thus, it intimately invests the entire surface of the brain, extending into the depths of the cerebral sulci and the cerebellar folia. In certain regions, it joins the ependymal tissue of the brain to form the tela choroidea.

Coverings of the Spinal Cord

Dura Mater (Figs. 4-9, 4-10.)

In the vertebral canal, the dura consists only of the meningeal layer, since each of the vertebrae has its own periosteal covering. Areolar connective tissue and a plexus of veins fill the epidural space. The subdural space contains a minute amount of fluid. The dura is attached firmly to the borders of the foramen magnum and also to the second and third cervical vertebrae. Below this level it sends fibrous slips to the posterior longitudinal ligament. At the level of the second sacral vertebra, the dura ends except for a rudimentary prolongation, the *filum terminale externum* which ensheaths the filum terminale

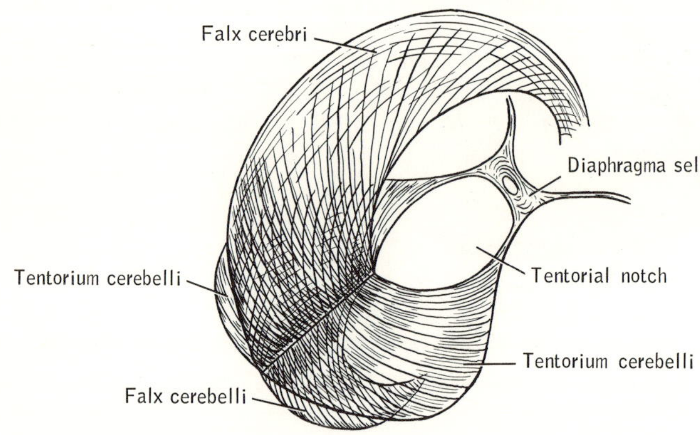

A

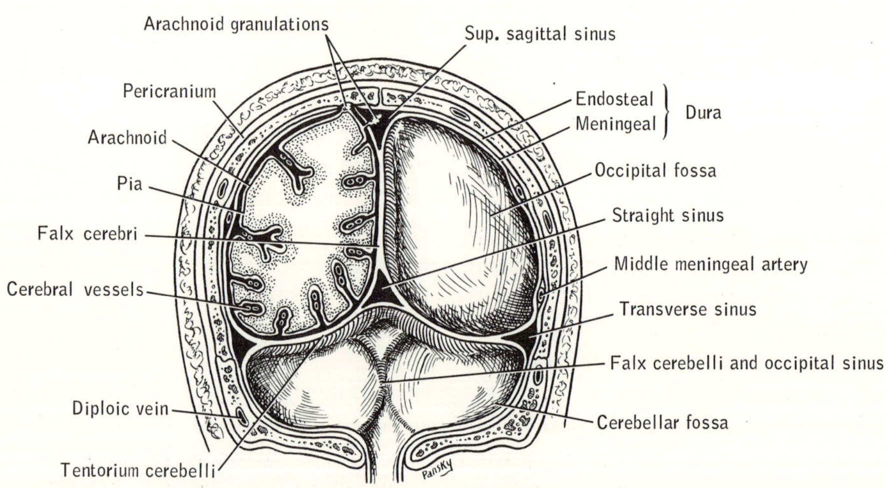

B

Fig. 4-3. A. Diagram of the reflections of the dura mater as seen from the right lateral aspect. B. Coronal section of the head at the level of the foramen magnum illustrating the relationships of the meninges, the venous sinuses and the blood vessels.

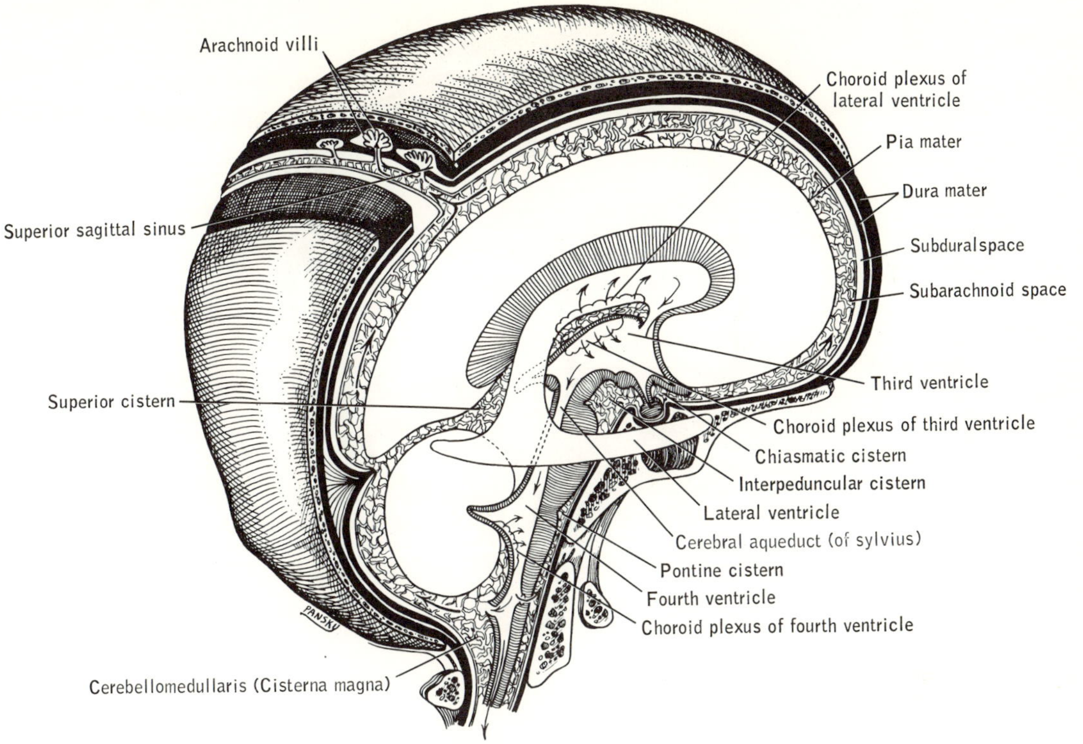

Fig. 4-4. Diagrammatic representation of the meninges, ventricles of the brain, and subarachnoid space. The direction of flow of the cerebrospinal fluid is indicated by arrows.

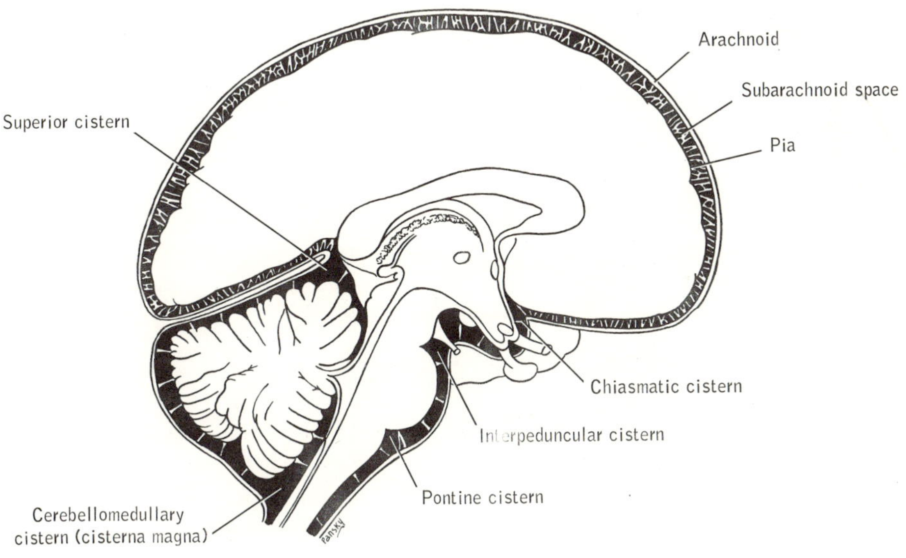

Fig. 4-5. Diagram of the principal subarachnoid cisterns seen in lateral view.

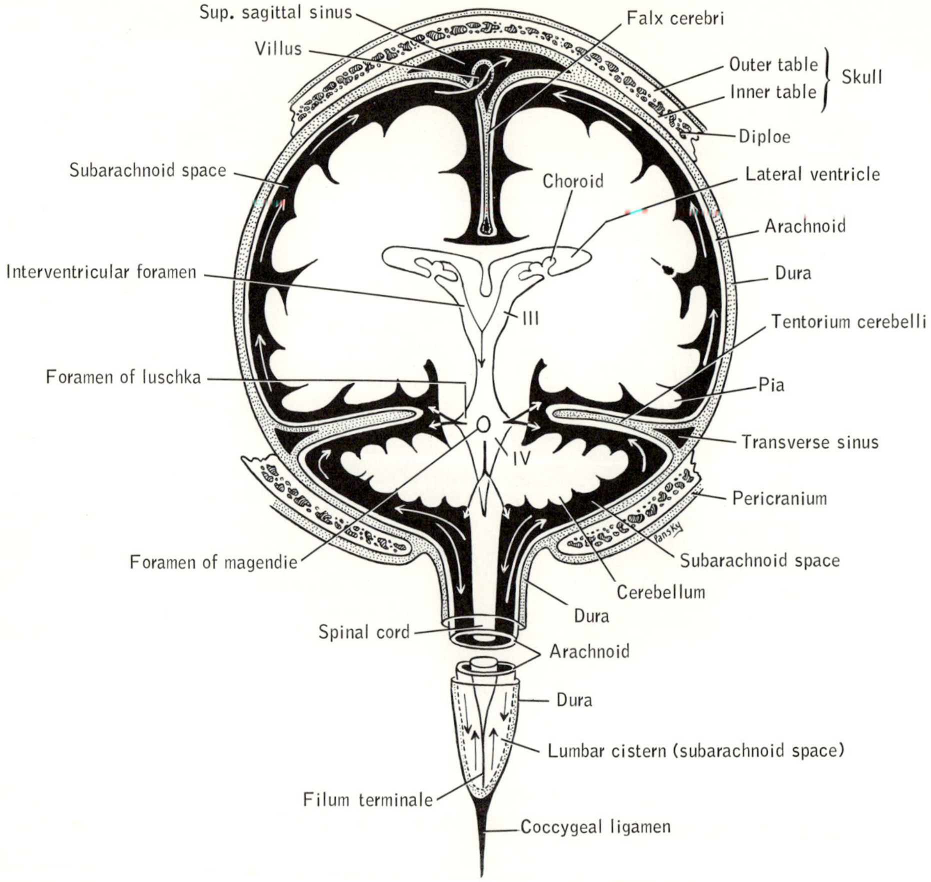

Fig. 4-6. Diagram to illustrate the essential points relating to the production, course, and absorption of cerebrospinal fluid. Meningeal layers are also shown.

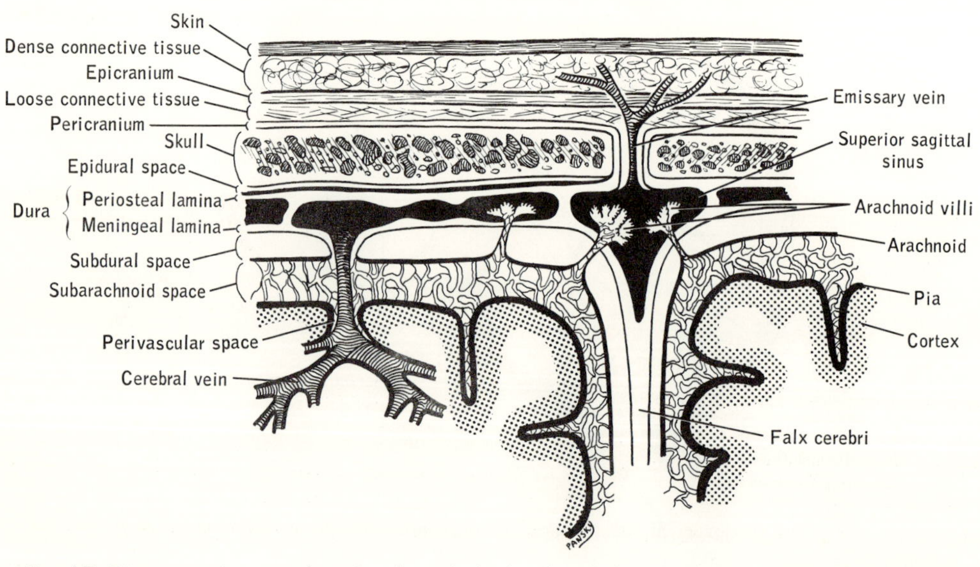

Fig. 4-7. Diagrammatic coronal section through the head, including the layers of the scalp and the superficial cerebral cortex. This shows the emissary veins and the relations of the arachnoid villi to the dural sinuses.

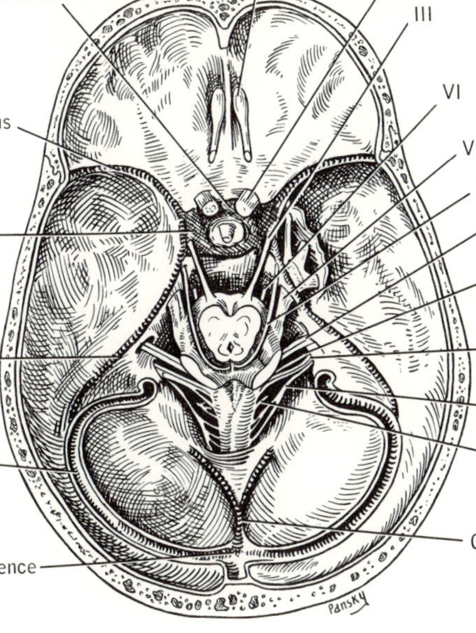

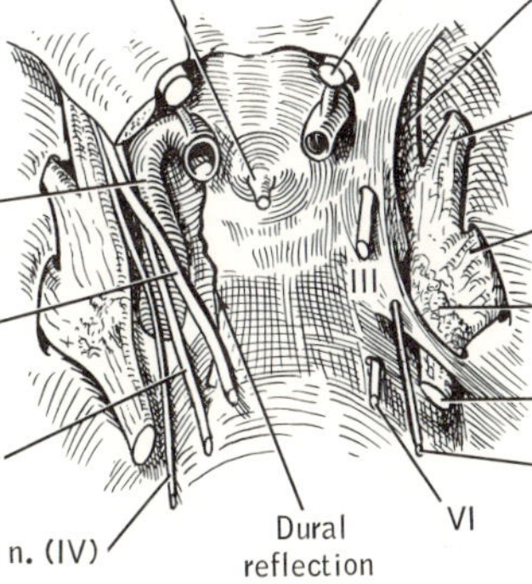

Fig. 4-8. Brain stem and base of skull viewed from above. The relations of the cranial nerves and internal carotid artery to the cavernous sinus are shown. The dura has been reflected on the left to better demonstrate the nerves and arteries.

internum to form the coccygeal ligament. This ligament continues caudalward to be attached to the coccyx. The spinal dura forms tubular prolongations along the spinal nerves where the latter pierce the dura. These sheaths pass with the nerves through the intervertebral foramina.

Arachnoid (Fig. 4-9, 4-10.)

The arachnoid is a thin, delicate, tubular membrane forming a loose investment for the cord, joined to the dura by connective tissue trabeculae. Through the foramen magnum, it is continuous with the cranial arachnoid, while in-

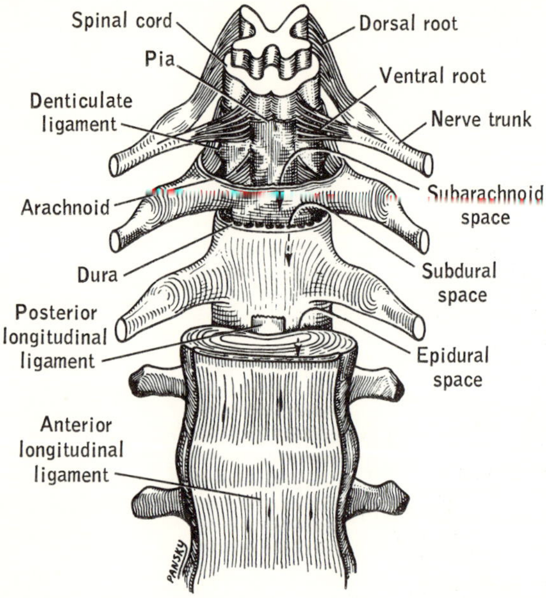

Fig. 4-9. The meninges and their associated spaces as shown through a longitudinal reconstruction of the spinal cord.

feriorly, it expands to surround the cauda equina. It forms tubular prolongations on the nerve roots, extending with each to their foramina of exit.

The subarachnoid space is widest caudally in the region of the cauda equina, ending at the level of the second sacral segment in the adult. The space is incompletely divided by a longitudinal, cribriform partition, the subarachnoid septum, which joins arachnoid and pia along the line of the posterior median sulcus of the cord. Laterally, it is also subdivided by the denticulate ligament. In addition, the space is traversed by a meshwork of delicate connective tissue trabeculae.

Pia (Figs. 4-9, 4-10.)

Along the cord, the pia is thicker, stronger, and less vascular than in the cranium. Ventrally, it is reflected into the ventral median fissure. In the midventral region it is a thickened, longitudinal band called the *linea splendens*. On either side, between the dorsal and ventral nerve roots is another band of longitudinal fibers, the *dentate ligament*. At intervals, the lateral aspect of the dentate ligament becomes attached to the dura. Below the conus medullaris of the cord, the pia continues as a slender filament along the filum terminale. At the level of the second sacral segment, it blends with the dura and continues caudally to insert into the dorsum of the coccyx.

CEREBROSPINAL FLUID (Figs. 4-4 to 4-7.)

This fluid is found within the ventricular system of the brain, the central canal of the spinal cord, and the subarachnoid space. Since it surrounds both the brain and cord, it helps to support the weight of the former and acts as a fluid cushion for the protection of both. This fluid may be formed in three ways: under hydrostatic pressure in the thin-walled, highly convoluted vessels of the choroid plexus; by a secretory mechanism inherent in the epithelial cells overlying the vessels of the plexus; or by a combination of both. The total amount has been estimated to be between 90 and 150 cc in adults. That formed in the lateral ventricles passes through the interventricular foramina (of Monro) into the third ventricle, where it is added to by the plexus of the latter. From here, the fluid courses caudally through the cerebral aqueduct into the fourth ventricle. Augmented by more fluid produced by the plexus in this cavity and by fluid ascending from the central canal of the cord, in which place it is formed by ependymal secretion, it finally leaves the ventricular system to enter the subarachnoid space through the foramen of Magendie and the foramina of Luschka. In the subarachnoid space, the fluid flows down and around the cord and up its ventral side to the basal part of the brain and then dorsally over the hemispheres, where it enters the arachnoid villi and is discharged through them into the venous system of the superior sagittal sinus or its lacunae. There is also evidence that at least a small amount of fluid is derived from the nervous tissue of the brain itself, passing outward into the subarachnoid space through the perivascular channels which occur along the penetrating blood vessels.

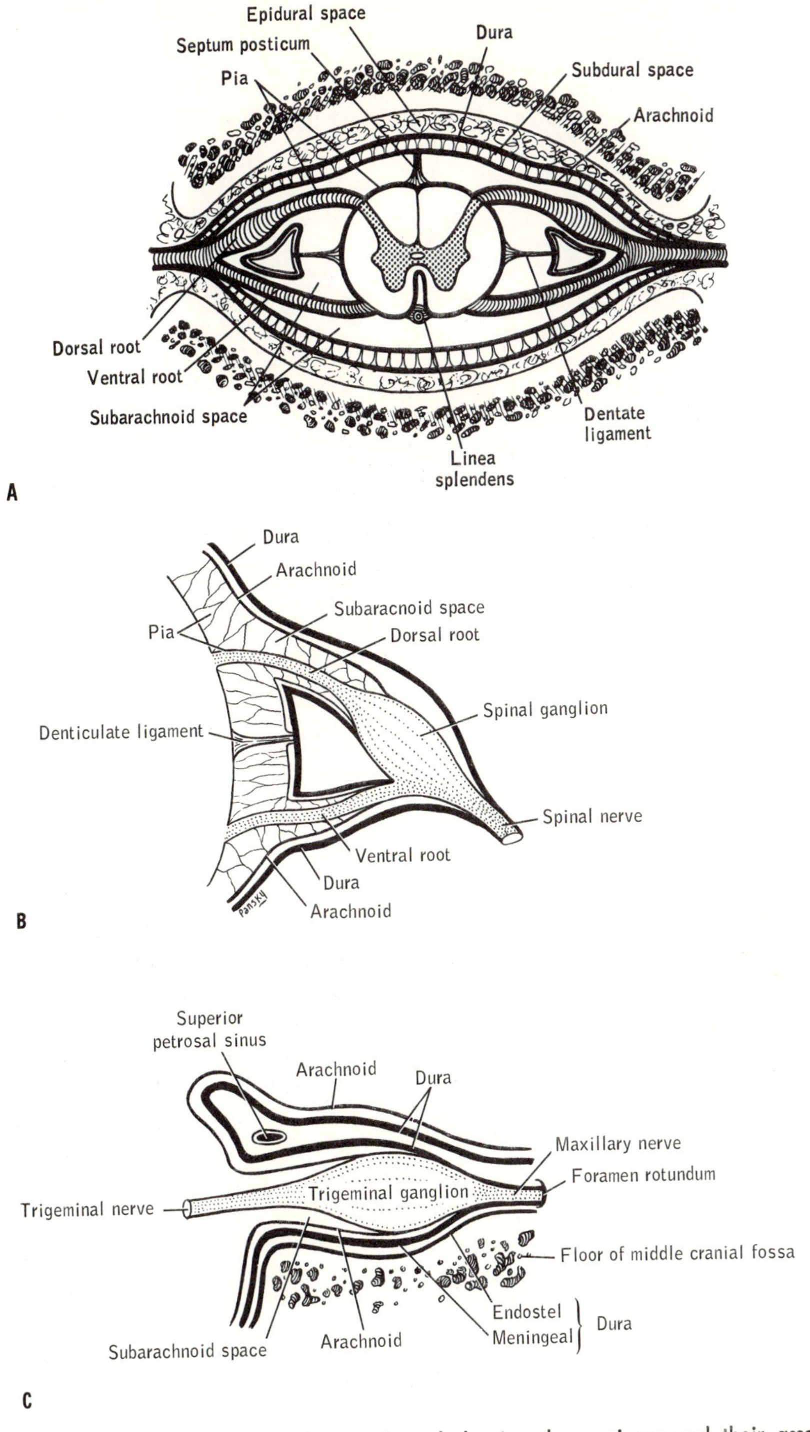

Fig. 4-10. A. Transverse section of the spinal cord showing the meninges and their associated spaces. B. The meningeal relations of a spinal nerve. C. Meningeal relations of the trigeminal ganglion in the cavum trigeminale. The dura is folded over the ganglion forming the floor of the middle cranial fossa. The cavum trigeminale has two layers of dura superior to it but otherwise the dural relations are the same as that in the dorsal root ganglion.

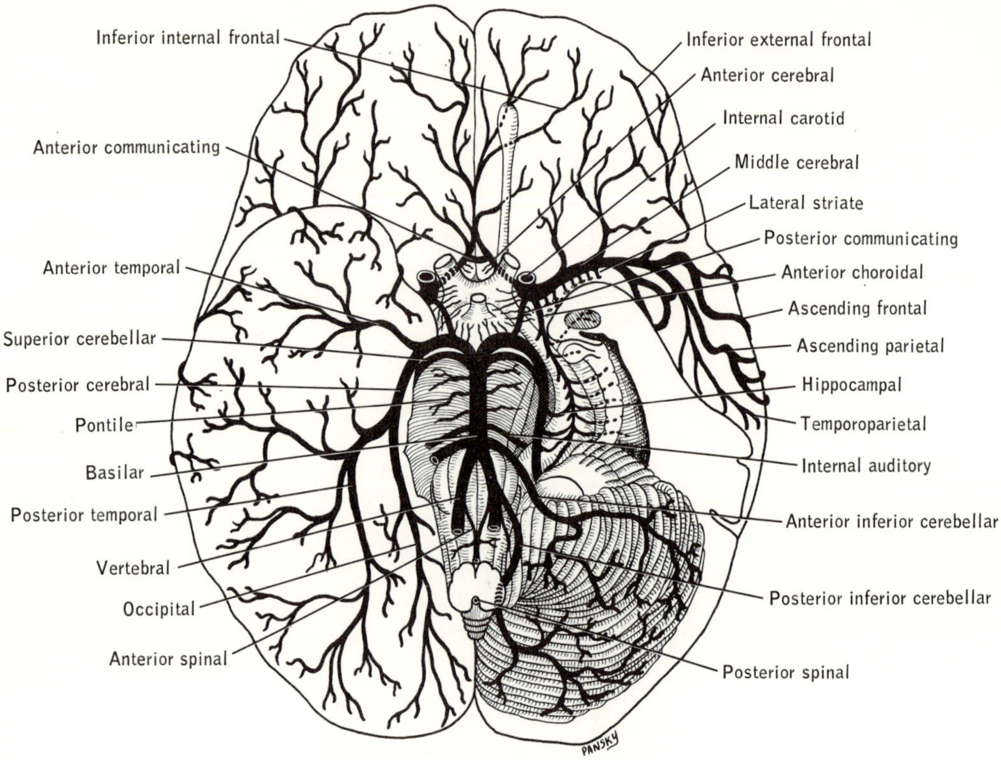

Fig. 4-11. Principal arterial vessels on the basal aspect of the brain.

BLOOD SUPPLY

Arterial Blood

Brain

Arterial blood is supplied to the brain through four main channels, namely, the two internal carotid and two vertebral arteries.

Internal Carotid Arteries. These channels (Figs. 4-8, 4-11, 4-13, 4-15, 4-19, 4-22) enter the skull via the carotid canal, cross the foramen lacerum, pass into the middle cranial fossa, and ascend in the carotid grooves on the sides of the sphenoid bone. At the level of the lateral cerebral fissure, they branch into several important divisions.[1]

Anterior Cerebral Arteries. (Figs. 4-11 to 4-17, 4-20 to 4-22.) These arteries course rostrally and medially across the anterior perforated substance and superior to optic tract to the beginning of the longitudinal fissure. Here, as the vessels from the two sides lie close together, an anastomotic branch called the *anterior communicating artery* is formed (Figs. 4-8, 4-13). Then each vessel continues upwards through the fissure, around the genu of the corpus callosum, and posteriorly along the dorsum of the latter, to terminate by joining branches of the posterior cerebral arteries. In its course, the anterior cerebral artery sends branches to the medial surfaces of the frontal and parietal lobes, the anterior perforated substance, the rostrum and the body of the corpus callosum, and the septum pellucidum. Frequently, a large recurrent branch, the *medial striate artery* (Heubner) is seen (Figs. 4-13, 4-19). It supplies the lower and rostral part of the caudate nucleus, the lower part of

[1] In this section, only those major branches giving direct blood supply to the brain will be included.

the rostral end of the putamen, and the anterior limb and genu of the internal capsule.

Middle Cerebral Arteries. (Figs. 4-11 to 4-13, 4-17, 4-19 to 4-21, 4-22.) These are the largest branches of the internal carotid arteries. They run in the lateral cerebral fissure, then curve posteriorly over the insula, where they are distributed to the lateral portion of the hemispheres. Near their origin, two sets of small vessels are given off which penetrate the anterior perforated substance. These are the *medial striate arteries,* which may also arise from the anterior cerebral (see above); and the *lateral striate* which supply a large part of the putamen, the lateral area of the glogus pallidus and adjacent parts of the internal capsule. Since the latter vessels, especially the so-called lenticulostriate are frequently disrupted in cerebrovascular accidents, the group is often referred to as the artery of cerebral hemorrhage.

Posterior Communicating Arteries. (Figs. 4-11, 4-13, 4-15, 4-19, 4-22.) These run posteriorly to join the posterior cerebral branches of the vertebral-basilar artery. Their branches run medially and enter the brain between the infundibulum and the optic tract. They supply the genu and anterior third of the posterior limb of the internal capsule; the rostral portion of the thalamus; and the walls of the third ventricle.

Anterior Choroidal Arteries. (Figs. 4-11, 4-18, 4-19, 4-22.) These usually arise from the internal carotid arteries just before their bifurcation. They pass backward along the optic tract and around the cerebral peduncle as far as the lateral geniculate body, where their main branches turn to enter the inferior border of the

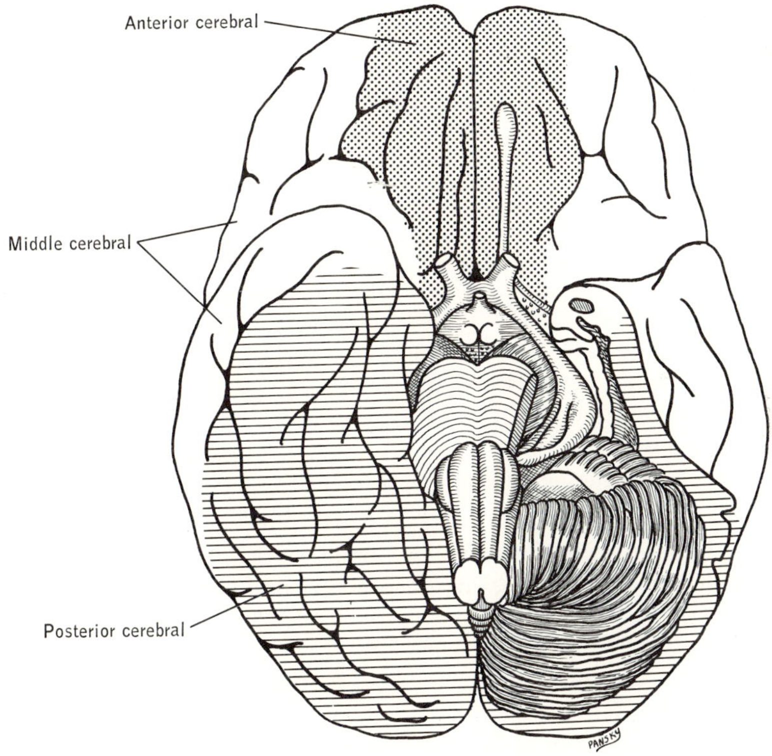

Fig. 4-12. Areas of distribution of the anterior, middle, and posterior cerebral arteries on the base of the brain.

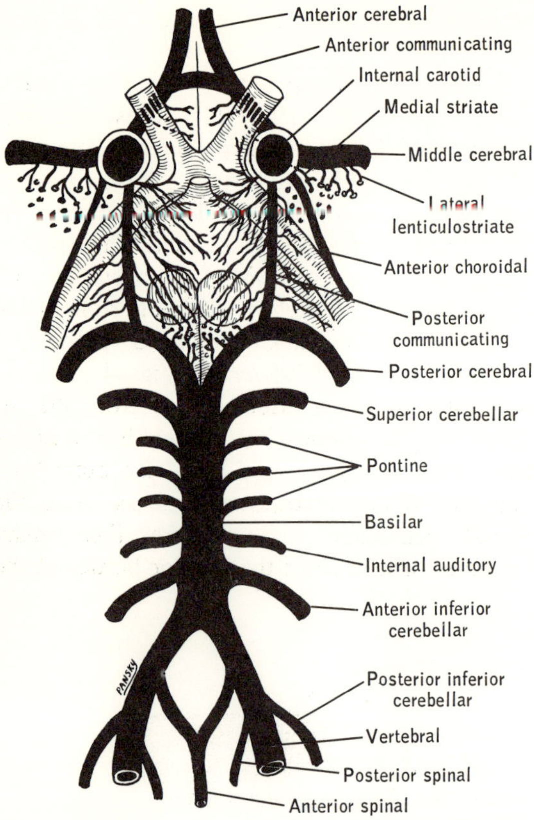

Fig. 4-13. Enlargement of the central portion of Fig. 4-11, showing some of the smaller branches in greater detail.

lateral ventricle. They supply the choroid plexus of that ventricle. In their course, branches are given to the optic tract, hippocampus, tail of the caudate nucleus, medial and intermediate portions of the globus pallidus; posterior two-thirds of the posterior limb of the internal capsule including its retro- and sublenticular portions; the middle third of the cerebral peduncle; and the external part of the lateral geniculate body.

Vertebral Arteries. (Figs. 4-11, 4-13, 4-15, 4-25.) These vessels enter the skull through the foramen magnum and ascend along the lateral ventral side of the medulla. Near the rostral end of the medulla, the two arteries join to form the *basilar artery*. In their intracranial course, the vertebral arteries give off several branches: the *anterior spinal* artery, which joins its fellow to form a single median vessel along the ventral side of the medulla and spinal cord; the *posterior spinal* artery, which descends onto the cord along the dorsal roots of the spinal nerves; the *posterior inferior cerebellar* artery, which usually comes off just below the union of the two vertebral arteries to form the basilar artery (occasionally, it is a branch of the basilar artery).

Basilar Artery. (Figs. 4-11, 4-13, 4-15, 4-18, 4-19.) This ascends on the ventral surface of the pons to terminate by dividing into the *posterior cerebral arteries.* Along its course the basilar artery gives several *pontine* arteries, to supply the pons; *internal auditory* artery, to the inner ear; *anterior inferior cerebellar* artery, to the rostral portion of the inferior surface of the cerebellum; *superior cerebellar* artery, to the upper surface of the cerebellum, where it branches to supply this region, as well as the corpora quadrigemina, pineal body, and choroid plexus of the third ventricle.

Posterior Cerebral Artery. (Figs. 4-11 to 4-21.) This vessel passes lateralward, receives the posterior communicating artery from the internal carotid artery, and bends around the cerebral peduncle to reach the inferior surface of the occipital lobe, where it branches out to supply both the inferior and medial surfaces of both temporal and occipital lobes. Posterior choroid branches of the posterior cerebral artery pass to the choroid plexuses of the third ventricle and the lateral ventricle.

Circle of Willis. (Figs. 4-11, 4-13, 4-14, 4-19.) The anastomosis of the internal carotid and vertebral circulation forms a circular pattern known as the circle of Willis. This anastomosis makes possible an adequate blood supply to the brain in case of occlusion of either the carotid or vertebral arteries.

Spinal Cord

Posterior Spinal Arteries. (Figs. 4-23 to 4-25.) These arise from the vertebral artery and run caudally either just medial or lateral to the dorsal roots of the spinal nerves. In their course, they are joined by small spinal branches of the vertebral, intercostal, lumbar, and sacral arteries.

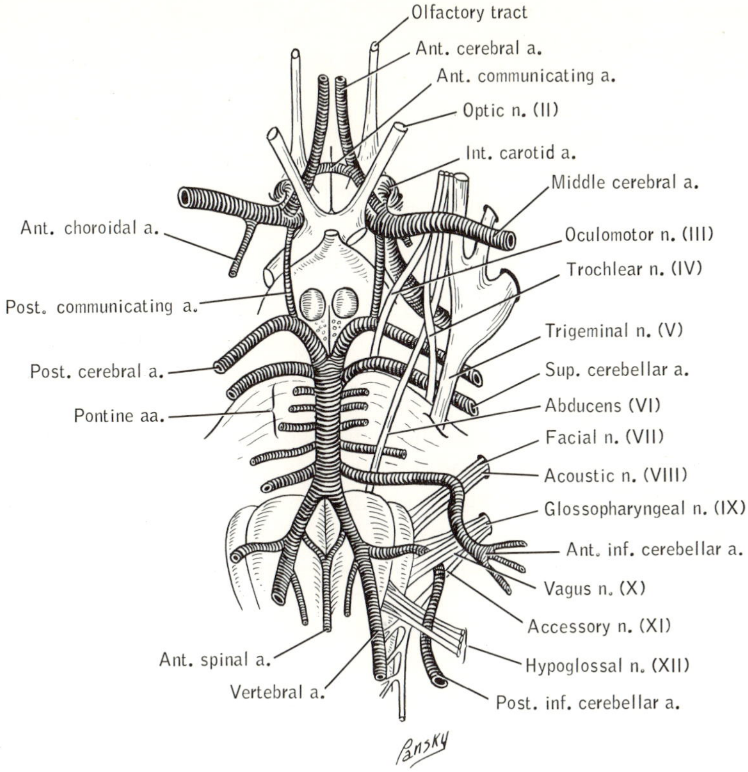

Fig. 4-14. Arteries at the base of the brain showing their relations to the cranial nerves.

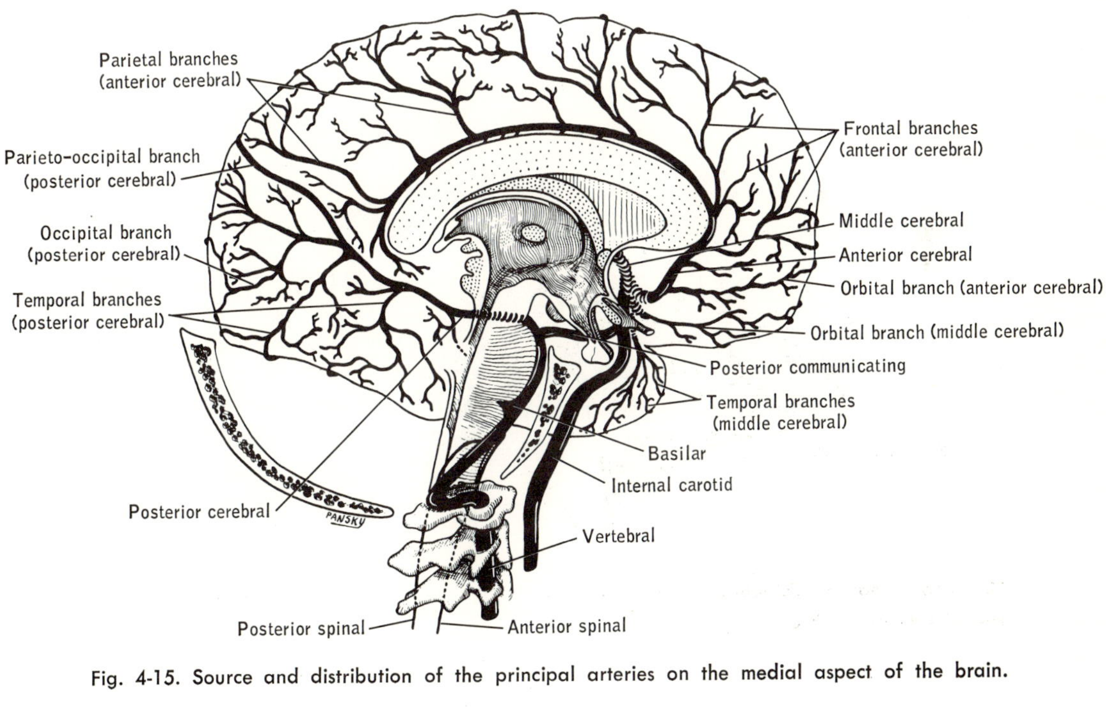

Fig. 4-15. Source and distribution of the principal arteries on the medial aspect of the brain.

Anterior Spinal Arteries. (Figs. 4-23 to 4-25.) These begin as medial branches from the vertebral arteries near their terminations and unite into a single trunk in front of the medulla at the level of the foramen magnum. This trunk descends to the lower end of the spinal cord, receiving contributions from spinal branches of the same vessels which contribute to the posterior spinal arteries.

Meningeal Arteries

Cranial. (Figs. 4-26, 4-37.) The meninges in the posterior cranial fossa are supplied by the posterior meningeal arteries, which are branches of the ascending pharyngeal arteries; and by posterior meningeal branches of the vertebral and occipital arteries.

The meninges in the middle cranial fossa are supplied by the middle meningeal and the accessory meningeal arteries, both branches of the internal maxillary arteries (branches of the external carotid arteries) and by the ethmoidal arteries from the ophthalmic branches of the internal carotid arteries.

Spinal. The spinal branches that supply the cord also supply its meninges.

Venous Drainage

Since the venous blood from both brain and meninges drains into the venous sinuses of the dura, a description of the latter, which are endothelium-lined spaces between the two layers of the dura, is essential.

Venous Sinuses of the Dura

Superior Sagittal Sinus. (Figs. 4-3, 4-7, 4-30, 4-37.) It begins at the foramen cecum, where it receives a vein from the nasal cavity, and courses dorsally and posteriorly in the attached border of the falx cerebri. Just above the internal occipital protuberance, in the majority of cases, it passes to the right, to enter the transverse sinus on that side. In its course, it receives the superior cerebral veins and cerebrospinal fluid from the arachnoid villi and the venous lacunae. The superior part of the dura also drains into this sinus.

Inferior Sagittal Sinus. (Figs. 4-1, 4-2, 4-6, 4-30.) This occupies the posterior half or two-thirds of the free margin of the falx cerebri. It receives a few veins from the medial surface of the cerebrum and ends in the straight sinus.

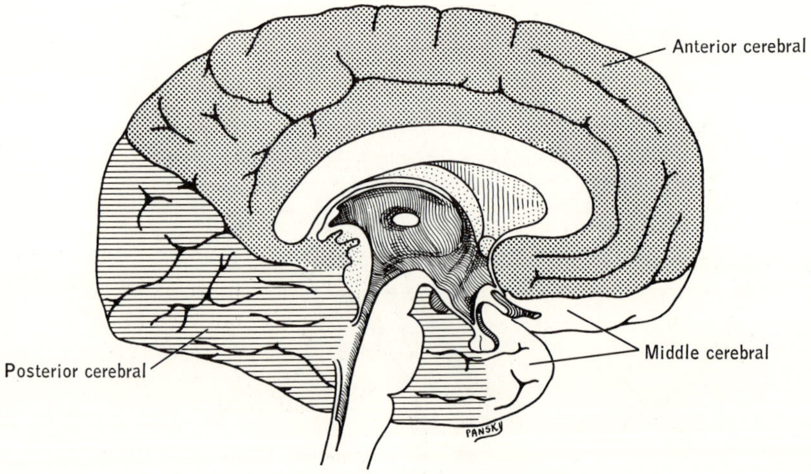

Fig. 4-16. Areas of distribution of the anterior, middle, and posterior cerebral arteries on the medial side of the brain.

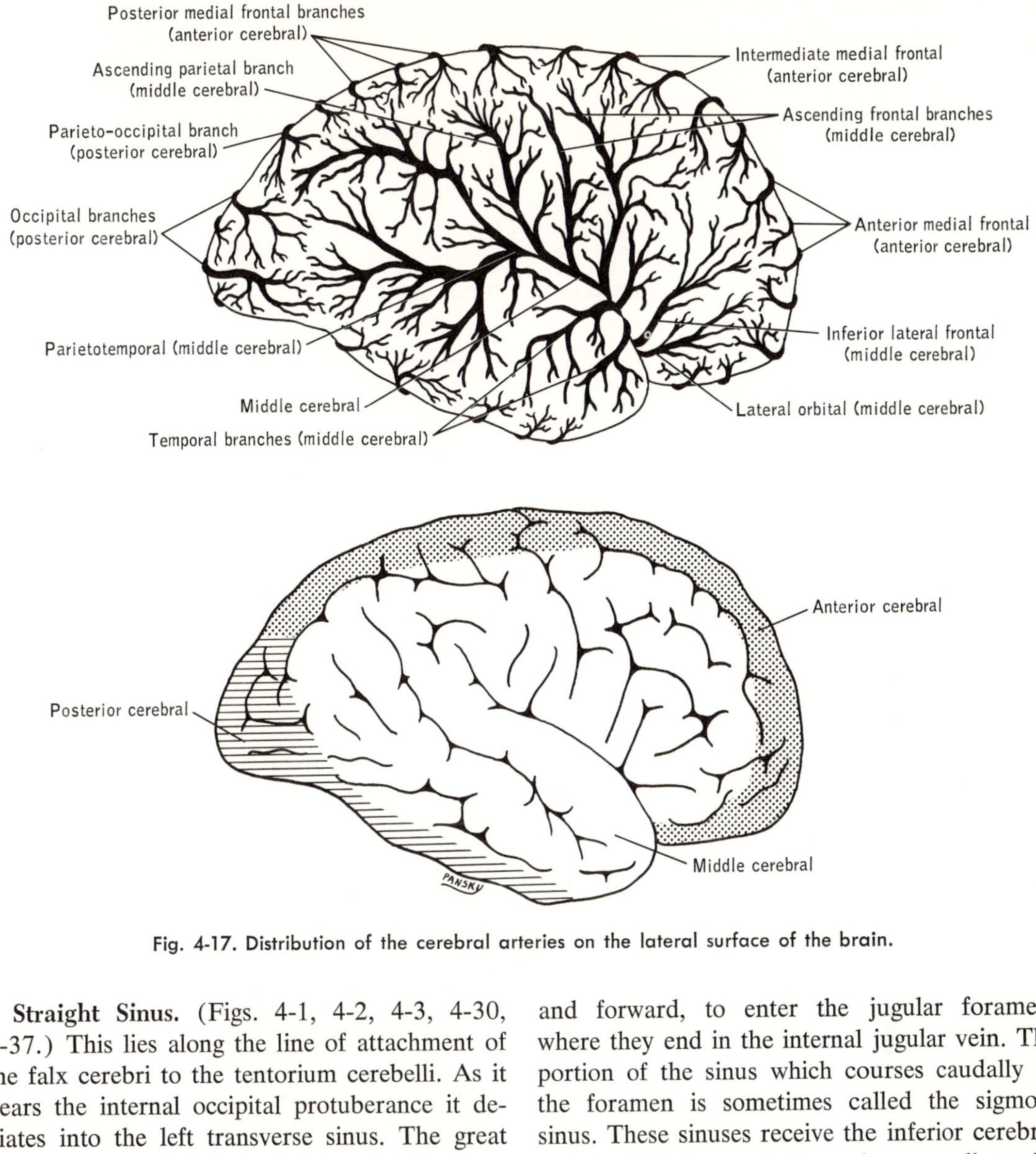

Fig. 4-17. Distribution of the cerebral arteries on the lateral surface of the brain.

Straight Sinus. (Figs. 4-1, 4-2, 4-3, 4-30, 4-37.) This lies along the line of attachment of the falx cerebri to the tentorium cerebelli. As it nears the internal occipital protuberance it deviates into the left transverse sinus. The great cerebral vein (of Galen) and the superior cerebellar veins also terminate in the straight sinus.

Transverse Sinuses (Lateral Sinus). (Figs. 4-1 to 4-3, 4-6, 4-8, 4-30.) These run laterally from the region of the internal occipital protuberance. The first part of their course lies in the attached border of the tentorium cerebelli. When they reach the base of the petrous temporal bone, they leave the tentorium and curve downward and forward, to enter the jugular foramen, where they end in the internal jugular vein. The portion of the sinus which courses caudally to the foramen is sometimes called the sigmoid sinus. These sinuses receive the inferior cerebral and the inferior cerebellar veins as well as the superior petrosal sinuses.

Occipital Sinus. (Figs. 4-1, 4-2, 4-30.) This is the smallest of the sinuses. It begins near the margin of the foramen magnum by the union of two tributaries, through which it may communicate with the sigmoid sinuses. It ascends in the attached margin of the falx cerebelli and ends at the confluence of the sinuses, a region overlying the internal occipital protuberance where the superior sagittal, straight, transverse, and occipital sinuses join. It also receives the inferior cerebellar veins.

Cavernous Sinuses. (Figs. 4-1, 4-2, 4-8, 4-30, 4-37.) These lie on either side of the body of the sphenoid bone between the superior orbital fissure and the apex of the petrous temporal bone. Their chief afferent vessels are the superior ophthalmic and the cerebral veins. Sometimes a division of the inferior ophthalmic vein also opens into the sinus. Blood leaves the cavernous sinuses by way of the intercavernous sinuses and the superior and inferior petrosal sinuses. Although separated from the blood of the sinus by an endothelial lining, the internal carotid artery, the ophthalmic and maxillary divisions of the trigeminal nerve, the oculomotor, trochlear, and abducens nerves are all intimately related to the cavernous sinuses.

Superior Petrosal Sinuses. (Figs. 4-2, 4-8, 4-30.) These leave the cavernous sinuses and pass posteriorly in the tentorium cerebelli along the superior angle of the petrous temporal bone to join the transverse sinuses. They receive blood from the cerebellum and cerebrum as well as the tympanic cavity.

Inferior Petrosal Sinuses. (Figs. 4-2, 4-30.) These begin in the cavernous sinuses and course caudally between the petrous temporal and the basilar part of the occipital bones, to terminate directly into the superior jugular bulb at the

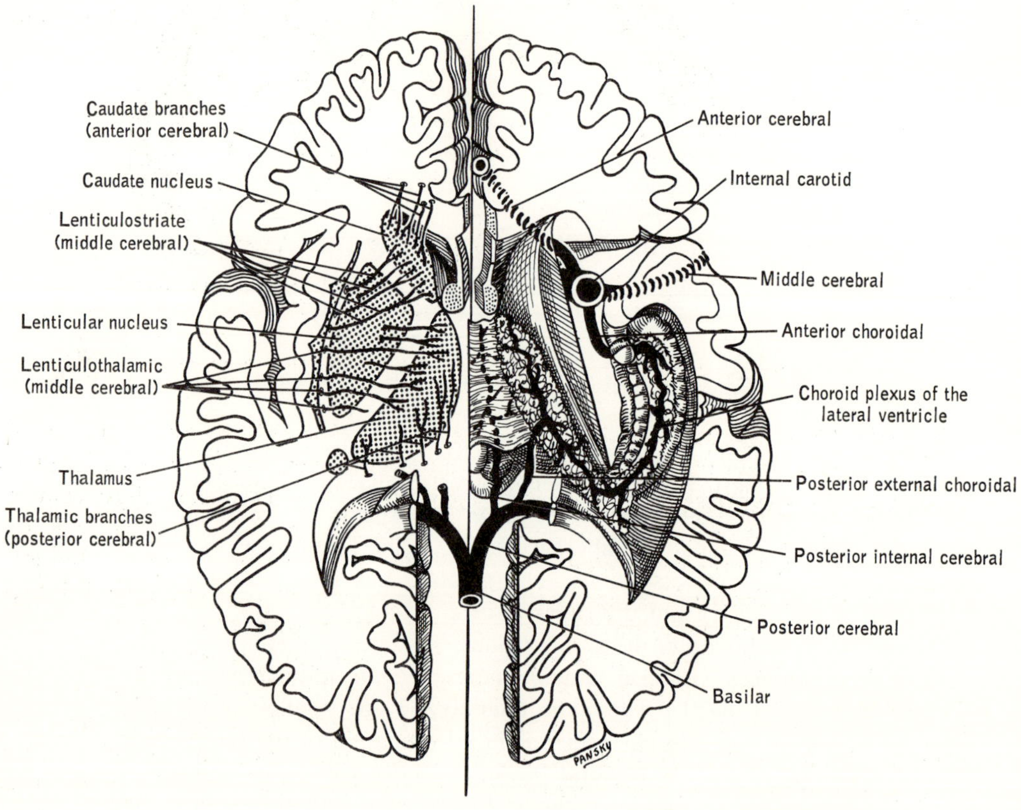

Fig. 4-18. Horizontal sections through the cerebrum: *right,* the lateral ventricle has been exposed to show the arteries supplying the choroid plexus; *left,* distribution of vessels to the basal ganglia and thalamus.

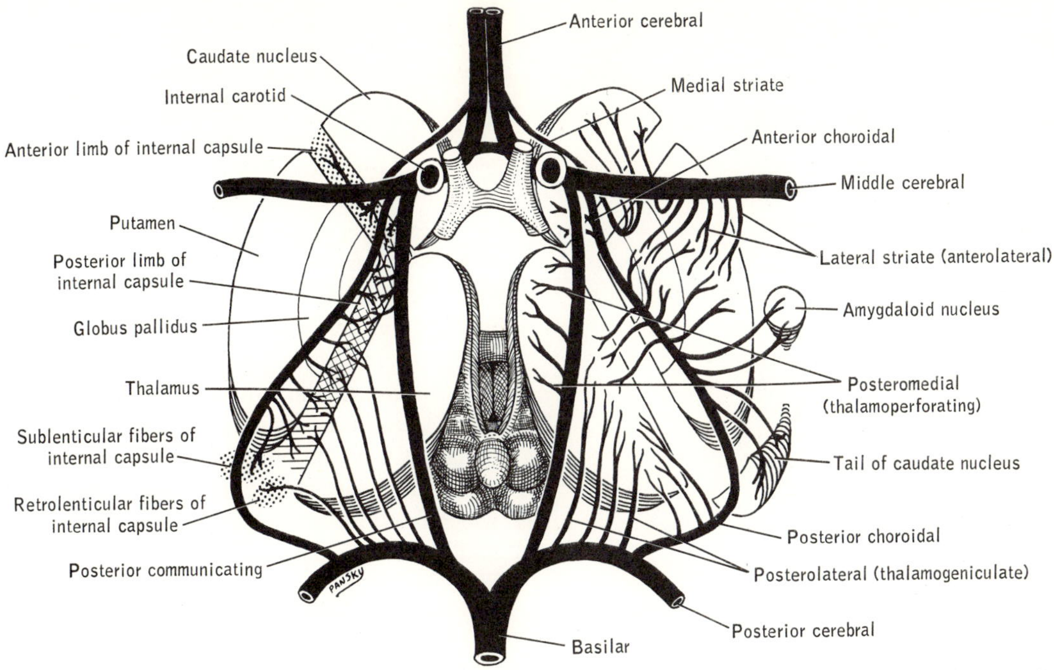

Fig. 4-19. Diagram of a horizontal section through the brain to show the arterial supply of the thalamus, internal capsule, and basal ganglia.

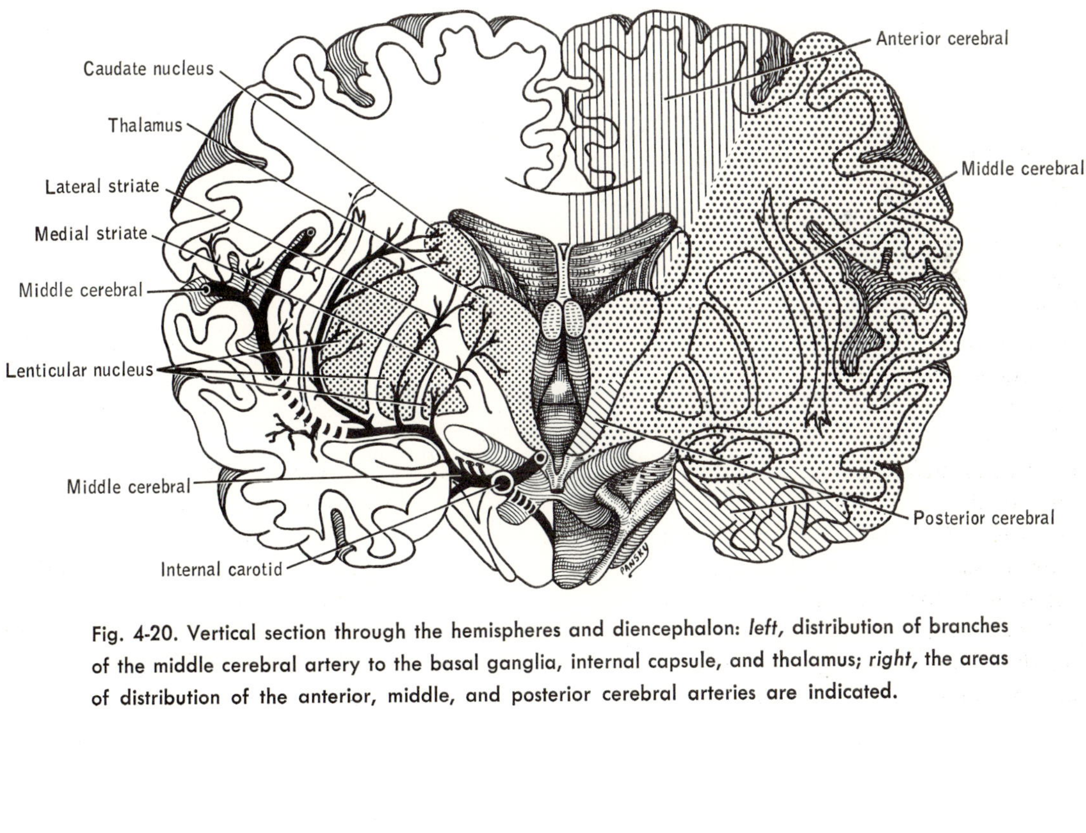

Fig. 4-20. Vertical section through the hemispheres and diencephalon: *left,* distribution of branches of the middle cerebral artery to the basal ganglia, internal capsule, and thalamus; *right,* the areas of distribution of the anterior, middle, and posterior cerebral arteries are indicated.

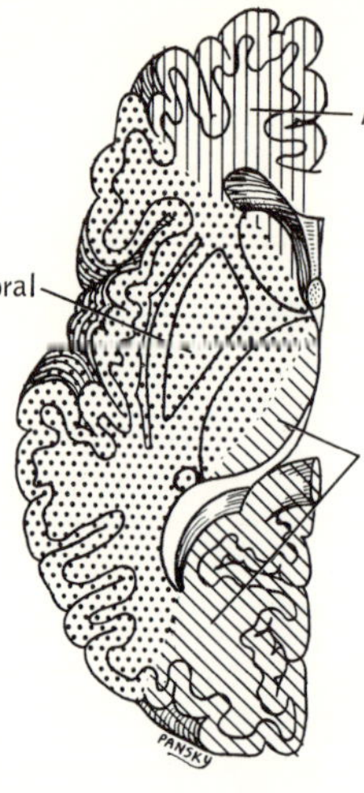

Fig. 4-21. Horizontal section through the left cerebral hemisphere, showing distribution of the anterior, middle, and posterior cerebral arteries.

jugular foramen. They receive veins from the medulla, pons, inferior portion of the cerebellum, and the inner ear.

Veins of the Brain (Figs. 4-27 to 4-29.)

The veins of the brain all terminate in the dural sinuses described above. They are classified as external and internal cerebral and cerebellar veins.

The *external cerebral veins* are usually described as (1) *superior cerebral veins* 8 to 12 of which drain the superior, lateral, and medial surfaces of the hemisphere and terminate in the superior sagittal sinus; (2) *middle cerebral veins,* beginning on the lateral surface of the hemispheres and ending directly or indirectly in the cavernous sinus (there are also intercommunications with the superior and transverse sinuses); (3) medial cerebral veins which drain part of the medial surface of the hemispheres and terminate in the inferior sagittal sinus; (4) *inferior cerebral veins,* which are small and drain the inferior surfaces of the hemispheres, those on the frontal lobe connecting via superior cerebral tributaries with the superior sagittal sinus, those on the temporal lobe joining either the middle cerebral or the basal venous system and terminating in the cavernous or superior petrosal sinuses; (5) *basal veins,* formed by the confluence of three small veins: the anterior cerebral vein, draining the frontal lobe; the deep middle cerebral vein, draining the insula and adjoining gyri; and the inferior striate veins, draining the corpus striatum. The basal vein receives tributaries from the interpeduncular fossa, the hippocampal gyrus, the inferior horn of the lateral ventricle, and the mesencephalon. It terminates in the great cerebral vein.

There are two *internal cerebral veins,* each in turn formed by the confluence of two veins: (1) the *terminal vein,* lying in the groove between the thalamus and the corpus striatum and receiving tributaries from both; and (2) the *choroid vein,* which runs the entire length of the choroid plexus and drains the hippocampus, fornix, and corpus callosum. When the internal cerebral veins reach the splenium of the corpus callosum, they are joined by the basal veins to form the great cerebral vein (of Galen).

The *cerebellar veins* are divided into two groups: (1) the *superior,* which passes rostrally and medially to end in the straight sinus, internal cerebral veins, transverse sinus, and superior petrosal sinus; and (2) the *inferior,* which ends in the transverse, superior petrosal, and occipital sinuses.

Emissary and Diploic Veins

The emissary veins (Figs. 4-2, 4-7, 4-30) connect the intra- and extracranial veins. Since blood can flow in either direction in these veins, the venous pressure in both the sinuses and the superficial veins can be equalized. The more important emissary veins are (1) the parietal, (2) the emissary veins of the foramen cecum, (3) the mastoid, and (4) the ophthalmic.

The diploic veins (Figs. 4-2, 4-30) form venous plexuses between the inner and outer tables of the skull. The veins form a plexus drained by four major venous trunks on each side: the frontal, anterior parietal (temporal), posterior parietal (temporal), and occipital. These trunks then drain into the sinuses of the cranium.

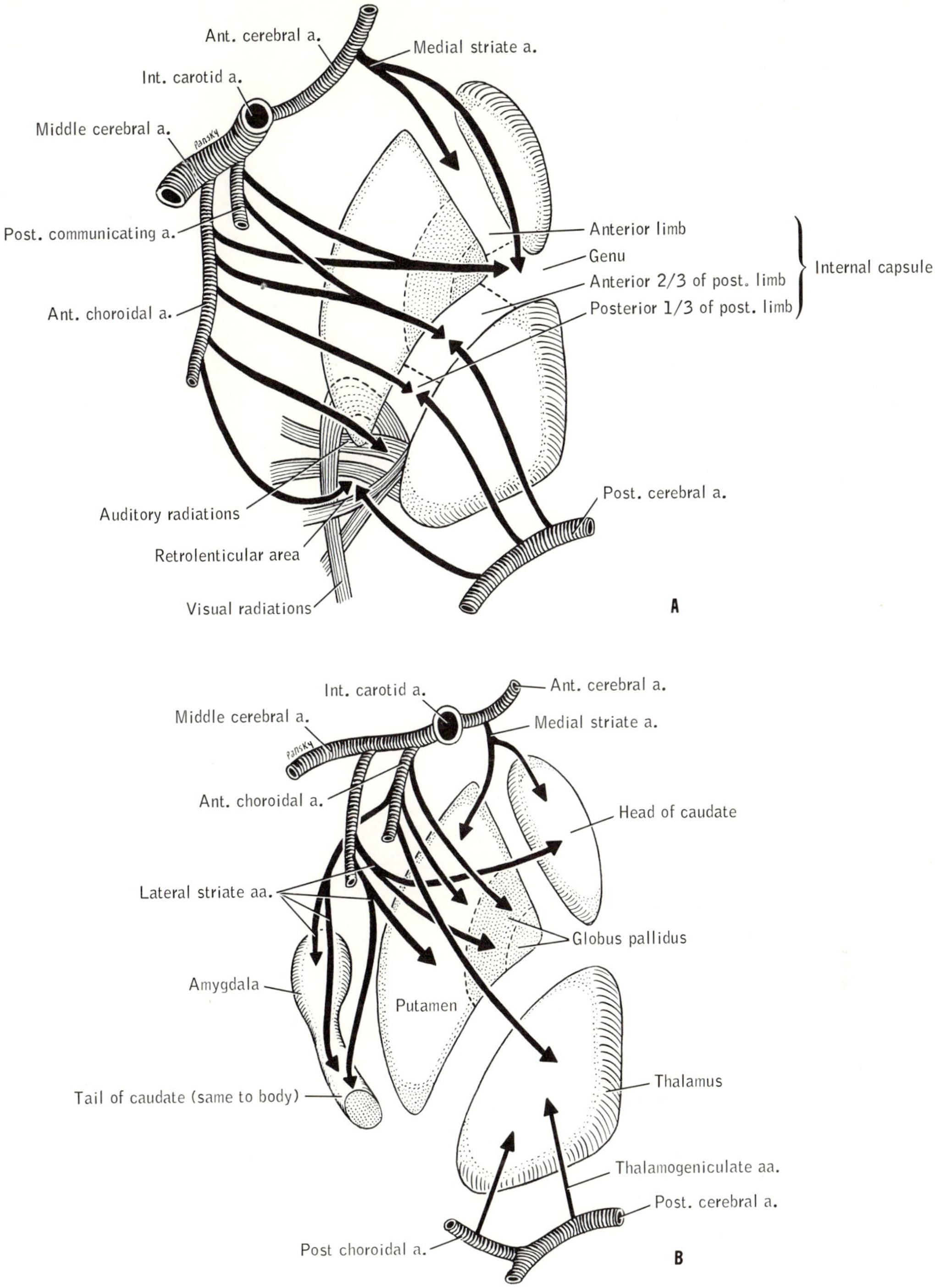

Fig. 4-22. Diagrams illustrating the arterial blood supply in the region of the basal nuclei and internal capsule. *A*. Vessels to the internal capsule. *B*. Vessels to the basal nuclei. (*Modified after Abbie*, 1937, *and Rubenstein*, 1944.)

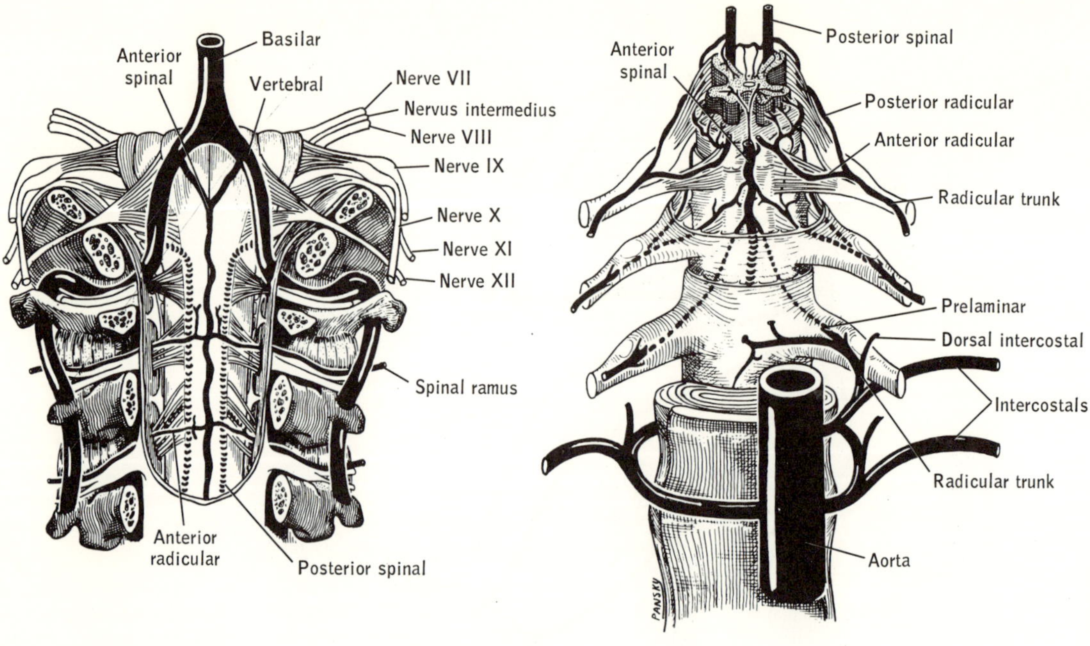

Fig. 4-23. Source, course, and distribution of the arteries supplying the spinal cord as revealed through longitudinal dissection: *left,* represents the cervical, *right,* the thoracic regions.

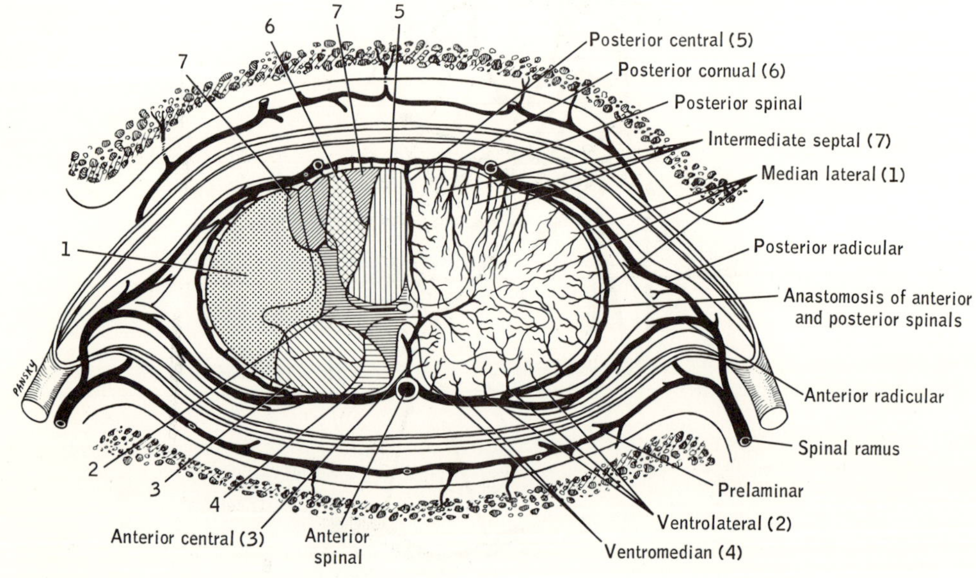

Fig. 4-24. Transverse section through the vertebral column and spinal cord showing: *right,* the finer branchings of the arteries; *left,* the areas of distribution of the arterial branches supplying the spinal cord.

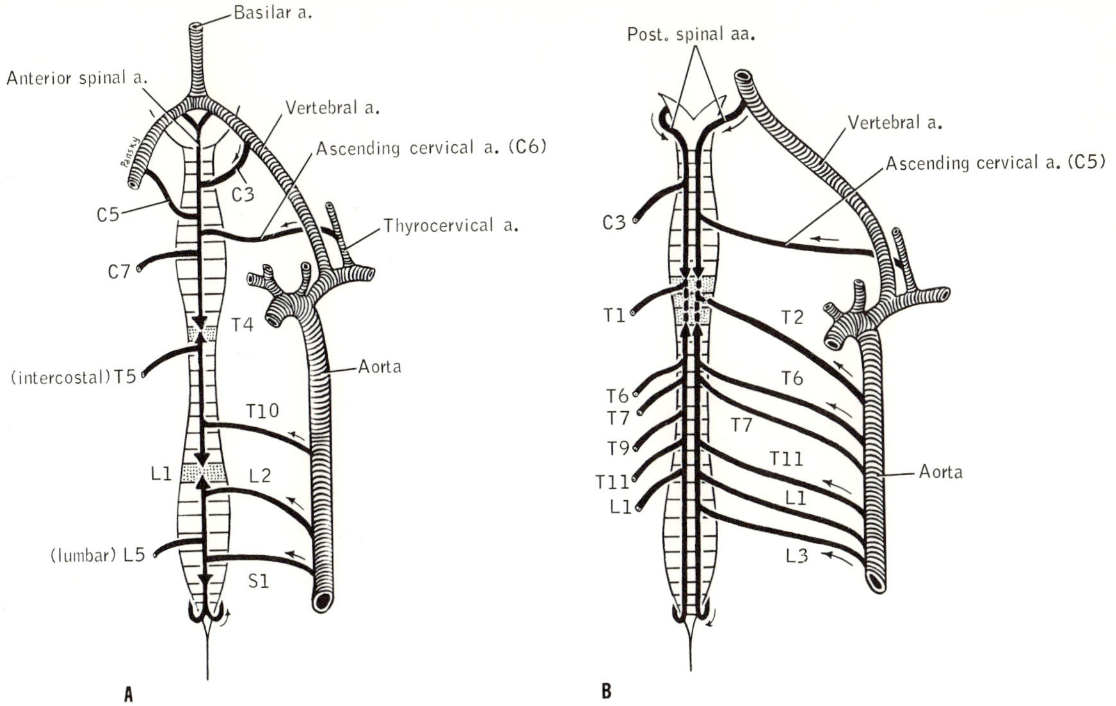

Fig. 4-25. Diagrams of the arterial vessels to the spinal cord. *A.* Anterior surface. Note that the chief sources are through radicular arteries of segments C-6, T-10, and L-2. The arterial bed at T-4 and L-1 (stippled) are said to be the weak points in the circulation since blood pressure is lowest there. Direction of flow is shown. *B.* Posterior surface. The region of poorest circulation (stippled) is thought to be from T-1 to T-3. Direction of flow is indicated. (*Modified after Bolton, 1939, and Zülch, 1954.*)

Veins of the Spinal Cord (Figs. 4-31, 4-32.)

The pia of the cord contains a minute and tortuous venous plexus, within which are found six or seven longitudinal channels. When six are present, one lies over the posterior sulcus, one in front of the anterior fissure while the remaining four are laterally disposed along the anterior and posterior surfaces of the cord. When seven are found, one vein overlies the posterior sulcus with one channel on either side just medial to the dorsal root fibers; those on the anterior side are arranged in pairs, lying between the anterior fissure and the anterolateral sulcus. In the upper cervical region near the skull, these units unite to form two or three small vessels which communicate with the vertebral veins and end either in the inferior cerebellar veins or in the inferior petrosal sinus. Below the cervical region, the veins communicate laterally with the intervertebral veins, which exit through the intervertebral foramina as tributaries of the vertebral, intercostal, lumbar, and lateral sacral veins.

In addition to the veins associated with the surface of the cord, there is a complex arrangement in the epidural space. This is the internal vertebral venous plexus, which communicates with veins about the exterior of the vertebral column. Around the foramen magnum, they communicate with the vertebral veins, and superiorly there are connections with the occipital sinus and the basilar plexus of veins.

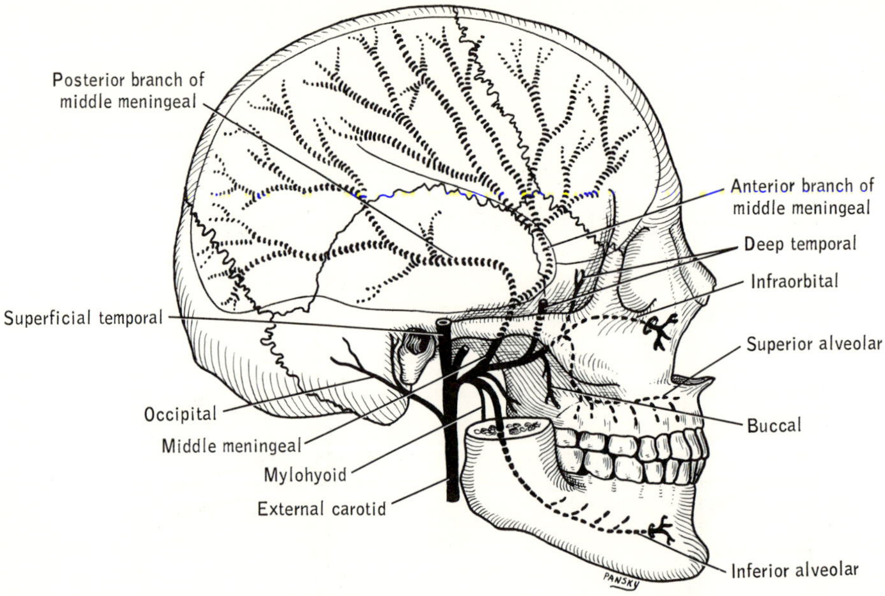

Fig. 4-26. Lateral view of the skull showing some of the branches of the external carotid and internal maxillary arteries. The surface projections of deep vessels embedded in bone or within the cranium are indicated.

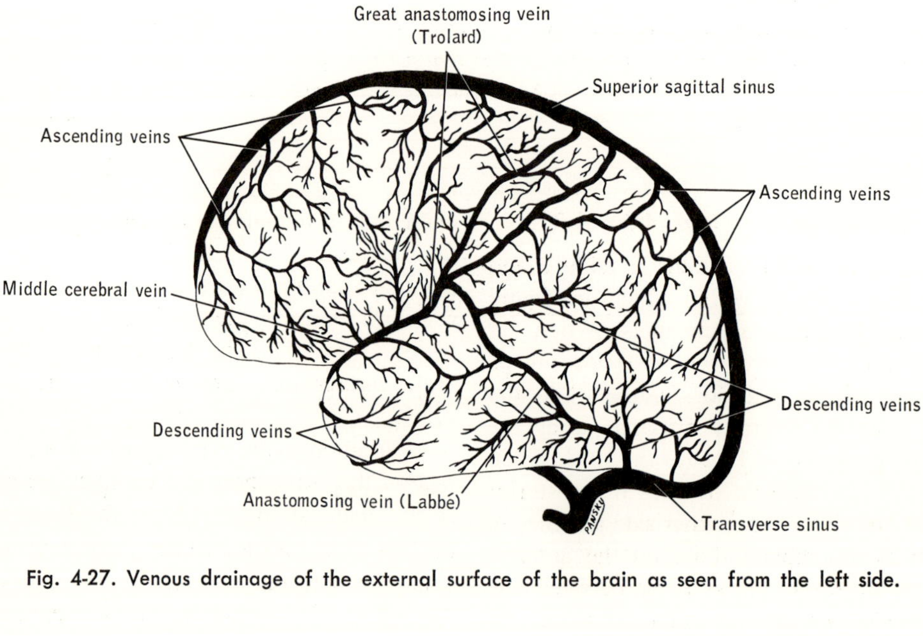

Fig. 4-27. Venous drainage of the external surface of the brain as seen from the left side.

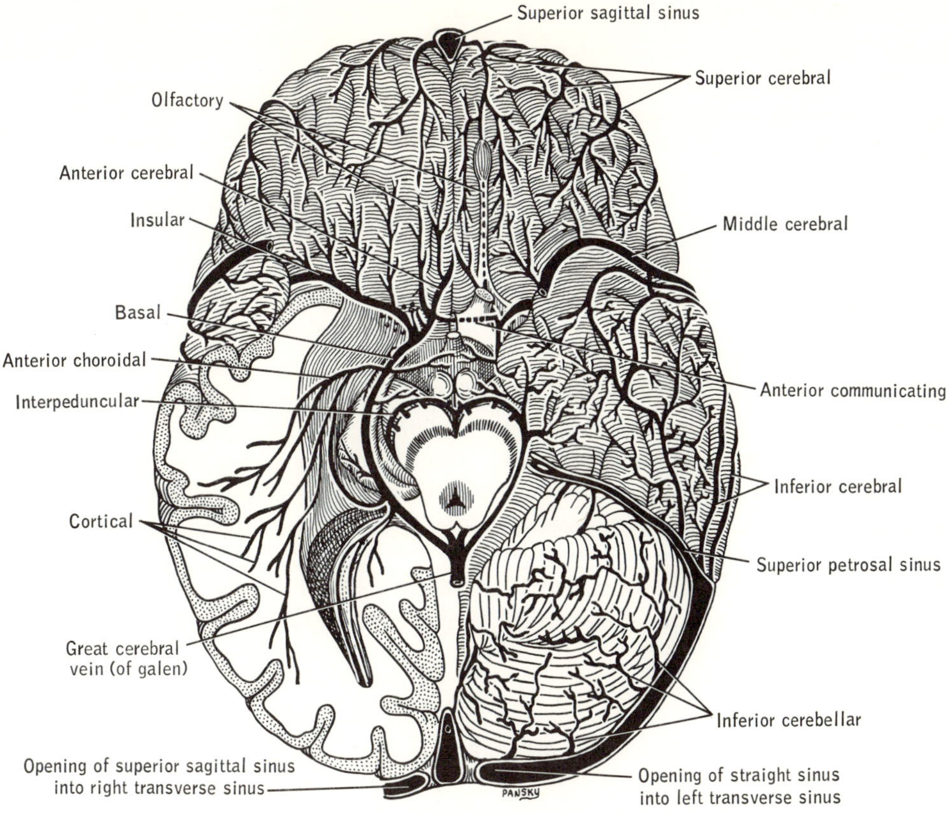

Fig. 4-28. Basal aspect of the brain showing its venous drainage.

CLINICAL CONSIDERATIONS

Surface Topography

Because of the frequency of injury to the vessels following fracture of the skull, it is essential to have an understanding of their relationships and to be able to delineate their position on the surfaces.

Arteriocranial Topography

Middle Meningeal Artery. (Figs. 4-26, 4-37.) The trunk of the vessel and its bifurcation can be found directly above the middle of the zygomatic arch. The *anterior branch* is located at a point about 3.75 cm behind the zygomatic process of the frontal bone and 4.5 cm above the zygoma. This locates the vessel as it crosses the pterion. The *posterior branch* is located 2.5 cm above the highest point of the external auditory meatus as it passes backward toward the lambda.

Sinocranial Topography

The *superior sagittal sinus* is indicated by a line in the median plane joining the naslon and inion.

The *transverse sinus* can be located by a line drawn slightly convexly upwards, from a point just above the inion to the top of the root of the auricle.

The *sigmoid sinus* is indicated by a line beginning at the top of the auricular root and extending downward behind the auricle toward the tip of the mastoid process. At the level of the lower border of the external meatus, the line turns rostrally to the margin of the meatus.

Cisternal Puncture (Figs. 4-5, 4-33.)

The spine of the second cervical vertebra is identified, and a point in the midline is taken immediately above it. The needle is then inserted forward and upward, paralleling an imaginary line joining the nasion and the external auditory meatus. The needle penetrates to a depth of about 4 to 5 cm to reach the posterior atlanto-occipital ligament. The cistern lies just in front of this ligament, with the medulla about 2.5 cm anterior to the ligament.

Pneumoencephalography (Fig. 4-40.)

This is also important, particularly in the localization of brain tumors. Following the technique for lumbar puncture described in the chapter on the spinal cord (Chap. 3), cerebrospinal fluid is removed in the lumbar region and replaced by up to 200 cc of air or oxygen. At the outset, the cerebrospinal pressure is measured, since this procedure must never be used when there is an increase in intracranial pressure.

Ventriculography (Figs. 4-34, 4-35, 4-40.)

This is important in diagnosis, particularly in the localization of tumors and obstruction of the ventricular system. This procedure is used in patients in whom pneumoencephalography is contraindicated, especially if there is evidence of increased intracranial pressure or suspicion of an expanding lesion in the posterior fossa.

The technique consists of making two small incisions in the scalp, 1 in. on either side of the midline and 2 in. above the lambdoid suture. Two small holes are drilled through the skull and a small incision is made in the dura. A ventricular needle is introduced through the incision, passing downward, forward, and inward to enter the lateral ventricle in the region of its collateral trigone. Fluid is removed and replaced by 50 to

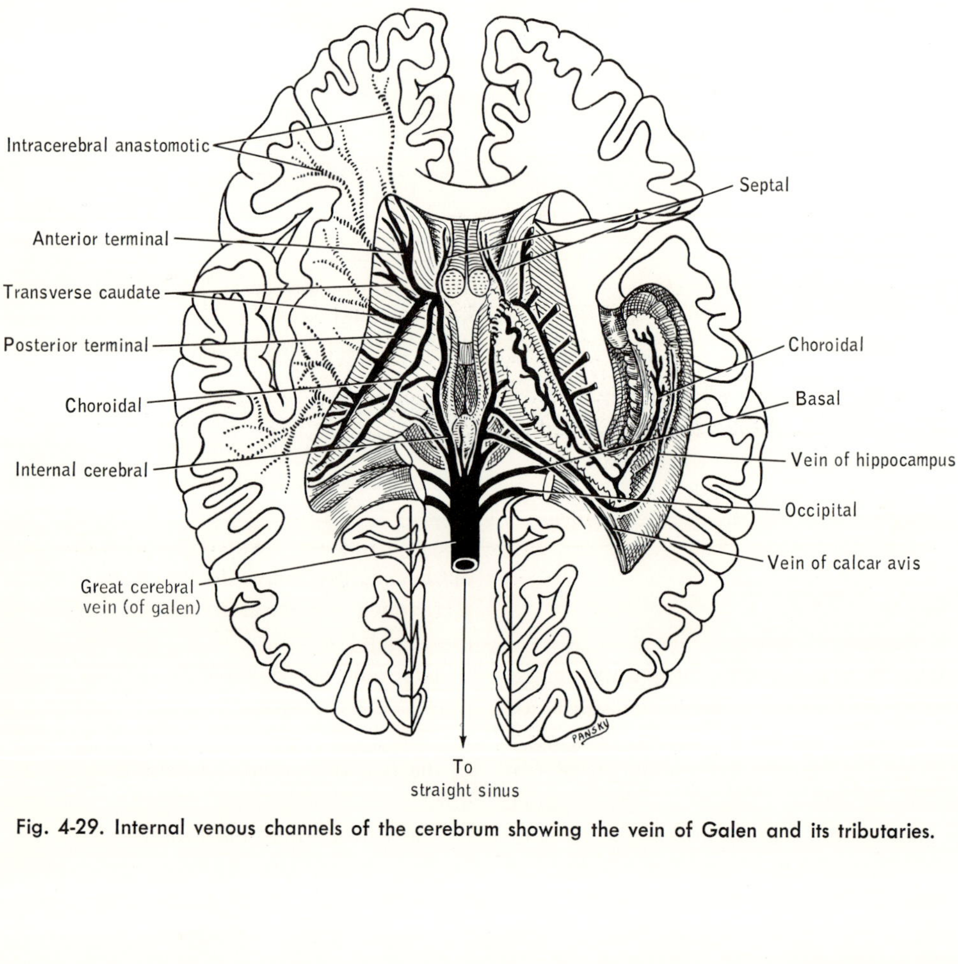

Fig. 4-29. Internal venous channels of the cerebrum showing the vein of Galen and its tributaries.

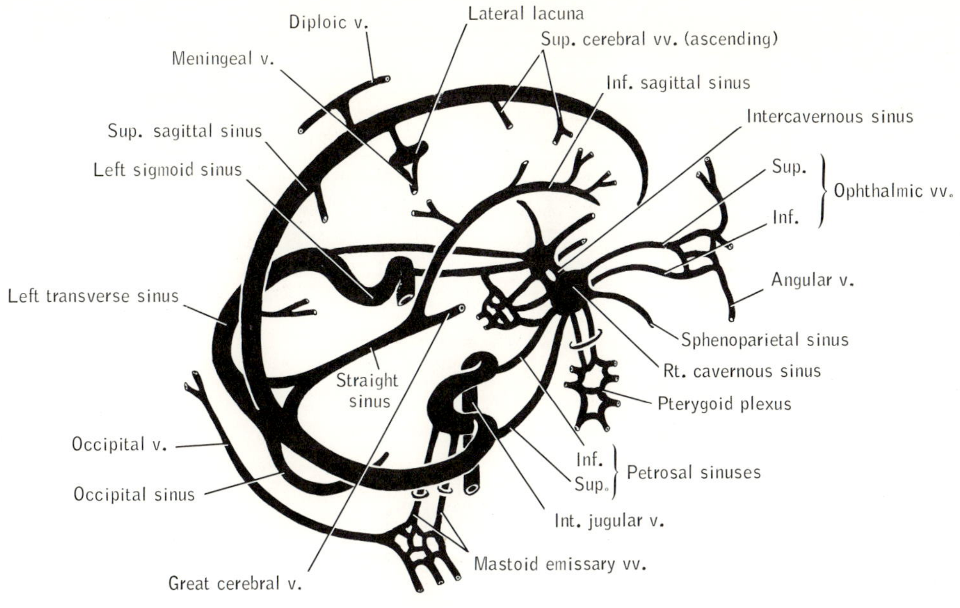

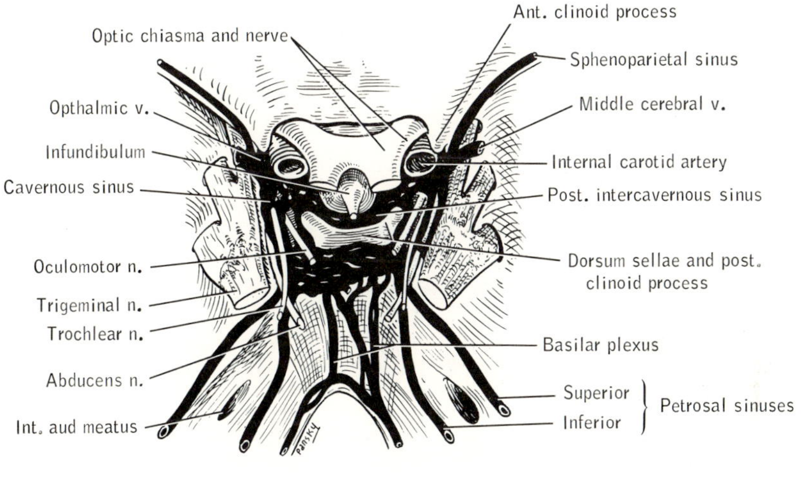

Fig. 4-30. *Upper figure.* Diagram of the dural venous sinuses showing their connections to the extracranial venous system. *Lower figure.* Detailed diagram of the cavernous sinus showing its relations to the pituitary gland, the internal carotid artery, and cranial nerves II, III, IV, V, and VI.

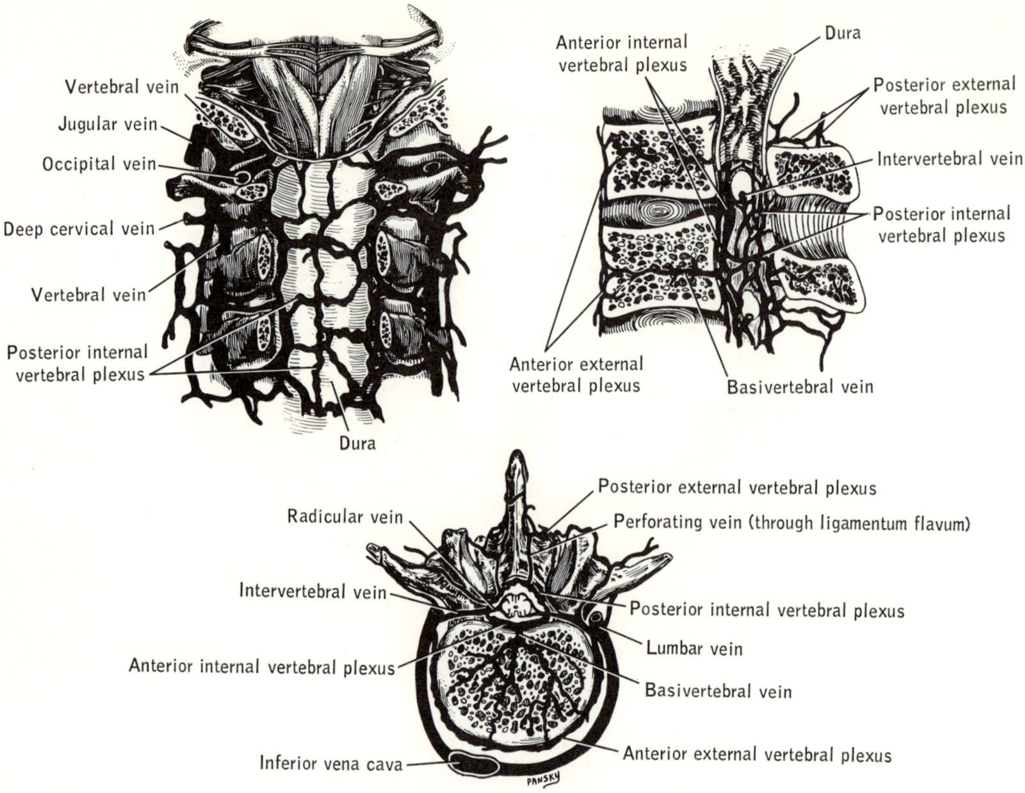

Fig. 4-31. Venous drainage of the vertebral column, spinal meninges, and cord: *above,* longitudinal arrangement; *below,* transverse section.

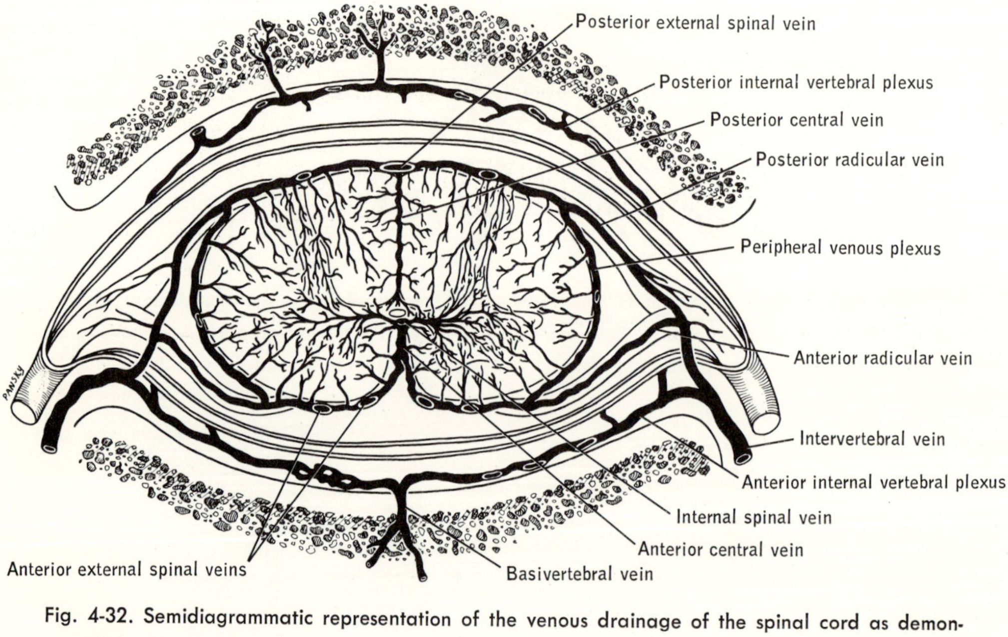

Fig. 4-32. Semidiagrammatic representation of the venous drainage of the spinal cord as demonstrated by transverse section.

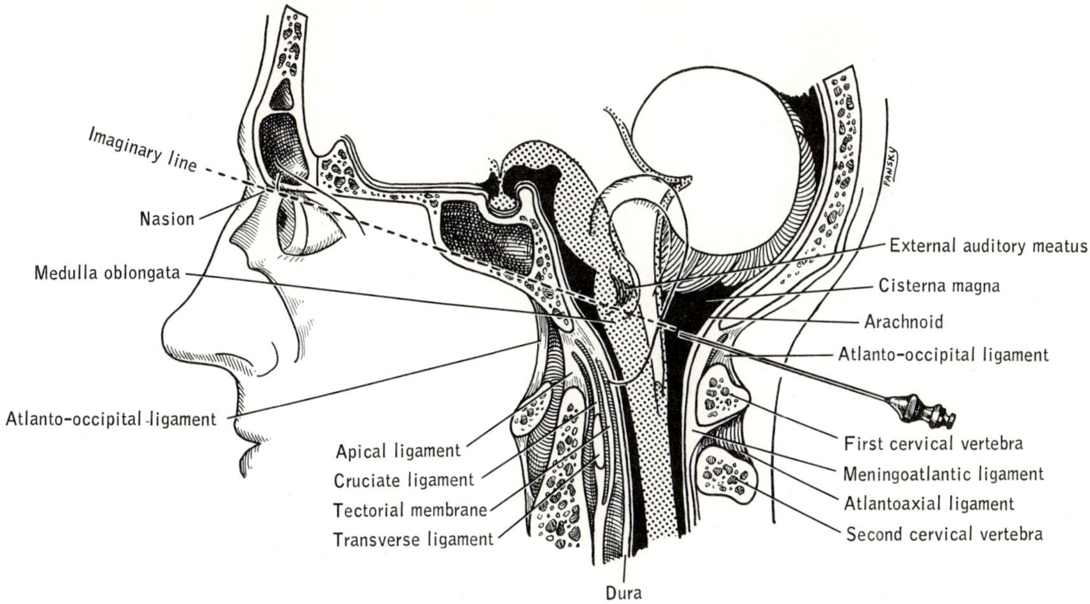

Fig. 4-33. Cisternal puncture, showing surface markings and structural relationships.

120 cc of air or oxygen. Lateral and anteroposterior roentgenograms are taken.

Specific Pathology

Meningitis

The meninges may be the seat of infection, hemorrhage, and tumor formation. Infection of the meninges is called meningitis; it may involve the dura (pachymeningitis) or the piarachnoid (leptomeningitis). Headache; neck stiffness; flexion at ankle, knee, and hip, when the neck is bent (Brudzinski's sign); inability to extend the leg completely when in the sitting position or when lying with the thigh flexed upon the abdomen (Kernig's sign); fever; mental confusion —all are indications of meningeal infection. Furthermore there is usually an increase of cells in the spinal fluid.

Meningeal Hemorrhages

These are more frequent as a result of causes not primarily vascular.

Extradural. This bleeding occurs between the dura and the skull. It is almost always *arterial* in origin, caused by trauma, and is usually due

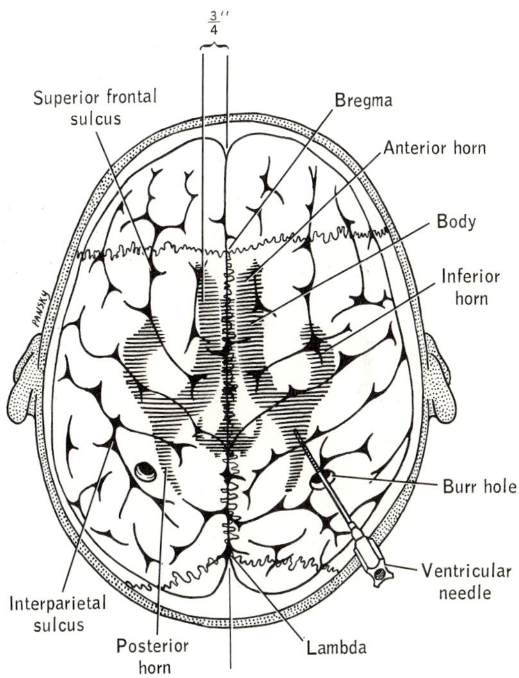

Fig. 4-34. Surface projection of the ventricular system of the brain related to the bones and sutures of the skull. The approach to the lateral ventricle is shown.

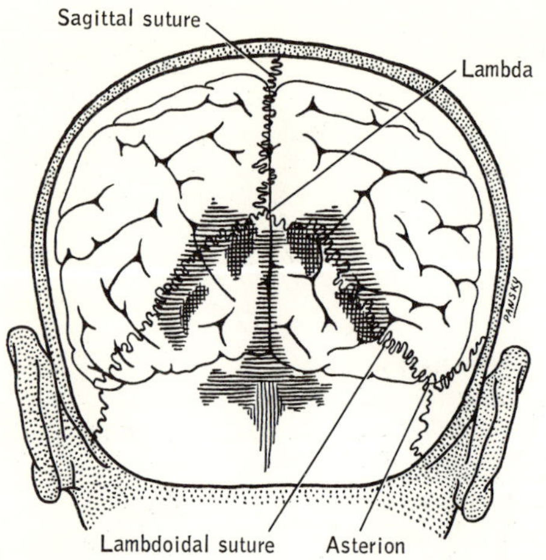

Fig. 4-35. The ventricular system related to the bones and sutures of the skull as seen from behind.

to a rupture of the *middle meningeal artery*.

Subdural. This is bleeding between the dura and arachnoid. It is predominantly *venous* in origin and may or may not be due to *trauma*.

Subarachnoid. This is bleeding between the arachnoid and pia and is usually *arterial*, involving the cerebral vessels. It may be *spontaneous* or *traumatic*.

Cerebral Vascular Pathology

Both hemorrhage and occlusion of the vessels in the central nervous system are of frequent occurrence. However, the symptoms presented involve many higher centers whose functions are, as yet, unknown to the beginning student. Therefore, the detailed account of pathology in specific vessels has been deferred until the study of the entire system has been completed. (See Appendix.)

Cerebral Hemorrhage

This occurs within the brain substance, is arterial in nature, and is usually spontaneous (nontraumatic).

Ventricular Hemorrhage

This may be primary or secondary and usually results from the rupture of a cerebral hemorrhage into the adjacent ventricle.

Cerebral Embolism and Thrombosis

These conditions lead to vascular occlusions of the cerebral arteries (sometimes even of the internal carotid or vertebral arteries), resulting in symptoms or signs that depend upon the area involved.

Hydrocephalus (Fig. 4-36.)

These cases may be placed into two general categories, communicating and noncommunicating. The former is the result of obstruction of the arachnoid villi and perivascular spaces by blood, serum, or an inflammatory process. The latter is caused by blocking or various portions of the

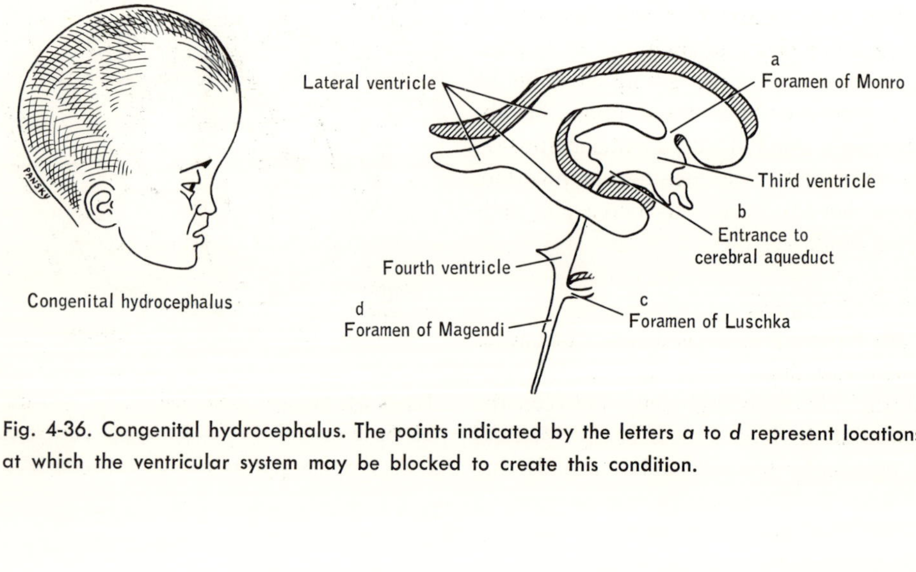

Fig. 4-36. Congenital hydrocephalus. The points indicated by the letters *a* to *d* represent locations at which the ventricular system may be blocked to create this condition.

ventricular system by tumors or other growths. If the block is located at the interventricular foramen, distention of the ventricle on the side of the block occurs: if the block is in the cerebral aqueduct, there is distention of both the lateral and third ventricles; if the block occurs near the opening of the fourth ventricle, all the ventricles are distended.

Intracranial Tumors (Figs. 4-38, 4-39.)

Unless they contain calcium, intracranial tumors are difficult to localize by roentgenography. However, using either pneumoencephalography or ventriculography, the position of a tumor (and some conception of its size) can be visualized. An examination of a pneumoencephalogram viewed from in front (Fig. 4-39) shows no trace of the right lateral ventricle while both the third and left are clearly circumscribed. It should also be noted that the tumor in the right hemisphere is so large that it has caused the deviation of the third ventricle to the left.

Another tool that sometimes proves useful in diagnosing and localizing tumors is arteriography (angiography). In this procedure a radiopaque substance such as thorium dioxide is injected into the internal carotid artery which is usually exposed just above the clavicle. Two or three x-rays are made as quickly as possible as the injection is being made. If the normal and abnormal arteriograms are compared (Figs. 4-37, 4-38) a shift in pattern can be observed in the area of the growth. In addition, a large number of small vessels which vascularize the tumor are also evident. There is slight calcification in this particular growth.

Another method, also making use of the high vascularity of tumors consists of the use of radioisotopes. After injection the head is "scanned" both photographically and mechanically. The soft parts surrounding the cranium show up as heavy shadings due to heavier uptake while the brain remains relatively clear in the normal condition. A tumor will appear as a dark area against the pale, normal background. (The use of the EEG and the echogram will be discussed in Chapter 23.)

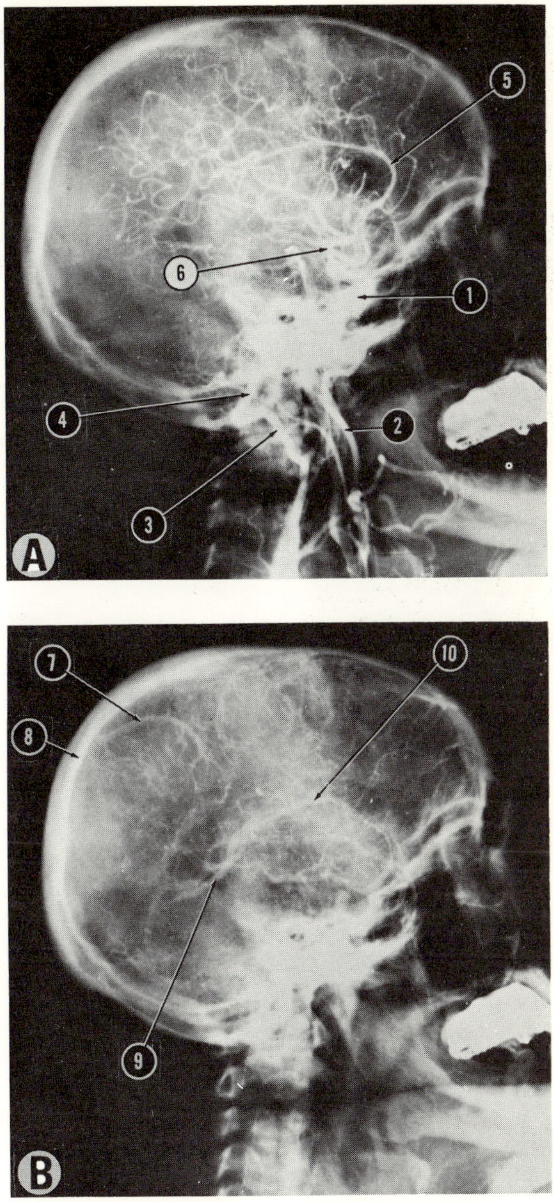

Fig. 4-37. A. Right brachial arteriogram-normal. (1) Internal carotid artery; (2) external carotid artery; (3) vertebral artery; (4) basilar artery; (5) anterior cerebral artery; and (6) middle cerebral artery. B. Right venagram-normal. (7) Great anastomotic vein (of Trollard); (8) superior sagittal sinus; (9) straight sinus; and (10) inferior sagittal sinus. (*Figs. 4-37, 4-38 and 4-39, through the courtesy of Drs. Frank Borrelli and Rita Girolamo, Dept. of Radiology, New York Medical College.*)

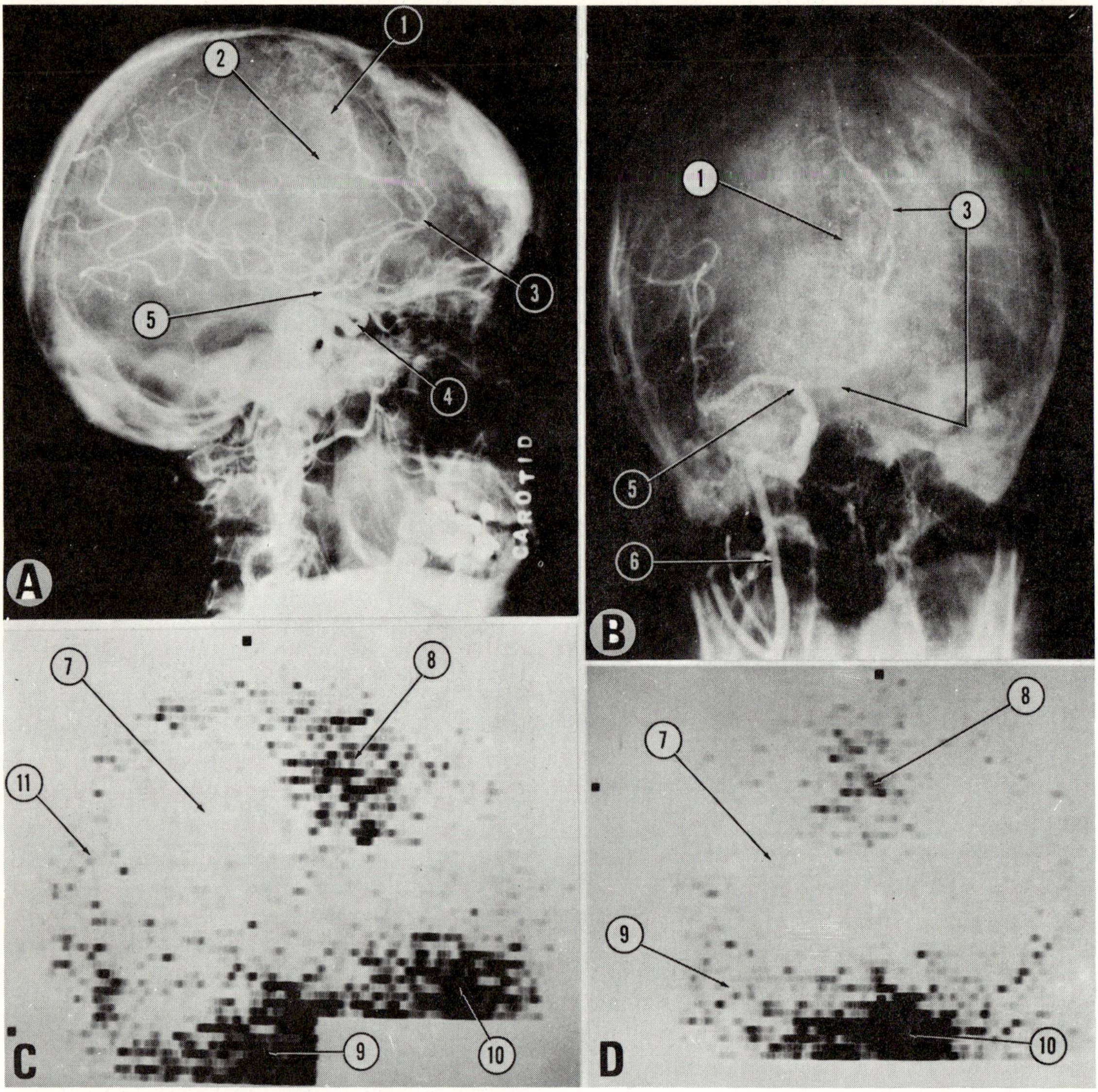

Fig. 4-38. Arteriogram and brain scan-abnormal. *A.* Right carotid arteriogram-lateral view. (1) Area of the tumor showing excess of arterial branches in region of the growth; (2) anterior cerebral artery flattened in region of tumor; (3) anterior cerebral artery; (4) internal carotid artery; (5) middle cerebral artery (compare with figure 4-37, A). *B.* Right carotid arteriogram of same patient in anterior-posterior view. (1) Area of tumor; (3) anterior cerebral artery deflected toward the left due to a tumor; (5) middle cerebral artery; and (6) internal carotid artery. C. Brain scan of same patient shown in *A* above, lateral view. (7) Background activity of normal brain; (8) abnormal activity in area of tumor; (9) activity of occipital and temporal muscles; (10) paranasal sinuses; and (11) scalp and soft tissues (compare with Fig. 2-53, *B*). *D.* Brain scan of same patient in anterior-posterior view. (7) Background activity of normal brain; (8) abnormal activity in area of tumor; (9) temporal muscles; and (10) paranasal sinuses.

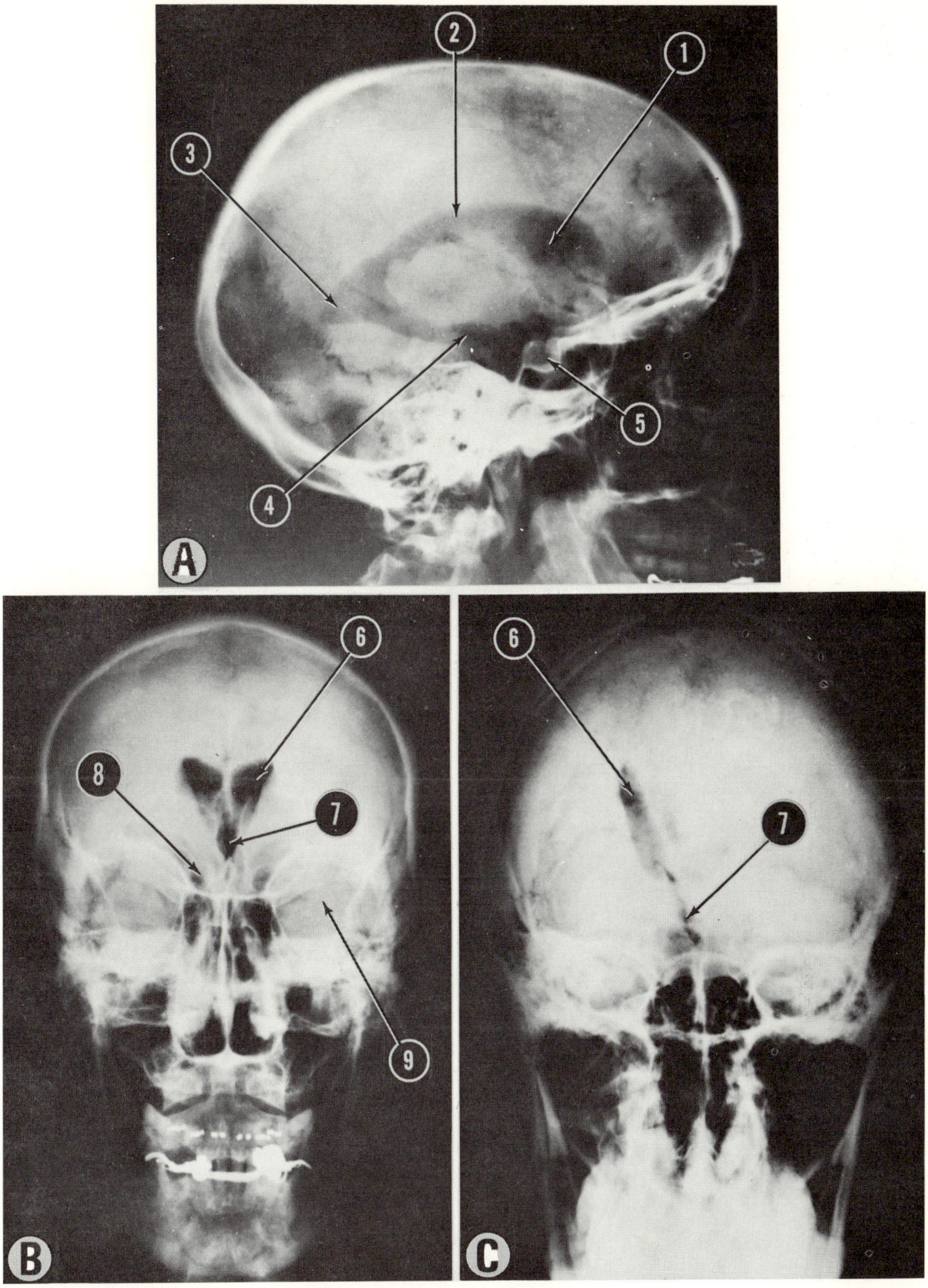

Fig. 4-39. *A.* Normal ventriculogram, right lateral view: (1) anterior horn; (2) body; (3) posterior horn; (4) inferior horn of lateral ventricles; (5) sella turcica. *B.* Normal ventriculogram, anterior-posterior view; (6) left lateral ventricle; (7) third ventricle; (8) frontal paranasal sinus; (9) orbit. C. Abnormal ventriculogram, anterior-posterior view. Large tumor on left side; (6) right lateral ventricle is compressed, while that on the left is completely blocked out; (7) the third ventricle is deviated toward the right.

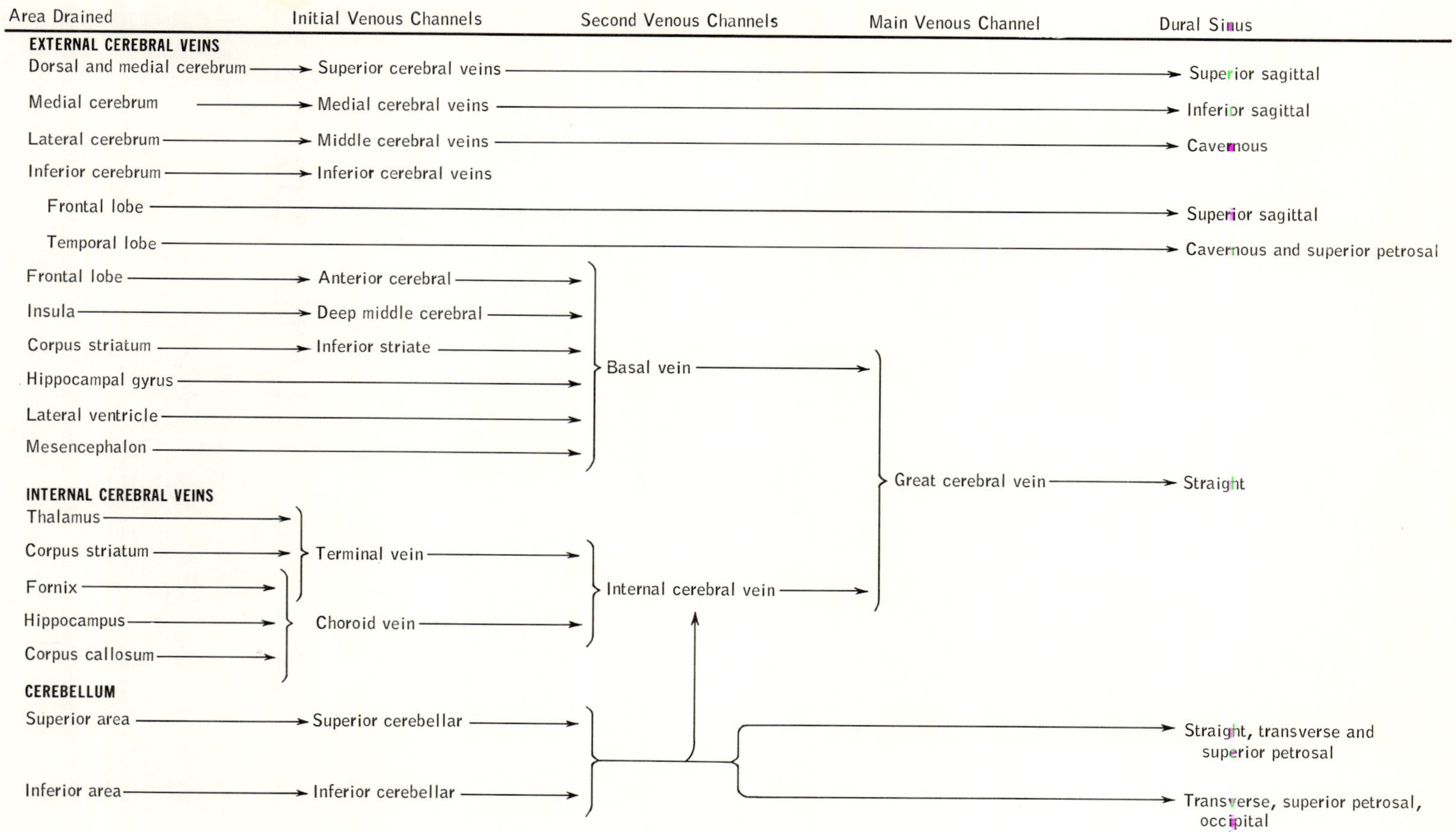
Area Drained
Initial Venous Channels
Second Venous Channels
Main Venous Channel
Dural Sinus
EXTERNAL CEREBRAL VEINS
Dorsal and medial cerebrum
Superior cerebral veins
Superior sagittal
Medial cerebrum
Medial cerebral veins
Inferior sagittal
Lateral cerebrum
Middle cerebral veins
Cavernous
Inferior cerebrum
Inferior cerebral veins
Frontal lobe
Superior sagittal
Temporal lobe
Cavernous and superior petrosal
Frontal lobe
Anterior cerebral
Insula
Deep middle cerebral
Corpus striatum
Inferior striate
Hippocampal gyrus
Lateral ventricle
Mesencephalon
Basal vein
Great cerebral vein
Straight
INTERNAL CEREBRAL VEINS
Thalamus
Corpus striatum
Terminal vein
Fornix
Hippocampus
Corpus callosum
Choroid vein
Internal cerebral vein
CEREBELLUM
Superior area
Superior cerebellar
Inferior area
Inferior cerebellar
Straight, transverse and superior petrosal
Transverse, superior petrosal, occipital

SUMMARY

VENOUS SINUS DRAINAGE

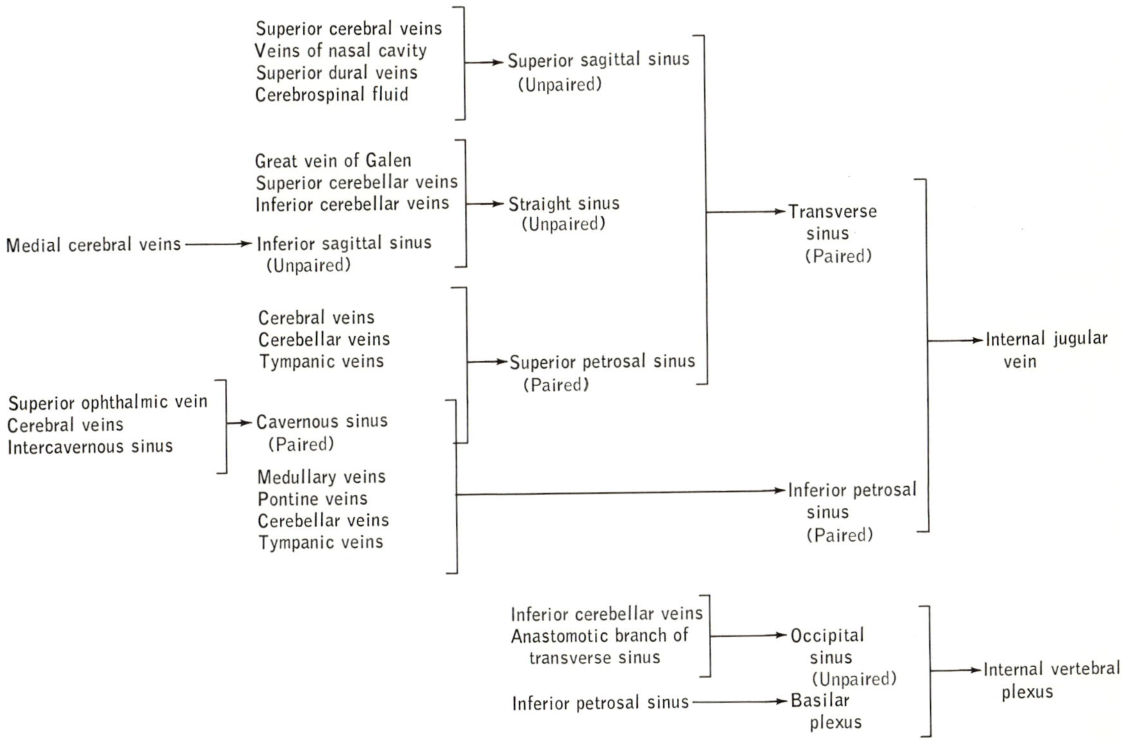

SUMMARY

ARTERIAL SUPPLY

- Brain →
  - Internal carotid →
    - Anterior cerebral →
      - Anterior communicating
      - Middle branches
      - Posterior branches
      - Medial striate
    - Middle cerebral →
      - Lateral striate
      - Inferior lateral frontal
      - Ascending frontal
      - Ascending parietal
      - Parietotemporal
      - Temporal
    - Anterior choroidal
    - Posterior communicating →
      - Hippocampal
      - Medial thalamic
  - Vertebral →
    - Basilar →
      - Posterior cerebral →
        - Posterior medial central
        - Posterior lateral central
        - Posterior choroidal
        - Anterior temporal
        - Posterior temporal
        - Calcarine
        - Parieto-occipital
      - Posterior communicating
      - Superior cerebellar
      - Pontine
      - Internal auditory
      - Anterior inferior cerebellar
    - Anterior spinal
    - Posterior spinal
- Cord →
  - Vertebral → Anterior spinal, Posterior spinal → Intramedullary branches to white matter and ventral gray
  - Intercostal, Lumbar, Sacral → Radicular branches to dorsal and ventral gray
- Meninges →
  - Cranial →
    - Ascending pharyngeal → Posterior meningeal
    - Occipital → Meningeal branches
    - Internal maxillary →
      - Middle meningeal →
        - Posterior branch
        - Anterior branch
      - Accessory meningeal recurrent branch
    - Lacrimal
  - Spinal → Same as cord

- Meninges
  - Brain
    - Membranes
      - Dura
        - Endosteal (outer)
        - Meningeal (inner)
          - Falx cerebri
          - Tentorium cerebelli
          - Falx cerebelli
          - Diaphragma sellae
      - Arachnoid
        - Granulations (Pacchionian bodies)
      - Pia
        - Choroid plexus
        - Choroid tela
    - Spaces
      - Subarachnoid cisterns
        - Magna
        - Pontine
        - Interpeduncular
        - Chiasmatic
        - Lateral
      - Subdural
      - Epidural
  - Cord
    - Membranes
      - Dura
        - Only meningeal
      - Arachnoid
      - Pia
        - Denticulate ligament
    - Spaces
      - Subarachnoid
      - Subdural
      - Epidural

5 DEVELOPMENT OF THE NERVOUS SYSTEM

GERM LAYER ORIGIN

Both central and peripheral nervous systems arise from the *ectoderm* of the embryo.

Neural Plate (Fig. 5-1.)

By the nineteenth day of embryonic life, the ectoderm has begun to thicken dorsally. This is the neural plate, which even at this stage shows a longitudinal groove along the middorsal line—the *neural groove*. The anterior end of the plate is much broader. This portion becomes the brain, while the narrower, caudal part forms the spinal cord. From the beginning, the prospective brain region shows subdivisions suggestive of the three primary brain vesicles (Fig. 5-2). The most rostral gives rise to the *forebrain* (prosencephalon); the middle and smallest represents the *midbrain* (mesencephalon); the most caudal becomes the *hindbrain* (rhombencephalon).

As the neural plate thickens and expands, its lateral edges are carried dorsally. These are the *neural folds*. During the third week the neural folds begin to meet and fuse along the middorsal line, forming the *neural tube* (Fig. 5-1). For a time, the neural tube is open at both extremities. However, by the end of the fourth week, the tube is completely sealed.

Neural Crest (Fig. 5-1.)

During the time that the neural folds are fusing, a proliferation of cells occurs along the boundary between the neural and general surface ectoderm. This is the *neural crest,* which forms two longitudinal bands on either side of the line of fusion of the neural folds.

EXTERNAL MORPHOGENESIS OF THE SPINAL CORD

For a time, the spinal cord is a simple, thick-walled tube completely filling the neural canal. Very early, before definite skeletal parts are formed, spinal nerves become associated with each of the adjacent mesodermal segments (somites). In this way, all the skeletal muscle derived from this mesoderm will be supplied by these nerves.

In the first 3 months of development, the spinal cord and the vertebral column grow at the same rate. Shortly thereafter, body growth exceeds that of the CNS, particularly in the caudal half of the fetus. Thus, at birth, the cord no longer fills the canal but ends near the lower border of the third lumbar vertebra (Fig. 5-3).

This growth phenomenon also has a profound effect upon the direction of spinal nerve fibers. Originally, nerve fibers leave at right angles to the cord. With the formation of the vertebrae, these nerves exit from the neural canal firmly held between the edges of adjoining vertebrae. Therefore, as the body grows caudally, the foramina containing the nerves are carried along (Fig. 5-3). As a consequence, the roots of the

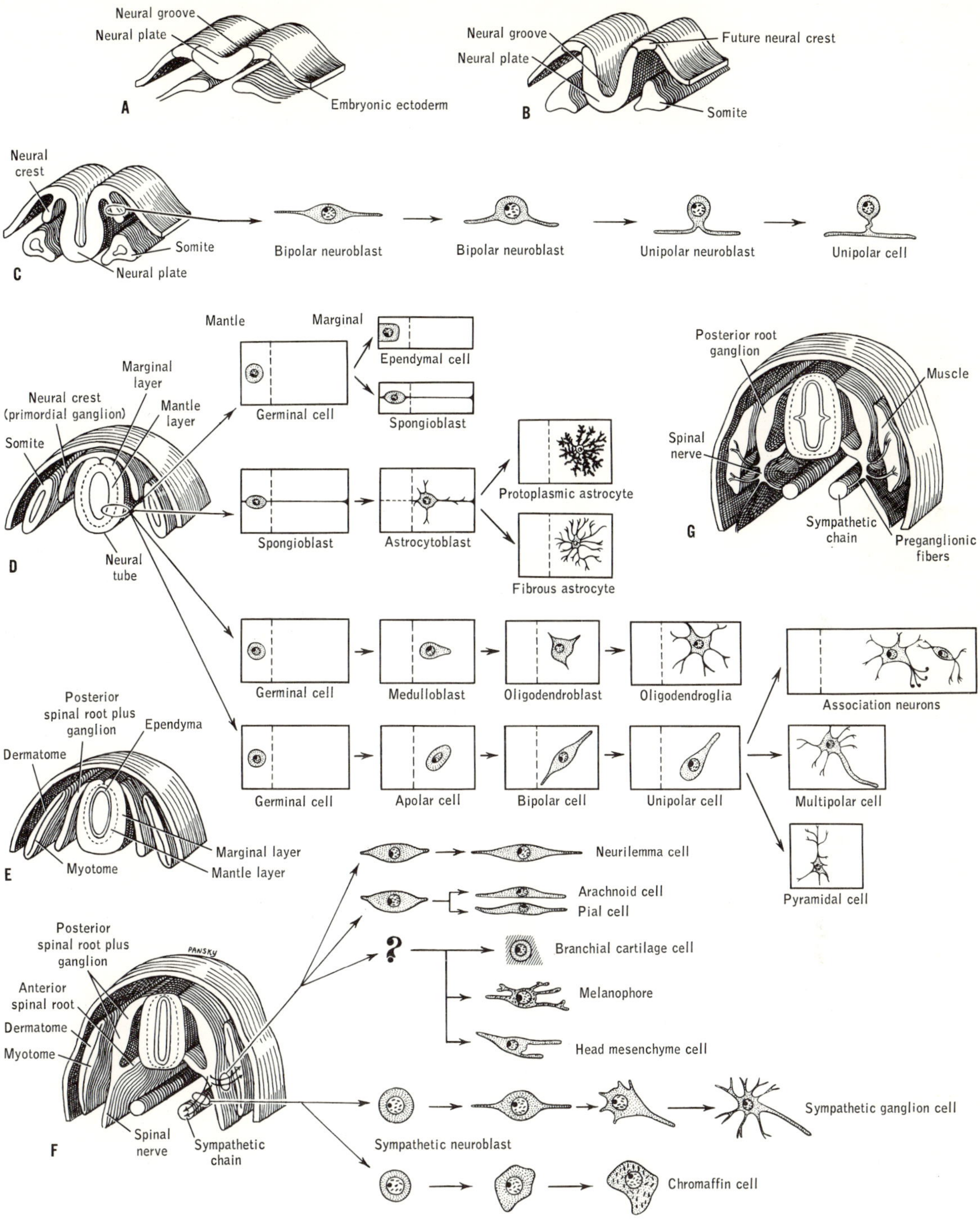

Fig. 5-1. Semidiagrammatic representation of the development of the neural tube from the neural plate, showing the histogenesis of the central nervous system as well as the differentiation of the neural crest.

nerves, especially those derived from the lower third of the cord, become greatly elongated and may extend considerable distances within the vertebral canal before exiting through the proper intervertebral foramina. In this way, the *cauda equina* is formed

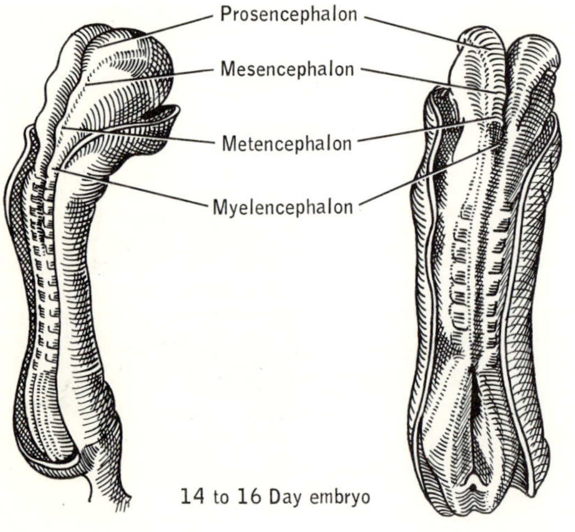

Fig. 5-2. Human embryos, 14 to 16 days of age, showing the development of the neural tube and the establishment of body segments.

In addition to changes in length, the cord shows regional increases in diameter to accommodate the large nerves passing to the extremities. In the fourth fetal month, a cervical enlargement for the brachial plexus and a lumbosacral enlargement for the plexus to the lower extremity appear.

EXTERNAL MORPHOGENESIS OF THE BRAIN (Figs. 5-4 to 5-7.)

In the fourth and fifth weeks, changes occur in the primary brain vesicles. From the prosencephalon appear two lateral evaginations. These are the *telencephalon,* later to become the cerebral hemispheres. That portion of the forebrain which remains medial is now called the *diencephalon.* The mesencephalon undergoes no radical changes. The rhombencephalon, however, subdivides. The rostral part becomes the *metencephalon,* the more caudal part the *myelencephalon.* Later, the metencephalon differentiates into the dorsal *cerebellum* and the ventral *pons.* The myelencephalon becomes the medulla oblongata.

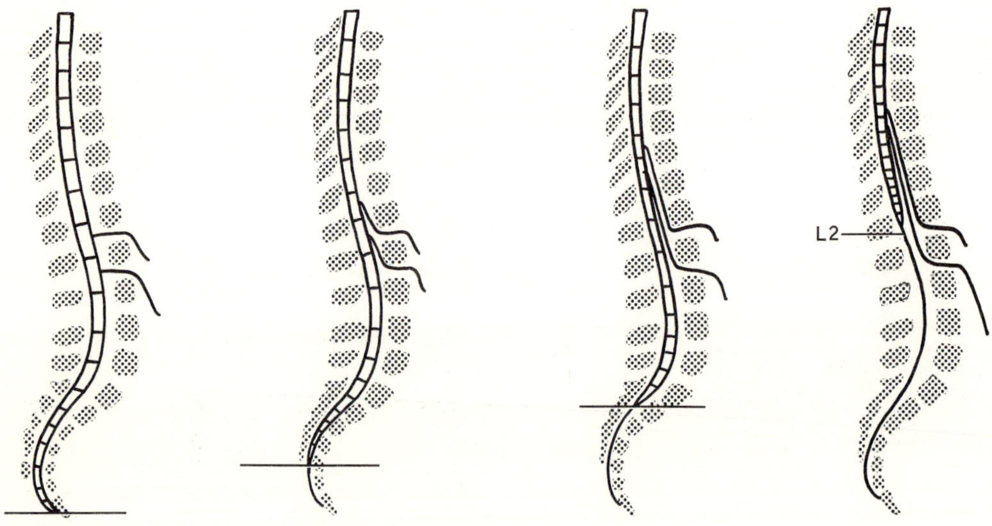

Fig. 5-3. Diagram showing the relation of growth of the spinal cord to that of the vertebral column. Stages represent embryos from 30 to 221 mm in length.

During the third week, the growth rate of the neural tube is so much more rapid rostrally and dorsally that a ventral bend occurs, first in the region of the midbrain. This is the *cephalic* or *midbrain flexure*. At about the same time, the *cervical flexure* forms at the junction of the hindbrain and spinal cord. Between 5 and 6 weeks, a third flexure appears in the region of the metencephalon. This is the *pontine flexure*. Eventually, both pontine and cervical flexures tend to straighten out. However, evidence of the cephalic bend remains.

STRUCTURE OF THE NEURAL TUBE

Macroscopic (Fig. 5-8.)

In cross section of the tube, certain portions are clearly indicated. In the dorsal midline is the thin *roof plate*. In the ventral midline lies the *floor plate*. Both roof and floor plates are continuous with the thickened lateral walls. Near the midpoint of each lateral wall is a shallow, longitudinal groove, the *sulcus limitans*. The latter serves as a boundary between the dorsal part of

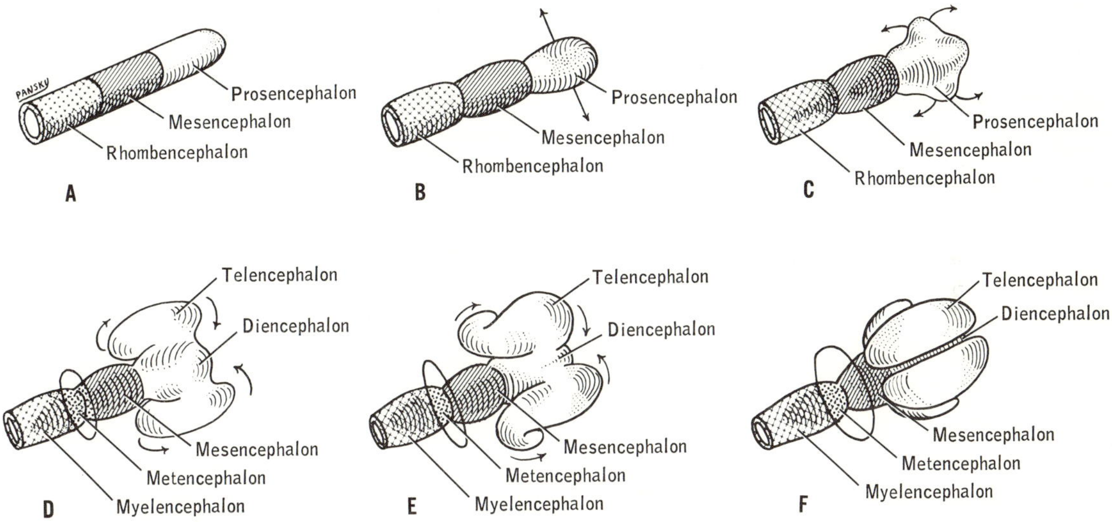

Fig. 5-4. Development of the brain, with special emphasis on the prosencephalon, as seen from the dorsal aspect.

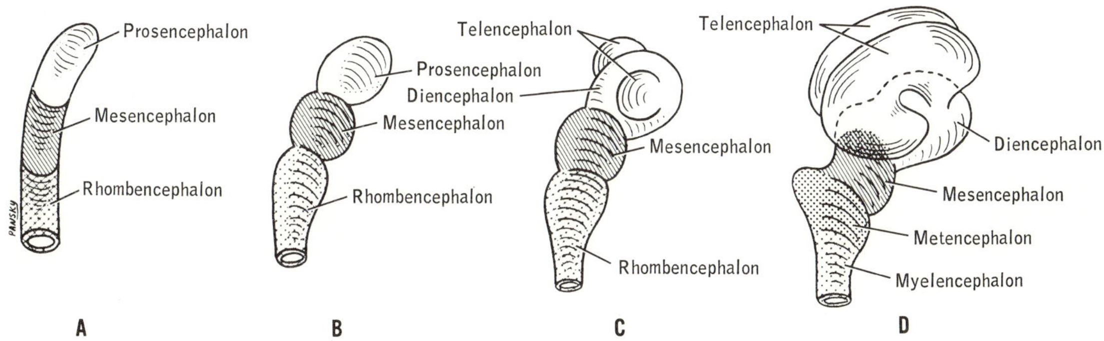

Fig. 5-5. Approximately the same stages as shown in Fig. 5-4, seen from the side.

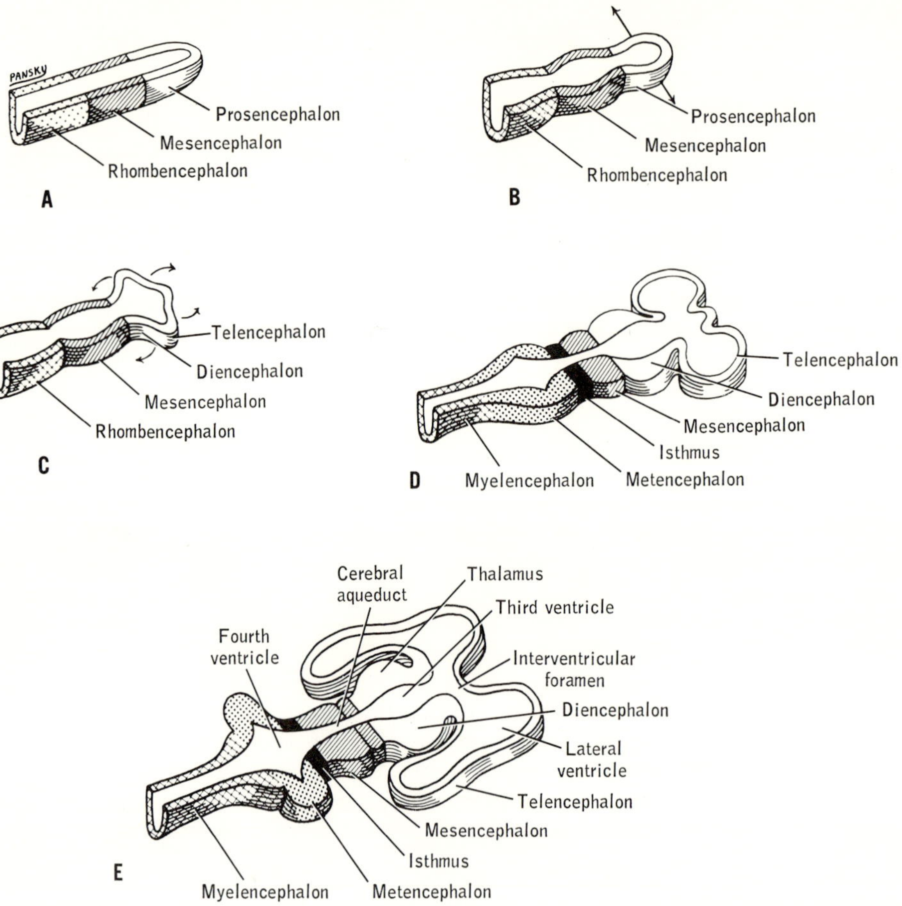

Fig. 5-6. Early development of the brain as demonstrated by horizontal sections of progressively older stages.

the wall, called the *alar plate,* and the ventral part, the *basal plate.*

Microscopic (Fig. 5-8.)

Although originally the ectoderm is but one cell layer in thickness, rapid proliferation produces many layers by the time the neural tube has formed. Soon, two limiting membranes are discernible, an internal one, which lines the cavity of the neural tube (neurocele), and an external one, lying at the periphery.

The cells adjoining the neurocele are at first most active in proliferation. Eventually, the mitotic activity among them becomes greatly reduced and the cells next to the lumen elongate, giving the appearance of a columnar epithelium. This layer is the *ependyma.* Surrounding the ependyma is a very cell-rich, heavily nucleated zone, the *mantle layer.* External to the mantle layer, a narrow, pale, almost cell-free area called the *marginal layer* can be seen. All these layers are present by the end of the fourth embryonic week.

DIFFERENTIATION OF THE SPINAL CORD (Fig. 5-9.)

The ependyma remains as the lining epithelium for all the cavities of the CNS and is an important component of both the roof and floor plates.

The marginal layers of the lateral walls increase in size by the accumulation of processes of nerve cells. Some supporting cells also migrate here. The marginal layer is destined to become the white matter of the cord.

One must not lose sight of the fact that the mantle layer, like the other two, is continuous in its longitudinal extent from one end of the primitive neural tube to the other. In that part of the lateral wall dorsal to the sulcus limitans, the mantle layer gives rise to the cell bodies which are functionally associated with the sensory mechanism. Thus arise the *dorsal gray columns* (horns). The mantle layer of the basal plate also gives rise to gray matter. Here, however, are found the cell bodies of motor neurons. Thus, the mantle layer of the basal plate forms the *ventral gray columns* (horns).

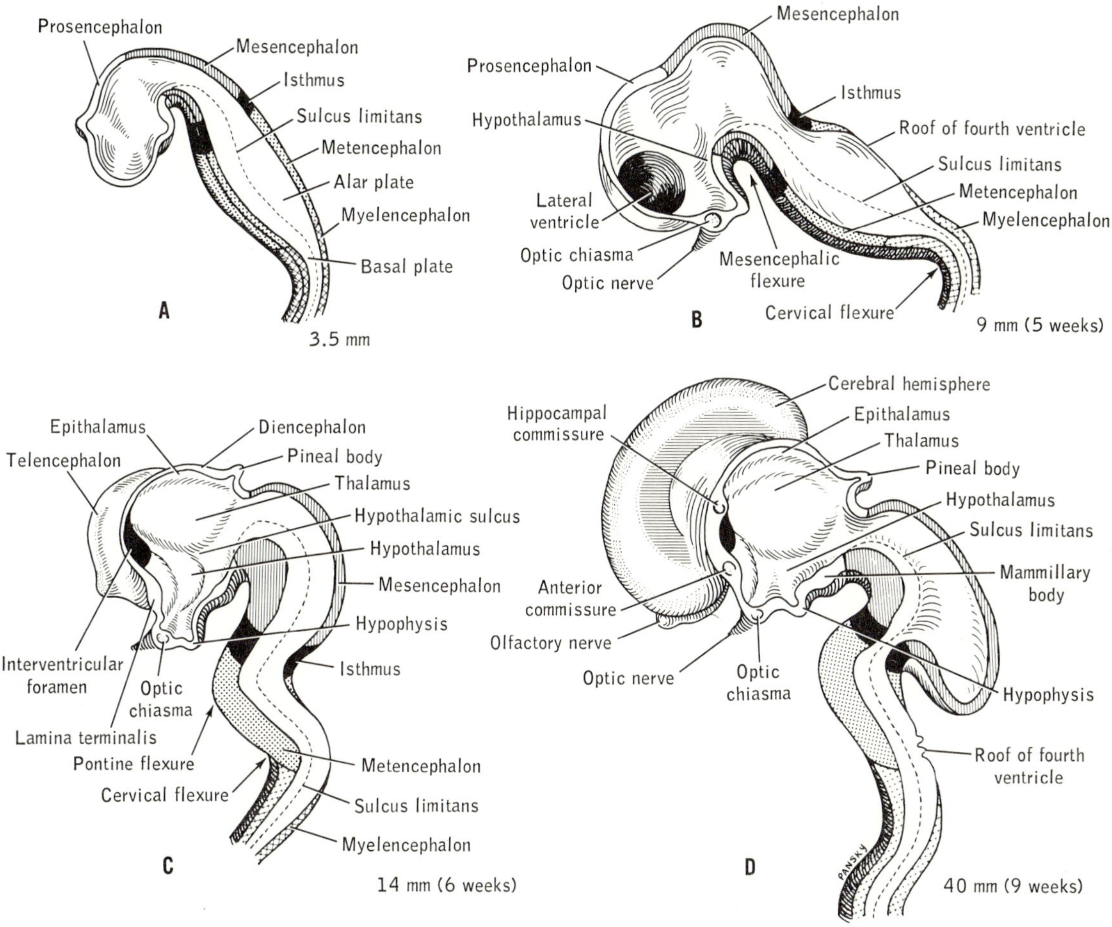

Fig. 5-7. Sagittal reconstructions of the brain, including the cerebellum, in embryos ranging in age from 3 to 4 weeks to fetuses of 5 months (3.5 to 150 mm).

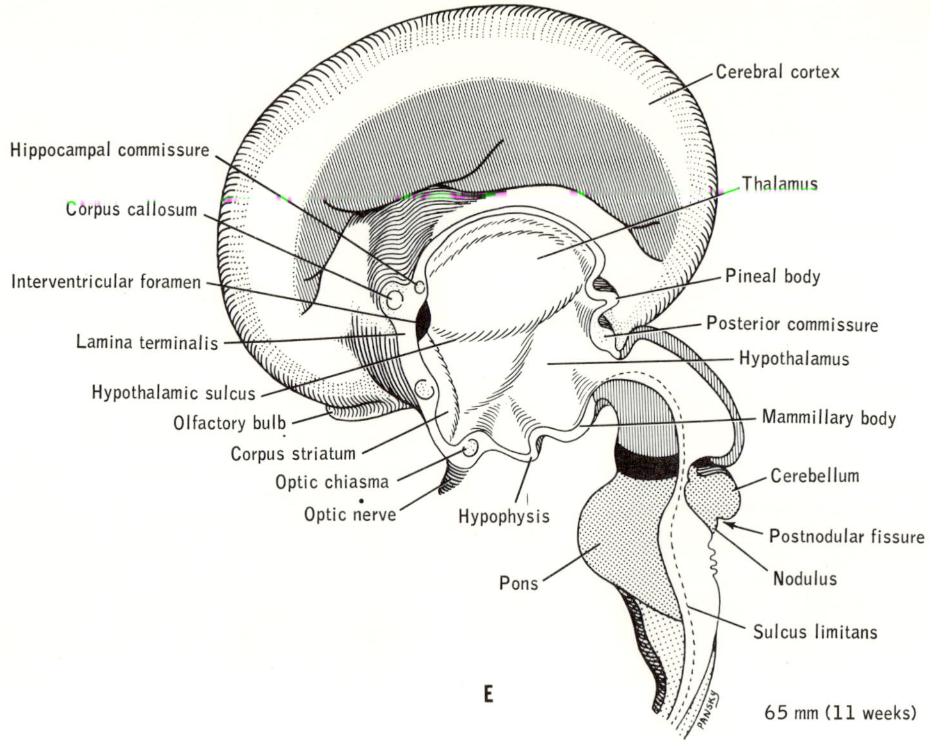

E

65 mm (11 weeks)

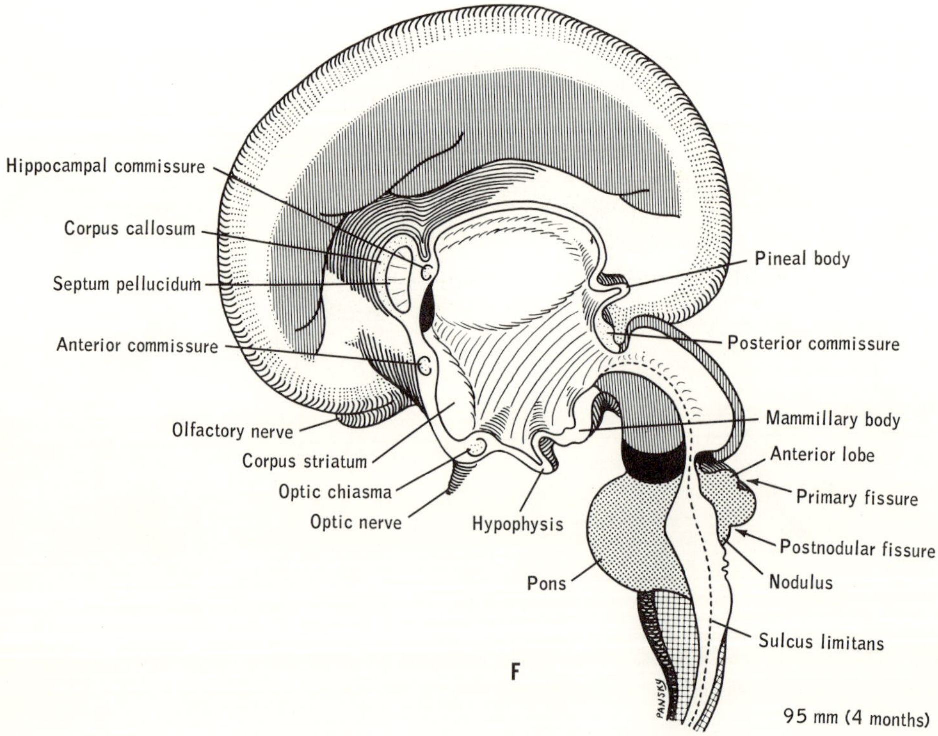

F

95 mm (4 months)

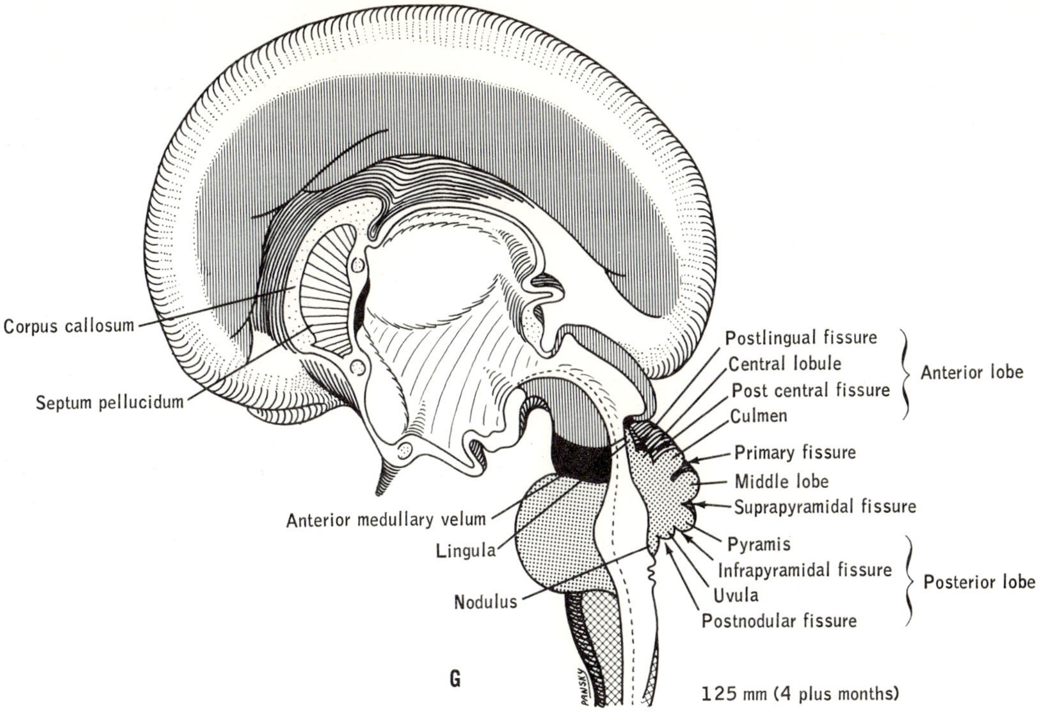

G

125 mm (4 plus months)

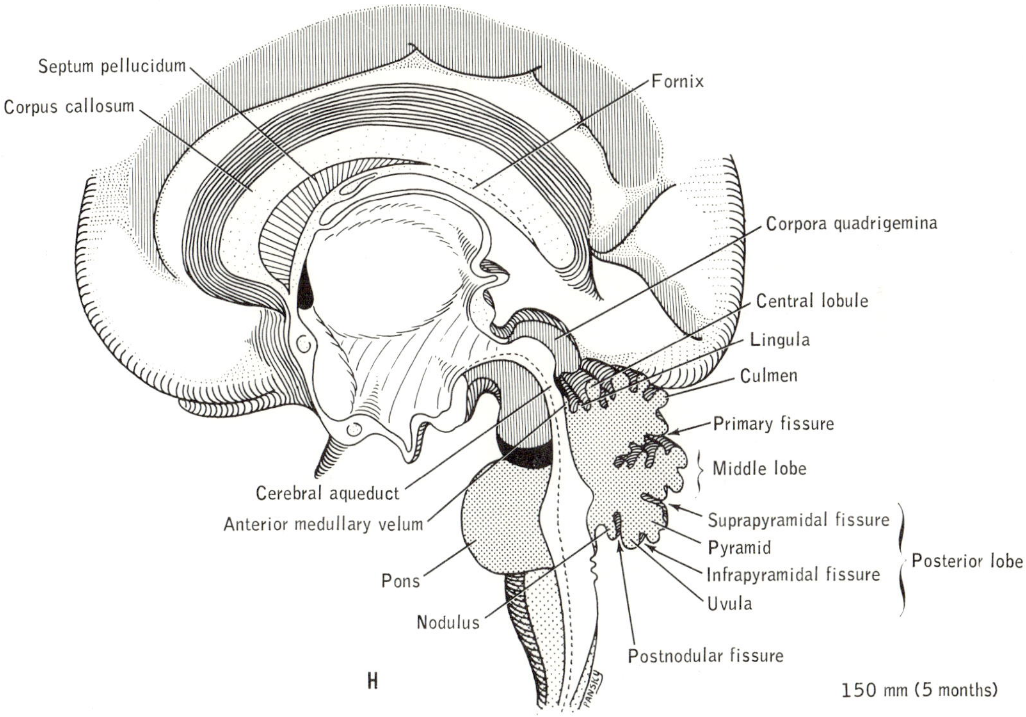

H

150 mm (5 months)

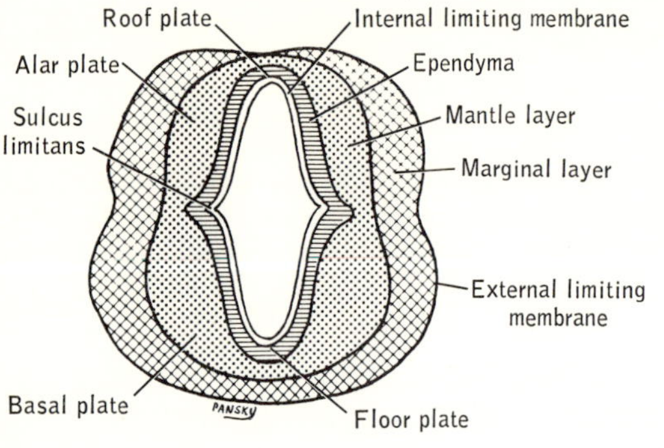

Fig. 5-8. Schematic cross section of the spinal cord showing its primitive divisions and layers.

DIFFERENTIATION OF THE BRAIN

Myelencephalon (Figs. 5-7, 5-10.)

There are differences between the differentiation of the brain and the cord even though they both develop from the same basic layers. This is probably because of several factors. First, in the cord, there is a definite relationship between neural and body segments. In the brain, existence of such a definite segmental arrangement is controversial. Therefore, since there is no need for a continuous chain of dorsal and ventral roots attaching to the myelencephalon, breaks in the continuity of the dorsal and ventral gray substance occur here. A second difference is related to the branchial arches. Since these differentiate into striated muscle related to viscera, new motor centers to supply these arches develop. The appearance of organs of special sense found in the head also results in structural differences and is associated with the formation of still other new cell masses. Further, the appearance of higher brain centers, which provide for better integration of sensory impulses and improved control of motor function, leads to structural changes in the medulla because of the establishment of long fiber bundles to and from these new centers.

One of the most striking events in the development of the myelencephalon is the tremendous enlargement of the neural tube cavity. This expansion does not involve all the walls equally. The floor plate remains fixed. The two lateral walls migrate laterally and ventrally, stretching the roof plate between them. The latter forms the thin roof, composed chiefly of ependyma, for the fourth ventricle. Thus, the two lateral walls are now in a nearly horizontal plane, the median sulcus indicating the region of the primitive floor plate. In this position, the lateral walls of the tube now form the floor of the fourth ventricle.

Surrounding the brain wall at this time mesenchymal tissue is becoming highly vascularized, giving rise to the *pia mater*. The latter becomes intimately related to the ependymal roof of the fourth ventricle. The two tissues combined are known collectively as the *choroid tela* (tela choroidea). Near the center, where the ventricle is broadest, vessels in the tela invaginate into the ventricle. This vascular mass is the *choroid plexus*.

Although the plane of the lateral walls has changed, the primitive sulcus limitans is still evident and acts as a boundary between alar and basal plates.

The marginal layer forms white matter here, also, but its appearance has altered because it is now interspersed with gray substance and contains fibers running in many planes.

The important consideration here is the fate of the mantle layer. As in the cord, the alar plate is sensory, but here in the myelencephalon, it lies lateral, rather than dorsal, to the motor area. In the medulla, the sensory zone is usually subdivided, although not by any visible, anatomic structures. Investigation has proved that the most medial part, next to the sulcus limitans, is concerned with visceral sense, while more laterally lies the area for the reception of somatic impulses. The extreme lateral portion is devoted to special somatic sense (Fig. 5-10).

The basal plate gives rise to efferent neurons. In the cord, the ventral gray columns supply skeletal muscle while the intermediolateral columns, when present, lie more laterally and supply smooth and cardiac muscle and glands. Similarly, in the medulla, the most medial portion of the basal plate differentiates into nuclei supplying skeletal muscle of somite origin, including the muscles of the tongue and eyes. Lateral to the

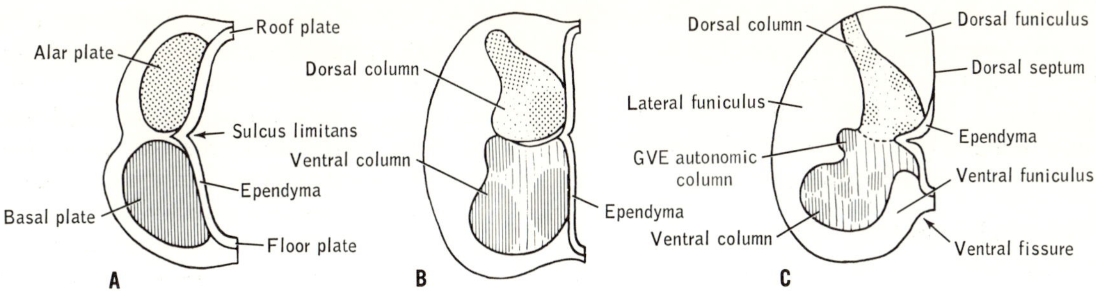

Fig. 5-9. Cross sections of the spinal cord at different stages of development, showing the differentiation of the alar and basal plates.

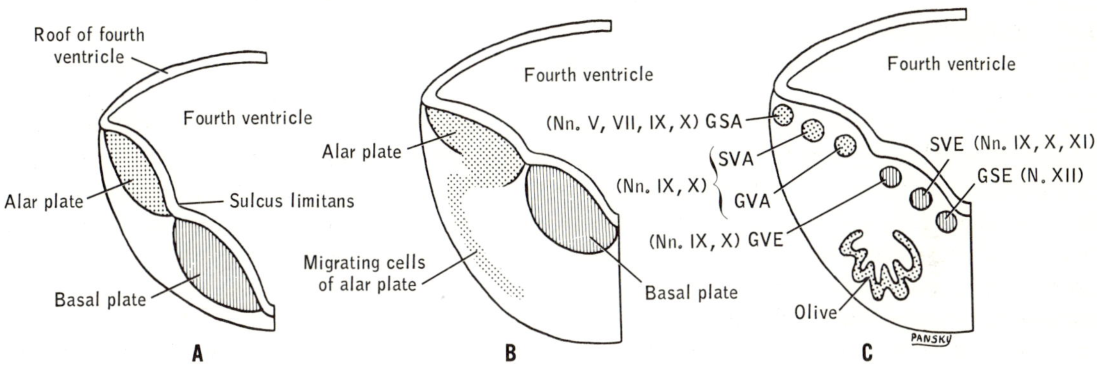

Fig. 5-10. Same as Fig. 5-9 except that these sections are through the myelencephalon.

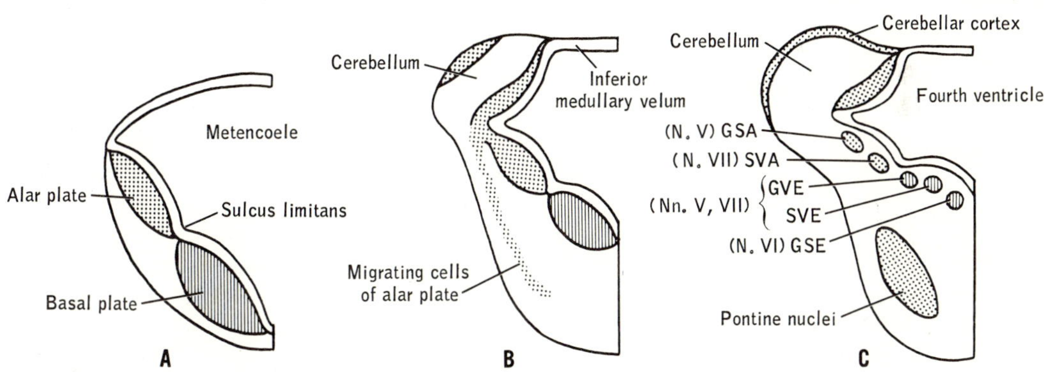

Fig. 5-11. Same as Fig. 5-9 but here the sections are through the metencephalon.

somatic column lies the visceral area, the neurons of which pass to autonomic ganglia. Because of the addition of skeletal muscle derived from the branchial arches, a portion of the basal plate lying intermediate between the somatic and visceral columns differentiates to supply this.

Metencephalon (Figs. 5-7, 5-11.)

This region has three zones. The first, and oldest, is the axial portion, or *tegmentum,* which is merely the rostral continuation of the myelencephalon. The second and largest, is the *cerebellum,* while the third is the *basal portion of the pons.*

The roof plate here, although thin, acquires some neurons and is known as the *anterior medullary velum.* The ependymal layer is present but inconspicuous.

Cerebellum (Fig. 5-7*E to H.*)

Viewed from above, the fourth ventricle is seen to be lozenge-shaped. When the pontine flexure occurs, its transverse plane is through the broadest portion of the ventricle. Here, at the zone of transition between the thick-walled alar plate and the thin roof, lies the so-called "rhombic lip." It is from a proliferation of this lip, just caudal to the lateral recess, that the oldest part of the cerebellum, the flocculonodular lobe, arises.

Rostral to the lateral recess, the rhomboid fossa is narrower, so that the alar plates of the lateral walls approach each other. The most dorsal parts of these plates begin to enlarge, at first inward toward the ventricle. In the third fetal month, these paired enlargements become obvious. Soon these swellings fuse in the midline. The medial portions, in the region of fusion, do not grow so markedly as the areas on either side. Thus, the central portion, or *vermis,* of the cerebellum is overshadowed by the expanding cerebellar hemispheres.

Subsequently, fissures and other local differentiations occur. The primary fissure appears in the fourth fetal month. By the end of the seventh month, all parts are recognizable.

Basal Pons

This is a much later development, serving to connect the cerebral and cerebellar hemispheres. The massive bundles of fibers which account for the bulk of this region have been secondarily wrapped about the ventral and lateral aspects of the original tegmentum.

Mesencephalon (Figs. 5-7, 5-12.)

The mesencephalon shows the least specialized differentiation of any part of the brain. It consists of three major zones. The dorsal portion is the *tectum;* the intermediate part is the *tegmentum;* the ventral portion is the *peduncular area.* Primitively, roof, alar, and basal plates are

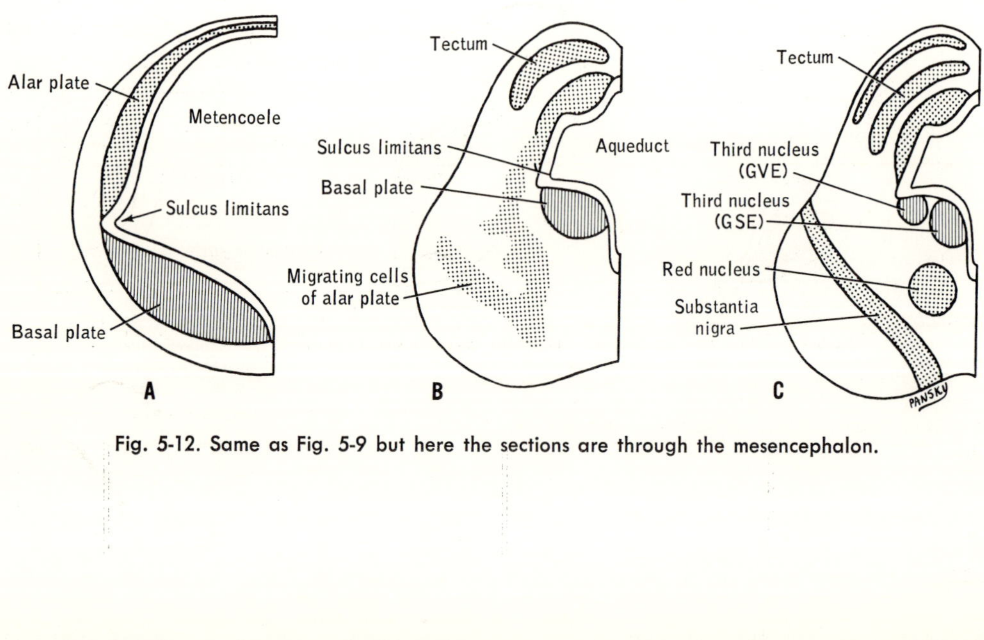

Fig. 5-12. Same as Fig. 5-9 but here the sections are through the mesencephalon.

present. The floor plate is said to be missing, having terminated in the metencephalon.

The cavity of the mesencephalon remains narrow and is known as the *cerebral aqueduct* (aqueduct of Sylvius), for which the ependyma forms a lining.

The roof plate is a narrow band joining the two alar plates, through which commissural fibers pass.

A major portion of the alar plates thickens to form the *tectum*. This consists of four paired swellings, the *corpora quadrigemina*. A small, ventral portion of the alar plate gives rise to at least one sensory nucleus, the *mesencephalic* of the *trigeminal* nerve. Some cells of the alar plate migrate ventrally to become the *red nucleus* and *substantia nigra*.

The basal plate differentiates into the remainder of the tegmental area. This includes the rostral continuation of the motor cell columns begun at lower levels.

The peduncular region is a recent acquisition laid down on the ventral surface of the midbrain as the long fiber tracts descend from the forebrain to lower levels of the brain stem and spinal cord.

Diencephalon (Figs. 5-4 to 5-7, 5-13.)

The diencephalon is that portion of the prosencephalon which remains medial after the telencephalon has evaginated. Certain peculiarities set this portion of the brain apart from the caudal levels thus far studied. First, there are no typical nerves attached to it. Second, not only is the embryonic floor plate missing, but the basal plates are also absent.[1] Thus, only the roof and alar plates remain; the former is composed chiefly of ependyma, while the latter has the three typical layers.

At first, the diocoele or cavity of the tube, is broad. However, with the enlargement of the two alar plates, the cavity becomes the slitlike *third ventricle*.

[1] Some investigators feel that the hypothalamic sulcus is a continuation of the sulcus limitans and therefore the hypothalamus would differentiate from the basal plate.

The roof plate becomes intimately associated with the pia mater, forming a *choroid tela*. This, with the enlargement of some of its vessels, invaginates into the third ventricle, forming the choroid plexus.

The remainder of the diencephalon develops from a differentiation of the alar plates. By the tenth fetal week, three main regions can be distinguished: the epithalamus, dorsally; the thalamus laterally; and the hypothalamus ventrally.

Epithalamus (Fig. 5-7.)

This lies at the junction between roof and alar plates. Near its inferior border adjoining the midbrain, the roof plate develops a caudal evagination called the *epiphysis,* or *pineal body*. A small thickening of the alar plates lateral to the pineal body represents the chief epithalamic differentiation, the *habenula.*

Thalamus (Figs. 5-7, 5-13.)

The walls of the third ventricle undergo such extensive growth that in most brains, the two sides meet and form a bridge, the *massa intermedia,* across the ventricle. A sulcus, the hypothalamic sulcus, appears as a longitudinal groove separating the thalamus from the ventral hypothalamic region.

Hypothalamus (Fig. 5-7.)

The lateral walls of the hypothalamic region thicken, but not to the degree seen in the thalamus. In addition to the nuclei, the optic chiasma is found associated with its rostral end. Other parts of the hypothalamus which arise ventrally include the tuber cinereum; the infundibulum, which gives rise to the neural hypophysis; and the mammillary bodies.

Telencephalon (Figs. 5-4, 5-6, 5-7, 5-13, 5-14.)

The telencephalon begins as a pair of lateral evaginations just behind the rostral limit of the forebrain. At first, the cavities (telencoele) open widely into the third ventricle, but later they become reduced in diameter. These are the *interventricular foramina* (of Monro).

As the hemispheres expand rostrally and then

dorsally, to rise above the diencephalon, the roof plate of each side is stretched vertically and fuses with the pia, forming the *choroid tela* (Fig. 5-13) of the lateral ventricles. This invaginates into the ventricles to create the *choroid plexus*. Later, as the hemispheres increase in mass, the region through which the blood vessels enter the plexus becomes very narrow but persists as the *choroid fissure*.

The telencephalon has three principal parts: the neopallium; the rhinencephalon; and the corpus striatum.

Corpus Striatum (Fig. 5-13.)

This begins as an enlargement of the floor of the telencephalon just lateral to and below the interventricular foramina, in direct line with the thalamic portion of the diencephalon. In each of these masses, two major nuclei, the *caudate* and *lenticular*, differentiate. The largest portions of these nuclei remain fixed. However, the caudal part of the caudate nucleus, the tail, is caught up in the growth and migration of the hemisphere, accounting for its adult shape and position.

Because of the extensive development of fibers to distant parts of the hemispheres, in particular those ascending from the thalamus, the internal capsule appears between the thalamus and the lenticular nucleus. Descending fibers from the hemispheres follow the same path, accompanying the ascending groups. Later, a portion of the internal capsule, created by descending fibers (but later acquiring some ascending fibers), appears anteriorly, between the caudate and len-

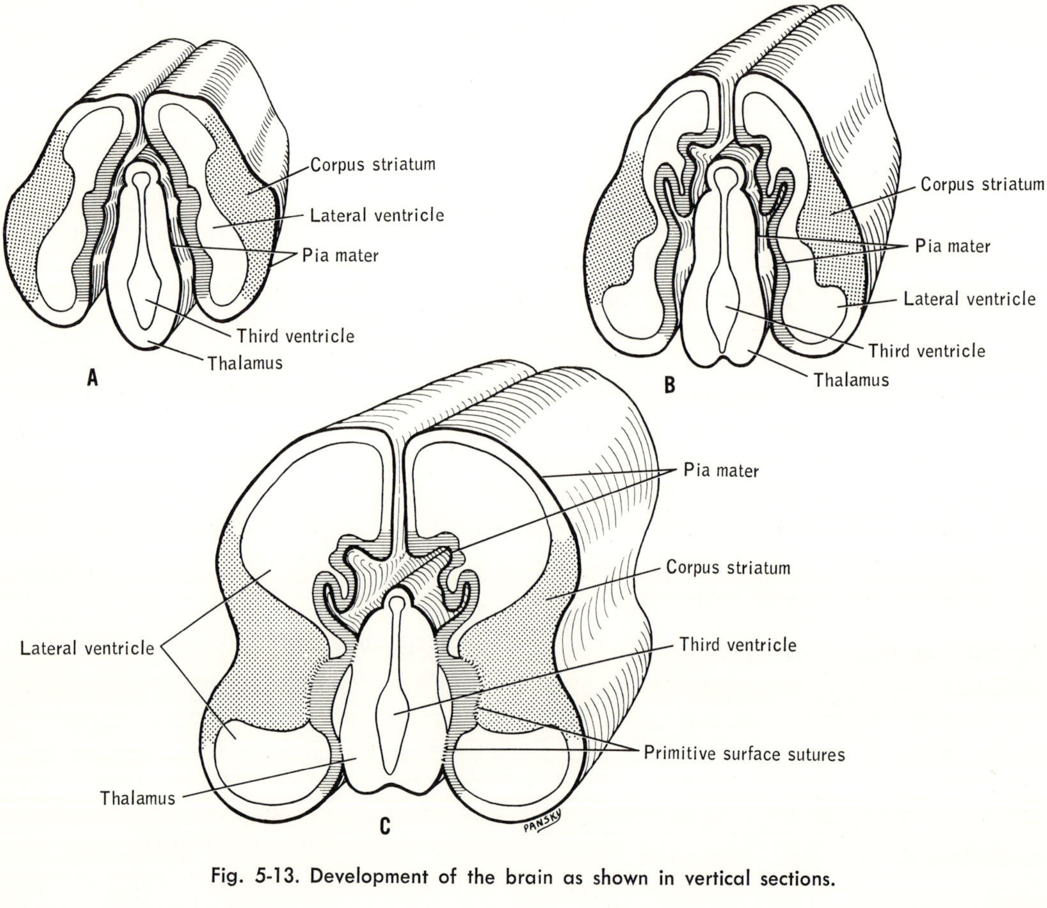

Fig. 5-13. Development of the brain as shown in vertical sections.

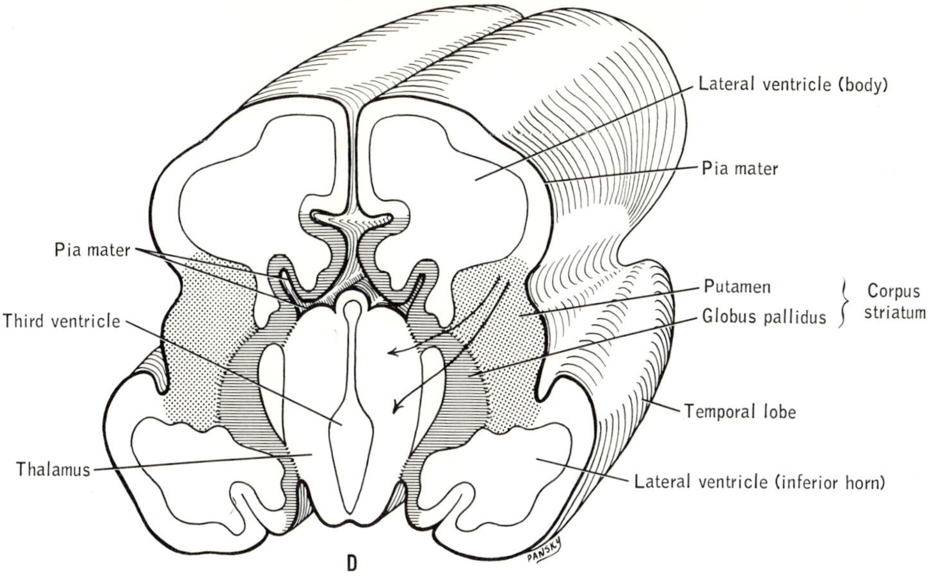

Fig. 5-13. D.

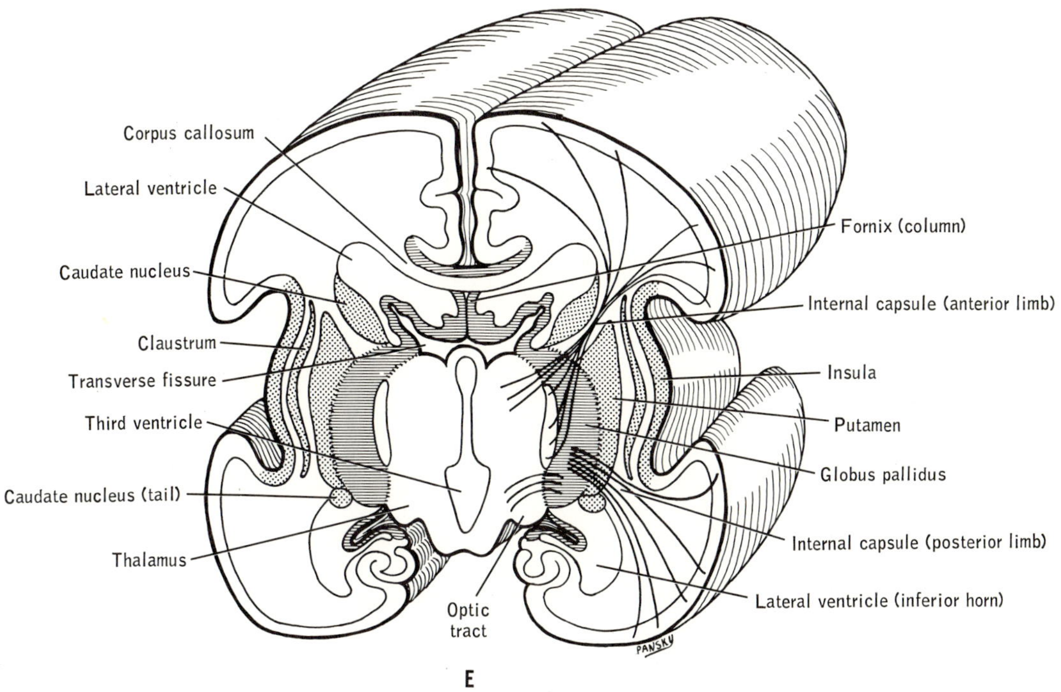

Fig. 5-13. E.

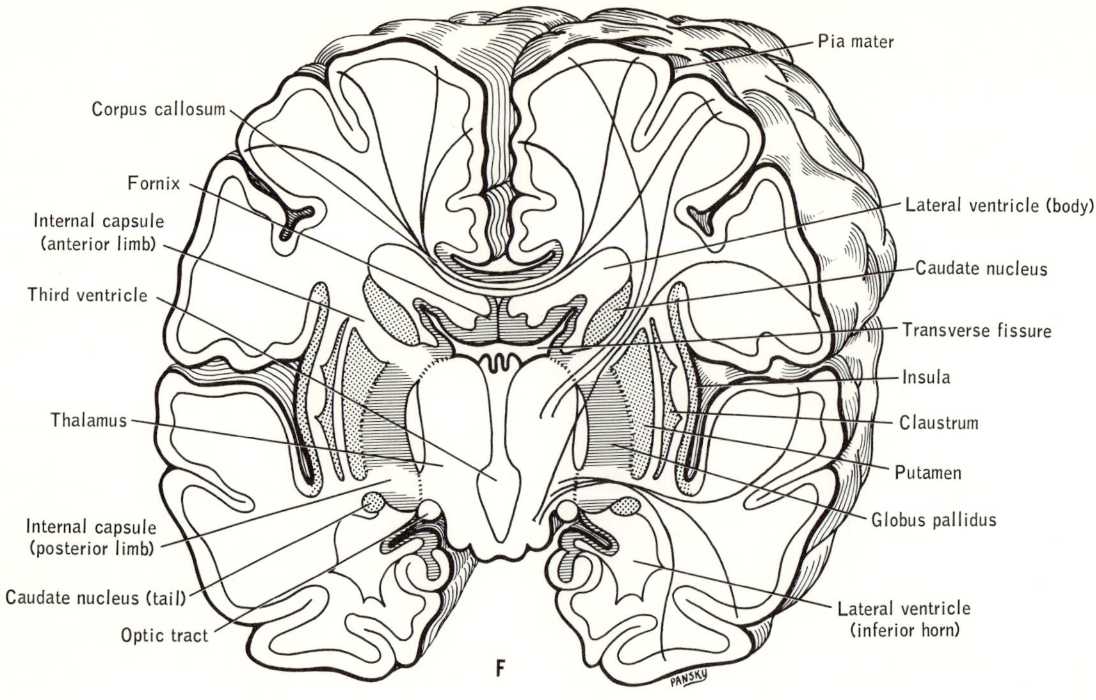

Fig. 5-13. F.

ticular nuclei. This is the *anterior limb of the capsule.*

Rhinencephalon (Figs. 5-14, 5-15.)

This begins as paired swellings on the ventral surface of each hemisphere which enlarge to become the *olfactory lobes*. These have two divisions: the more rostral becomes the *olfactory bulb* and *tract;* the more caudal differentiates into the *anterior perforated substance* and the *parolfactory area.*

Because of growth, posterior migration, and lateral expansion, the olfactory lobe becomes bent and partially obscured. Further, two pallial areas differentiate, the *archipallium* and *paleopallium* (the *hippocampal formation*).

Neopallium

During the first 4 months, the outer surface of the hemisphere is smooth. At about this time, the external gray substance begins to grow faster than the underlying white. This results in the cortex at the surface being thrown into folds or convolutions (*gyri*) separated by furrows (*fissures and sulci*).

The largest fissures appear first, the region for the *sagittal fissure* being indicated almost from the beginning, when the telencephalon first evaginated. The *rhinal* (Fig. 5-15) and *hippocampal fissures* appear in the fourth month. About the same time, a suggestion of the *lateral* (*sylvian*) *fissure* may be found, but this is not complete until after birth. This fissure is due, at least in part, to the fact that the cortex overlying the striatum, the *insula* (island of Reil), grows more slowly than surrounding regions (Figs. 5-13, 5-14). Thus, opercular coverings from frontal, parietal, and temporal lobes begin to overgrow it. The continued rostral advance of the temporal lobe serves to elongate this fissure still more. The *central fissure* (of Rolando) is evident at 6 to 7 months. The parieto-occipital, calcarine, and collateral fissures come into being at about the same time.

A word should be added here concerning the inversion of the layers of the cortex. In its orig-

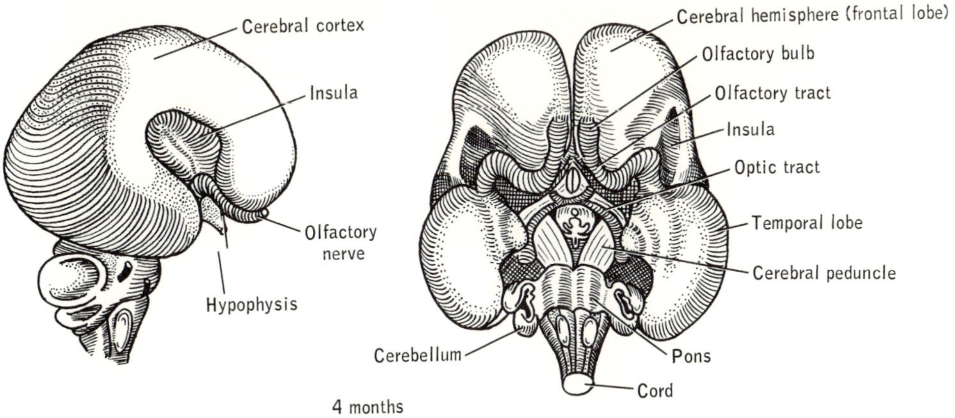

Fig. 5-14. Human brain at 4 months: *left,* seen from the side and *right,* from below, showing the development of the insula and parts of the rhinencephalon. (*Adapted from H. K. Corning.*)

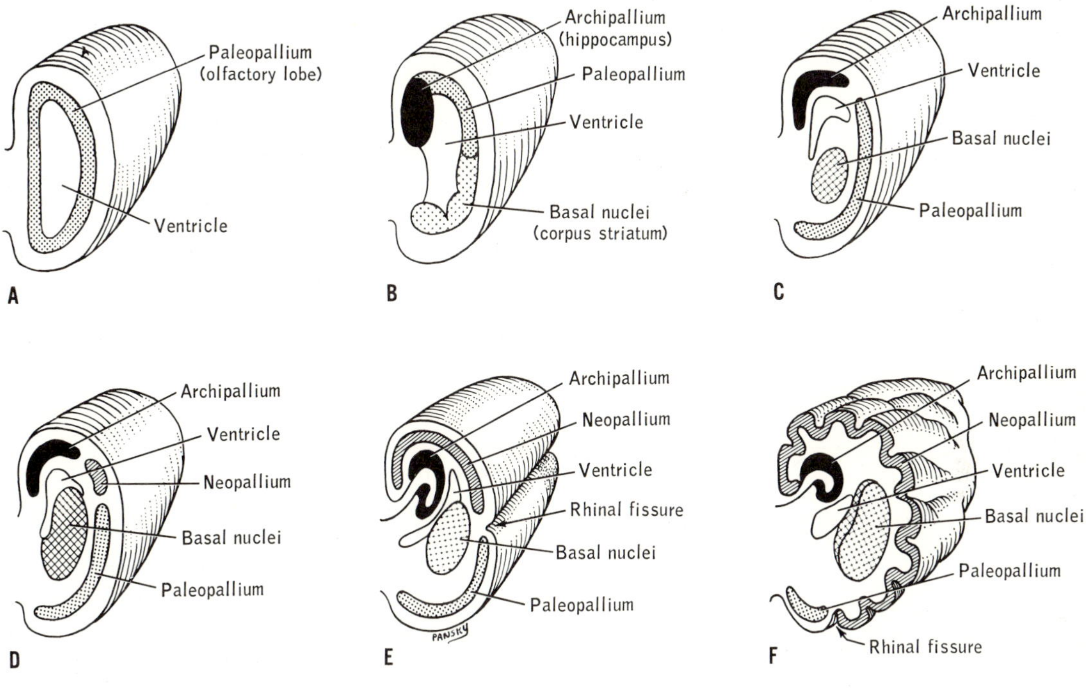

Fig. 5-15. Diagrammatic representation of vertical sections through the right cerebral hemisphere showing the evolution of the basal nuclei together with the archi- and neocortex. (*Adapted from Romer, The Vertebrate Body, W. B. Saunders Company, Philadelphia,* 1949.)

inal condition, the alar plate consists of the three typical layers. In the hemispheres, there is little change in the ependyma. However, there occurs a mass migration of cells outward from the mantle layer into the relatively cell-free marginal zone. Thus, the cortical gray substance comes to lie on the outside, while fibers going to or coming from it form the underlying white matter.[2]

COMMISSURES (Figs. 5-7, 5-13.)

From the begining, the lamina terminalis, representing the most rostral end of the prosencephalon at the time the hemispheres first appear, serves as a bridge, linking the two sides. It is natural, then, that commissural fibers, subsequently developed, would utilize this bridge. The commissures to be discussed here are the anterior and hippocampal, associated with the archipallium, and the corpus callosum, belonging to the neopallium.

Anterior Commissure

This is the most rostral and ventral of the commissures. Its fibers pass through the lamina terminalis, uniting the anterior portions of the olfactory apparatus.

Hippocampal Commissure

This also has its origin in the lamina terminalis, but with the subsequent development of the corpus callosum and the caudal migration of the hippocampi, it comes to lie a considerable distance behind its site of inception, now being associated with the crura of the fornix.

Corpus Callosum

It begins in the roof region of the lamina terminalis rostral and dorsal to the hippocampal commissure and almost directly dorsal to the anterior commissure. This area is extended caudally and is further enlarged by the growth and fusion of the medial walls of the hemispheres.

[2] The same inversion is also seen in the cerebellum.

HISTOGENESIS

Myelination in CNS

The deposition of myelin sheaths is of physiologic importance for it appears that fiber tracts in the CNS begin to function at about the time they acquire myelin. Myelination begins in the spinal cord at cervical levels during the middle fetal months but is not completed until the first and second years after birth with the myelination of the corticospinal [3] and tectospinal tracts.

In the brain, myelination begins about the sixth fetal month and is not actually completed until adolescence. Only the fibers in the corpus striatum and the tracts ascending from lower levels are myelinated at birth. Among the last fibers to become ensheathed are the commissures.

Peripheral Nervous System (PNS) (Fig. 5-1.)

Afferent Fiber

In the region of the cord, each of the columns of the neural crest breaks up into small, spherical masses corresponding to each pair of somites, beginning with the first cervical and extending to the first coccygeal. They lose their longitudinal interconnections and slip down along the cord so that their position is more lateral than dorsal. These are the primordia of the spinal ganglia.

In the cranial region, the crest also breaks up but the arrangement is irregular.

Within these primordia, two types of cells differentiate. One of these is the *neuroblast,* the other is the *spongioblast.*

The neuroblast elongates, forming a spindle-shaped cell, which sprouts a process at either end. This is the bipolar neuron. The central process of this cell grows toward the neural tube and enters the marginal layer of the spinal cord, terminating about a cell in the dorsal part of the mantle layer. The peripheral process of the bi-

[3] It is possible that at least some of the fibers of the corticospinal tracts are not completely myelinated until the twenty-first year.

polar neuron grows ventrally and aligns itself with the efferent fibers of the ventral root to form the spinal nerve trunk. Later, the original bipolar cell undergoes a series of transformations to become a unipolar (monopolar) cell. These morphologic changes are underway in some ganglia by the tenth fetal week.

At first, the spongioblasts in the ganglia form a syncytial net around the ganglion cells. Some of the spongioblasts remain close to the neuron cell body to become *capsule cells*. Others migrate along both central and peripheral processes, giving rise to the *sheath cells of Schwann*.

Efferent Fiber

Within the mantle layer of the basal plate two types of cells differentiate, *neuroblasts* and *spongioblasts*.

The neuroblasts multiply by typical mitosis, the rate of which gradually slows down until, during the first postnatal year, the ability to reproduce is lost entirely. At first the neuroblast is spindle-shaped. Gradually, it becomes more pear-shaped, with a thin process growing out of its more slender end. This is the axon, which elongates, penetrates the marginal layer, and leaves the spinal cord to become a part of the ventral root. The details of development are the same whether these fibers terminate in skeletal muscle or in autonomic ganglia. After the axon is well-established, many shorter processes, the dendrites, sprout from the broader portion of the neuroblast. Thus, the typical multipolar neuron develops.

Many of the spongioblasts remain within the CNS to form *neuroglia* (Fig. 5-1), both *astrocytes* and *oligodendroglia*. Others migrate outside the CNS to become *Schwann's sheath* for efferent fibers.

Myelination in PNS

Myelin begins to be deposited on many afferent fibers in the fourth fetal month and continues for 3 months after birth. On efferent fibers, myelination begins slightly earlier.

DISTRIBUTION OF PERIPHERAL NEURONS

Afferent Fibers (Fig. 5-16.)

There is one pair of spinal nerves to each pair of somites. As growth continues, bringing sensory fibers to the surface, a nerve-to-skin relationship is established. This is the *dermatome*. In certain body areas, where there has been little shifting or migration during development, this relationship is easy to follow, e.g., in the upper portion of the thorax. However, the evolution of the limbs and their subsequent rotation have complicated the picture.

The development of sensory neurons from cranial ganglionic masses is essentially the same.

Efferent Fibers (Figs. 5-16 to 5-18.)

Very early, efferent nerve rootlets become intimately associated with the myoblasts (of the somites), which become skeletal muscle. This basic relationship is maintained regardless of the size of the muscle or the distance it may have migrated from the original site of formation. This same general principle holds true for efferent fibers of the cranial nerves.

GANGLIA

Sensory

See Afferent Fiber, under Peripheral Nervous System, above (Fig. 5-1).

Motor (Figs. 5-16 to 5-18.)

It was originally believed that neuroblasts which give rise to all postganglionic neurons of the autonomic nervous system arose from migrations of the neural crest. More recently, the evidence indicates that at least some of the autonomic ganglion cells arise through a migration from the basal plate of the neural tube. In the thoracic and lumbar regions, the migration is regular and on a segmental basis, groups of crest cells accumulating in series along the lateral aspects of the vertebral column. These represent

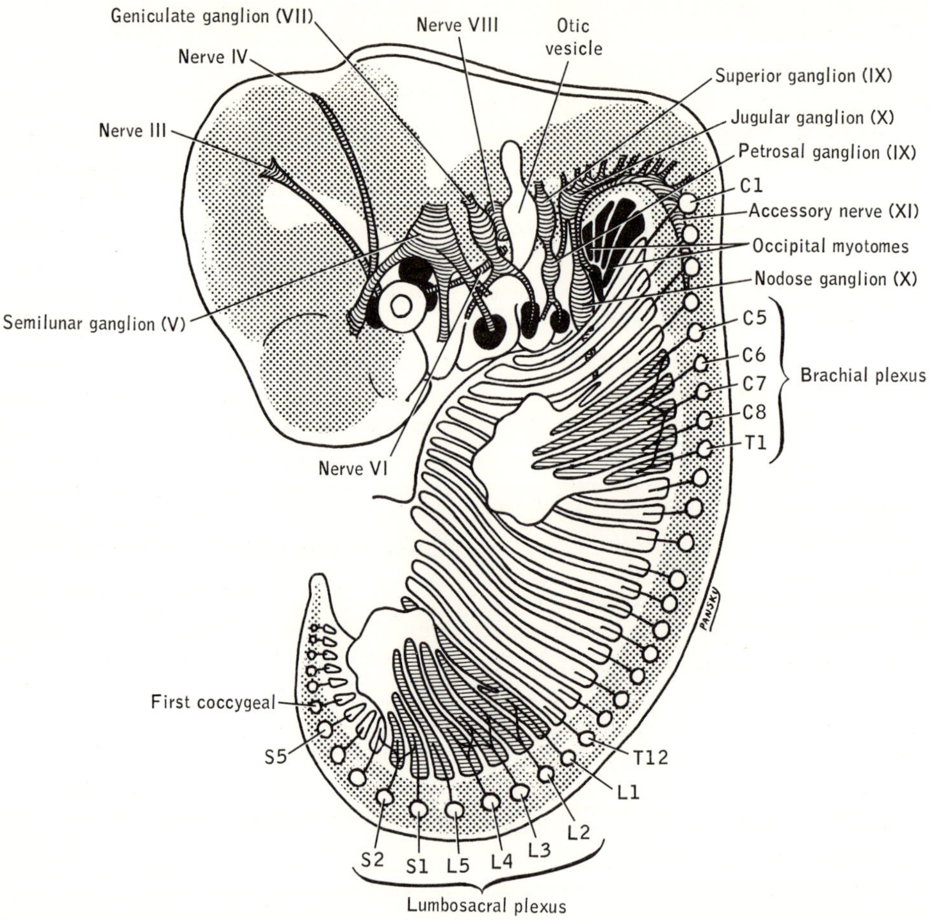

Fig. 5-16. Relationship between the body musculature and the nerves. *(Adapted from Patten, Human Embryology, 2d ed., McGraw-Hill Book Company, Inc., Blakiston Division, New York, 1953.)*

the chain ganglia. Here, neuroblasts become the multipolar *postganglionic* neurons of the *thoracolumbar outflow*. Spongioblasts give rise to the *Schwann sheath* for these fibers. Here, myelin fails to appear.

There is still further ventral migration of the crest cells, some of which become localized anterior to the aorta, becoming closely associated with the origins of arteries arising from the aorta. These are the *collateral autonomic ganglia,* i.e., the *celiac* and *superior mesenteric*. Some of the migratory cells differentiate into the *adrenal medulla.*

A scattering of crest neuroblasts migrates still further toward the viscera, forming ganglia in or near the walls of individual organs. These are the *terminal ganglia,* the cell bodies of which may be arranged in the *intermuscular plexus* (*Auerbach's*) or *submucosal plexus* (*Meissner's*).

Terminal ganglia also develop from the neural crest in the sacral and cranial areas for the craniosacral outflow of the autonomic system, i.e., the ganglia of the prostatic and vesical plexuses of the pelvis, and the otic, ciliary, sphenopalatine, and submaxillary ganglia of the head.

CLINICAL CONSIDERATIONS

General

In addition to the obvious conditions to be discussed below, there are many factors in the development and histogenesis of the nervous system of which a thorough understanding is of great value to the clinician. Among these are the following:

1. The difference in growth rate between the spinal cord and body length, which accounts for the fact that during the third fetal month the cord completely fills the vertebral canal; at birth the cord terminates at the lower border of the third lumbar vertebra, while in adults the caudal end of the cord lies near the upper border of the second lumbar vertebra. This is likewise why cord segments, particularly in the lower half of the body, do not lie adjacent to vertebral segments of the corresponding number.

2. The constant relationship between the nerve and the mesoderm giving rise to muscle, whether somite or branchial arch, is maintained. Hence, knowing the embryonic origin of a muscle, it can be assumed that the nerve supply will be the same as that established in the embryo.

3. The early nerve-to-surface relationship, with the establishment of the dermatomes, is an

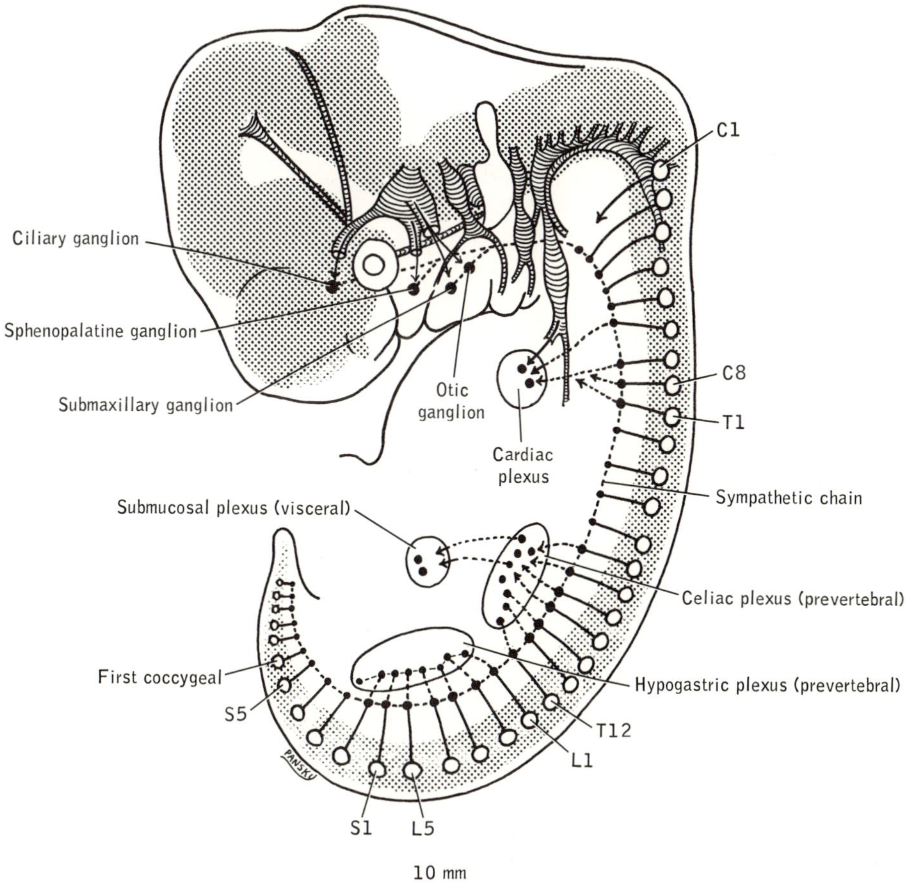

Fig. 5-17. Sagittal reconstruction showing the migration of autonomic cells, the primary migration being linked together longitudinally in the neck and trunk to form the sympathetic chain, while the second and third migrations give the prevertebral and visceral plexuses, respectively.

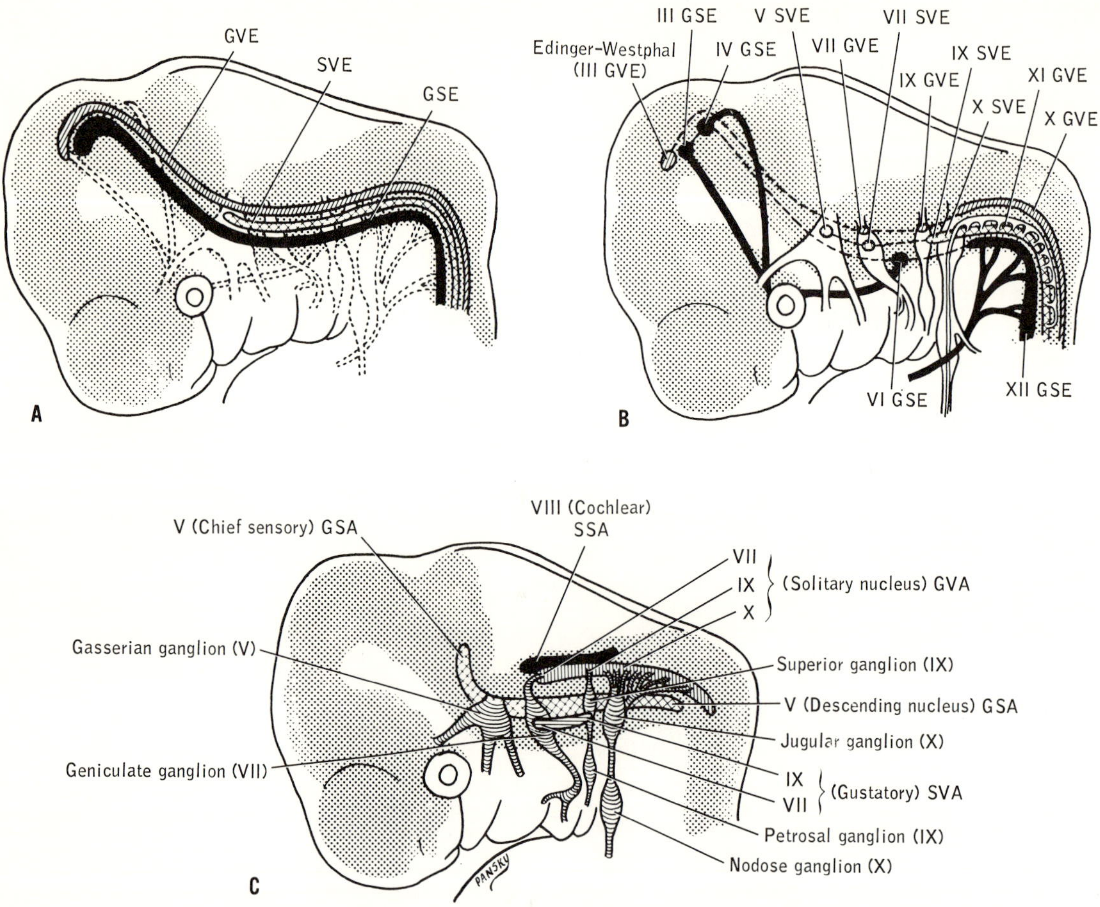

Fig. 5-18. Sagittal reconstruction of embryos to show the development of the motor columns of the brain stem (*A*); their differentiation into nuclei (*B*); and the sensory columns and nuclei (*C*).

invaluable aid in localizing the level of a lesion in the CNS. Even on the appendages, the development of which interrupted the trunk dermatomal segmentation, this primitive relationship still can be seen.

Specific Pathology

Congenital Deficiencies

A partial or complete agenesis or hypoplasia is not a problem peculiar to the nervous system but is encountered throughout the development of all viscera. One of the most common manifestations, *microcephalus,* is a condition in which there is defective development of the whole brain and premature ossification of the skull. Whether cerebral maldevelopment is due to the premature ossification, or vice versa, or to pre- or postnatal meningeal involvement is not known. Microcephalic persons are usually idiots or imbeciles and are often epileptic. *Cerebral palsy* may also result from a hypoplastic condition involving certain motor centers of the brain.

Cranioschisis

This is caused by the failure of the neural tube to close in the brain region. This defect further results in a massive deficiency of the skull, thus leaving the inside of the CNS exposed

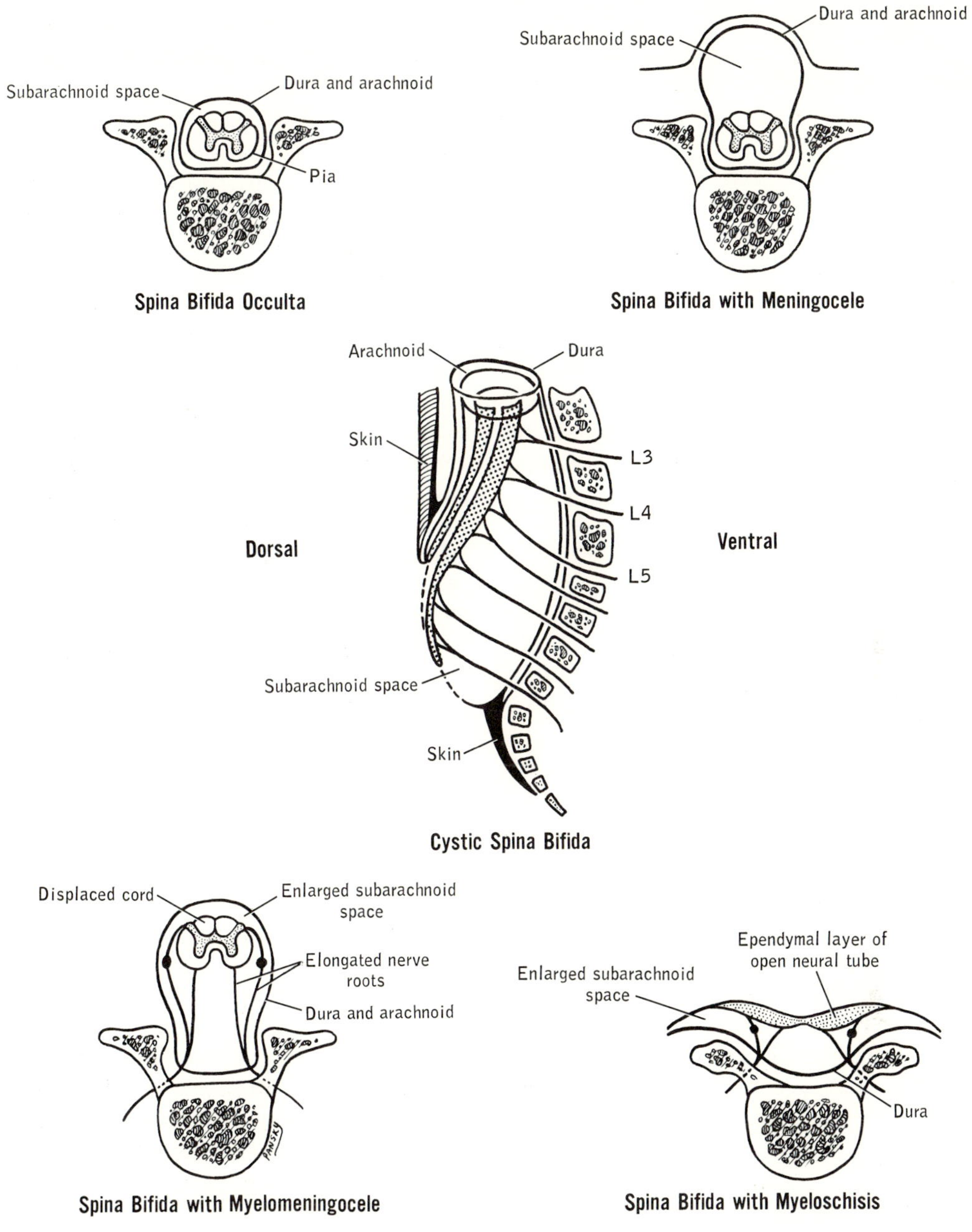

Fig. 5-19. Diagrammatic representation of the various types of spina bifida. (*Adapted from Patten, Human Embryology, 2d ed., McGraw-Hill Book Company, Inc., Blakiston Division, New York, 1953.*)

to the exterior. In most cases, the remainder of the brain does not develop to even close-to-normal proportions, and for this reason the term *anencephaly* is often applied. Because of the combination of little development and exposure to infection, death usually ensues shortly after birth.

Myeloschisis (Fig. 5-19.)

In such cases, the neural tube fails to close at spinal cord levels. This, too, is associated with a secondary condition in which the neural arch of the vertebra also fails to form, again leaving the inside of the CNS exteriorized. The defect in the spine is called *spina bifida.* The latter condition can also occur without abnormalities of the spinal cord and is primarily a skeletal abnormality.

Spinal Bifida (Fig. 5-19.)

Unlike myeloschisis, this condition is not an inherent defect in the development of the cord. Fundamentally, it involves a failure on the part of the surrounding mesoderm to form normal or complete neural arches on one or more of the adjacent vertebrae. Thus, the spinal cord may become secondarily involved. In its simplest form -*spina bifida occulta*- the neural arch is missing but there is no protrusion of either meninges or spinal cord through the hiatus. Thus, the skin lies flat over the surface and, except for a lack of a protective lamina of bone, the cord and spinal nerves are normal. When the bony deficiency is greater, the pressure of the cerebrospinal fluid in the subarachnoid space may cause a visible herniation of a meningeal sac filled with fluid. This is called *spina bifida with meningocele.* In this case the spinal cord and its attached nerves is also normal but the cord is left without the protection usually afforded by hard tissue. Again, when the bony deficiency is great, fluid pressure building up ventral to the cord may cause it, too, to protrude dorsally through the hiatus. In such cases, a variable extent of the cord has been distorted and the spinal nerves in the area are greatly stretched. Furthermore, the cord is now in a superficial position making it extremely vulnerable to trauma. This condition is *spina bifida with myelomeningocele.* A final anomaly belonging in this category is *cystic spina bifida.* In this type, it appears that the caudal end of the neural tube does not quite close off from the skin, leaving an opening from the central canal of the cord to the body surface. At the same time, the subarachnoid space fills up with fluid forming a kind of cyst anterior and caudal to the lower portion of the spinal cord putting considerable stress on the spinal nerves in this area. In this instance, the cord has an abnormal curvature and even the normal portions are vulnerable. Perhaps the most serious consequence lies in the fact that the cord is open to bacterial invasion.

Hydrocephalus

In the course of development, an occlusion may form in the ventricular system, especially the interventricular foramina or cerebral aqueduct. This leads to the expansion of the brain and cranium under pressure from cerebrospinal fluid. This pressure causes poor development of other portions of the brain, the cortex in particular.

Arnold-Chiari Deformity

This condition is characterized by elongation of the cerebellar tonsils; a small and deformed medulla; a small pons with degeneration of its transverse fibers; and herniation of the cerebellum into the vertebral canal.

SUMMARY

GENERAL DEVELOPMENT

- Neural ectoderm
  - Neural plate
    - Rostral
      - Neural tube
        - Wall
          - Prosencephalon
            - Telencephalon
              - Pallium
              - Basal nuclei
              - Rhinencephalon
            - Diencephalon
              - Thalamus
              - Epithalamus
              - Subthalamus
              - Hypothalamus
          - Mesencephalon
            - Mesencephalon
          - Rhombencephalon
            - Metencephalon
              - Cerebellum
              - Pons
            - Myelencephalon
              - Medulla
        - Cavity
          - Prosocoele
            - Lateral ventricle
            - Third ventricle
          - Mesocoele
            - Cerebral aqueduct
          - Myelocoele
            - Fourth ventricle
    - Caudal
      - Neural tube
        - Wall
          - Spinal cord
        - Cavity
          - Central canal

HISTOGENESIS

- Neural ectoderm
  - Neural crest
    - Neuroblast
      - Afferent neuron
      - Postganglionic efferent
      - Adrenal medulla
    - Spongioblast
      - Capsule cell
      - Schwann cell
  - Ependyma
    - Mantle layer of neural tube
      - Neuroblast
        - Motor
          - Somatic
          - Visceral
        - Association neurons
      - Spongioblast
        - In the CNS
          - Astrocyte
          - Oligodendroglia
        - In the PNS
          - Schwann cells

DIFFERENTIATION OF NEURAL TUBE

- Wall of neural tube
  - Rostral (brain)
    - Roof plate
      - Prosencephalon
        - Choroid tela and plexus of lateral ventricle
        - Choroid tela and plexus of third ventricle
      - Mesencephalon
        - Commissures of corpora quadrigemina
      - Rhombencephalon
        - Anterior medullary velum
        - Posterior medullary velum
        - Choroid tela and plexus of fourth ventricle
    - Alar plate
      - Prosencephalon
        - All of telencephalon
        - All of diencephalon
      - Mesencephalon
        - Corpora quadrigemina
        - Red nucleus
        - Substantia nigra
        - Mesencephalic nucleus of V
        - Chief nucleus of V
      - Rhombencephalon
        - Metencephalon
          - Cerebellum
          - Sensory nuclei V and VIII
        - Myelencephalon
          - Sensory nuclei V, VII, VIII, IX, and X
    - Basal plate
      - Prosencephalon
        - Missing
      - Mesencephalon
        - Motor nuclei III and IV
        - Reticular nuclei
      - Rhombencephalon
        - Metencephalon
          - Motor nuclei V, VI, and VII
          - Reticular nuclei
        - Myelencephalon
          - Motor nuclei IX, X, XI, and XII
          - Reticular
    - Floor plate
      - Prosencephalon
        - Missing
      - Mesencephalon
        - Missing
      - Rhombencephalon
        - Metencephalon — Region of median raphe
        - Myelencephalon — Region of median raphe
  - Caudal (cord)
    - Roof plate
      - Region of posterior median sulcus and septum
    - Alar plate
      - Dorsal columns
    - Basal plate
      - Ventral columns
    - Floor plate
      - Region of ventral median fissure

6 BASIC STRUCTURE AND FUNCTION OF THE NERVOUS SYSTEM

STRUCTURE

The Neuron in the Central Nervous System

Definition

A neuron is the unit of structure and function of the nervous system, composed of a cell body and one or more processes.

Classification of the Neuron Processes

From a functional standpoint, *axons* conduct impulses *away* from the cell body and *dendrites* conduct impulses *toward* the cell body.

Morphologic Classification of Neurons

Neurons are classified on a morphologic basis according to the number of their processes or upon the length and disposition of the axons.

Classifications According to Number of Processes. *Unipolar* (*Monopolar*). (Figs. 6-1, 6-2.) The cell is spherical and has a single process. A short distance from the cell, the process splits into two branches which travel in opposite directions. Most authorities agree that the single-stem process and its branches are structurally similar to axons. However, it is preferable to speak of a peripheral process leading toward the stem of the cell and a central branch leading impulses away from the stem toward the CNS. Neurons of this type are predominantly sensory and are found almost exclusively in the peripheral system.

Bipolar. (Fig. 6-2.) Neurons of this type have two processes, a dendrite and an axon attached to opposite ends of a fusiform cell body. Bipolar elements are found in the retina, cochlear and vestibular ganglia, and in certain places in the central system.

Multipolar. (Figs. 6-1, 6-2.) The cell has several poles, each representing the point of attachment of a process. Although occasionally a cell may have only one dendrite, there are usually several, each of which may give off secondary branches. The dendritic network makes contact with the terminations of other neurons possible. Each neuron has only one axon (axis cylinder). This arises from a small conical elevation of the cell body, the *axon hillock*. The axon may travel considerable distances (from a fraction of an inch to several feet) and may give off branches. However, near its termination, a considerable arborization occurs. These branches, the *telodendrons,* vary greatly in number, shape, and distribution. Multipolar neurons comprise the bulk of the neurons whose cell bodies lie within the CNS. They are also typical of the autonomic division of the peripheral nervous system.

Classification on the Basis of Axon Length (*Golgi Classification*). Morphologically, these neurons are all of the multipolar type.

Golgi Type I. (Fig. 6-1.) These neurons have long axons, most of which leave the CNS through the ventral roots of spinal nerves or through the main trunks of the cranial nerves.

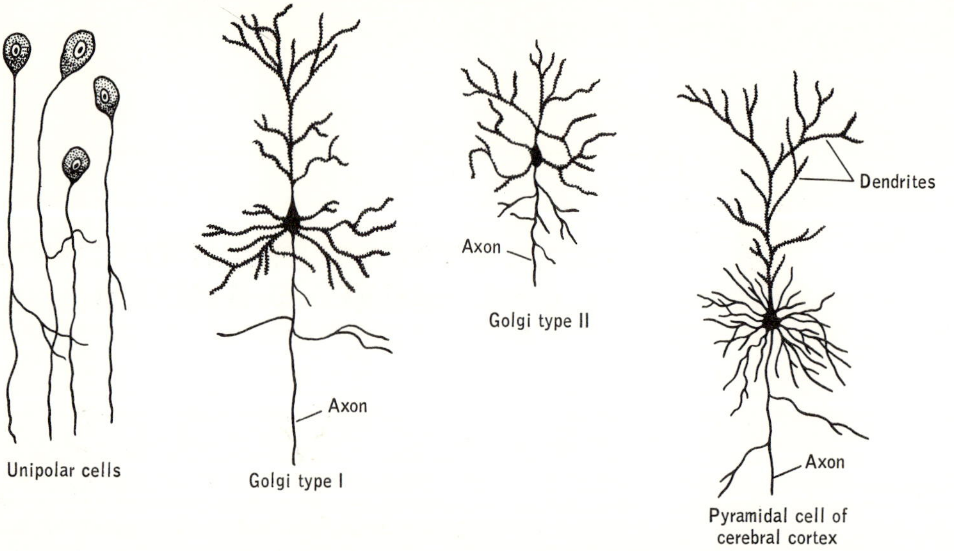

Fig. 6-1. Neuron types found in the nervous system.

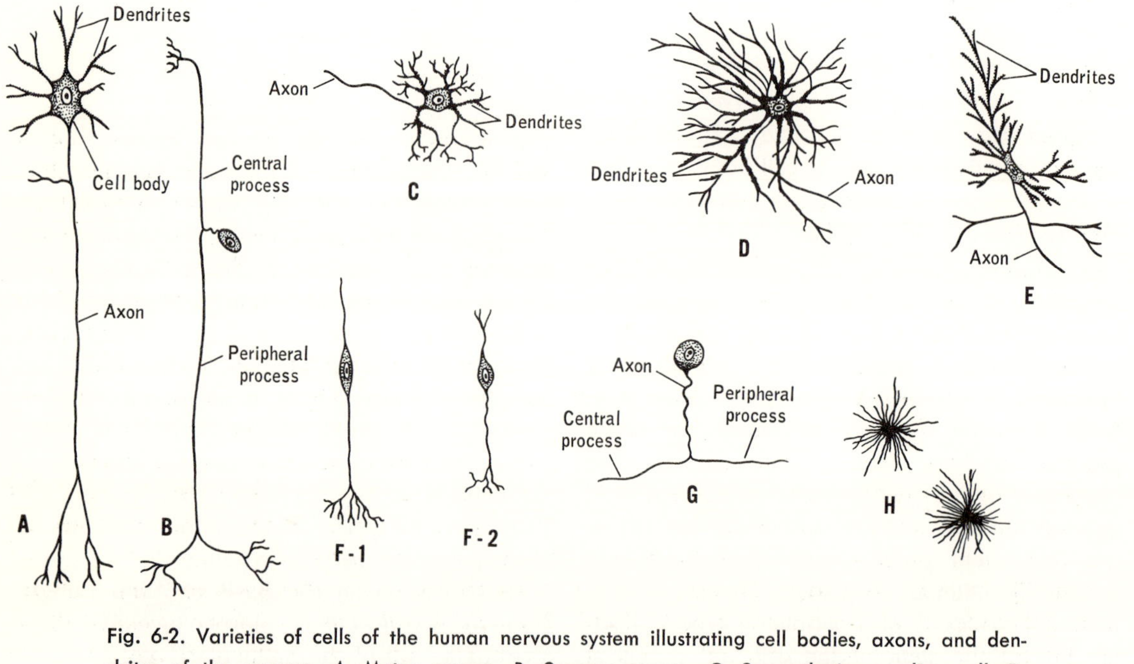

Fig. 6-2. Varieties of cells of the human nervous system illustrating cell bodies, axons, and dendrites of the neurons. *A.* Motor neuron. *B.* Sensory neuron. C. Sympathetic ganglion cell. *D.* Ventral horn cell. *E.* Fusiform cell of the cerebral cortex. *F*-1. Olfactory bipolar cell. *F*-2. Retinal bipolar cell. G. Spinal ganglion cell. *H.* Neuroglia cells of the cerebral cortex.

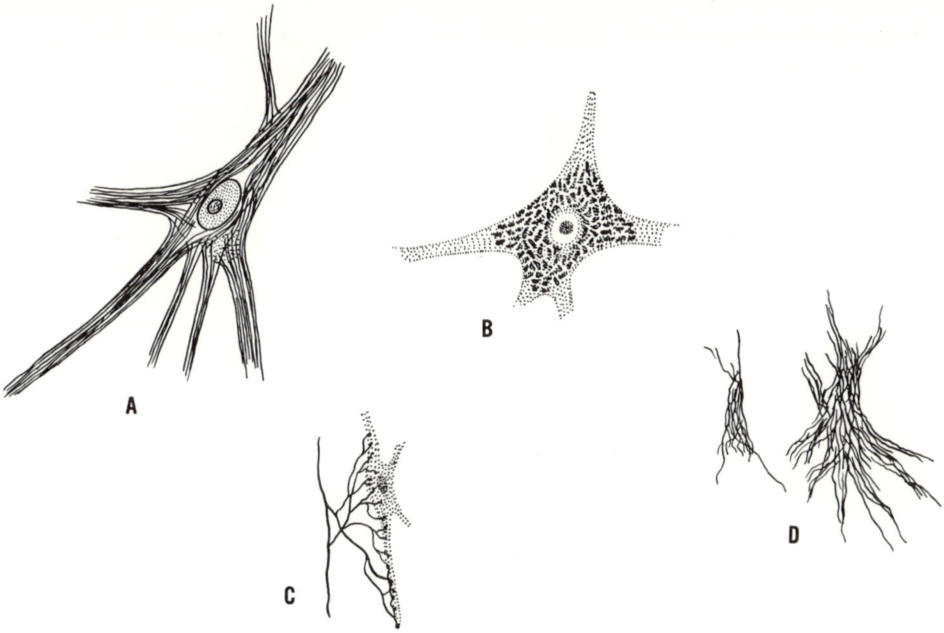

Fig. 6-3. Diagrammatic representation of structural details of several nerve cells. (*After Cajal.*) *A.* Neurofibrillar network of a pyramidal cell of the human motor cortex. *B.* Nissl bodies of an anterior horn cell from the human spinal cord. C. Nerve fiber endings on a nerve cell. *D.* Golgi network (pericellular).

Golgi Type II. (Fig. 6-1.) These are neurons having short axons, all of which stay within the CNS. The majority of association neurons are of this type.

Microscopic Structure of the Neurons

The Cell Body. This is the portion of the neuron which contains the nucleus and is frequently called the *perikaryon.* These cells assume different shapes (round, oval, fusiform, and pyramidal) and vary in size from 4 to 120 micra. An outer cell membrane is present and plays a part in the transmission and conduction of impulses.

The Cytoplasm. This is differentiated into several components: neurofibrils, neuroplasm, Nissl bodies, mitochondria, Golgi apparatus, and centrosome.

NEUROFIBRILS. (Fig. 6-3.) These are fine cytoplasmic fibrils distributed in a complex network throughout the cell body. Electron microscopy indicates that they consist of aggregates of minute filaments 60 to 100A thick which extend into all the cell processes. Those found in dendrites are finer than those in axons. They may represent an internal supporting structure. It is no longer thought that they are concerned with conduction.

NEUROPLASM. This is the semiliquid, undifferentiated cytoplasm surrounding neurofibrils. In dendrites, it is sometimes referred to as *interfibrillar substance;* in axons, as *axoplasm.*

NISSL SUBSTANCE. (Figs. 6-3, 6-12.) This substance, also called Nissl bodies, chromophil, chromidial substance and tigroid bodies, is the most conspicuous element in the cytoplasm when sections are stained with basic aniline dyes. It takes the form of irregular clumps or finely granular particles. Although these blocks (or particles) may vary in size from cell to cell, they tend to have the same appearance in cells which have similar functions, for example—in large motor neurons, the blocks are of considerable size while in large sensory neurons they are fine and dustlike. Electron microscope studies reveal that these bodies are composed of parallel cytoplasmic lamellae, possibly vesicular in nature, among which are scattered numerous granules, thought to be ribonucleic acid. It has been shown that the ratio of lamellae to granules varies considerably. No evidence for a limiting membrane has been found. Generally, Nissl bodies lie in the interstices between neurofibrils. They are absent beneath the cell membrane and immediately surrounding the nucleus. They extend into the dendrites but not into the axon hillock or axons. It is believed that Nissl bodies are directly concerned in the continuous synthesis of new cytoplasm which flows continuously down the axon (axoplasmic flow). They change in appearance under different physiologic conditions: in extreme fatigue, or in pathologic conditions where there is injury (either trauma or disease) to the cell body or axon, they disappear almost completely (chromatolysis). Temporary chromatolysis, together with a shift of the nucleus to one side, is noted when an axon is cut. These phenomena comprise the "axon reaction."

PIGMENTS such as lipochrome and melanin also appear in nerve cells. The significance of these pigments is not completely understood.

GOLGI NET AND MITOCHONDRIA. Both of these organelles are found in neurons. The Golgi is a network of irregular threads or bands, heavier than the neurofibrils. They vary morphologically in neurons of different types. Filamentous mitochondria are scattered freely between the Nissl bodies and the neurofibrils. Their function here is probably similar to that in other body cells, i.e., they act in protein synthesis, respiration and in the production of secretions. There is evidence for the presence of a continuous distal flow from the region of the perikaryon. This flow is responsible not only for the maintenance of the ultimate branches of the cell but also bring to their terminations the substances required for the chemical transmission of nerve impulses. Thus, the neuron can perform as a type of gland cell in which the axon serves as a duct and whose secretions are released in small quantities into contact with the tissue to be affected.

The Nucleus. (Figs. 6-1, 6-2, 6-12.) This is relatively large, generally round, and centrally placed. Both relative size and position may appear to vary considerably when seen in different parts of the nervous system, because of the great irregularity and size of the many cells. There is a definite nuclear membrane which is not often outstanding in ordinary preparations. The nucleus is predominantly made up of pale-staining nucleoplasm. The linin framework is prominent but sparse. The basichromatin granules are fine and greatly dispersed. There is usually one large, very distinct, oxyphilic nucleolus in each nucleus. A smaller, round basophilic body lies so close to the nucleolus that it is referred to as a nucleolar satellite (sex chromatin). This is said to be present in the nuclei of females but not in males.

Support

Ependyma. This is a term applied to the epithelial cells lining the ventricles of the brain and the central canal of the spinal cord. In the latter location and over the choroid plexuses, these cells are important for reasons other than lining or support for there they may play a role in the production of cerebrospinal fluid.

Neuroglia. (Fig. 6-4.)

Astrocytes. These are found throughout the central nervous system. Their nuclei are oval and contain little chromatin. Nucleoli are usually absent. In general, astrocytes may be divided into two classes, *protoplasmic* and *fibrous*. Both types have many processes, one of which is larger than the others. This process extends to adjacent blood vessels, terminating there in an "end foot." The protoplasmic astrocytes with their numerous and relatively heavy branches predominate in the gray matter. The fibrous astrocytes are found in the white matter. Their longer, thin and less numerous branches are seen to contain minute fibrillae. These cells tend to be arranged in rows parallel to the nerve fibers among which they lie. Their end feet form a complete layer outside the endothelium of the capillaries within the CNS and, together with the endothelium, are responsible for the "blood-brain barrier" which may serve to prevent certain substances from passing from the blood to the nervous tissue. At the surface of the CNS is found a layer of small astrocytes which is adherent to the overlying pia. Internally, the processes of these cells join the processes of other astrocytes lying deeper in the tissue. The external membrane is continued as a sleeve around the blood vessels entering the CNS from the pia and there becomes continuous with the layer of end feet around the intraneural capillaries. After injury to the nervous tissue, astrocytes are capable of rapid proliferation, forming a kind of "scar tissue" which interferes with the regeneration of neurons by blocking the path of growing cell processes.

Oligodendroglia. These cells are smaller than astrocytes and their nuclei contain more chromatin. Their nuclei also lack nucleoli. Oligodendroglia may be found in both gray and white matter of the CNS. They appear to help hold the gray matter together but they are not so important in this respect as are the astrocytes. Since they are often seen closely surrounding neuron cell bodies they are sometimes spoken of as *perineural satellites.* In the white matter they tend to align themselves between the axis cylinders of neuron, their processes forming incomplete sheaths for the nerve fiber. They appear to be the counterparts of the Schwann cells of the peripheral nerves and, like them, are responsible for the formation of myelin in the white matter. Unlike the Schwann cells, each oligodendrocyte forms myelin segments on several different axons rather than on one, as is the case in the peripheral system.

Microglia. These are the smallest of the neuroglia. Their nuclei are also smaller than those of other types, they stain more darkly and may be irregular in shape. They are only moderately branched. Unlike the other glia, they are highly mobile as can easily be demonstrated under pathological conditions. Thus, they may serve as macrophages. Microglia are more common in gray than in white matter. In the former, they also appear in limited numbers as perineural satellites but are more often arranged along blood vessels as *perivascular satellites.* In the white matter they are distributed among the nerve fibers.

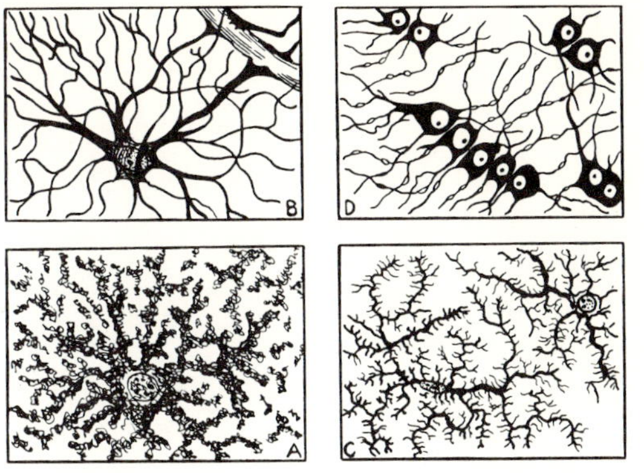

Fig. 6-4. Neuroglial cells of the central nervous system. *(Adapted from del Rio-Hortega in Maximow and Bloom, A Textbook of Histology, 7th ed., W. B. Saunders Company, Philadelphia, 1957.)*

Insulation (Fig. 6-10.)

Myelin. During the fourth fetal month, an insulating substance begins to be laid down in the white matter of the cervical spinal cord. It is, however, absent or scarce around the cell bodies and dendrites. This material is known as myelin. Since myelin, when seen grossly in the CNS, appears a glistening white, the regions occupied by these fibers are called *white matter*. Myelin is a fatty substance containing cholesterol, cerebrosides, and certain phospholipids, the most important of which is sphingomyelin. The lipid is said to be in the form of a lipid-protein complex. Apparently, myelin develops under the influence of nerve fibers in collaboration with neuroglia. The persistence of myelin, however, is dependent upon the integrity of the axis cylinder. Although myelin is not essential for the conduction of nerve impulses, it does seem to be required if impulses are to be conducted to such a degree that delicate and precise movements may result from the conduction.

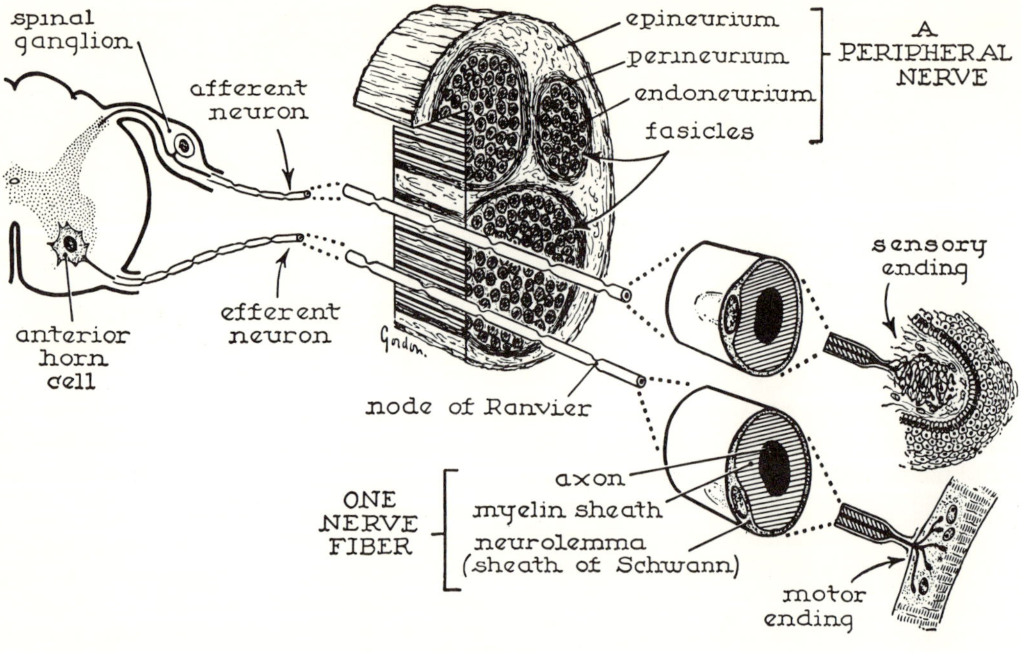

Fig. 6-5. Diagram showing the parts of a peripheral nerve. (*From Ham, Histology, 3d ed., J. B. Lippincott Company, Philadelphia,* 1957.)

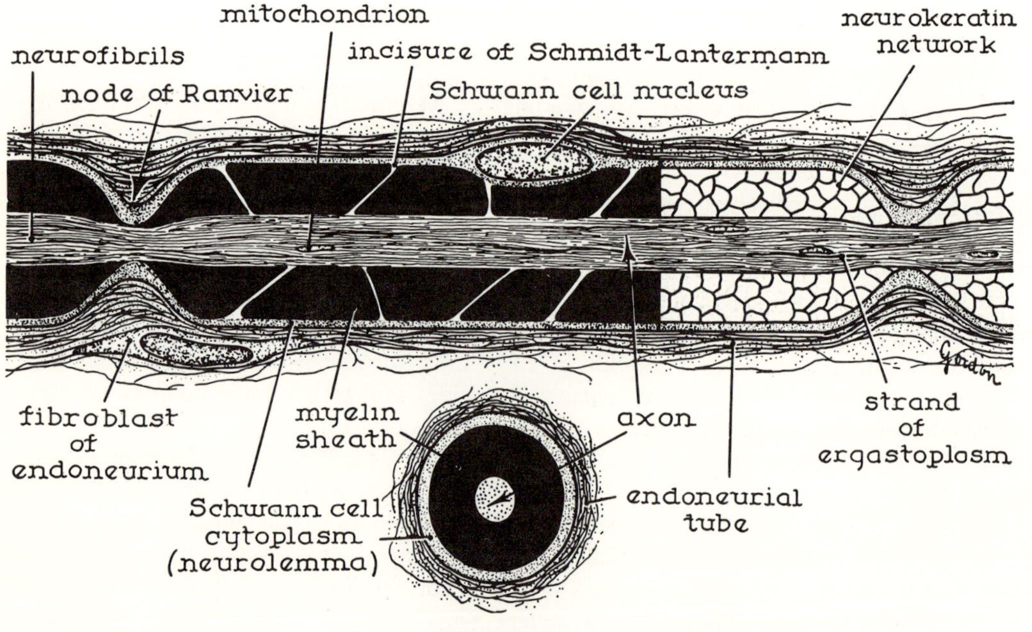

Fig. 6-6. Semidiagrammatic drawing of a longitudinal and cross section of a myelinated nerve fiber and its endoneural sheath. On the left side of the upper drawing, the myelin has been preserved and blackened by osmium tetroxide; on the right, the fatty portion of the myelin has been dissolved away. (*From Ham, Histology, 3d ed., J. B. Lippincott Company, Philadelphia,* 1957.)

The Neuron in the Peripheral Nervous System

In the peripheral nervous system (PNS), axons carrying impulses away from the CNS are mingled with the peripheral processes of neurons carrying impulses toward the CNS. This combination of fibers is called a *nerve*. Each nerve contains a variable number of fibers, together with their supporting elements.

Components of a Nerve

Axis Cylinder. (Figs. 6-5 to 6-8, 6-10.) This consists of bundles of neurofibrils set in axoplasm. There is no Nissl substance, but mitochondria have been demonstrated. Although the periphery of the axoplasm shows no anatomic membrane when observed by classical methods, the electron microscope reveals a thin but definite *axolemma*. It is differentially permeable to ions and possesses certain electrical properties, both factors important in nerve conduction. The diameters of the axis cylinders are subject to much variation (from one to several micra).

Myelin. (Figs. 6-5 to 6-8, 6-10, 6-11.) The vast majority of the peripheral nerve fibers are myelinated, at least to a small but demonstrable degree. However, a certain group of fibers, belonging to the autonomic portion of the peripheral nervous system, their cells of origin lying in ganglia, show no myelin and are referred to as nonmyelinated or nonmedullated fibers. The term *Remak fiber* is also applied to them. The

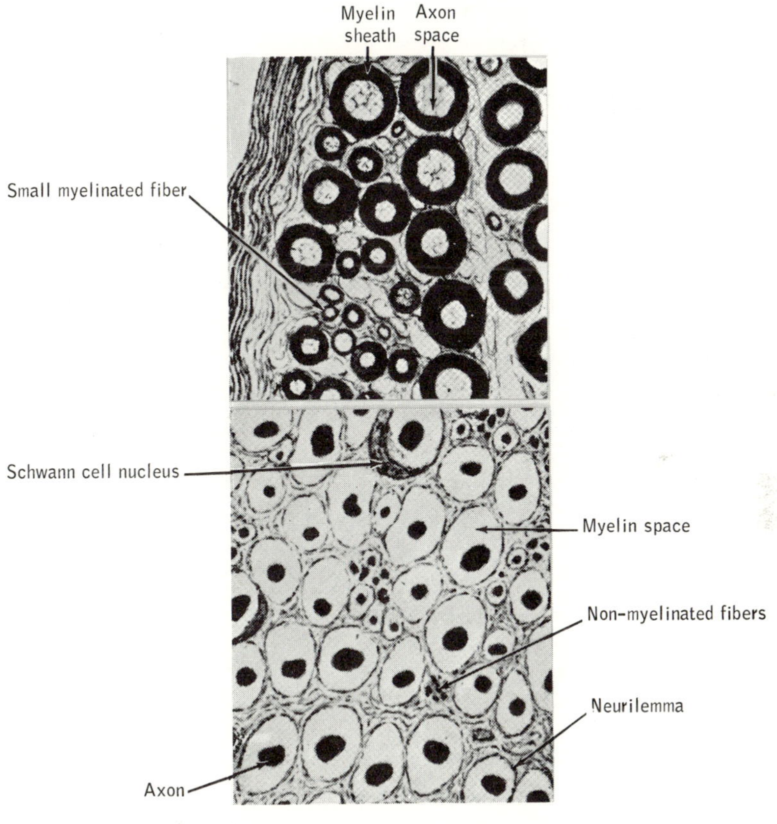

Fig. 6-7. Cross section of a nerve. Upper figure after fixation in osmic acid which stains myelin black. Lower figure has been stained according to the Cajal silver technic. In this case the axis cylinders are black.

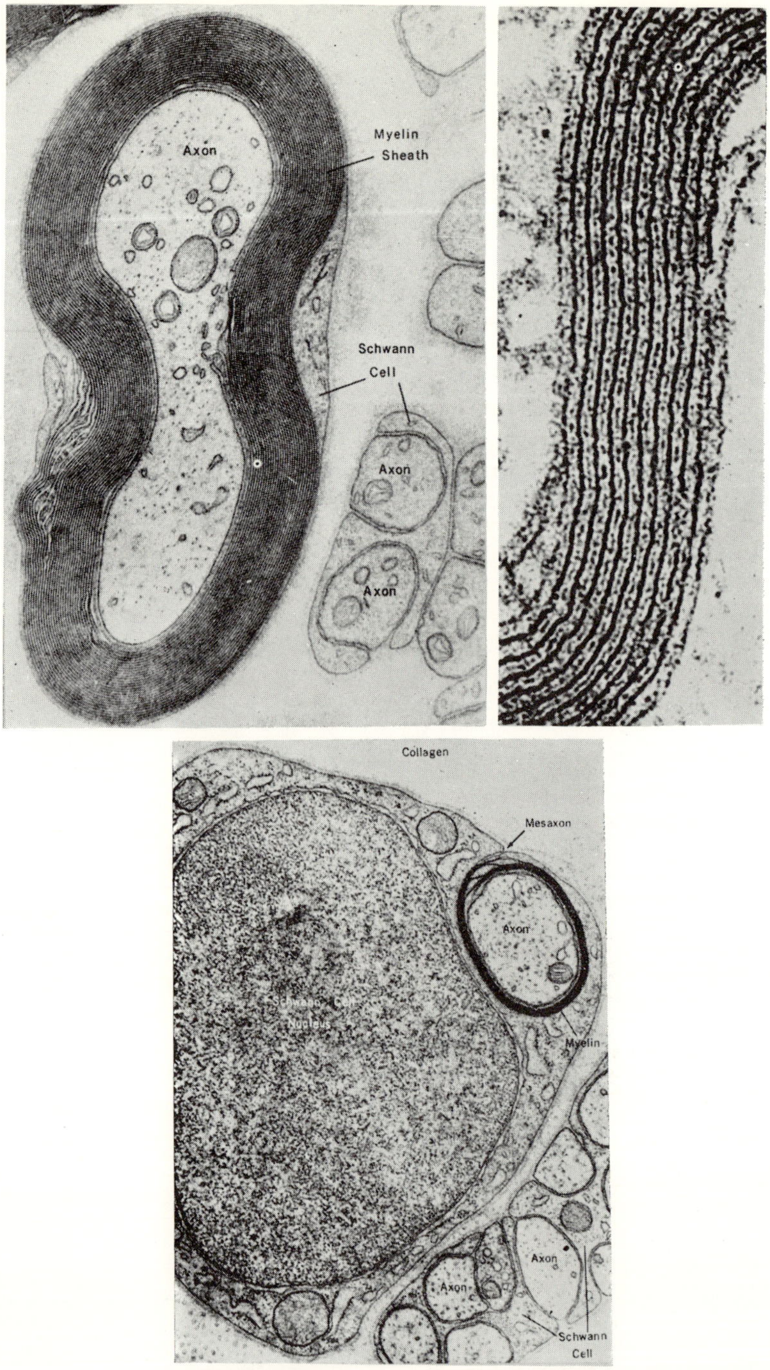

Fig. 6-8. Electron micrographs of nerve fibers. *Upper left.* This is a section through a fiber showing the lamination of the myelin and the relations of the myelin to the Schwann cell. Several nonmyelinated fibers appear on the right side of the figure. *Upper right.* Higher magnification of a small portion of the myelin sheath showing the alternating major dense lines with the intraperiod lines. *Lower figure.* This shows the relations of several nonmyelinated fibers and one lightly myelinated fiber to a single Schwann cell. (*Courtesy of Drs. Bloom, Webster, and Fernandez-Moran in Bloom and Fawcett: A Textbook of Histology, 8th ed., W. B. Saunders Co., Philadelphia,* 1962.)

peripheral myelin is of the same general composition as that found in the CNS. It is apparently supported by a protoplasmic neurokeratin net, which, in part, may be intrinsic to the myelin or may represent trabeculae penetrating from the overlying layer. However, the myelin sheath is not continuous but is interrupted at intervals by constrictions or *nodes of Ranvier*. The internode, or the distance between nodes, varies in different fibers from 50 to 1,000 micra. The greater the diameter of the fiber, the longer the internode. In addition, certain preparations show that the myelin is broken up by little oblique clefts known as the *incisures of Schmidt-Lantermann*. The existence of the latter as real structures and not artefacts has been confirmed by electron microscopy.

Neurilemma. (Figs. 6-5, 6-6, 6-10.) Although some authorities prefer to separate the sheath external to the myelin into two layers, the sheath of Schwann and the neurilemma (also spelled neurolemma), the terms will be used synonymously in this book. This covering is found on all peripheral nerves, whether myelinated or not. It is a delicate, transparent membrane composed of Schwann cells. Each of the latter contains a flattened, oval nucleus surrounded by protoplasm in which a Golgi net and mitochondria are found. The remainder of the cytoplasm extends in both directions along the fiber. In myelinated nerves, the edges of these cells dip into the nodes, there joining the edge of another Schwann cell (Figs. 6-6, 6-10.) Thus, there is one such cell per segment, the nucleus lying near the center of the internode. In nonmyelinated fibers, from one to a dozen axis cylinders may invaginate the surfaces of Schwann cells (Figs. 6-8, 6-9). This sheath not only is important for support but apparently is essential to the normal metabolism of the axon.

The descriptions of the myelin and neurilemma given above follow the established classical line. However, more recent evidence indicates that these two sheaths must be considered together, as a single unit. It is now clear that the myelin sheath (myelin lamella) is formed by the plasma membrane (neurilemma) of the Schwann cells

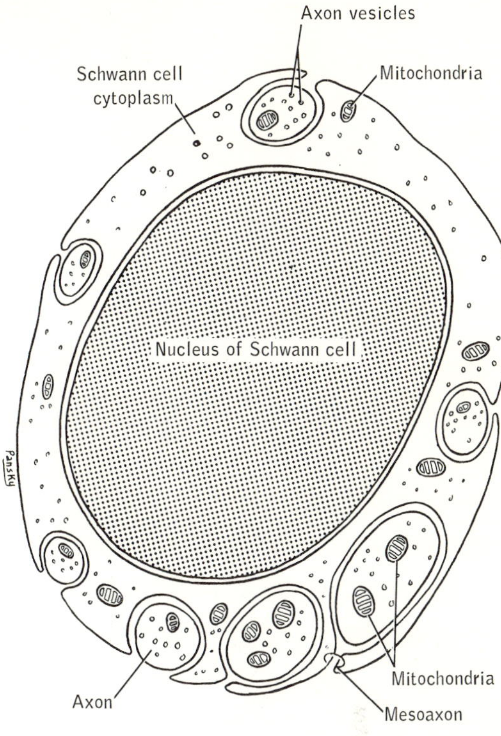

Fig. 6-9. Diagrammatic representation of an electron micrograph illustrating the relations of unmyelinated fibers to a single Schwann cell.

(neurolemma). In the process of myelination, the first step appears to be the settling of a naked axon into a groove on the Schwann cell surface. Gradually, the cytoplasm and plasma membranes of the latter completely envelop the axon. Where the two enveloping cell ends meet along the opposite side of the axon, a double-layered membrane, the mesaxon, is formed. If the fiber is to remain unmyelinated, several axons may thus "invaginate" a single Schwann cell. If myelination is to occur, there is a one to one relationship between axon and Schwann cell. After the stage of envelopment, there follows a growth and elongation of the mesaxon which spirals around the axon—the "jelly roll" effect. At first the coils of the mesaxon are separated from each other by neurolemma cytoplasm. However, in time, this layer is almost completely obliterated so that the inner surfaces of the Schwann cell

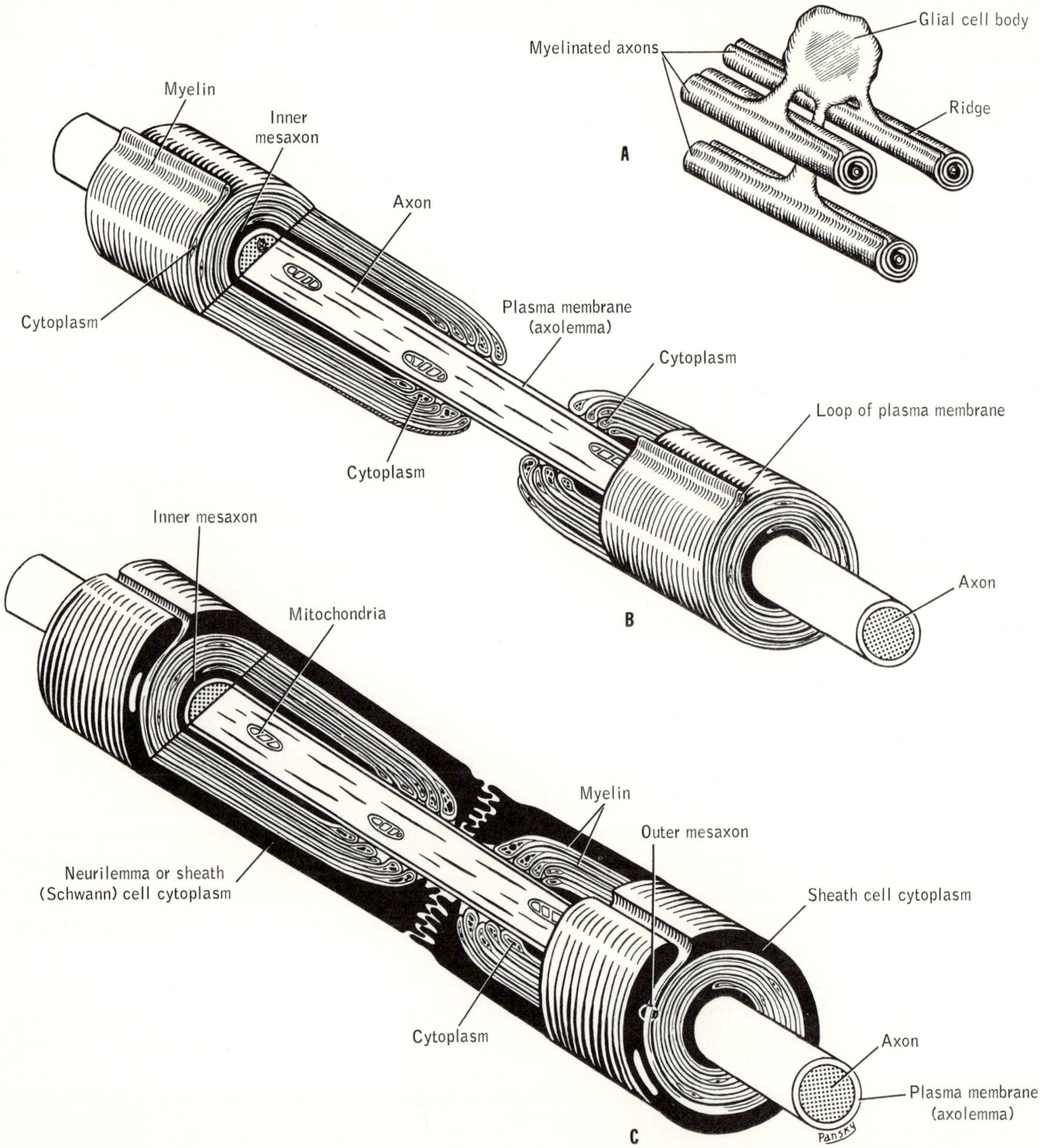

Fig. 6-10. *A.* Myelin-glial relationship in the central nervous system. *B.* Myelinated fiber in the central nervous system. The inner mesaxon completes its initial turn around the axon. Small regions of cytoplasm are occasionally trapped in the layers of laminated myelin. C. Myelinated fiber in the peripheral nervous system.

membrane are in close contact. The fusion of these membranes becomes the dense line of the definitive myelin sheath. Where the outer or contact surfaces fuse is represented by the intermediate (intraperiod) line of mature myelin. If it is assumed that the unit membrane of the Schwann cell consists of a bimolecular layer of lipids with their polar groups overlaid by proteins, this would account for the fact that adult myelin is seen to consist of many lamellae made up of two bimolecular leaves of lipid sandwiching a protein monolayer.

Endoneurium. (Figs. 6-5, 6-6.) This consists of fine strands of connective tissue which extend

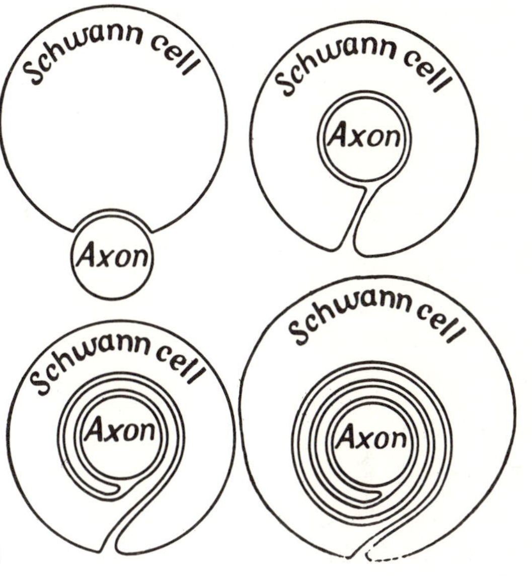

A

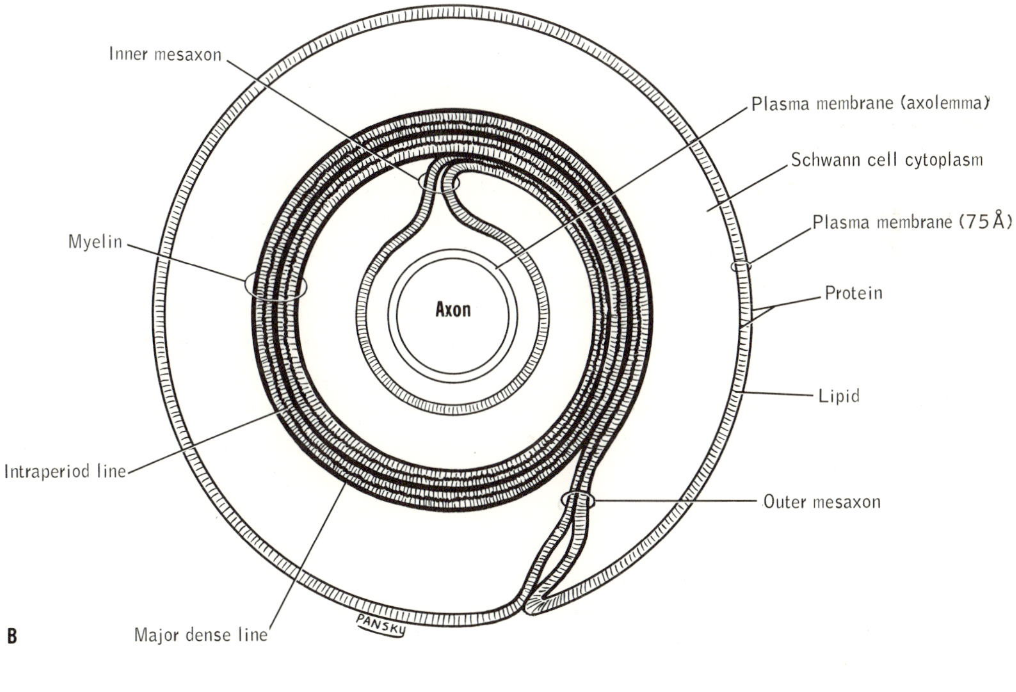

B

Fig. 6-11. *A.* Diagram to show the "jelly-roll" hypothesis of myelination. (*Courtesy of B. Geren-Uzman in Maximow and Bloom: A Textbook of Histology, 7th ed., W. B. Saunders Co., Philadelphia, 1957.*) *B.* Diagram of an electron micrograph showing the relations of myelin to the Schwann cell. The plasma membrane (unit membrane) of the Schwann cell consists of outer and inner layers of protein separated by lipids. The major dense lines are formed by the fusion of the inner layers of the plasma membrane after the cytoplasm is squeezed out of the cell during rotation about the axon.

inward to fill the spaces between individual nerve fibers. Some histologists describe an extremely delicate network of connective tissue filaments, the sheath of Henle, derived from the endoneurium, which surrounds each fiber and may actually be attached to the neurilemma. The sheath of Henle is also called the *neurolemma* or the sheath of *Key and Retzius.*

Perineurium. (Fig. 6-5.) This is a connective tissue sheath located external to the endoneurium which surrounds groups of nerve fibers, thus dividing the entire nerve into bundles or fascicles. In the course of a given nerve there apparently is much communication between fascicles where nerve fibers pass from one to another. It also appears that individual nerve fibers may branch within fascicles.

Epineurium. (Fig. 6-5.) The entire nerve trunk is surrounded by this covering of dense connective tissue.

The Ganglia

Definition

A ganglion is an aggregation of neuron cell bodies outside the CNS.

Classification

Ganglia are divided into two major classes, sensory and motor.

Sensory Ganglia. These are described as belonging to two groups: spinal or cranial. The spinal ganglia, also called dorsal or posterior root ganglia, are found on the posterior roots of the spinal nerves. Certain of the cranial nerves—V, VII, VIII, IX, and X—have cell bodies in cranial ganglia located near the attachment of the nerves to the brain stem.

Motor Ganglia. These are part of the autonomic nervous system. Here originate all the fibers which terminate in the heart, glands, or smooth muscle (Chap. 15).

Structure of the Ganglia

Sensory. The cell bodies in such ganglia, except those in cranial nerve VIII, which are bipolar, are all of the monopolar type. The nucleus is round and large with a distinct nucleolus. The cytoplasm contains finely granular Nissl substance. The cells themselves tend to be peripherally placed in the ganglion. Each nerve cell is surrounded by a single layer of flattened cells which form a capsule (Fig. 6-12). Because of this arrangement, the term *satellite* is sometimes applied to them. Actually, the capsule cells become continuous with the sheath of Schwann down along the single process of the nerve cell body. The internal (central) portion of the ganglion is occupied by myelinated fibers. The fibrous coverings of the peripheral nerve are continued on to the ganglion. The epineurium, in particular, forms a dense connective tissue capsule for the ganglion.

Motor. The cell bodies are multipolar. When compared with dorsal root ganglia, the cells look smaller, with nuclei which "seem" eccentric and are more scattered throughout the ganglion. Because these cells have many dendrites their capsules may appear to be incomplete or lacking. Both myelinated and nonmyelinated fibers are present.

FUNCTION

Activation of the Neuron

The nerve impulse is the unit of response (or activity) of the neuron. Under physiologic conditions, the neuron is activated either by a stimulus applied to a receptor and transmitted toward the cell body, or by a stimulus applied to it by another activated neuron.

Mechanism of Transmission of the Impulse (Membrane Theory) (Fig. 6-13.)

The membrane of the nerve cell body, together with the axolemma, is the seat of an electromotive force which is responsible for the resting potential of the cell. This potential is determined by the properties of the membrane, which maintains an ionic distribution within the cell different from that of the surrounding media (tissue fluid). That is, the membrane is polarized, but when it is at rest there is no longitudinal flow of

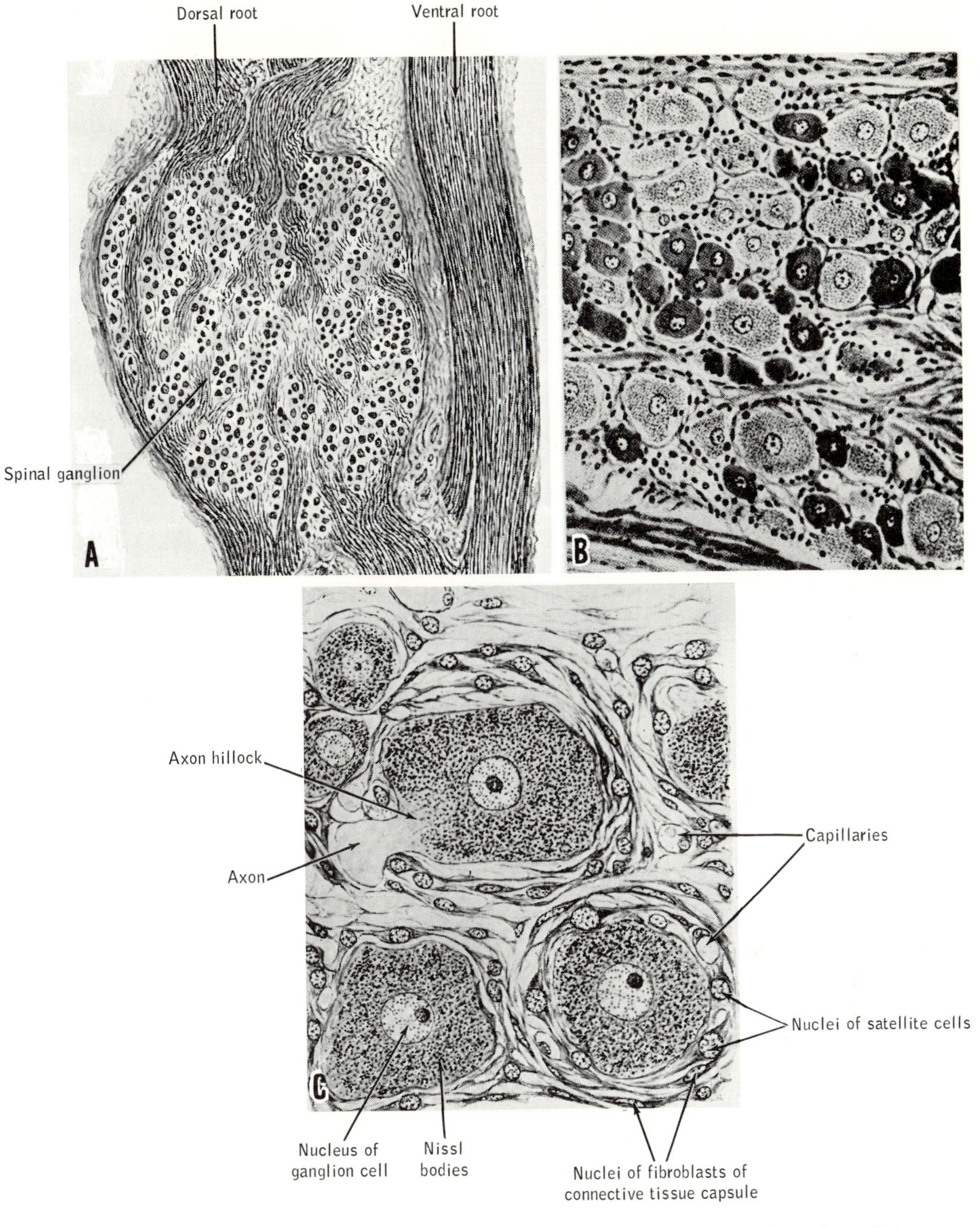

Fig. 6-12. A. Low power photomicrograph of a spinal nerve showing the relationship of the ganglion to the dorsal and ventral roots. *B.* A higher power photomicrograph through the peripheral part of a dorsal root ganglion showing variations in cell size and in the density of the Nissl substance. C. A high power photomicrograph of several ganglion cells.

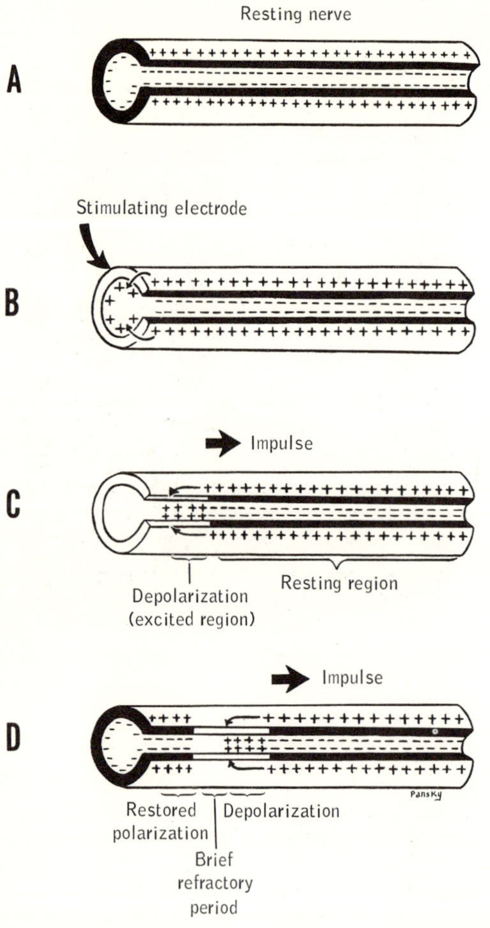

Fig. 6-13. Diagram to illustrate the membrane theory of nerve conduction.

current, since the potential is the same along all parts of the axolemma. When a stimulus is applied to the nerve, a breakdown occurs on the membrane at the point of application which locally abolishes the membrane charge (depolarizes). Thus, a difference in potential between the depolarized point and the surrounding, normal regions is created. This "draws" the charge from the adjacent polarized region of the membrane, causing it to become depolarized, while the initial point regains its polarity. This leads to the formation of a local current. This process spreads along the entire length of the fiber. Thus, the impulse is said to be a "self-propagating, depolarization wave." It is also spoken of as a wave of negativity, since the depolarized point is negative to the inactive, polarized region. It is thought possible that a chemical substance, acetylcholine, may play a part in conduction of the impulse by altering ionic permeability of the nerve membrane, particularly to ions of sodium and potassium.

Refractory Period

The passage of an impulse is followed by a refractory period considered to have two parts: the first is absolute, the second relative. In the absolute period no stimulus whatever can elicit a response. In the relative refractory period an impulse is started, but a stronger-than-usual stimulus is required to produce it. The duration of these refractory periods varies with the size and structure of the fiber but is of the order of milliseconds.

Frequency

The frequency of transmission along a fiber depends upon the absolute refractory period. Thus, the action current flowing along the neuron is discontinuous. It has been shown that these currents pass with frequencies of from 5 to 50 per second, but they have been recorded at rates of 100 per second.

Strength

The strength of the nerve impulse is not dependent upon the strength of the activating stimulus. It has been demonstrated to follow the all-or-none law. In other words, a stimulus strong enough to activate the neuron is strong enough to produce an impulse of maximum strength for the condition of the fiber at that time.

Rate

The rate of transmission is directly related to both the diameter of the axon and the thickness of the myelin. The speed of conduction has been found to vary from a fraction of a meter in small fibers to 120 meters per second in the largest. Conduction has also been found to be slower in unmyelinated fibers.

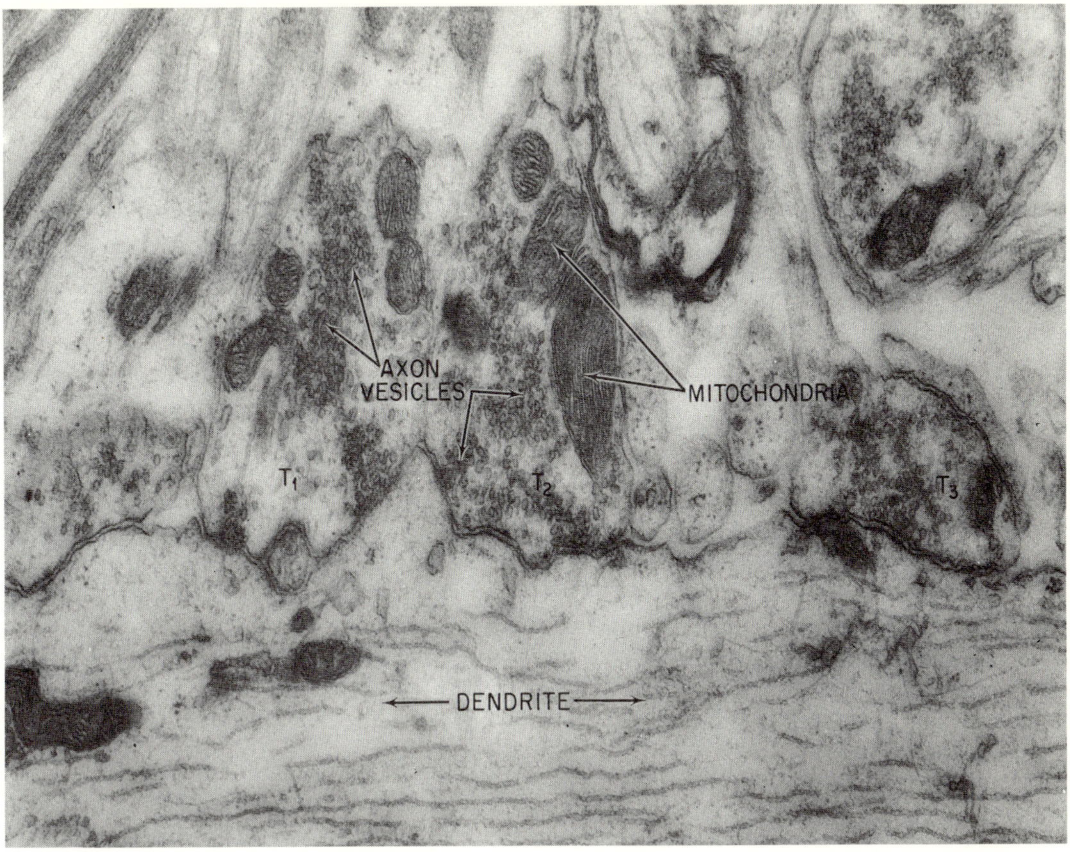

Fig. 6-14. Electron micrograph (×43,000 through axodendritic synapse. Three axon terminals (telodendria T_1, T_2, T_3) are seen in upper part of figure. Note that the axon terminals have many mitochondria and numerous small vesicles. The opposing synaptic membranes, consisting of the membrane of the axon and the membrane of the dendrite, are separated by a narrow space only about 200A in width. (*Courtesy of S. Palay, in Maximow and Bloom, A Textbook of Histology, 7th ed., W. B. Saunders Company, Philadelphia, 1957.*)

Influence of Environment on Excitability

The properties of excitability and conductivity of a nerve can be greatly altered by the chemical composition of the surrounding fluid. This is particularly true of the concentrations of sodium and calcium. For example, a calcium-free solution increases excitability, while increased calcium reduces excitability. Prolonged treatment in low-calcium or calcium-free solution actually leads to spontaneous neuron activity. Clinically, increased nervous excitability, called *tetany,* is observed in cases of calcium deficiency.

Transmission of Impulses from Neuron to Neuron or to Muscle (Figs. 6-14, 6-15, 6-16.)

The transfer of impulses from neuron to neuron occurs across the synapse which may take many forms. Their ultrastructure has recently been revealed through electron microscopy. First, whether the synapse occurs between axon and dendrite or axon and cell body, their structure is similar. Basically, the two plasma membranes are separated by a gap ranging from 60 to 200 Å. In some instances, peculiar electron-dense areas may be seen in the gap. Sometimes one or both of the membranes show zones of increased density. The termination of the axon enlarges and shows groups of small vesicles which measure from 300 to 500 Å. These are the synaptic vesicles. In some terminals, larger vesicles measuring up to 1,000 Å are found and these contain a dense substance in their centers. When these appear at the ends of autonomic fibers, they are thought to be concerned with the catecholamines. Small mitochondria are also observed.

The passage of impulses from neuron to muscle occurs across the myoneural junction. The electron microscope has also revealed the ultimate details of these junctions. Fundamentally, the axon terminal is much the same as described at the synapse except that small granular elements and tube-like components of the endoplasmic reticulum appear in the axoplasm. Contrary to earlier beliefs, the nerve termination does not lie within the sarcoplasm but rather in deep grooves (synaptic gutter) formed by the infolding of the sarcolemma. There is actually a small gap (synaptic gap) between the opposing axolemma and sarcolemma. In the depths of the grooves numerous invaginations of the sarcoplasm are found. The entire myoneural ending is covered by the cytoplasm of Schwann cells. However, the neurolemma, axolemma and sarcolemma are never fused but remain separated by gaps which are said to be filled by "gap substance" which some have likened to basement membrane material. This substance extends out into the extracellular space surrounding the ending.

There is a difference of opinion as to just how transmission is accomplished, but it is agreed that flow occurs in one direction only: in the synapse, from the axon of one neuron to the dendrites or cell body of another; in the myoneural junction, from the axon of a neuron to the muscle. There are two major theories concerning this problem of transmission: electrical and chemical.

Electrical

According to this theory, the second neuron or the muscle fiber is stimulated in a manner similar to that described in the membrane theory.

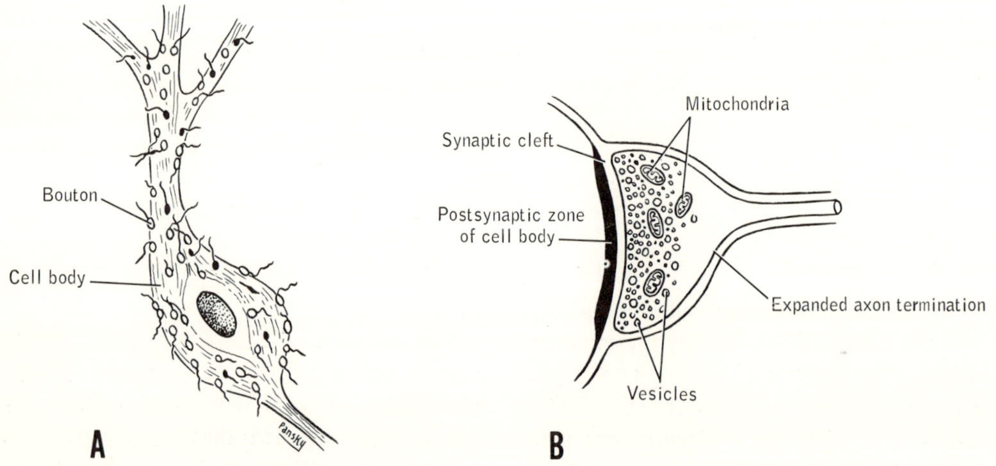

Fig. 6-15. *A.* Enlarged cell body showing the neuropodia or boutons of other neurons in a typical synaptic relationship. *B.* Diagram of an electron micrograph through a bouton showing the expanded axon termination with its mitochondria and vesicles. The postsynaptic zone of the cell is also shown.

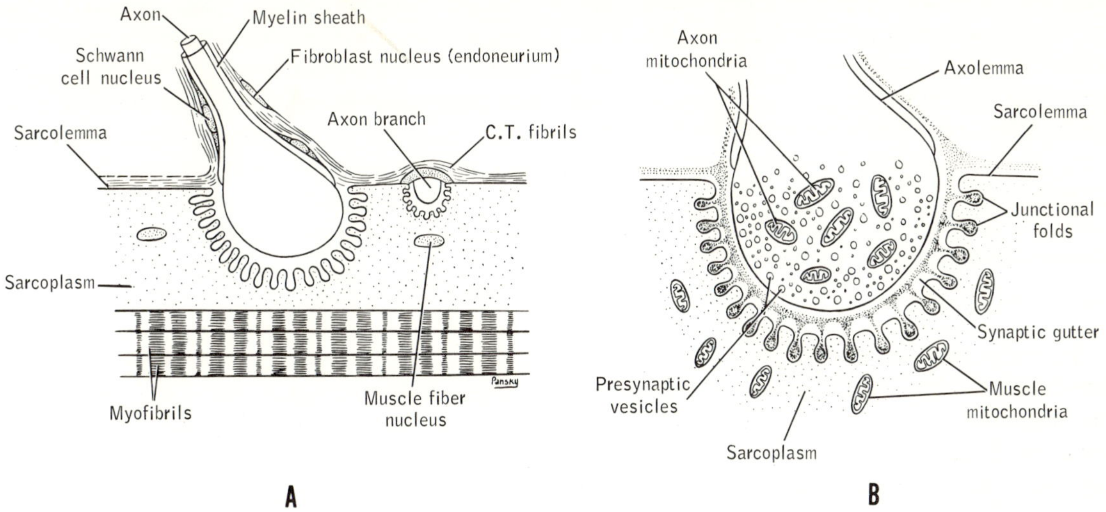

Fig. 6-16. *A.* Diagram of a motor nerve ending on skeletal muscle as observed through the electron microscope. The myelin is seen to end just before the axon reaches the muscle fiber. Schwann cells end at the same point except for "teloglia" which continue onto branches of the axon. Axon branches are seen to lie in invaginations of the sarcolemma known as "synaptic gutters" or primary synaptic clefs. *B.* Enlarged diagram showing greater details at the synaptic junction. The space between axon and sarcolemma contains an amorphous material which is continuous with the basement membrane substance around the muscle.

Chemical

Transmission occurs as a result of the liberation of chemical substances around the termination of the activated axons. There are thought to be two such substances: acetylcholine and sympathin (Chap. 15).

It is also possible that under physiologic conditions, these two processes are combined. Thus, acetylcholine is liberated at the end of the presynaptic fiber or at the end of an efferent neuron. This leads to the creation of electrical currents. The currents cross the synaptic "space" to reach the membrane of the postsynaptic neuron or muscle. As a result, acetylcholine is formed there, causing a change in permeability of the postsynaptic membrane which leads to the setting up of action currents in the second neuron or muscle. Enzymes such as acetylcholinesterase appear to be necessary for this process.

CLINICAL CONSIDERATIONS

Since both central and peripheral neurons are frequently interrupted through trauma, the problems of degeneration and regeneration are important to the clinician.

Degeneration and Regeneration of Neurons in the CNS

It is well-established that as long as the neuron cell body is alive all the processes still attached to it will also live. Further, since protoplasmic synthesis is continually going on, such processes are capable of growth. Thus, axis cylinders interrupted through trauma should theoretically once more reach the destination formerly attained by the damaged axon. However, certain difficulties arise which, as yet, have proved insurmountable. First, when the axis cylinder is cut, the myelin insulation surrounding that portion of the axon lying distal to the point of interruption disintegrates along with the axon itself. Secondly, the processes of the supporting neuroglia soon fill the space once occupied by the fiber and its sheath, becoming such a dense tangle that it is impossible for new growth to get through.

Degeneration of Neurons in the PNS

Nerve Damage

In nerve damage, certain points of reference are important. First, the location of the site where the nerve is interrupted must be determined; second, the location of the cell bodies of the damaged neurons should be established. Two terms are used in connection with nerve interruption. The first of these is *proximal portion,* used when speaking of that portion of the nerve still attached to the cell body between the CNS and the site of the trauma. The second is *distal* or *peripheral,* referring to that portion of the severed nerve which is no longer attached to the cell body, lying between the cut and the peripheral termination of the nerve. With these concepts in mind, it is now possible to classify degeneration into two types: retrograde and Wallerian.

Retrograde Degeneration. (Fig. 6-17.) This usually involves the proximal few millimeters of a severed nerve closely adjoining the site of trauma. The extent of degeneration toward the CNS is to some degree determined by the nature of the wound. When the site of trauma lies close to the cell body, the latter may also become involved in degenerative changes which eventually result in death of the cell. In any event, one should recall the "axon reaction" which occurs when nerve fibers are damaged, the degree of reaction diminishing as the injury site approaches the periphery. At any time, there is a small amount of breakdown in both axis cylinder and myelin. The Schwann cells comprising the neurilemma remain alive and may actually proliferate.

Wallerian Degeneration. (Fig. 6-17.) This involves the entire length of the distal portion of the severed nerve. The axis cylinder, cut off from its metabolic center, soon dies. Actually, within a few days, the axon consists merely of scattered debris. Furthermore, it is equally certain that disintegration of the axon will lead to the disappearance of myelin. This disappearance occurs a little more slowly, although changes have been observed within 24 hours after injury. The Schwann cells remain viable and even proliferate, forming a syncytium with longitudinally disposed slits. Phagocytes formed in the surrounding connective tissue pass through the spaces in the mesh to clean up fragments of disintegrated myelin and axons, after which they disappear. Thus, if the two ends of the severed nerve are close enough together, the neurilemma soon becomes once more continuous. Degeneration of the axis cylinders often has profound effects upon the end organs supplied by them. In the case of somatic motor fibers to skeletal muscle, nerve death leads to complete atrophy of the muscle fibers. Certain sensory receptors are also affected. This is especially true of the taste buds on the tongue, which degenerate almost immediately after denervation.

Degrees of Nerve Injury

Although nerve injuries have been classified according to the severity of the damage, only a brief and general discussion will be attempted here.

First Degree. This is usually due to pressure strong enough to prevent action currents from passing into the part of the nerve fiber distal to the point of applied pressure. There is no degeneration.

Second Degree. This is also usually due to pressure, but here the axon has been destroyed at the point of pressure and all the axons distal to that point degenerate. All the supporting structures remain intact. The term *axonotmesis* is applied to this phenomenon.

Third, Fourth, or Fifth Degrees. In each of these degrees of injury, the axon is completely severed, together with variable amounts of its supporting structure. For this type of injury the general term *neurotmesis* is often used. In third-

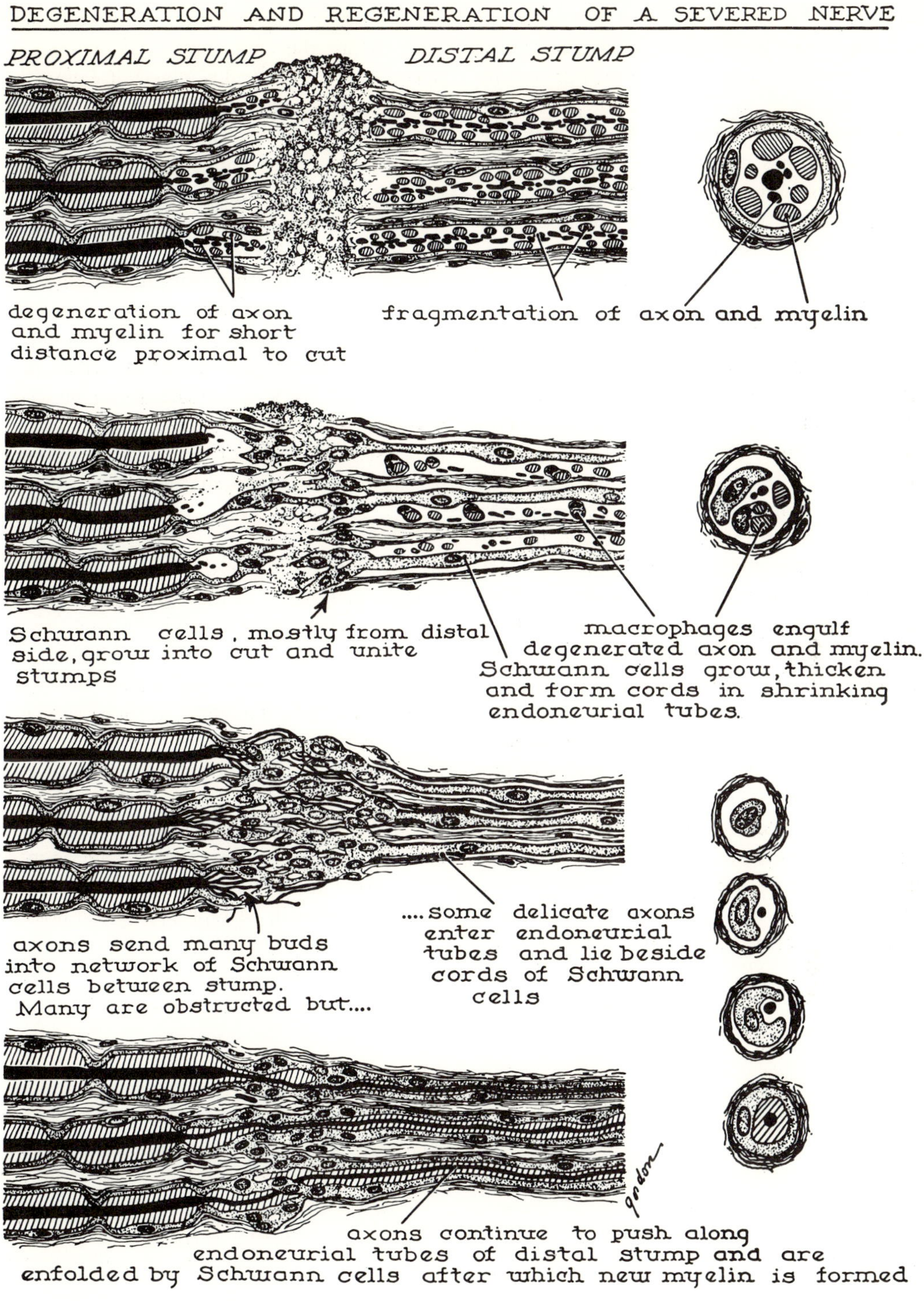

Fig. 6-17. Diagram showing the changes that occur in a nerve when it is severed and regenerates. (*From Ham, Histology, 3d ed., J. B. Lippincott Company, Philadelphia, 1957.*)

degree cases, the injury involves not only the axon but also the endoneurium, the fascicles of the nerve being still intact. In fourth-degree injuries, the fascicles are also severed. In fifth-degree injuries, the entire nerve trunk, including the epineurium, has been cut through.

Any of these injuries will lead to at least a temporary loss of sensation in the area of distribution of the involved nerve and to paralysis of the muscles supplied by it.

Regeneration of Neurons in the PNS

Axons still attached to their cell bodies are viable and capable of growth. Unlike the discouraging situation encountered in the CNS, the possibility of restoring function to the peripheral nerve is greater for several reasons. First, the presence of significant connective tissue sheaths makes it possible to bring together and hold in approximation the cut ends of the nerve. Next, the fact that debris from degeneration has been cleared away leaves a relatively open field. Further, the living, proliferating neurilemma has left channels through which growth of axons from the proximal portion can pass toward the end organ (Fig. 6-13). Under good conditions, growth is said to occur at the rate of 1 to 2 mm per day. The rate of growth of the regenerating fiber, directly related to axoplasmic flow, is influenced by many factors, including the abovementioned degrees of injury.

One should not be misled into believing that regeneration described above will eventually result in 100 per cent return of normal function. Such is not the case, since even when severed nerve ends are carefully joined, it cannot be expected that each axon will find its own proper path. Thus, many may be wasted by going to the wrong type of end organ. Fortunately, this waste may be to some extent circumvented by the fact that growing axis cylinders tend to form many branches as they pass through the maze of slits in the neurilemma. Another disadvantage is the tendency of connective tissue to overproliferate when damaged. Thus, there is the everpresent possibility that fibroblasts which produce collagenous fibers will create a scar between the severed ends. Scar formation can be minimized by close, firm union of the severed ends and the use of measures to combat possible infection.

Nerve Grafts

The nature of the damaging agent and the longitudinal extent of the traumatized area influence regeneration. Occasionally, an area of a nerve is damaged to such an extent that the two ends cannot be joined. An area of a nerve may even be deleted completely. In such cases, a piece of nerve taken from a storage bank or removed from the body of someone who died recently is sutured in to close the gap. It should be understood that this is a "scaffold graft" which will act as a bridge over which axons may pass to reach the neurilemma in its own distal portion. Gradually, the graft will be replaced by the host's own tissue.

SUMMARY

- Neuron
  - Components
    - Cell body
      - Cytoplasm
        - Mitochondria
        - Neuroplasm
        - Neurofibrils
        - Golgi
        - Nissl substance
        - Cell membrane
      - Nucleus
        - Nucleoplasm
        - Chromatin
        - Nucleolus
        - Nuclear membrane
    - Processes
      - Axon
        - Axolemma
        - Neurofibrils
        - Axoplasm
      - Dendrites
        - Same as in cytoplasm
  - Classification
    - Morphologic
      - Number of processes
        - Monopolar
        - Bipolar
        - Multipolar
      - Axon length
        - Golgi I (long)
        - Golgi II (short)
    - Physiologic (functional)
      - Afferent
      - Efferent
      - Internuncial (associational)
  - Coverings
    - Myelin
    - Neurilemma
    - Endoneurium
    - Perineurium
    - Epineurium
- Ganglia
  - Components
    - Cell bodies outside CNS
  - Classification
    - Sensory
      - Cranial
      - Spinal
    - Motor
      - Autonomic
- Support
  - CNS
    - Glia
      - Astrocyte
        - Fibrous
        - Protoplasmic
      - Oligodendroglia
      - Microglia
    - Myelin
  - PNS
    - Same as coverings for neuron

7 FUNCTIONAL CLASSIFICATION OF SYSTEMS AND REFLEXES

It is essential to have a definite understanding of the descriptive terms used in connection with the functional components of the nerves and the systems to which they belong.

SYSTEMS

Afferent (A)

Afferent means that the conduction current is traveling toward the brain or spinal cord. The terms *afferent* and *sensory* are often used synonymously. However, in the strict sense of the word, sensory implies consciousness. Thus, not all afferent impulses can be classed as sensory, since many of them never reach the level of consciousness. The letter "A" will be used to designate afferent.

Afferent fibers are placed in three major categories, depending upon the region where the impulse originates: somatic, visceral, or proprioceptive.

Somatic (S)

This term can be thought of as pertaining to the framework of the body as distinguished from the viscera or organs. Embryologically, it is concerned with those parts derived from the somatopleure. Thus, somatic afferents carry information concerning changes in the external environment. The letter "S" will be used for somatic.

The somatic afferent fibers are of two principal classes, general and special.

General (G). This refers to those impulses which begin at or near the body surface. The letter "G" will be used for general.

Within the *GSA* system are three sensory modalities or types of sensation. In other words, three different environmental changes can be detected by receptors: *pain; temperature,* both warm and cold; and *touch.* The latter is often regarded as being of two sorts: *light touch,* requiring stimulation by very slight surface changes, and *deep touch,* which is synonymous with pressure. This requires stronger stimulation to activate the receptors, most of which lie in the deeper tissues below the surface.

Special (S). The receptors in this case are highly specialized. Instead of having the widespread distribution of the general receptors, they are concentrated in relatively small areas or organs, no longer located directly on the surface. They are usually contained within a framework of nonnervous tissue and are often associated with accessory structures (as in the eye and ear) which may enhance or modify the stimulation. Another characteristic of the organs of special sense is that they are activated by environmental changes which may occur at some distance from the receptor. The letter "S" will serve as an abbreviation for special.

Within the *SSA* system are two modalities: *vision,* the stimuli for which are short, high-frequency waves called light; *hearing,* for which the stimuli are long, low-frequency waves known as sound.

Visceral (V)

This term implies afferent impulses arising in or around the viscera. These impulses are essential in the reflex regulation of all visceral activity. The letter "V" is used for visceral afferents, which are also described as being of two sorts, general and special.

General (G). These receptors are found in or on mucous membranes and in the walls of most organs.

The *GVA* system carries impulses which arise as a result of physical or chemical composition of the substances contained within the organ and the amount of distention of their walls.

Special (S). There is no general agreement among neuroanatomists as to the existence of this category. However, the receptors for this system do answer, at least in part, the structural and functional requirements of organs of special sense. The stimuli are chemical in nature, and the impulses initiated by these substances have profound effects upon the activity of certain organs.

The *SVA* category also includes two modalities: *taste,* whose receptors are taste buds located chiefly on the dorsum of the tongue and inside the cheeks and lips, as well as on the palate and pharynx; *smell,* the olfactory receptors being found in the roof of the nasal cavity.

Proprioception (P)

The division of the afferent system designated as proprioceptive is peculiar in many respects. Although its receptors often lie deep in the body tissue and, in this respect, are similar to visceral receptors, this system is concerned not with the internal adjustment of viscera but with the position and movement of the body. The letter "P" will symbolize this system.

General (G). The receptors for this system are widely dispersed throughout the body: in muscles, together with their fasciae; in tendons; and in or around articular capsules.

The *GP* system prossesses receptors of the pressure or tension type, activated by changes in tension of muscles or tendons and by movements at joints. In general, the activity of this system takes place outside consciousness, the impulses making possible normal walking, balancing (in part), regulation of head position, and the adjustment of the proper amount of muscle contraction to perform a specific act.

Special (S). The receptors for this system are in the inner ear, particularly in the ampullae of the semicircular canals, the utricle, and the saccule.

The *SP* system consists of a group of cells related to a fluid medium in such a way that the slightest movement of the head will cause a current to flow, thus stimulating the receptors. Impulses beginning here carry information concerning the position of the head at rest; any changes in position of the head; and the plane in which movement occurs.

Efferent (E)

Efferent impulses originate in the CNS and flow outward, away from the brain or spinal cord. The term *motor* can justly be applied to this system, since its conduction currents result in activity.

Somatic (S)

The tissue activated through these motor fibers is skeletal muscle which traces its origin to the embryonic somites. As in the afferent systems, the letter "S" will be used as a symbol for somatic.

General (G). Since there is no "special" category, the use of the term "general" in this connection is almost superfluous. However, since the terminations of all these fibers lie in the motor end-plates of skeletal muscle derived from somites, and since they have a very general distribution, the term is not inappropriate.

In the *GSE* system, most of the efferent fibers originate in the ventral gray columns of the spinal cord, pass through the ventral roots, join the spinal nerve trunks, and run directly to the myoneural junction (motor end-plate) of skeletal muscle. Fibers of this system also originate in the nuclei of cranial nerves III, IV, VI, and XII, the first three supplying the extrinsic muscles of the eye, the last innervating the muscles of the tongue.

Visceral (V)

This is a system of efferent fibers the conduction current of which activates organs. The letter "V" will be used to designate visceral.

The visceral motor division consists of two parts, a general and special.

General (G). The distribution of these fibers is widespread; they pass to all smooth muscle, to cardiac muscle, and to all glands.

The *GVE* system is concerned with the maintenance of body homeostasis, including the regulation of heart rate and blood pressure; temperature; glandular secretion; peristalsis; sphincter tension; and pupil size.

Special (S). This group of fibers has a relatively small distribution. Peculiarly enough, the tissue activated is, histologically, typical striated muscle. However, this muscle is not derived from somites but from the embryonic branchial arches.

The muscles innervated by the *SVE* system include those of facial expression; of mastication; of the pharynx and larynx. Since these muscles are actually related to the rostral end of certain visceral systems, the digestive and respiratory, and to such organs of special sense as the eye and ear, the term visceral is applicable to them. The cells of origin for these efferent fibers lie in groups or nuclei in the special visceral efferent column limited to the brain stem and send their impulses out over certain of the cranial nerves (V, VII, IX, X, XI).

REFLEXES

Although reflex arcs have been previously defined and their parts described, it is frequently useful to classify reflexes according to the functional systems which form the limbs of these arcs. Thus, the afferent components may be either somatic or visceral. The efferent limbs may be similarly grouped. Therefore, the entire mechanism may be described in terms of variable combinations of these functional systems, for example: *somatosomatic,* where the afferent limbs belong to the GSA or SSA systems while the efferent limbs are part of the GSE apparatus. In like fashion the other reflexes may be designated. The *somatovisceral,* where the sensory limb is again either GSA or SSA, utilizes fibers belonging to either the GVE or SVE system for its efferent limb. In the *viscerosomatic* type, the receptors lie in or around viscera and send their impulses over fibers belonging to either the GVA or SVA system while the effectors are skeletal muscles of the trunk, limbs, eyes, or tongue supplied by way of GSE fibers. In *viscerovisceral* reflexes, the afferent limbs are in the GVA or SVA systems and the efferent limbs are a part of the GVE or SVE apparatus. In this text, some of the above designations are occasionally prefaced with the term *general* or *special.* By this means the efferent limb is further characterized. Thus, general somatovisceral means that the motor component of the arc belongs to the autonomic system (GVE) and involves smooth muscle, glands, or heart muscle. A special somatovisceral reflex would be one in which the muscles of branchial arch origin are activated through the SVE fibers.

SUMMARY

I. Neurons
- *A.* Afferent
  1. Somatic
     - *a.* General—pain, temperature, touch
     - *b.* Special—hearing, vision
  2. Visceral
     - *a.* General—organ content and distention
     - *b.* Special—taste, smell
  3. Proprioception
     - *a.* General—muscle, tendon, joint capsule
     - *b.* Special—equilibrium
- *B.* Efferent
  1. Somatic
     - *a.* General—to skeletal muscle of somite origin
     - *b.* Special—none

2. Visceral
   a. General—smooth muscle, heart, glands
   b. Special—to muscles of branchiomeric origin

II. Reflexes
   A. Somatosomatic: afferent, GSA or SSA; efferent, GSE
   B. Somatovisceral: afferent, GSA or SSA; efferent, GVE or SVE
      1. General somatovisceral: afferent, GSA or SSA; efferent, GVE
      2. Special somatovisceral: afferent, GSA or SSA; efferent, SVE
   C. Viscerosomatic: afferent, GVA or SVA; efferent, GSE
   D. Viscerovisceral: afferent, GVA or SVA; efferent, GVE or SVE

8 GENERAL SOMATIC AFFERENT SYSTEM (GSA)

PAIN AND TEMPERATURE

Trunk

Reflex Pathways (Fig. 8-1.)

Receptors. Pain appears early in phylogenesis at reflex levels. Pain receptors are the most primitive of all receptors, being naked, free, unembellished terminations of the peripheral nerve which have sprayed out among the epithelial cells of the epidermis and are distributed quite uniformly over the body surface.

Temperature mechanisms also differentiate early. The probable receptors, the bulbs of Krause for cold and the organs of Ruffini for warmth, consist of nerve endings covered with a capsule of some complexity. These receptors are located at various distances from the skin surface, in the dermis.

Afferent Neuron. Nerve fibers for both pain and temperature are of small caliber. Their cell bodies, lying in the dorsal root ganglia, are of the small, unipolar variety. As the central process of the afferent neuron approaches the *spinal cord,* it joins others belonging to the same system on the lateral side of the dorsal root of the spinal nerve and enters the dorsolateral fasciculus (Lissauer's tract). Within this fasciculus, each fiber bifurcates into an ascending and descending branch. Unlike the fibers belonging to other systems, these branches are very short, the longest probably ascending no more than two segments. Each branch gives off collaterals which terminate, together with the main branches, in that portion of the dorsal gray column nearest to the fasciculus, the *substantia gelatinosa* (Fig. 3-4). Herein lie the cell bodies for both the associational neurons and the secondary neurons in the circuit to consciousness.[1]

Associational Neuron. Associational neurons in the reflex arcs are numerous. However, because of their diverse courses, scattered throughout the reticular formation rather than accumulated in distinct bundles, their very existence, let alone their exact positions, has never been proved experimentally. Therefore, in many instances it must be admitted that the reflexes described are purely hypothetic, suppositions being based almost exclusively on observed reactions. Some of these neurons pass from the substantia gelatinosa at one level, through the fasciculus proprius, to the dorsal column at other levels. Such connections may occur many times. Eventually, some of these associational neurons will make contact with secondary neurons in a conscious pathway at a point far removed from the level of original entry.

In addition to the strictly intersegmental con-

[1] Some investigators believe that collaterals or terminals of the first order neurons end in both the substantia gelatinosa and the proper sensory nucleus. On this basis, the latter nucleus gives rise to the second order neuron in the pathway to consciousness while the former is concerned mainly with the reflex mechanism.

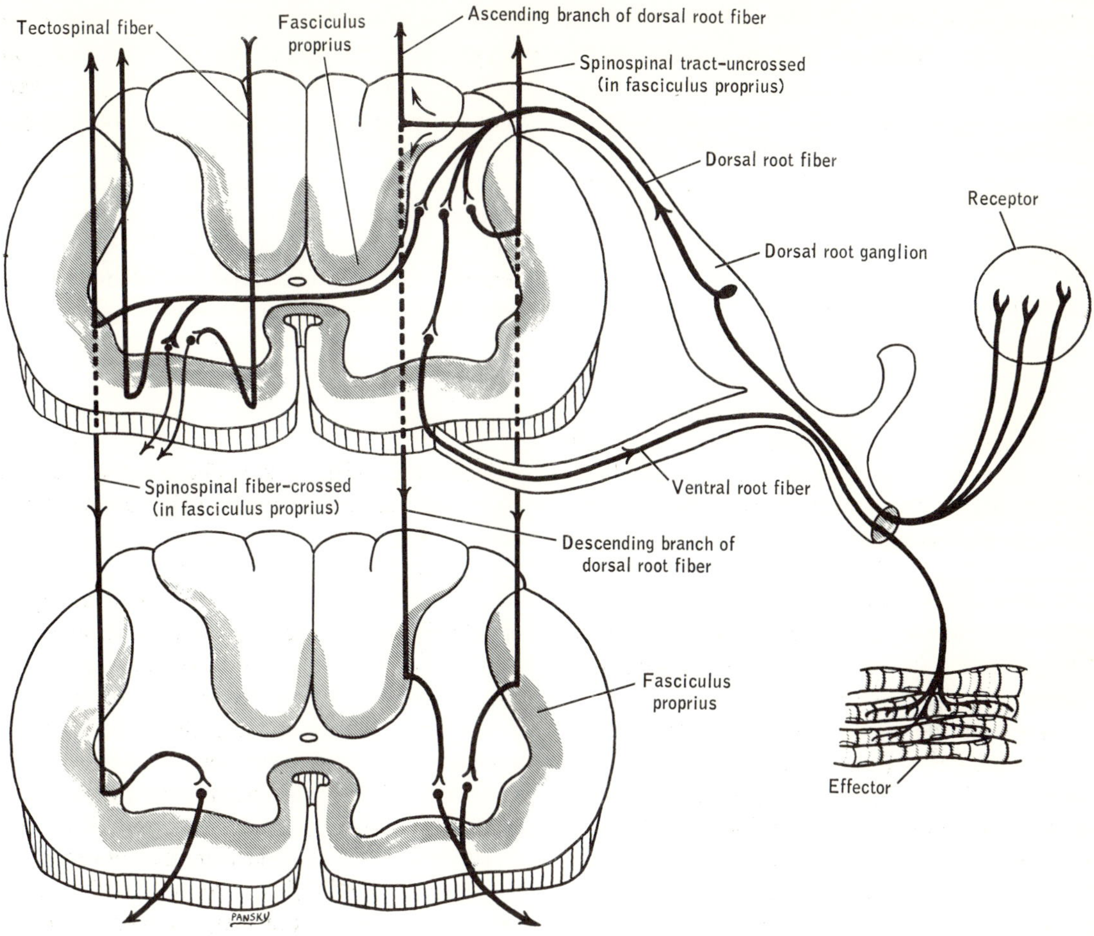

Fig. 8-1. Intersegmental (intraspinal) reflex connections.

nections, another circuit exists which implements reflex action for the *entire* body. In this pathway, axons from the substantia gelatinosa pass ventrally, cross the cord in the anterior gray commissure, enter the lateral funiculus of the opposite side, and bend rostrally to form a part of the *spinotectal tract* (Fig. 3-5). This tract ascends to the roof of the mesencephalon. From this region, a second associational neuron descends in the *tectospinal tract* (Chap. 9) to synapse around the primary motor cells in the anterior gray columns of the cord.

Efferent Neuron. Only the efferent neurons concerned with the somatosomatic and somatovisceral reflexes will be discussed here. In the former, associational neurons synapse with cells of the anterior gray columns of the cord. On activation of these cells, impulses leave the cord via the ventral roots of spinal nerves to end in the skeletal muscle of trunk and limbs (Chap. 14). In the somatovisceral type of reflex, the association fibers synapse in the intermediolateral gray columns of the cord. From here, efferent neurons pass ventrally and leave the cord with the ventral roots of the spinal nerve. Such efferent neurons eventually leave the main nerve trunk and terminate in various autonomic ganglia. Second efferent neurons arise in the latter ganglia and are distributed to smooth muscle, glands, and heart. Among the more commonly observed reflexes of this type are sweating, flushing, blanching, and the appearance of "goose flesh," all in response to raising or lowering the temperature; and sweating and dilation of the pupil in response to pain. Other such reflexes, e.g., changes in blood pressure, respiration rate, and heart rate, will be discussed later (Chap. 15).

Conscious Pathway (Fig. 8-2.)

Neuron I. This neuron, together with its receptors, is identical with the afferent neuron described under Reflex Pathways, above.

Neuron II. These neurons arise from cells in the substantial gelatinosa [1] very close to the level at which the primary fiber enters the cord. Each of the secondary fibers tends to cross the cord immediately. The crossing occurs just ventral and in close proximity to the central canal. After reaching the periphery of the lateral funiculus of the opposite side, these fibers bend rostrally in the *lateral spinothalamic tract* to terminate in the *posterolateral ventral nucleus* of the thalamus (Chap. 22). Within the tract there is a definite layering of fibers, those representing the most caudal regions of the body lying most lateral while those for more cephalic levels are more medial in position (Figs. 8-2, 8-3). It is also held that pain fibers are more ventral and somewhat medial than those fibers mediating temperature. In addition, some fibers of the spinothalamic tracts either terminate in or send collaterals into the reticular formation of the brain stem in both medulla and pons (Fig. 25-1). Further rostrally, before the spinothalamic fibers terminate in specific thalamic nuclei (i.e., posterolateral ventral nuclei), still others enter such nuclei as the medial intralaminar of the thalamus (Chap. 22). In any event, whether ascending all the way to the cortex in the reticular system through some as yet undetermined route or passing through the "diffuse thalamic system" (Chap. 22), they form an integral part of the so-called "reticular activating mechanism" of the cerebrum. Throughout its extent in both cord and brain stem, the lateral spinothalamic tract lies close to the lateral surface of the CNS. Those fibers which enter the tract from lower levels of the body are located most laterally in the tract and are, therefore, more superficial than fibers entering at progressively higher levels (Fig. 8-3).

Neuron III. From the posterolateral ventral nucleus of the thalamus, a third neuron arises which passes through the posterior limb of the internal capsule (Chap. 23) to terminate in the postcentral gyrus of the cerebrum.

Head

Reflex Pathways

Receptors. (Fig. 8-2.) The receptors are the same type as those found in the spinal mechanism.

Afferent Neuron. These occur in all divisions of the trigeminal nerve, their typical monopolar cells lying in the semilunar (Gasserian) ganglion. The central processes of these cells form a large part of the sensory root (portio major) of the nerve. After entering the brain stem, the primary pain and temperature fibers bend caudally to form a distinct bundle known as the spinal trigeminal (spinal V) tract (Figs. 8-3, 25-1 to 25-8). The latter extends from mid-pons as far caudally as the third or possibly fourth cervical segment, there merging with the dorsolateral fasciculus of the cord. Apparently, the fibers which comprise the spinal trigeminal tract are arranged according to their peripheral root of entry and also according to functional considerations. Thus, fibers from the ophthalmic division lie most ventrally in the tract and extend farthest caudally (C3 and C4); those from the maxillary division are more centrally placed, just posterior to fibers from the ophthalmic division and ending near the upper limit of C1; those from the mandibular division are most dorsal in the tract and extend caudally in the brain stem only to the level of the nucleus of the glossopharyngeal nerve. Regardless of root of entry, pain fibers lie more medially than do those for temperature. Within the spinal trigeminal tract, many collaterals arise; together with the terminals of all primary neurons, they enter

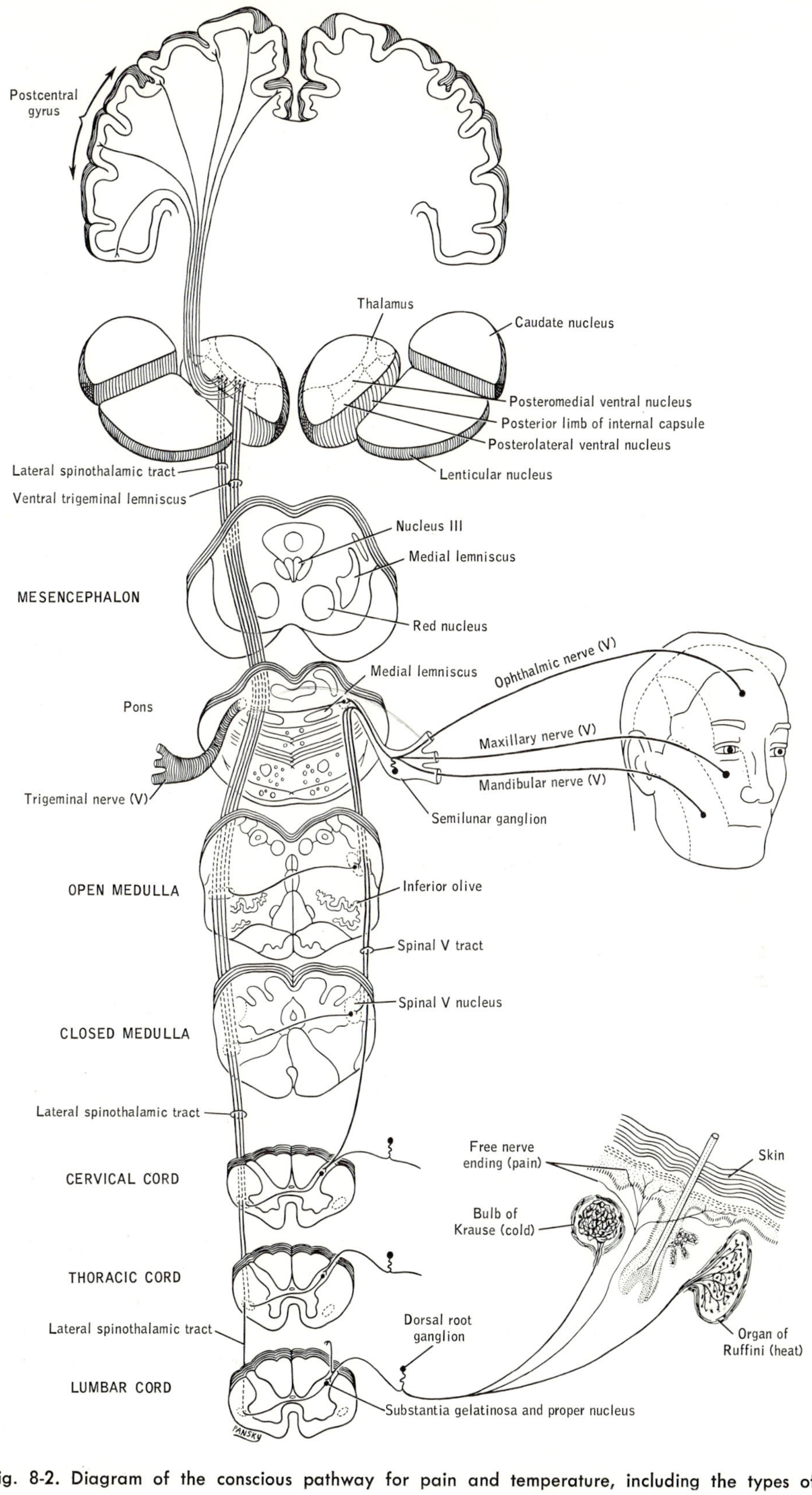

Fig. 8-2. Diagram of the conscious pathway for pain and temperature, including the types of

the elongated nuclear mass which adjoins the tract on its medial side. This nucleus, known as the *spinal* or *descending* nucleus, is continuous with the substantia gelatinosa of the cord and contains the cell bodies of both the associational neurons of the reflex circuit and the secondary neurons in the pathway to consciousness (Fig. 8-3).

Associational Neuron. These are given off along the entire medial and ventromedial borders of the spinal trigeminal nucleus. They pass into the surrounding reticular formation, where some of them aggregate into longitudinal bundles, passing cranially and caudally to synapse directly in the cranial motor nuclei. Others pass into the cord through the reticulospinal tract to end around cells of the anterior and intermediolateral columns. It is also believed that chains of associational neurons are formed from a series of synapses among the cells of the reticular formation, with eventual terminations similar to the direct route just described.

Efferent Neuron. For the *somatosomatic reflex,* the efferent limb for the trunk musculature is the same as that described above. An example of such a reflex reaction is striking at an insect which has stung the face. There are also somatosomatic reflexes which involve cranial nerves. In these cases, the efferent neuron leaves the brain by way of cranial nerves III, IV, VI, and XII. Such a reflex could be exemplified by the retraction of the tongue from a hot or cold object, or the movement of the eyes toward a site of injury on the face.

The *somatovisceral* reflex can be of two types, depending upon the origin of the efferent neuron. Those concerned with the general variety originate in the intermediolateral cell column of the cord or in the cranial autonomic nuclei. Efferent fibers for special somatovisceral reflexes have their cells in the nuclei of cranial nerves V, VII, IX, X, and XI, leaving the brain by way of these nerves. An example of this general type would be the dilation of the pupil resulting from a severe toothache; blinking the eye as a result of painful stimuli applied to the cornea exemplifies the special type.

Conscious Pathways (Figs. 8-2 to 8-4.)

Receptors. These are the same as those described under Reflex Pathways, above.

Neuron I. This neuron is identical with the afferent neuron of the reflex mechanism. It should be noted that cranial nerves VII, IX and X carry some general somatic afferent fibers which join the spinal V tract and terminate in the nucleus of that tract. The cell bodies of these primary neurons lie in the geniculate, petrosal and nodose ganglia respectively.

Neuron II. These fibers are given off along the length of the spinal trigeminal nucleus. They pass ventromedially across the midline at about their level of origin in the nucleus and approach the lateral spinothalamic tract of the opposite side. Here, they turn rostrally along the medial border of the latter as the *ventral trigeminal lemniscus* (ventral secondary ascending V) (Fig. 8-3). Thus, these two functionally similar bundles accompany each other to the thalamus. In the thalamus, the trigeminal lemniscus enters the *posteromedial ventral nucleus* (Chap. 22). There are also contributions from the trigeminal lemniscus to the reticular system.

Neuron III. These fibers, arising from cells in the posteromedial ventral nucleus, pass through the posterior limb of the internal capsule to terminate in the inferior portion of the postcentral gyrus of the cerebrum.

Clinical Considerations

Testing

Pain. The integrity of the pain pathway is determined by pricking the skin with a pin, pinching a fold of skin, or applying a faradic current. The sensibility is described as analgesia (absence); hypalgesia (diminution); hyperalgesia (exaggeration).

Temperature. The integrity of this system is determined by having the patient distinguish between cold or warm objects, e.g., tap water with ice or water warmed to 50° placed in separate test tubes and applied to various areas of the skin. The sensibility is described as thermoanesthesia (absence); thermohypesthesia (dimi-

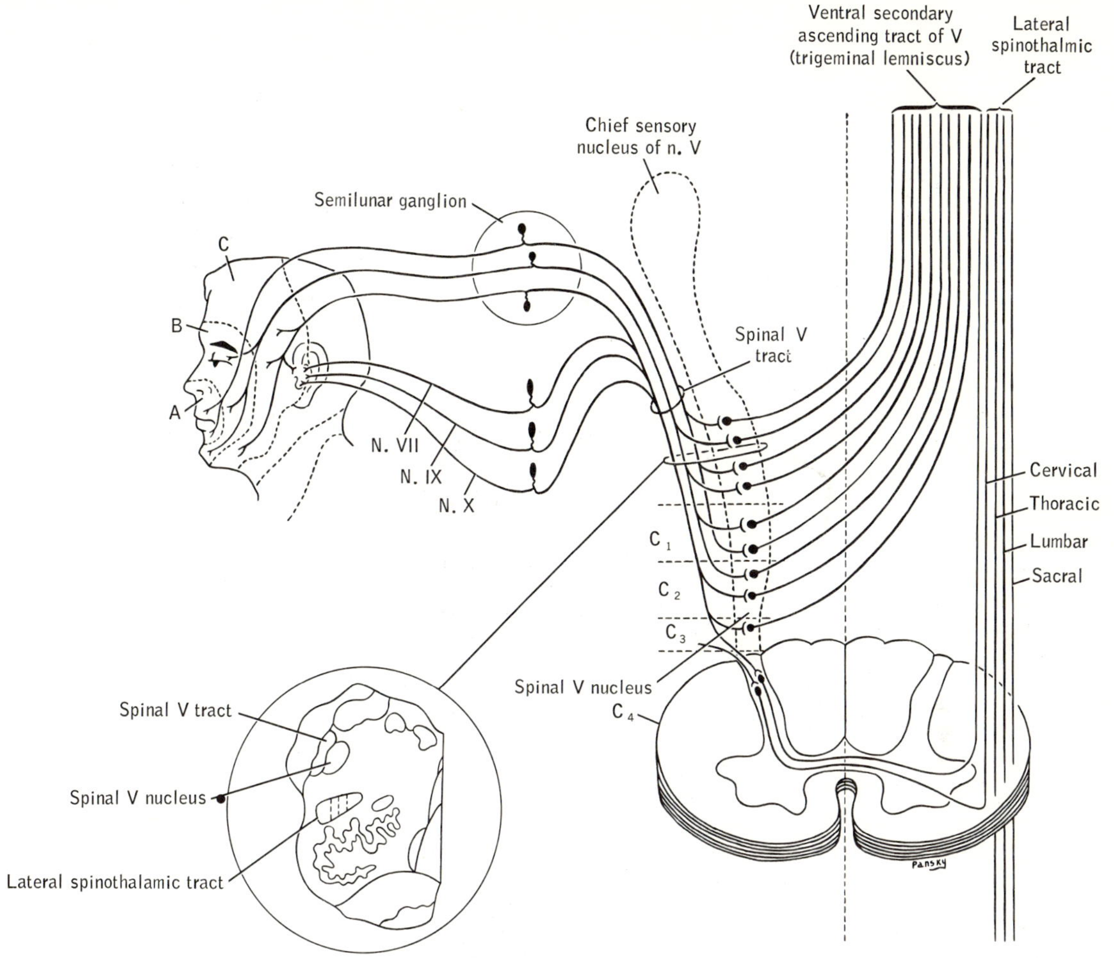

Fig. 8-3. Diagram showing the distribution of pain fibers from the cranial nerves to the nucleus of the spinal V tract; the origin of the ventral secondary ascending tract of V (trigeminal lemniscus) mediated from the caudal part of this nucleus.

nution); and thermohyperesthesia (exaggeration).

Specific Pathology

Referred Pain. (Fig. 8-6.) Technically, the consideration of sensory phenomena associated with internal organs belongs in another chapter (Chap. 10). However, since pathologic conditions in many organs exhibit symptoms in the form of pain directly related to specific skin areas and are so characteristic that they are useful in clinical diagnosis, an account of referred pain seems justified at this point.

As is the case at the body surface, viscera are supplied with nerve endings of variable complexity (Chap. 10), distributed particularly among the smooth muscle cells of the muscularis. These endings are stimulated by overdistention (as stones in the ureter or biliary ducts), abnormal contraction (spasm), inflammation (as in appendicitis), or impaired blood supply (ischemia). Peripheral fibers from these visceral receptors usually accompany the visceral motor system all the way to the spinal nerve trunk. This occurs particularly in the thoracic, upper lumbar, and midsacral levels. Thus, from

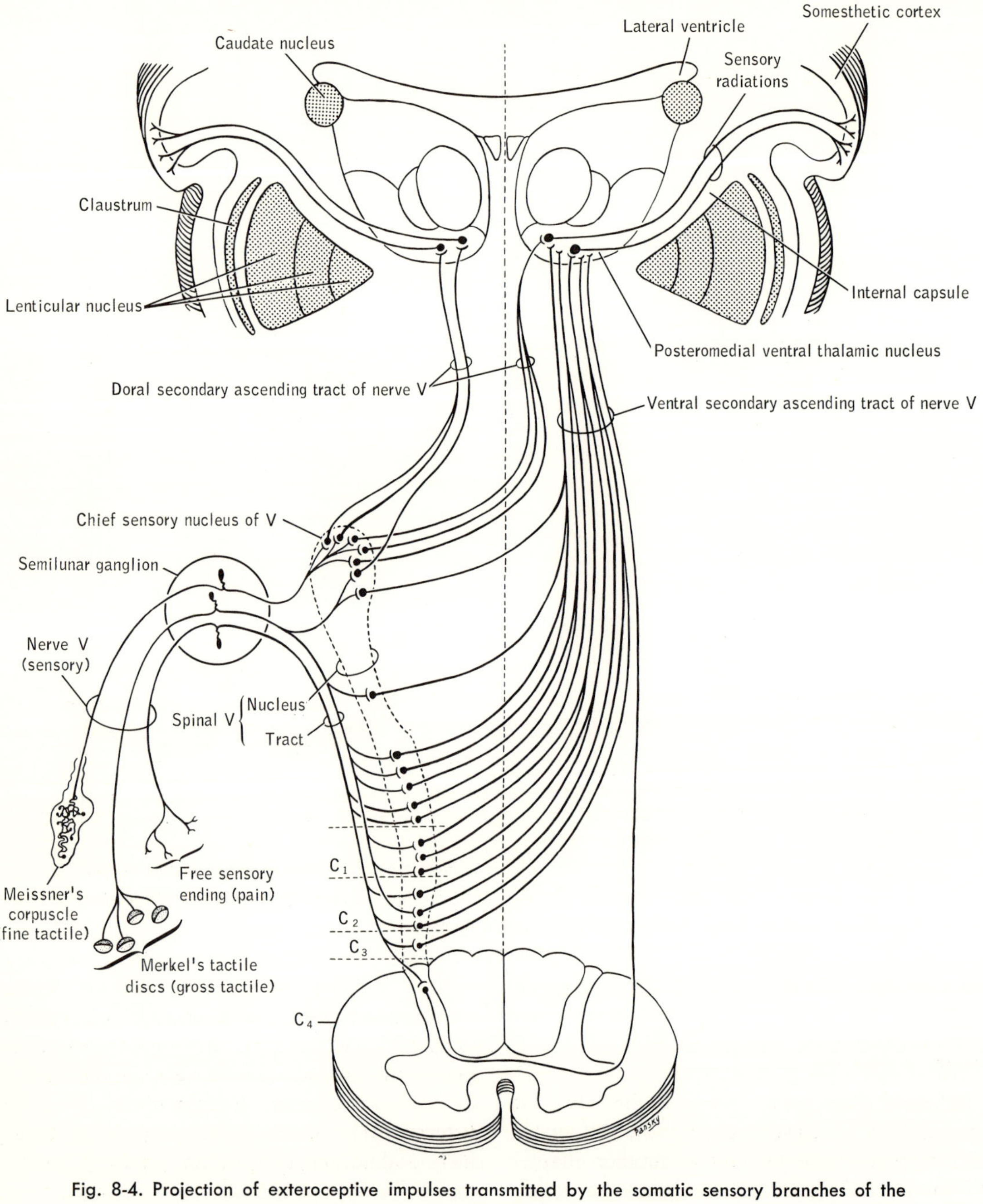

Fig. 8-4. Projection of exteroceptive impulses transmitted by the somatic sensory branches of the trigeminal nerve. Note: the chief sensory nucleus transmits only impulses of gross and fine tactile stimuli; pain is transmitted only via the caudal part of the spinal nucleus. Gross tactile impulses are transmitted throughout all parts of the nuclear complex. (*Modified after Crosby, Humphrey, and Lauer, 1962.*)

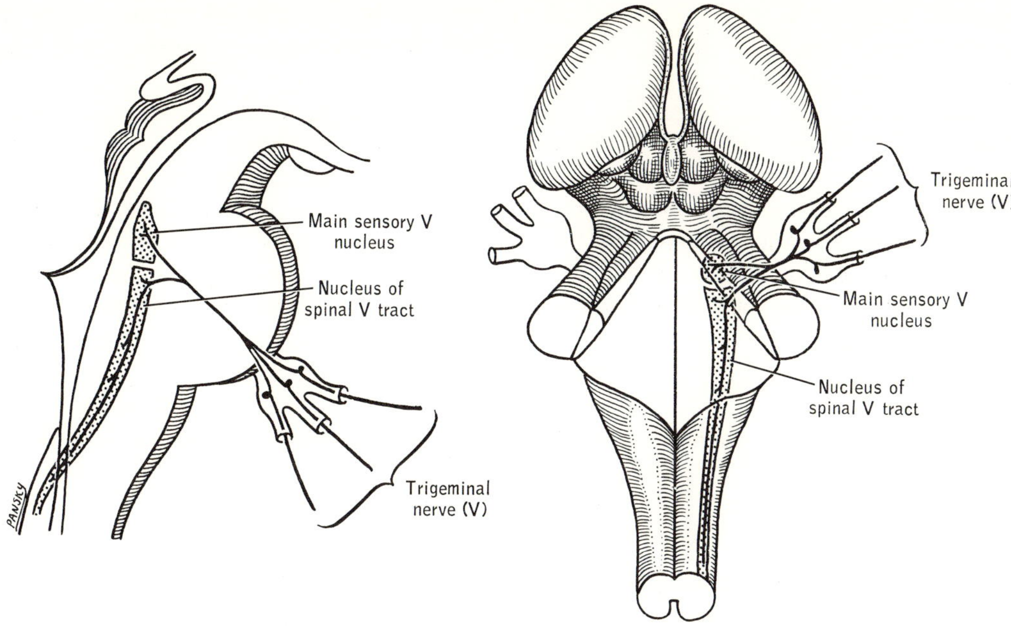

Fig. 8-5. The spinal (descending) and chief sensory nuclei of the trigeminal nerve. *Left,* lateral view; *right,* dorsal view.

the heart, afferent fibers enter levels T1 to T5; from the liver and gallbladder, fibers go to T6 to T9; from the stomach, the distribution is similar to that for the liver and gallbladder; the small intestine sensory fibers enter the cord from T9 to T11; the colon afferent fibers join the last two thoracic segments as well as L1, S2, and S3; the kidney afferent fibers to T11, T12, and L1; the ureter afferent fibers reach the cord at L1 and L2; the bladder and uterus afferent fibers enter the cord at T11, T12, L1, S2, and S3. These visceral afferent fibers follow the dorsal roots of spinal nerves having their cell bodies in the dorsal root ganglia. After entry into the cord, their disposition is identical with that of afferent fibers arising from receptors at the body surface. Potentially, too, the secondary neurons are similar. The chief difference may lie in the fact that there are no specific thalamic nuclei or cortical areas for individual organs. Therefore, the brain is only able to interpret the stimulus as occurring at the body surface in the neighborhood of the receptors belonging to those nerve trunks which the visceral fibers join and in the dorsal roots of which they pass.

Another explanation is also given. Here, of course, the impulse from an organ follows the same path as that described above, but in this case, the emphasis is placed upon the fact that the visceral fibers terminate in the same region of the substantia gelatinosa and proper sensory nucleus as do the fibers from the surface area of the nerve trunks which the visceral fibers join. Thus, when there is disease in a particular organ, so many impulses pass into the substantia gelatinosa that its threshold for painful impulses from that particular surface territory is so greatly reduced that even light touch at the periphery may seem painful.

Still a third explanation may be that some neurons in the posterior or sensory root of the spinal nerve may bifurcate, one branch arising in receptors in the skin, the other having its terminals in the walls of viscera.

One of the best-known and most specific examples of referred pain is angina pectoris, in which the pathologic condition is in the heart but the pain rediates from the upper chest down the medial side of the arm, forearm, and hand. This is because the visceral afferents carrying pain fibers from the heart join the upper thoracic nerves, which carry somatic sensory fibers from the chest and the medial aspect of the upper extremity. Other visceral pains, frequently encountered but often poorly localized, are intestinal colic, labor pains, heartburn, and injuries to the testicles or celiac plexus.

Trigeminal Neuralgia (Tic Douloureux, Facial Neuralgia). This is a severe neuralgia of the trigeminal nerve associated with intense pain along one or more of its divisions. The ophthalmic division is rarely at fault, but involvement of the maxillary and mandibular portions is common. This disease is apparently caused by

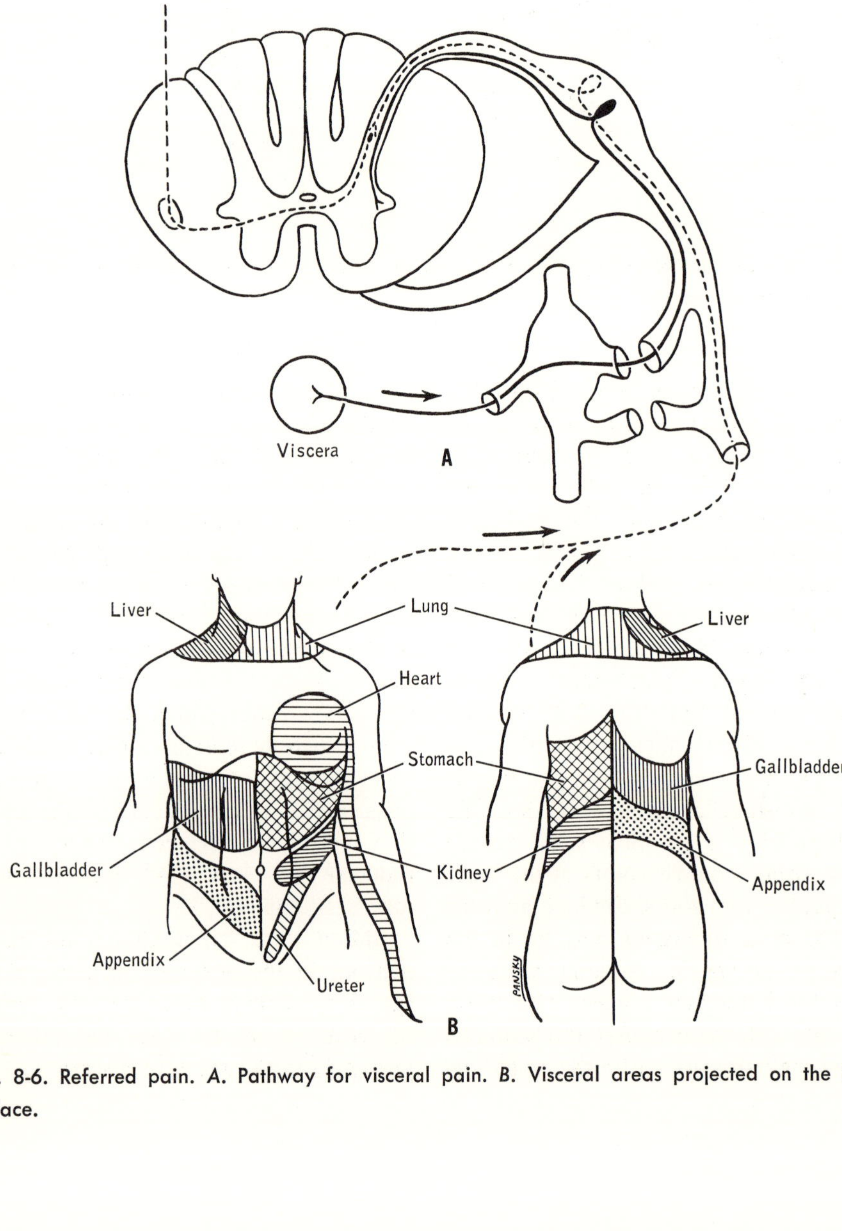

Fig. 8-6. Referred pain. *A.* Pathway for visceral pain. *B.* Visceral areas projected on the body surface.

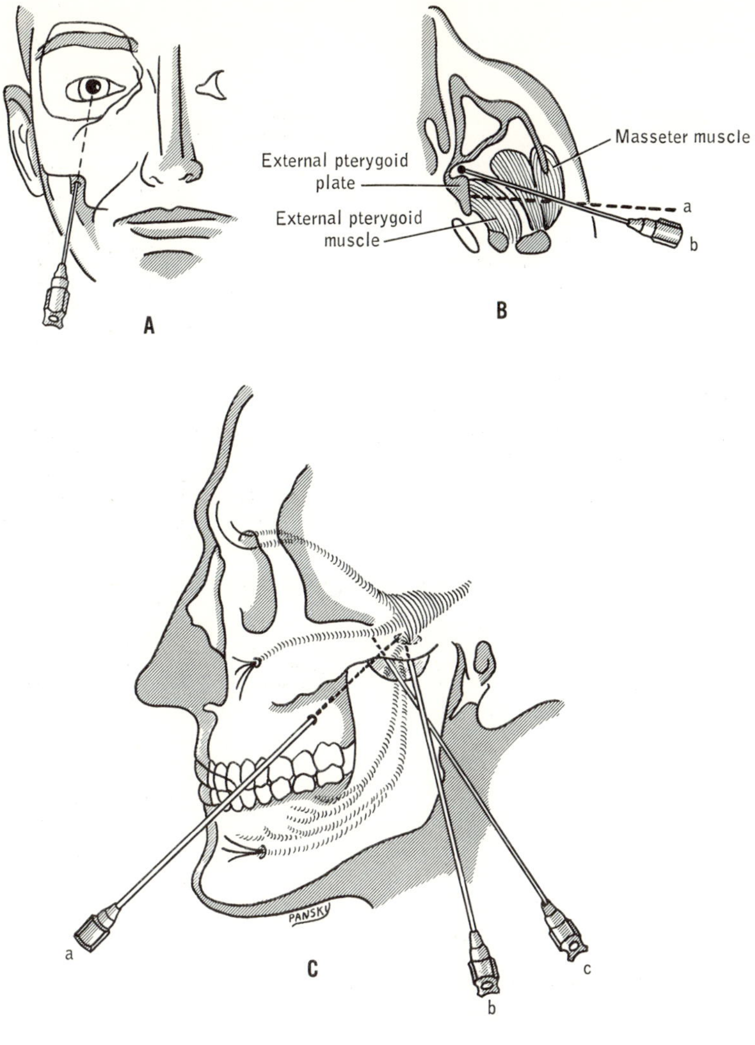

Fig. 8-7. Injection treatment for trigeminal neuralgia. A. Needle in line with pupil, directed forward. *B. a,* Needle directed to external pterygoid; *b,* needle directed to foramen ovale. C. *a,* injection of Gasserian ganglion; *b,* injection of mandibular nerve; *c,* injection of maxillary nerve.

an irritative lesion, of unknown etiology, localized in or near the semilunar ganglion. Certain surgical measures have been adopted to alleviate the symptoms, among them the injection of alcohol into peripheral parts of the nerve or the ganglion (Fig. 8-7). If this fails, section of the sensory root (portio major) near its attachment to the pons may be resorted to. Medullary tractotomy, involving section of the spinal trigeminal tract in the medulla, is sometimes used to alleviate the painful symptoms of this disease.

Occasionally, pain may arise from blood vessels of the face and may be confused with trigeminal neuralgia.

Syringomyelia.[2] (Fig. 8-8.) This is a chronic, slowly progressive disease, mainly of the cord but sometimes seen in the brain stem. The essen-

[2] Hydromyelia, due to localized accumulations of cerebrospinal fluid in the central canal, might be expected to produce similar symptoms.

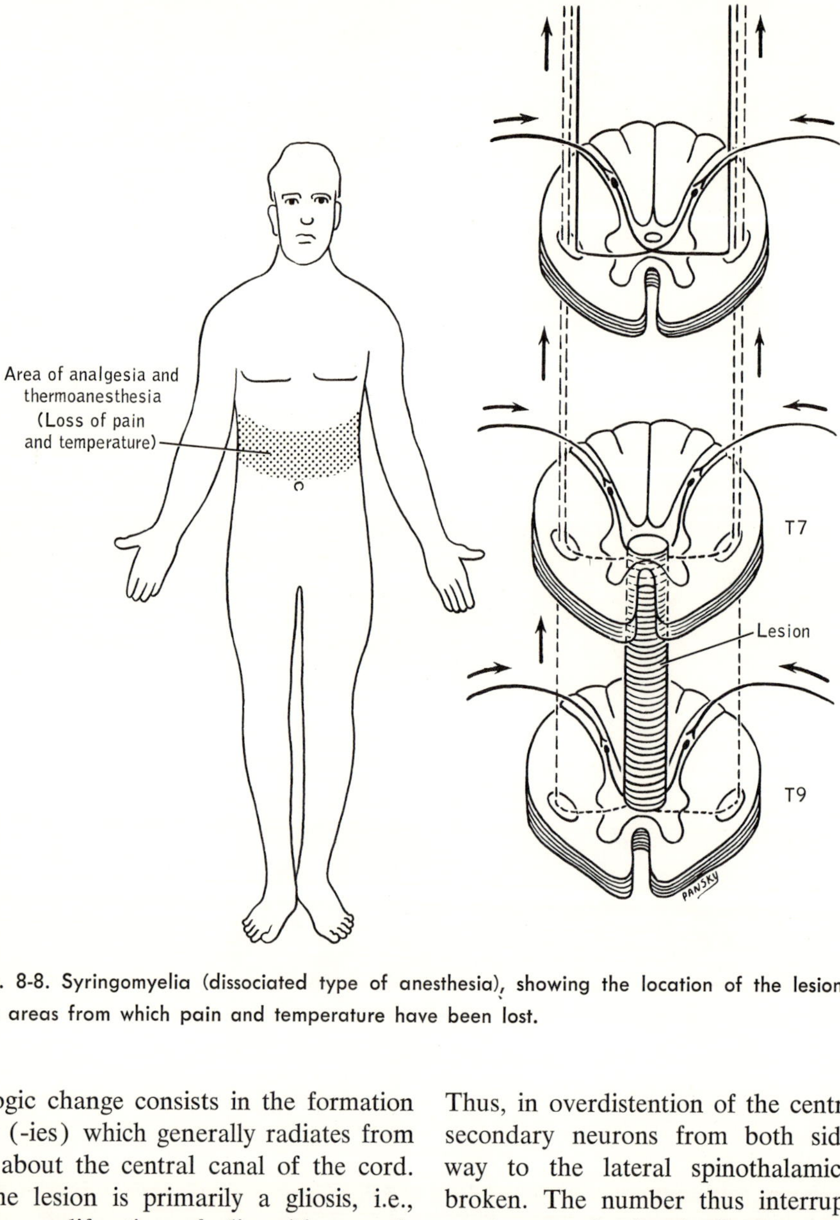

Fig. 8-8. Syringomyelia (dissociated type of anesthesia), showing the location of the lesion and the areas from which pain and temperature have been lost.

tial pathologic change consists in the formation of a cavity (-ies) which generally radiates from or centers about the central canal of the cord. Whether the lesion is primarily a gliosis, i.e., a tumor-like proliferation of glia with secondary cavity formation, or a primary cavitation, the clinical findings are generally the same.

To understand the clinical findings, one must recall that secondary pain fibers arise and pass across the cord close to the level of entry of the primary fibers and that, in crossing, the secondary fibers are in the anterior white commissure which lies just ventral to the central canal. Thus, in overdistention of the central canal, the secondary neurons from both sides, on their way to the lateral spinothalamic tracts, are broken. The number thus interrupted will depend upon the longitudinal extent of the enlarged canal. As a result, there will be analgesia and thermoanesthesia on both sides of the body in the areas supplied by the spinal nerves in the territory of the lesion. The amount of the sensory disturbance will be proportional to the size of the lesion. When this condition occurs in the low cervical or upper thoracic region, the area of anesthesia will cover the shoulders and arms and is referred to as *jacket-type anesthesia.*

Cordotomy. (Fig. 8-9.) This is a surgical procedure which makes use of the knowledge of the location and function of the lateral spinothalamic tract. It is used in cases where some pathologic condition (e.g., cancer) has progressed to such a stage that the control of pain with drugs is difficult or impossible. If the lesion is peripheral, as in the skin or connective tissue, a unilateral section of the lateral spinothalamic tract at a level about two segments above the entrance of the highest spinal nerve involved in the area and on the side opposite to the lesion, is performed. If the disease involves an organ, bilateral section of the tract must be made.

It has been noted, however, that, if a patient lives long enough after tract section, a return of the sensation of pain may occur. This is doubtless owing to those long chains of associational neurons passing into the dorsal gray columns at levels well above the cordotomy site where contact is eventually made with a secondary neuron of the conscious pathway. Since this course would involve such a large number of synapses, long exposure to a constant flow of impulses is required to open it up, for under normal conditions, impulses would follow the course of least resistance and bypass the more complex fiber system.

Phantom Limb. Although the authors have tried to point out that each fiber belonging to the sensory component of every nerve has a receptor at its peripheral end while its central process is followed by a series of fibers which lead to consciousness, it should be understood that if some physical shock or chemical substance were applied anywhere along this chain

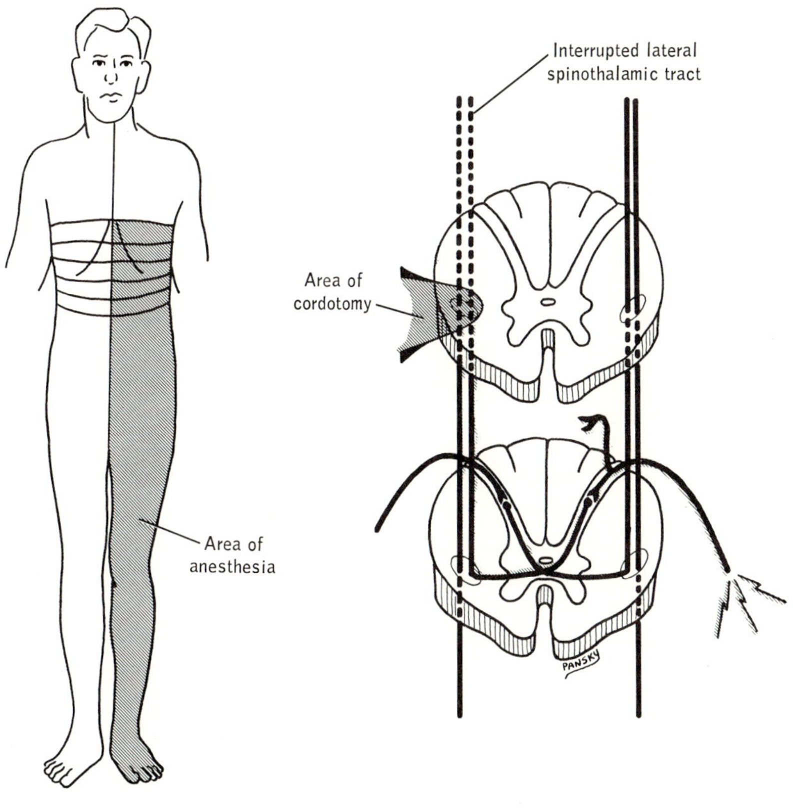

Fig. 8-9. Tractotomy (cordotomy) for treatment of intractable pain.

of conducton, the brain would interpret the point of stimulation as being at the skin surface where the receptors belonging to the stimulated fibers are located. Thus, a patient who has had an amputation of one of his extremities may state that he feels pain from a particular area on a limb he no longer possess. This is possibly because some of the pain fibers have been pinched in the scar tissue of the limb stump. It is immaterial that the portion of the fiber attached to the receptor is missing, for there is still a region in the cerebral cortex particularly for that portion of the extremity. All that is required is that an impulse reach the cortex for that area.

Hemisection of the Cord. Since this type of lesion involves many pathways other than those for pain and temperature sensation, no discussion of the *Brown-Séquard syndrome* will be attempted now.

LIGHT (CRUDE) TOUCH AND PRESSURE

Trunk

Reflex Pathways (Fig. 8-1.)

Certain reflexes are particularly associated with light touch, e.g., scratching; blinking and lacrimation at the slightest touch on the cornea; and sneezing after inhalation of small, irritating particles which come in contact with the nasal mucosa.

Receptors. (Fig. 8-10.) The receptors belonging to this system are of several types. *Merkel's disks* are platelike expansions of nerve fibers associated with specialized epithelial cells in the epidermis. Over most of the body surfaces, fine nerve fibrils entwine themselves around hair follicles, the *peritrichial arborizations*. These are sensitive to the slightest movements of the hair. In the dermal papillae, particularly over the volar surface of the fingers and hand, as well as on the soles of the feet, are the encapsulated tactile *corpuscles of Meissner*. Lying deep in the dermis, around tendons and joints and in the mesenteries and walls of the body cavities, are nerve terminals enclosed within numerous lamellae of connective tissue, the *Pacinian corpuscles. Genital corpuscles,* also encapsulated, are found in the connective tissue portions of the external genitalia.

Afferent Neuron. The peripheral process leading from the receptor is large and well myelinated. The cell body, located in the dorsal root ganglia of the spinal nerves, is of considerable size and unipolar in type. The central processes of the primary tactile fibers tend to aggregate into the medial division of the dorsal root as the latter joins the spinal cord along the dorsolateral sulcus. After entry, all fibers of this medial division becomes a part of the posterior funiculus of the same side. In the funiculus, each fiber divides into a very long ascending portion and a short descending branch, both of which give off collaterals to the gray matter. Fibers in the posterior funiculus have a definite orientation, those entering from caudal levels lying most medially, while those added from more cranial segments take a progressively more lateral position (Fig. 8-11). This tendency toward regional separation becomes grossly visible above the midthoracic cord when a thin septum appears running obliquely ventromedially from the dorsal intermediate sulcus. The division of the posterior funiculus medial to this sulcus and septum is the *fasciculus gracilis* (Goll's column) and contains fibers from the lower half of the body. The more lateral portion of the dorsal funiculus is made up of fibers from the upper half of the body and is known as the *fasciculus cuneatus* (Burdach's column). All the descending branches, all the collaterals, and some of the ascending branches of the primary afferent neuron end in the dorsal gray column around cells of the proper sensory nucleus. Many of the ascending fibers continue upward into the lower medulla, where they terminate in the *nucleus gracilis* and *cuneatus*.

Association Neuron. From the cells in the dorsal columns, axons of the association neurons have a wide distribution, i.e., to the ventral column on the same side of the cord; to the ventral column on the opposite side of the cord by way of the anterior white commissure; to the ventral column of the cord on the same side but at levels far removed from the point of origin, by way of ascending and descending bundles in the fasciculus proprius; and to the ventral columns on the opposite side at levels some distance from that of origin, by way of the anterior white commissure and the fasciculus proprius. Since there are characteristic changes, such as erection of the penis in response to touch, which involve the activation of the autonomic nervous system, some of the associational neurons traveling in the fasciculus proprius must terminate in the intermediolateral cell column. The spinotectal-tectospinal pathway (see under Pain and Temperature, above) may also assist in spreading reflex activity over the entire body.

Efferent Neuron. Only the somatosomatic and somatovisceral types of reflex will be considered here. In the former, the cells of the anterior gray columns of the cord give rise to axons which leave the CNS through the ventral roots of the spinal nerves to be distributed to the skeletal muscles of the trunk and extremities. In the latter, efferent fibers arise from small, multipolar cells in the intermediolateral cell column of the thoracic, upper lumbar, and midsacral cord. The axons pass through the ventral column, cross the ventral funiculus, and follow the fibers of the ventral root to beyond the point of union with the nerve trunk. Then, the visceral motor fibers diverge from the trunk through white rami communicantes to terminate in ganglia of the autonomic nervous system.

Conscious Pathway (Fig. 8-10.)

Neuron I. This neuron, together with the receptors, is identical with that described as the afferent neuron in the reflex pathway.

Neuron II. The cells of this second neuron, like those of the association fibers, are located in the body of the dorsal column. From here, their axons pass across to the opposite side of the cord through the anterior white commissure into the anterior funiculus. As they approach the ventral margin of the cord they bend sharply rostrally as the *ventral spinothalamic tract* (Fig. 3-7). Fibers added to the latter at successively higher levels would occupy more dorsal positions within the tract. There is a general feeling that few of these secondary neurons go all the way to the thalamus without interruption. Many terminate among cells adjoining the tract, particularly in the medulla and pons. These in turn give rise to other fibers which reenter the tract. Since such synapses may occur repeatedly, the entire tract is actually composed of a series of short relays. Eventually, all the fibers end in the *posterolateral ventral nucleus of the thalamus* (Chap. 22). In its course, the ventral spinothalamic tract may give off collaterals which are involved both in reflex activity and in the reticular activating mechanism.

The course of the ventral spinothalamic tract, particularly in the medulla and pons, has not been definitely established. Some investigator believe that it joins the lateral spinothalamic tract to form a single spinothalamic lemniscus. Others feel that it becomes associated with the medial lemniscus, and still others place it in a position intermediate between the two.

Neuron III. This originates in cells of the posterolateral ventral nucleus of the thalamus, from which axons pass laterally into the posterior limb of the internal capsule to terminate in the postcentral gyrus of the cerebrum.

Head

Reflex Pathway

Receptors. Reflexes activated by appropriate stimuli applied to the facial area, including the cornea, conjunctival sac, and the mucous membranes of the nose and mouth, begin with receptors of the same type described for the trunk.

Afferent Neuron. The peripheral processes follow all the divisions of the trigeminal nerve and have their cell bodies in the semilunar (Gasserian) ganglion, while the central processes make up a part of the sensory root (portio major) of that nerve. The sensory root joins the lateral aspect of the pons where the tactile fibers

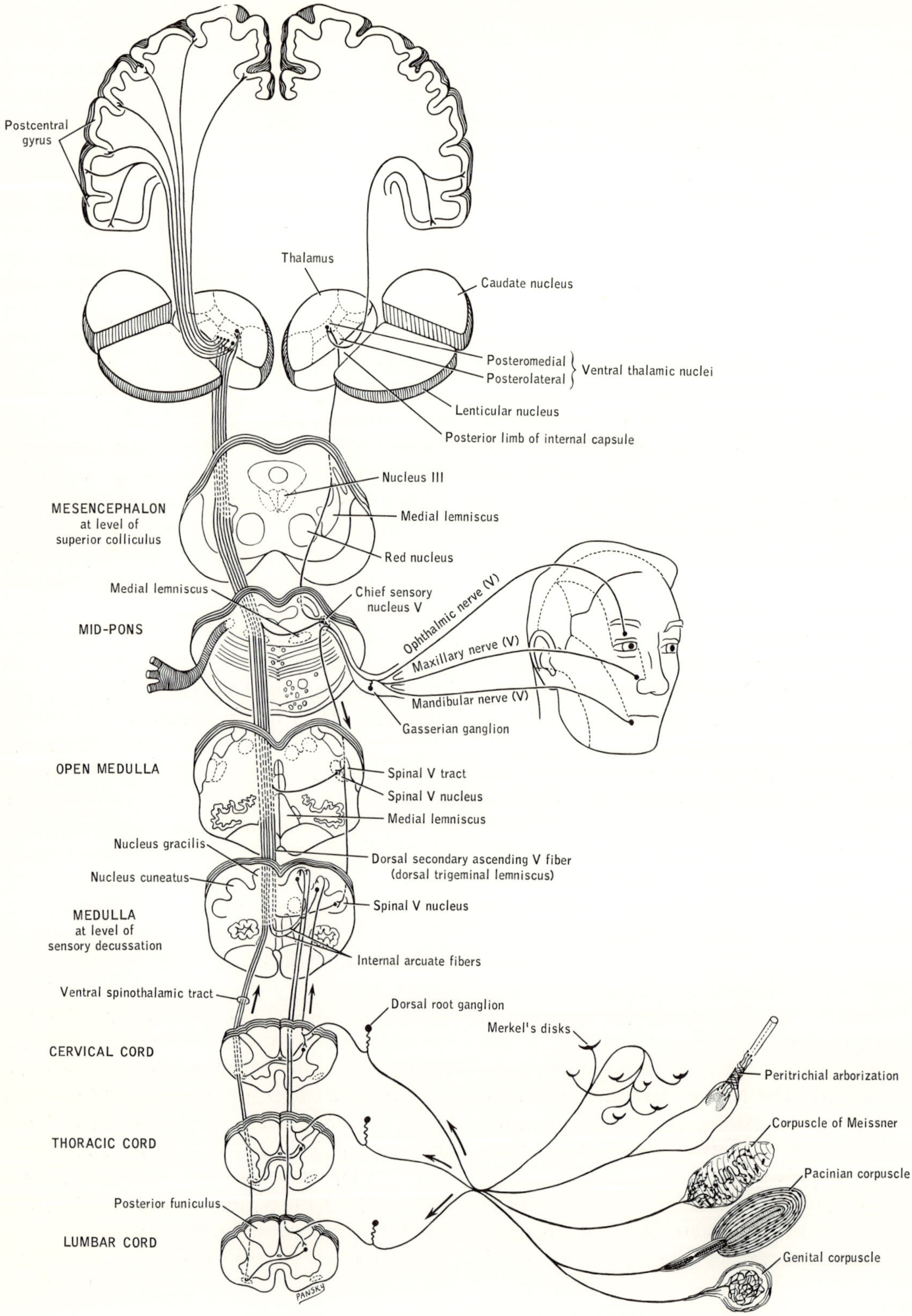

Fig. 8-10. Diagram of the conscious pathway for light (crude) touch.

pass obliquely dorsomedially across the brachium pontis into the ventrolateral portion of the tegmentum. Here, these fibers bifurcate into short ascending and longer descending branches. The former end in the chief (main) sensory nucleus of the trigeminal nerve (Figs. 8-3 to 8-5, 25-9), while the latter enter the descending (spinal) V tract to end around cells lying in the medial portion of the descending (spinal) V nucleus. Tactile fibers are apparently not well localized in the spinal V tract and probably do not extend as far caudally as do the pain and temperature fibers.

Association Neuron. These originate in either the spinal V or main sensory nucleus of the trigeminal nerve and pass almost immediately into the adjacent reticular formation. Through the latter they extend in any direction to end in any of the cranial motor nuclei (somatic or special or general visceral) and also in the ventral column of the spinal cord, which is reached by way of trigeminospinal fibers in the reticulospinal tract.

Efferent Neuron. Efferent neurons of the somatosomatic type of reflex may originate in such cranial motor nuclei as III, IV, VI, or XII, or in the anterior gray columns of the cord. Thus, tongue movements in response to touch, or eye movements toward the side of the face that has been stroked are examples of this mechanism. Another familiar reaction is sneezing. This is initiated by irritation of the nasal mucosa. The excitation spreads over the reticulospinal tract to the phrenic nucleus (diaphragm) in the midcervical cord and to the anterior horn cells at other cervical and thoracic levels.

Efferent neurons involved in the somatovisceral type of reflex have various origins, depending upon the region to be activated. These neurons ultimately will terminate in muscles of branchial arch origin, such as the SVE components of nerves V, VII, IX, X, or XI, or in smooth muscles or glands, such as the GVE portions of nerves III, VII, IX, or X. Twitching of the face as it is lightly stroked and blinking the eye as the conjunctiva is touched are examples of the former. Reflex salivation resulting from the presence of an object in the mouth (not taste) and lacrimation as the cornea is touched exemplify the latter.

Conscious Pathway (Fig. 8-10.)

Consciousness of even the slightest touch upon the facial area, particularly about the eyes, lips, and nasal mucous membrane, is extremely acute.

Neuron I. The receptors and the first neuron in the cerebral circuit are identical with the receptors and the afferent neuron, respectively, described under Reflex Pathway, above.

Neuron II. The cell bodies of secondary neurons lie in the medial aspect of the descending (spinal) V nucleus and in the chief sensory nucleus (Figs. 8-3 to 8-5, 25-9). From the former, fibers stream ventromedially toward the midline. Beyond this point, the exact distribution of these fibers is in dispute. Some may join the opposite medial lemniscus, while others may accompany the ventral spinothalamic tract in whatever location the latter may be. It is believed that fibers pass obliquely dorsomedially, across the midline directly below the hypoglossal nucleus, and turn rostrally in the dorsolateral portion of the tegmentum, just below the lateral side of the fourth ventricle. This bundle is the *dorsal secondary ascending V* or the *dorsal trigeminal lemniscus* (Figs. 25-10 to 25-12).

The vast majority of secondary neurons in the conscious pathway arise in the chief sensory nucleus. From here, part of the fibers run medially across the midline to join the dorsal trigeminal lemniscus of that side. Others ascend in this tract on the same side. Thus, the tactile mechanism here is both crossed and uncrossed. Throughout the pons and midbrain, the dorsal trigeminal lemniscus remains dorsal in position, staying medial to the brachium conjunctivum proper and dorsal to the decussation of the latter. Near the caudal end of the diencephalon, however, this lemniscus slopes ventrally to approach the ventral trigeminal and medial lemnisci, with which it enters the thalamus, terminating in the *posteromedial ventral* nucleus.

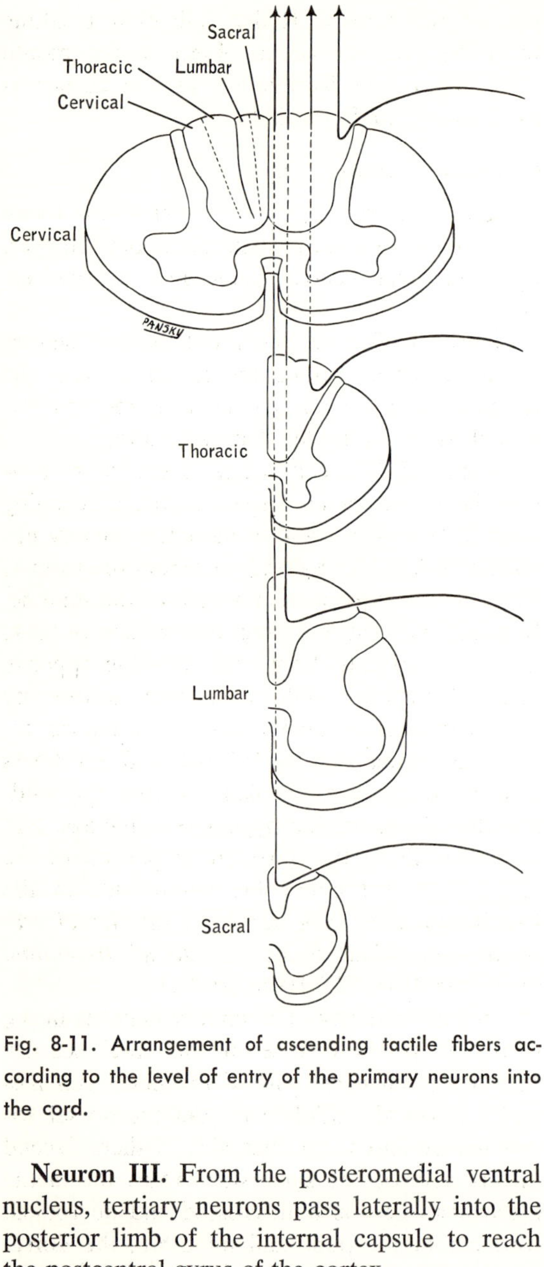

Fig. 8-11. Arrangement of ascending tactile fibers according to the level of entry of the primary neurons into the cord.

Neuron III. From the posteromedial ventral nucleus, tertiary neurons pass laterally into the posterior limb of the internal capsule to reach the postcentral gyrus of the cortex.

TACTILE DISCRIMINATION—STEREOGNOSIS

Tactile discrimination is the ability of the individual to recognize separately two distinct points of contact (Fig. 8-12) and to identify an object by its size, shape, weight, and texture. Although tactile localization is primarily a function of the cortex, tactile discrimination requires much greater cortical involvement. The latter is not solely a function of the tactile system alone, since the judgment of size and shape depends on movements at joints, while judgment of weight depends upon tension in muscles and tendons. Such discrimination requires the function of the proprioceptive system.

Similarly, *pallesthesia* (*vibratory sense*), the perception of repetitive mechanical stimuli, goes beyond simple touch or pressure, since the element of time must be taken into account. Thus, it is not possible to complete the entire picture of the stereognostic mechanism at this time.

Since tactile discrimination is primarily a cortical problem, reflexes need not be considered. Furthermore, since the primary function of this system is associated with the extremities, only passing attention will be given to pathways beginning in facial receptors. Although the ability to recognize as distinct entities two contact points separated from each other by variable distances is a function of the tactile apparatus, it should again be emphasized that much of discrimination involves more than simple touch. This, unfortunately, may be misleading when the term "two-point touch" is used to include all of discrimination. At this point, only the data pertinent to the tactile system will be considered. For additional material, see Proprioception, in Chap. 12.

Trunk

Conscious Pathway (Fig. 8-13.)

Receptors. (Fig. 8-10.) The receptors, *Meissner's corpuscles,* are located in dermal papillae closely applied to the surface epithelium. They are placed close together on the volar areas of the fingers and hands and on the plantar surface of the feet. Elsewhere, they tend to be much farther apart.

Neuron I. The peripheral process of the primary neuron, running centrally from the receptors, is heavily myelinated. The cell bodies are large and unipolar, located in the dorsal

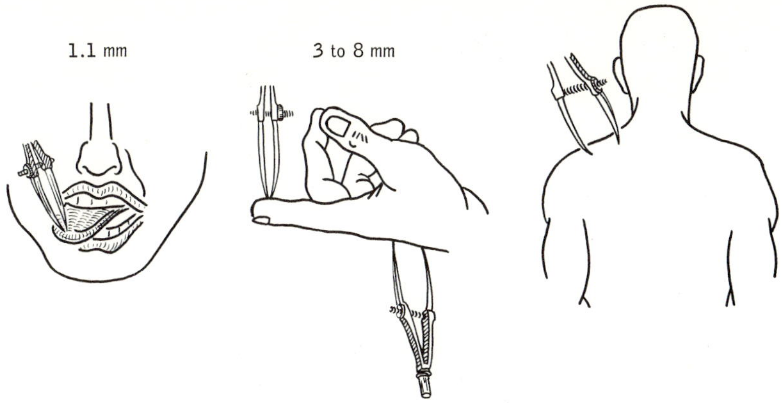

Fig. 8-12. Two-point touch. Separation of receptors on different body areas.

root ganglion. The central process joins others belonging to the same system in the medial division of the dorsal root and enters the cord along the dorsolateral sulcus.

Within the cord, these fibers enter the posterior funiculus and are oriented in a manner similar to that of the fibers of light touch. Likewise, each fiber bifurcates, the long ascending branches being most essential to the system. The latter continue rostrally in the posterior funiculus of the same side of the cord, enter the lower medulla, and terminate in the nucleus gracilis or nucleus cuneatus (Figs. 2-49, 25-3).

Neuron II. The secondary neurons have their cell bodies in the nuclei mentioned above. From the ventral aspects of both, axons sweep ventrally and medially, forming an inverted arc around the central gray matter. As a result of this course and their depth within the medulla, they are called the *internal arcuate fibers* (Figs. 25-2, 25-3). All these arcuate fibers cross the midline, the fibers of the two sides interlacing as they cross. This is the *sensory decussation* (Figs. 25-2, 25-3). Almost immediately after reaching the contralateral side, all fibers turn rostrally, forming the *medial lemniscus* (Figs. 2-49, 25-3 to 25-13).

Within the lemniscus there is a definite anatomic lamination. Fibers representing lower levels of the body lie more ventrolaterally, while those from succeedingly higher regions are piled on dorsally. Throughout the medulla, the medial lemniscus is seen to be compressed from side to side, its long axis being in the dorsoventral plane. In the pons, the configuration changes so that its long axis lies in the horizontal plane. With this shift, fibers from the lowest body levels come to occupy the most lateral position, while those from the neck region, for example, are most medial. In the mesencephalon, the lemniscus moves outward toward the surface of the brain stem. Here, the lateral extremity of the lemniscus joins the lateral spinothalamic tract, which, in this part of the brain stem, lies quite superficially. All secondary neurons terminate in the *posterolateral ventral nucleus* of the thalamus but at a level more rostral and dorsal than that which receives the endings for crude touch, pain, and temperature. (Figs. 2-37 to 2-39, 2-45 to 2-49.)

Neuron III. These begin with cells in the posterolateral ventral nucleus of the thalamus, pass laterally into the posterior limb of the internal capsule, and terminate in the postcentral gyrus and the adjacent parietal cortex.

Head

Conscious Pathway (Fig. 8-13.)

It is well-established that Meissner's corpuscles are abundant at the tip of the tongue,

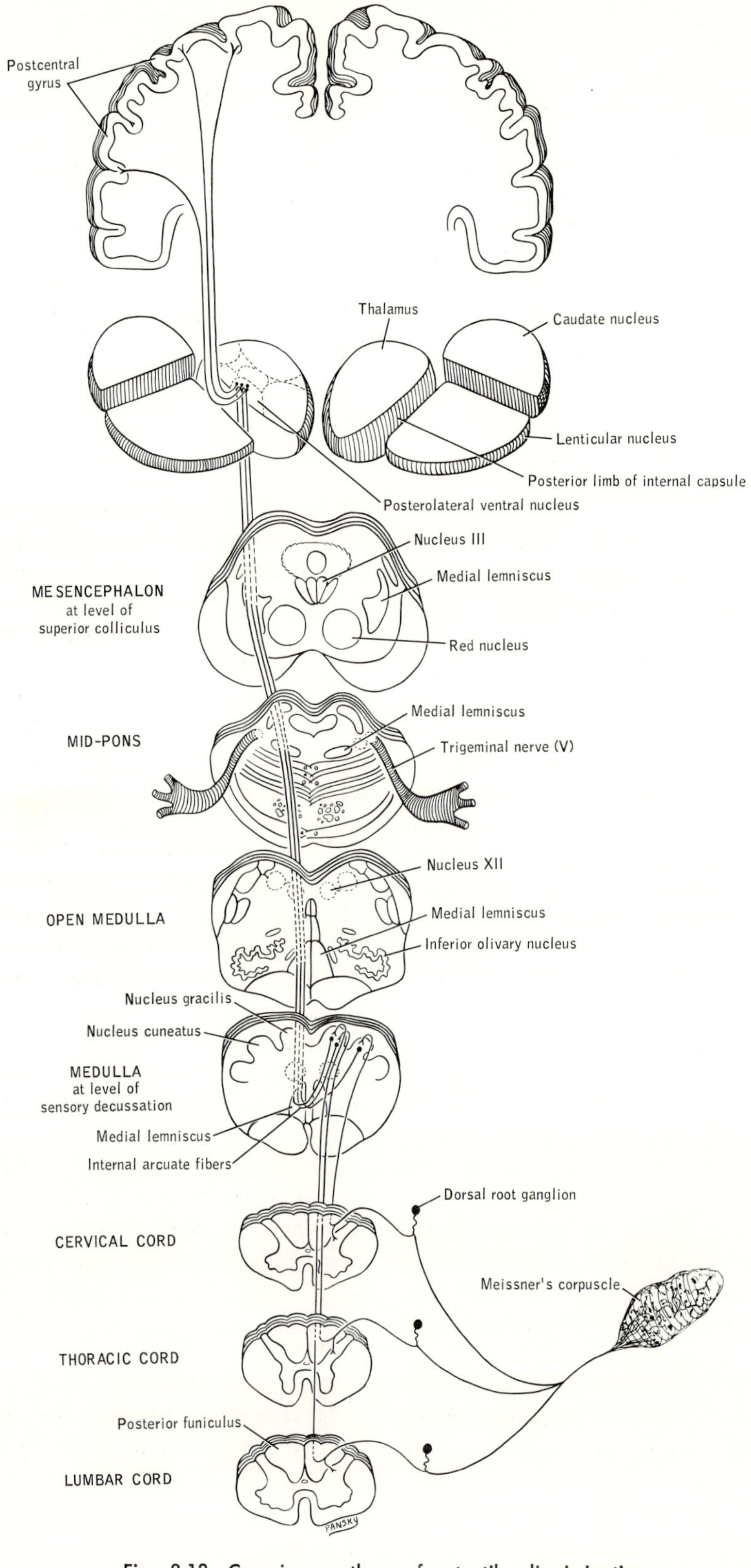

Fig. 8-13. Conscious pathway for tactile discrimination.

where two points are distinguishable as close together as 1.1 mm (Fig. 8-12). Meissner's corpuscles are associated with the mandibular division of the trigeminal nerve. Such receptors are also common on the lips, related to both the maxillary and mandibular divisions of nerve V. Impulses originating here would follow the same peripheral course and have the same terminations as those for crude touch in the corresponding area. The course of secondary neurons in the path to the thalamus is not clear, but it would not be illogical to speculate that they might lie close to similar neurons arising in the cord for the same purpose—in other words, near the medial lemniscus.

Clinical Considerations

Testing

Crude or Light Touch. The integrity of this system may be tested with a fine, soft paint brush, a wisp of wool, or even a piece of paper. The sensibility is described as tactile anesthesia (absence); tactile hypesthesia (diminution); tactile hyperesthesia (exaggeration).

Tactile Localization. Using the same materials, the patient must close his eyes and then indicate the exact spot that the examiner has touched.

Tactile Discrimination. (Fig. 8-12.) This may be tested in several ways. An area of skin is touched simultaneously with two points of a compass or calipers. The minimum distance between the points when felt separately, as two points, is noted. This may vary from 3 to 8 mm on the fingers to as much as 75 mm on the upper arm or thigh. Further, the patient is asked to discriminate between materials of different texture, such as silk, wool, linen, or emery cloth. The disturbance of sensibility may be described as *allocheiria* or *astereognosis*. The former concerns false localization, i.e., if one extremity is stimulated, the sensation is referred to the other side. The latter is a disturbance of discrimination in which the patient is unable to recognize, by feel, familiar objects when the eyes are covered.

Specific Pathology

Syringomyelia. This condition has been described previously. It is mentioned again here, since in these cases, the patient experiences *sensory dissociation*. In other words, sense of pain and temperature may be completely lost on both sides of the body in areas corresponding and in proportion to the lesion, while crude touch is not clinically diminished. The latter phenomenon is due to the fact that primary tactile fibers pass long distances before synapsing with secondary fibers. Actually, many of these primary fibers pass all the way into the medulla before making synapse with the second neuron.

Tabes Dorsalis. (Fig. 8-14.) This lesion is of neurosyphilitic origin and leads to the destruction of primary neurons in the dorsal roots

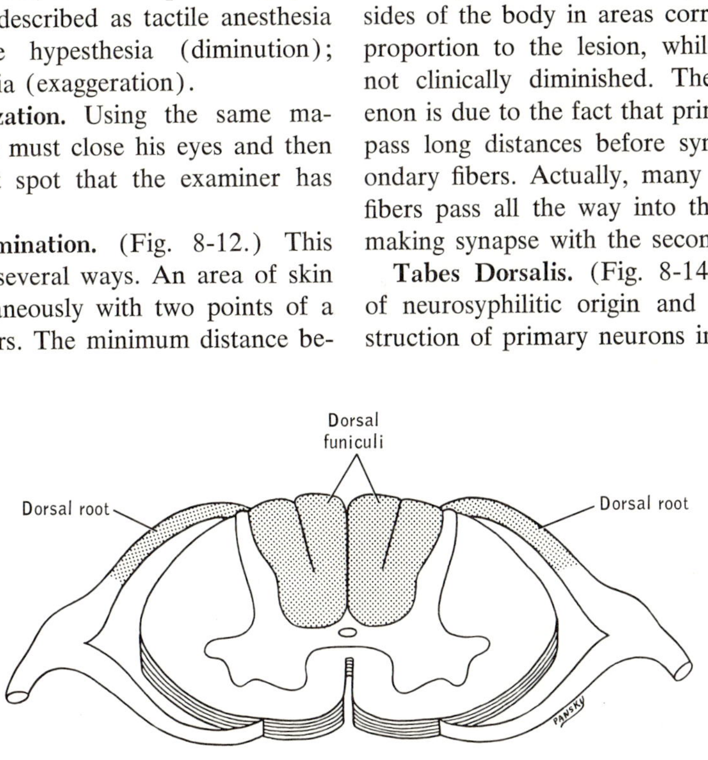

Fig. 8-14. Tabes dorsalis, showing the areas affected (degeneration of the dorsal funiculi and the dorsal roots).

of spinal nerves. Although the filaments of the medial divisions are apparently destroyed first, leading to the degeneration of the posterior funiculi, all sensory fibers of the dorsal root may eventually become involved. In the tabetic patient, there is loss of position and vibratory sense below the lesion on the same side of the body. However, the disease may spread to the other side. With destruction of the entire root, loss of pain and temperature perception will also be noted.

Traumatic Lesions of the Cord. In the cord, most tactile loss which is clinically detectable is that of discrimination which occurs on the same side of the body below the level of the lesion.

Traumatic Lesions of the Medulla. When the medial lemniscus of one side is involved, there results a complete loss of position, vibratory sense, two-point discrimination, and pressure sense over the entire contralateral side of the body. Because of the proximity of the two lemnisci, it is quite possible for a single lesion to involve both of them. Since the ventral spinothalamic tract also lies close to the medial lemniscus in the brain stem, this, too, is frequently involved in the same lesion. Because by this time the secondary neurons in the conscious pathway for light touch are grouped within this tract, a destruction of the ventral spinothalamic tract here would result in a noticeably diminished crude touch on the contralateral side.

Phantom Limb. After limb amputations, this phenomenon is also common, expressing itself as itching or tickling. The explanation is the same as that given under Phantom Limb (see Pain and Temperature, above).

SUMMARY
Pain and Temperature

REFLEX

Trunk		Head
1. Free endings (pain) Bulbs of Krause (cold) Organs of Ruffini (warmth)	Receptor	1. Same as for trunk
2. Through all spinal nerves, with cells in dorsal root ganglia, into dorsolateral funiculus, terminating in the substantia gelatinosa of the dorsal gray column	Afferent neuron	2. Through all roots of the trigeminal nerve, with cell bodies in the semilunar ganglion, into the brain stem via the portio major to terminate in the spinal V (descending) nucleus and chief sensory nucleus
3. From cells in the substantia gelatinosa to ventral gray column at the same level on the same side; ventral gray column at other levels of the same side through the fasciculus proprius; ventral gray column at the same and other levels of the opposite side through the anterior gray commissure and the fasciculus proprius From the substatia gelatinosa to the intermediolateral cell column, wherever found, by the routes described above	Association neuron	3. From cells, chiefly in the spinal V nucleus, fibers pass to all GSE nuclei of the brain stem (III, IV, VI, and XII); to the ventral gray columns of the cord via the reticulospinal tract; to all SVE nuclei of the brain stem (V, VII, IX, X, and XI); to all cranial autonomic nuclei (EW, superior and inferior salivatory, and dorsal motor nucleus of the vagus); to the intermediolateral cell column of the cord via the reticulospinal tract
4. *Somatosomatic* From the ventral column through the ventral roots of all spinal nerves to skeletal muscle of the trunk, neck, and extremities *Somatovisceral* (general) From intermediolateral cell column of the cord by way of preganglionics in the ventral roots of spinal nerves in the thoracic, upper lumbar, and midsacral regions through white rami to autonomic ganglia for synapse, thence through postganglionics to smooth muscle, heart, and glands	Efferent neuron	4. *Somatosomatic* From nuclei III, IV, and VI through respective nerves to extrinsic muscles of the eye From nucleus XII through hypoglossal nerve to muscles of the tongue From ventral column of the cord to skeletal muscle of the neck, trunk, and extremities *Somatovisceral* (general) From EW nucleus through preganglionics in nerve III to ciliary ganglion and thence by postganglionics to sphincter pupillae From superior and inferior salivatory nuclei by preganglionics in nerves VII and IX, respectively, to synapse in autonomic ganglia, thence by postganglionics to salivary glands From the dorsal motor nucleus of the vagus through preganglionics in vagus to autonomic ganglia, thence via postganglionics to heart, smooth muscle, and glands From the intermediolateral cell column by preganglionics running in the ventral roots of spinal nerves at thoracic, upper lumbar, and midsacral levels to autonomic ganglia, thence to heart, smooth muscle, and glands through postganglionics *Somatovisceral* (special) From nuclei V, VII, IX, X, and XI to skeletal muscle of branchial arch origin, (mastication, face, pharynx, larynx, sternocleidomastoid, and trapezius

CONSCIOUS

Trunk		Head
5. *Somatic* Same as in reflex *Visceral* Free endings in walls of viscera	Receptor	5. *Somatic* Same as in reflex *Visceral* Same as in reflex
6. *Somatic* Same as afferent neuron in reflex *Visceral* From viscera, then through white rami to spinal nerves, with cell bodies in dorsal root ganglia, to terminate in the substantia gelatinosa	Neuron I	6. *Somatic* Same as afferent neuron in reflex *Visceral* Same as afferent neuron in reflex
7. *Somatic and visceral* From cells in the substantia gelatinosa to the opposite side of the cord through the anterior white commissure into the lateral spinothalamic tract, thence rostrally to terminate in the posterolateral ventral nucleus of the thalamus	Neuron II	7. *Somatic and visceral* From cells in spinal V nucleus to opposite side of brain stem, entering the ventral trigeminal lemniscus and running rostrally to terminate in the posteromedial ventral nucleus of the thalamus
8. *Somatic and visceral* From the posterolateral ventral nucleus of the thalamus by way of the posterior limb of the internal capsule to terminate in the postcentral gyrus of the cerebrum	Neuron III	8. *Somatic and visceral* From the posteromedial ventral nucleus of the thalamus by way of the posterior limb of the internal capsule to terminate in the postcentral gyrus of the cerebrum

SUMMARY
Crude Touch

REFLEX

Trunk		Head
1. Merkel's disks Meissner's corpuscles Pacinian corpuscles Genital corpuscles Peritrichial arborizations	Receptor	1. Same as for trunk except that genital corpuscles are lacking
2. Through spinal nerves, with cells in the dorsal root ganglia, entering the posterior funiculus (fasciculus gracilis and cuneatus) to end in the dorsal gray column	Afferent neuron	2. Through all roots of the trigeminal nerve, with cells in the semilunar ganglion, into the brain stem to end mostly in the chief sensory nucleus of V
3. From cells in the dorsal column to the ventral gray column at the same level, same side; the ventral gray column at other levels of the same side through the fasciculus proprius; the ventral gray column at the same and other levels of the opposite side through the anterior white commissure and the fasciculus proprius; the intermediolateral gray column, wherever found, by the same paths	Association neuron	3. From cells in the chief sensory nucleus of V, through the reticular formation to all GSE nuclei of the head (III,IV, VI,and XII); all the SVE nuclei of the head by way of reticulospinal tract; cranial autonomic nuclei (especially the lacrimal and salivatory); the intermediolateral cell column of the cord by way of the reticulospinal tract
4. *Somatosomatic* From the ventral gray columns by way of the ventral roots of all spinal nerves to skeletal muscle of the neck, trunk, and extremities *Somatovisceral* (general) From the intermediolateral column through preganglionics in the ventral roots of spinal nerves in thoracic, upper lumbar, and midsacral regions and through white rami to synapse in autonomic ganglia, thence, via postganglionics to heart, smooth muscle, and glands	Efferent neuron	4. *Somatosomatic* From cranial nuclei III,IV, and VI through respective nerves to extrinsic muscles of eye; from nucleus XII by way of hypoglossal to muscles of tongue From the ventral gray columns through the ventral roots of all spinal nerves to skeletal muscles of neck, trunk, and extremities *Somatovisceral* (general) From lacrimal and salivatory nuclei through preganglionics in nerves VII and IX to synapse in autonomic ganglia, thence, by postganglionics, to lacrimal and salivary glands From the intermediolateral cell column of the cord by preganglionics in the ventral roots of spinal nerves in the thoracic, upper lumbar, and midsacral regions through white rami to autonomic ganglia, thence by postganglionics to smooth muscle and glands *Somatovisceral* (special) From nucleus V to muscles of mastication through the trigeminal nerve From nucleus VII through the facial nerve to muscles of face From nucleus IX and X (ambiguus) through the glossopharyngeal and vagus nerves to the muscles of the pharynx and larynx

CONSCIOUS

Trunk		Head
5. Same as in reflex	Receptor	5. Same as in reflex
6. Same as afferent neuron in reflex	Neuron I	6. Same as afferent neuron in reflex
7. From cells of the dorsal gray column, across the cord in the anterior white commissure, thence rostrally in the ventral spinothalamic tract to terminate in the posterolateral ventral nucleus of the thalamus	Neuron II	7. From cells in the chief sensory nucleus either across the brain stem to the dorsal trigeminal lemniscus, or rostrally on the same side in the dorsal trigeminal lemniscus, fibers ending, in either case, in the posteromedial ventral nucleus of the thalamus From cells in the spinal nucleus to the opposite side of the brain stem to pass rostrally in the ventral spinothalamic tract; in the medial lemniscus; or in the dorsal trigeminal lemniscus, all terminating in the posteromedial ventral nucleus of the thalamus
8. From cells of the posterolateral ventral nucleus of the thalamus through the posterior limb of the internal capsule to the postcentral gyrus	Neuron III	8. From the posteromedial ventral nucleus of the thalamus through the posterior limb of the internal capsule to end in the postcentral gyrus of the cortex

SUMMARY
Tactile Discrimination

CONSCIOUS

Trunk		Head
5. Meissner's corpuscles	Receptor	5. Same as for trunk
6. Through spinal nerves with cells in dorsal root ganglia into posterior funiculus (fasciculus gracilis and cuneatus), running rostrally to terminate in either nucleus gracilis or nucleus cuneatus	Neuron I	6. Essentially the same as neuron I in conscious pathway for crude touch in the head
7. From cells in either nucleus gracilis or nucleus cuneatus, through internal arcuate fibers, across to the opposite side in the sensory decussation, then rostrally in the medial lemniscus to the posterolateral ventral nucleus of the thalamus	Neuron II	7. About the same as neuron II in the concious pathway for crude touch in the head but the termination may be farther dorsally and rostrally in the posteromedial ventral nucleus
8. From cells in the posterolateral ventral nucleus of the thalamus through the posterior limb of the internal capsule to the postcentral gyrus and adjoining parietal cortex	Neuron III	8. Same as nueron III in the conscious pathway for crude touch in the head

9 SPECIAL SOMATIC AFFERENT SYSTEM (SSA)

VISUAL SYSTEM

Development (Fig. 9-1.)

The first trace of photoreceptors in the evolutionary process is found on the skin, particularly on the dorsal side of the trunk. In time, these receptors become concentrated near the rostral end of the animal and are enclosed within the developing neural tube. With further development, these receptors can be traced to the lateral evaginations of the neural tube called the *optic vesicles.* These appear in the human embryo between the third and fourth weeks and later lie in the *optic cup,* which develops from the vesicles. Essentially, at 7 months of development, the neural elements which lie in the retina of the eyeball are complete and perceptive of light.

Although the emphasis will be placed on the neural structure, it is essential to have an understanding of the anatomy of the eyeball, including the cornea, lens, iris, and ciliary body, since these are important for normal vision under changing conditions (Fig. 9-2). Although, the extrinsic muscles of the eye also play a part in vision, their specific anatomy will be dealt with in a later chapter (Chap. 14). Since the neural mechanism lies in the retina of the eyeball, a knowledge of the finer structure of this layer will help in comprehending its function (Fig. 9-4).

General Definitions

Before going into a detailed study of the nervous pathways, it is necessary to understand what is meant by optic axis, visual fields, retinal fields, retinal quadrants, and macular vision.

The central points of the anterior and posterior surfaces of the eyeball are its anterior and posterior poles (Fig. 9-2). A straight line connecting the two poles is called the *optic axis.* The optic axis can be considered a sagittal plane of cleavage which divides each eyeball into a medial, or nasal, half and a lateral, or temporal, half. Thus, the retina is divided into a nasal and temporal *retina field.* A horizontal cleavage plane through the middle of the eyeball, at right angles to the sagittal plane, further subdivides the retina into upper and lower nasal and temporal *retinal quadrants* (Fig. 9-5).

The term *visual field* refers to that part of space seen by a specific area of the retina; e.g., the nasal half of the retina of each eye receives light impulses from the temporal area in space, and the temporal halves from the nasal area in space (Figs. 9-4, 9-5).

The center of best vision is at the macula lutea of the retina, which is a little to the temporal side of the posterior pole of the eyeball. Vision here is called *central* or *macular vision* (Figs. 9-2, 9-5, 9-6).

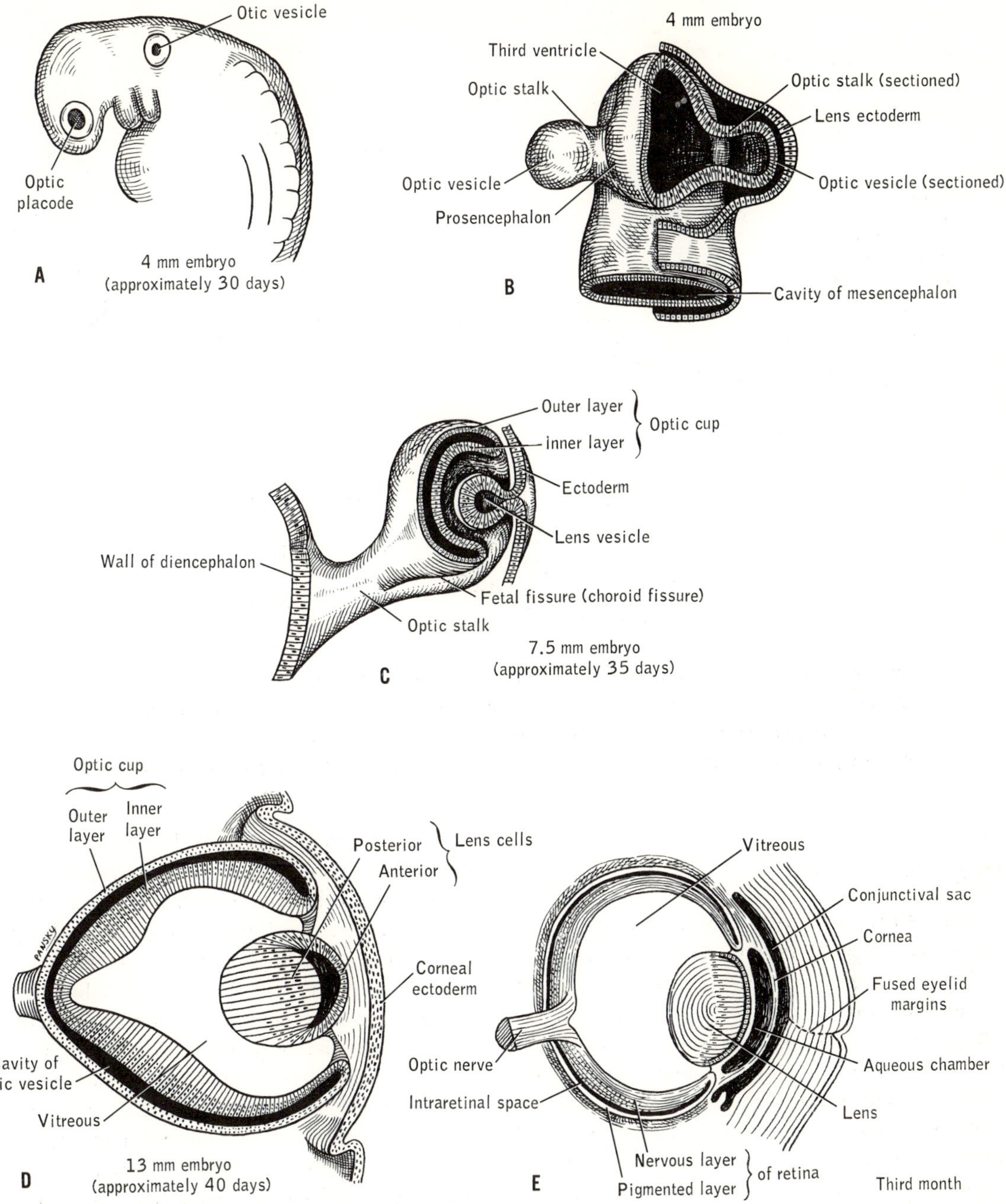

Fig. 9-1. Development of the eye. (*Adapted from Hamilton, Boyd, and Mossman, Human Embryology, 2d ed., The Williams & Wilkins Company, Baltimore, 1952.*)

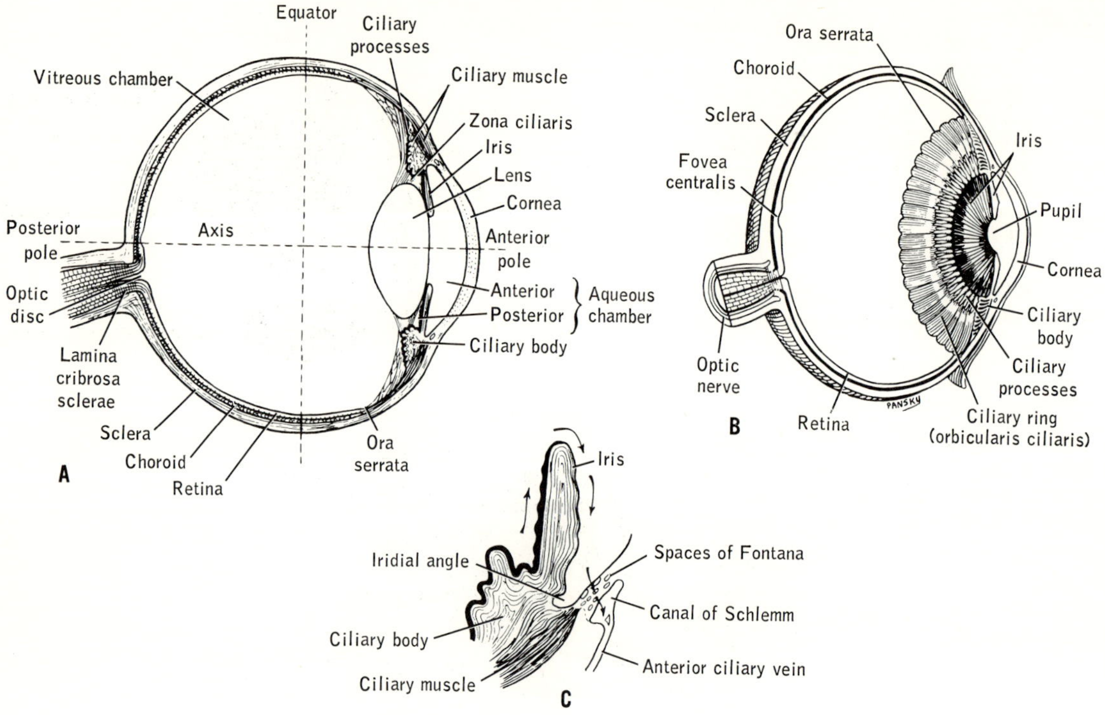

Fig. 9-2. Structure of the eye. *A.* Horizontal section of the left eyeball seen from above. *B.* Hemisection of the right eyeball seen from above and behind. C. Illustration of the filtration angle showing the path of flow of the aqueous humor. (*Adapted from Schaeffer (ed.), Morris' Human Anatomy, 11th ed., McGraw-Hill Book Company, Inc., Blakiston Division, New York, 1953.*)

Pathways

Reflex (Fig. 9-7, 9-8.)

Receptors. (Fig. 9-4.) Within the retina are two types of receptors, the *rods* and *cones.*

The rods are the most numerous (estimates range from 100 to 130 million). They are absent from the fovea centralis but gradually increase in number in areas of the retina farther removed from that point. The rods react to low-intensity illumination and are said to subserve twilight and night vision. They contain a substance known as *visual purple,* or rhodopsin, which is rapidly reduced and disappears when exposed to light. As long as the rods maintain contact with the pigment layer of the retina, rhodopsin regenerates. This reduction process is responsible for the production of an action current in the nerve fibers. The rod cell is also capable of changing length. In strong light, the cell lengthens and is pushed deep into the pigment layer which lies superficial to it. In dim light, it contracts, drawing away from the pigment, thus exposing a greater portion of the rod to what little light may be available.

The cones number 6 or 7 million. Except at the fovea, where they are the only cells found, their distribution is fairly even among the predominant rods. The cones have a higher threshold of excitability than the rods and are stimulated by light of relatively high intensity. They are important for clear vision and for color determination, adequate light being required for both. The cones do not contain visual purple but may possess a colorless substance which reacts in the same way. Cones are also thought to have the ability to extend or contract, perhaps to a greater degree than the rods.

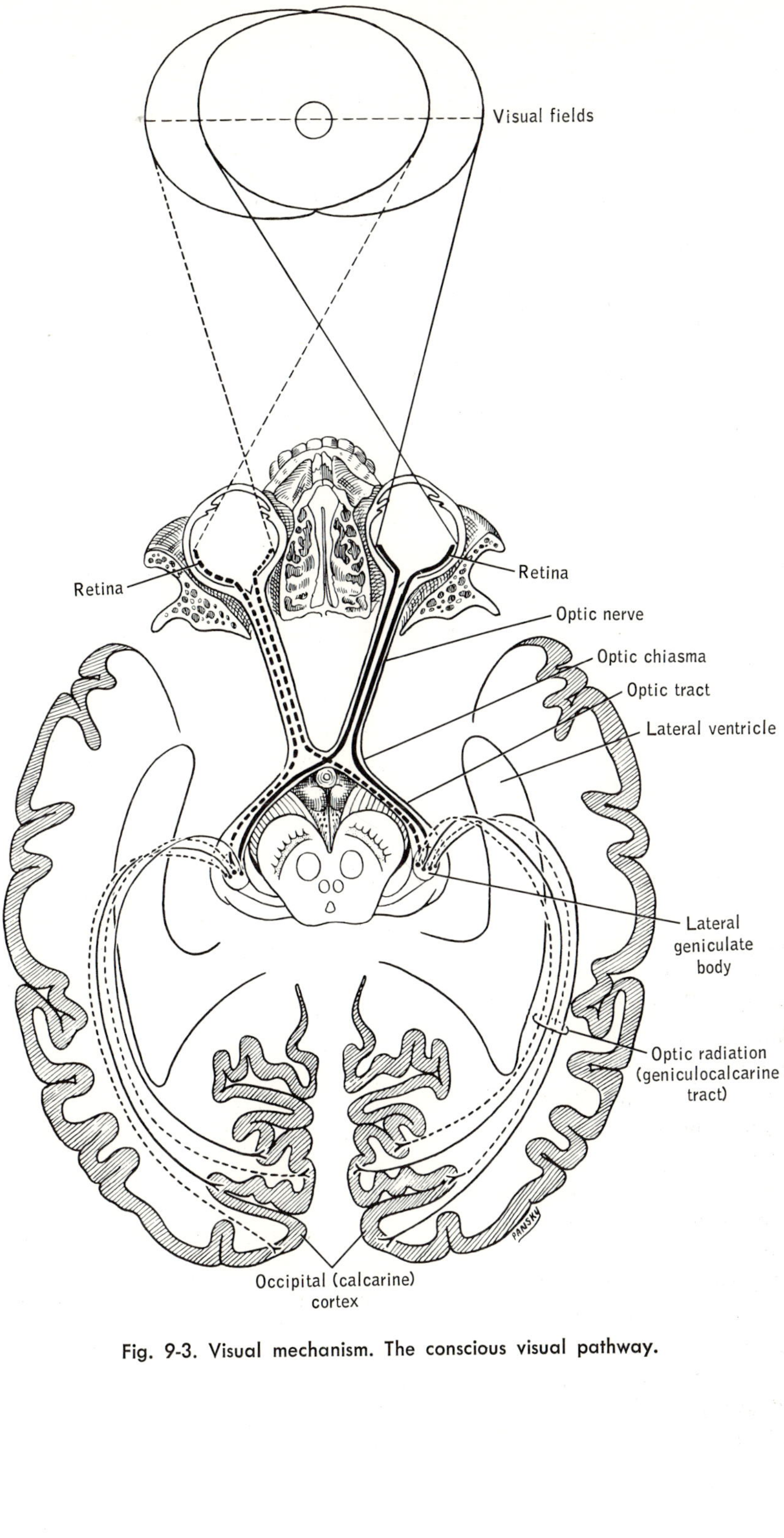

Fig. 9-3. Visual mechanism. The conscious visual pathway.

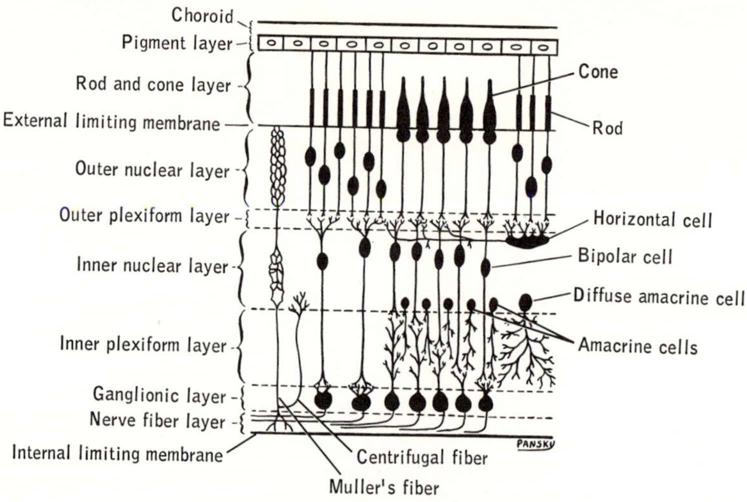

Fig. 9-4. Structure of the retina.

Both rods and cones are absent from the optic disk or blind spot, the point where the "optic nerve" fibers converge to leave the retina (Figs. 9-3, 9-6). The nuclei of the rods and cones lie in the outer nuclear layer of the retina, those of the cones being located next to the outer limiting membrane. Each also has a fibrous process which extends into the outer plexiform layer of the retina (Fig. 9-4). Here the terminals of these fibers contact the peripheral process of the afferent neurons and the dendrites of the association cells (horizontal cells), the latter interconnecting groups of cone cells in one area with both rods and cones of another.

Afferent Neuron. (Figs. 9-3, 9-4, 9-7.) The primary afferent neurons of this system are the shortest encountered anywhere, their entire extent lying within the retina. They are of the bipolar type. Their nuclei, covered by a thin layer of cytoplasm, are found in the *inner nuclear layer*. The peripheral process (functionally the dendrite) of each bipolar cell lies in the outer plexiform layer. They branch to receive the endings of several rod fibers. Cones more generally have a 1:1 relationship to the bipolar elements. The central process (axon) of the afferent neuron lies within the inner plexiform layer, where it synapses with the dendrites of the ganglion cells (Fig. 9-4).

First Association Neuron.[1] The ganglion cell layer must be thought of as a "nucleus of termination" for the afferent neurons, a feature common to all afferent mechanisms. This layer is composed of from one to several strata of large, multipolar cells. The dendrites of these cells spread out in the inner plexiform layer, where they synapse with the axons of the afferent neuron. The axons of the ganglion cells accumulate in the nerve fiber layer of the retina (Fig. 9-4). This layer is separated from the vitreous body by the inner limiting membrane. The axons of the ganglion cells then pass around the inside of the retina to approach the papilla or optic disk. At the disk, these fibers bend sharply to penetrate the outer coats of the eyeball. In order to permit passage of these fibers, the heavy scleral coat of the eye is perforated with many small holes. This region is known as the *lamina cribrosa* (Fig. 9-2), the weakest point in the ocular bulb.

When the axons of the association neuron emerge from the sclera, they form the optic nerve. However, if one recalls the connections

[1] There is a belief, held by some, that the rod and cone cells not only are receptors but also are the primary afferent neurons, as well. Thus, the bipolar cells could be considered the nucleus of termination and would represent the first association neuron.

made within the retina, it will be seen that this "nerve" more nearly fits the description of a fiber tract of the CNS.[2]

Within the nerve, the axons are arranged on the basis of origin (Figs. 9-3, 9-5). Fibers arising from the cells in the temporal side lie in the lateral portion of the optic nerve, while those from the nasal retina occupy the medial part.

The optic nerves pass dorsally through the orbit, exit through the optic foramina, and enter the middle cranial fossa. Here, they approach each other and enter the *optic chiasma* (Figs. 9-3, 9-5, 25-19, 25-20). In the chiasma the fibers from the nasal retinae undergo complete decussation. Those which arise in the lower nasal quadrant form short loops in the medial part of the opposite optic nerve before becoming a part of the optic tract. At the same time, fibers from the superior nasal segment send loops into the rostral end of the optic tract on the same side before they enter the contralateral optic tract. Fibers from the temporal halves do not cross at all (Figs. 9-3, 9-5). Dorsal to the chiasma, the large fiber bundles running along the lateral aspect of the diencephalon are known as the *optic tracts* (Figs. 9-3, 9-5, 25-15 to 25-18). These contain the fibers from the temporal retina of the same side (homolateral or ipsilateral) and the fibers of the opposite (contralateral) nasal retina. Thus it should be understood that, for example, the entire left field of vision is being projected centrally by the right optic tract.

The fibers of the optic tract sweep backward around the hypothalamus, cross the rostral portion of the cerebral peduncles, and curve upward. Some of these fibers pass dorsally and medially over the lateral geniculate body and approach the rostral end of the mesencephalon to terminate in either the *superior colliculus* or the *pretectal zone* (Figs. 9-7, 9-8). The latter is a small gray area lying between the anterior border of the mesencephalon and the caudal margin of the epithalamus. Some fibers also pass into the hypothalamus to terminate both in the supraoptic nucleus and among the cells in the medial portion of the tuber cinereum. By way of fibers descending through the infundibulum, the pituitary is reflexively related to the retina. In lower forms, this may be part of the mechanism involved in pigment distribution. In man, the function of this pathway is not clearly understood.

Second Association Neuron. (Fig. 9-7.) These neurons have a variety of terminations, depending upon the final distribution of the efferent limbs of the reflex arcs.

From some cells in the superior colliculus, axons pass ventrally and caudally, undergoing partial decussation. They then descend as the *tectospinal tract* (Figs. 25-1 to 25-11) near the midline throughout the brain stem and continue into the cord in the anterior funiculus. These fibers terminate in either the anterior or intermediolateral cell column.

From other cells in the superior colliculus, fibers pass ventrally and caudally but *do not* decussate. They descend in the reticular formation of the brain stem as the *tectobulbar tract*[3] and enter the cervical cord as a part of the *reticulospinal system.* These fibers terminate in the cranial motor nuclei of nerves III, IV, VI, and XI (Figs. 2-41, 2-47, 2-49, 2-52, 9-6) and in the anterior gray columns of the cervical cord.

From cells in the pretectal zone, axons pass ventrally and caudally around the cerebral aqueduct to terminate in the *Edinger-Westphal (EW) nucleus.* This nucleus lies in the mesencephalon surrounding the rostral end of the oculomotor nucleus.

Efferent Neuron. (Figs. 9-7, 9-8.) From cells in the anterior gray column of the entire cord, axons leave through the ventral roots of the spinal nerves to reach the skeletal musculature of the trunk and extremities, initiating a *somatosomatic reflex.*

[2] The fact that there is myelin without neurilemma; neuroglia rather than endoneurium; and dura in place of a typical epineural sheath, lends further support for the tract concept.

[3] Some fibers which technically should be classified as tectobulbar, since they terminate around nuclei of the brain stem, apparently cross with the tectospinal fibers and descend in this tract.

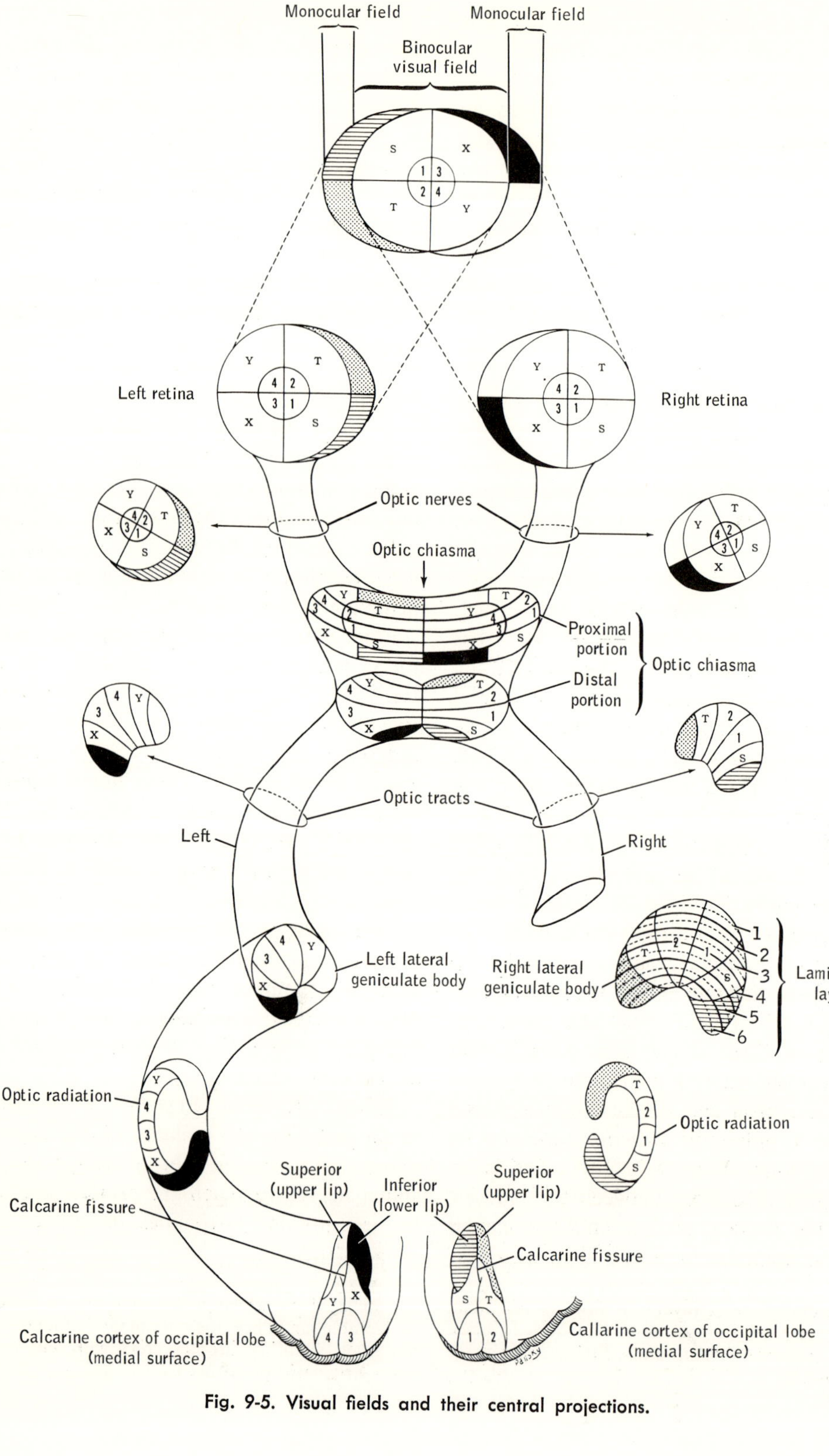

Fig. 9-5. Visual fields and their central projections.

From cells in the cranial motor nuclei of nerves III, IV, VI, and XI, axons pass by way of the roots of these nerves to certain muscles of the neck and eyes. This is also a *somatosomatic reflex,* enabling the coordinated movement of head, neck, and eyes.

From cells in the intermediolateral cell column, axons pass from the cord through the ventral roots of appropriate spinal nerves. These diverge from the nerve trunk as white rami communicantes, pass through the thoracic sympathetic chain, and terminate in the superior cervical sympathetic ganglia. These fibers are referred to as preganglionic fibers (Chap. 15). Postganglionic fibers from the superior cervical ganglia are then distributed to the dilator pupillae muscle of the eye. Thus, the *somatovisceral reflex* enables the pupil to dilate (enlarge) in dim light.

From the *Edinger-Westphal nucleus* in the mesencephalon, the axons pass ventrally and accompany the fibers of the oculomotor (III) cranial nerve. After the oculomotor nerve reaches the orbit, these fibers diverge to enter the ciliary ganglion, in which they synapse. Thus, these fibers are also referred to as preganglionic fibers. From the ciliary ganglion, postganglionic fibers pass by way of the short ciliary nerves to the sphincter pupillae muscle. This *somatovisceral reflex* constricts the pupil in the presence of strong light. (Fig. 9-8.)

Conscious (Figs. 9-3, 9-5.)

Receptors. These are the same as described under Reflex, above.

Neuron I. These, too, are the same as the afferent neurons described under Reflex, above.

Neuron II. This is the same as the first association neuron, described above, up to the point where the optic tracts enter the thalamus. Here, the fibers to consciousness terminate in the *lateral geniculate nucleus* (*body*) of the thalamus.

In the optic tract, fibers arising from the macular region of the retina occupy an intermediate position between those arising from the upper quadrants which lie in the anteromedial area of the tract and those originating in the

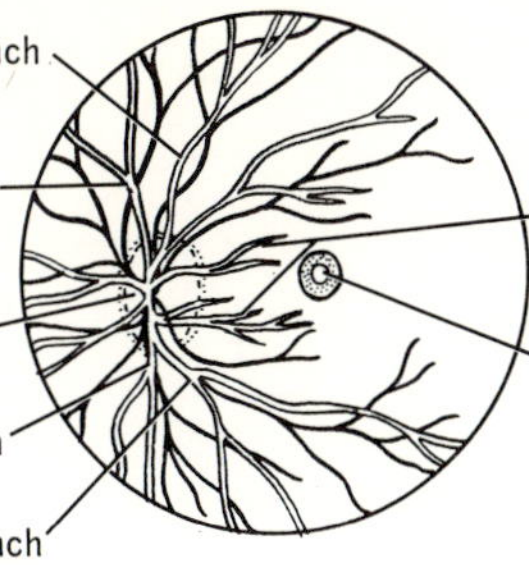

Fig. 9-6. Blood vessels (arteries labeled) of the left retina.

lower quadrants which run in the posterolateral part. There is also apparently a very exact relationship between points in the retina and specific parts of the lateral geniculate nucleus. Fibers arising in the upper quadrants of the retina terminate in the medial part of the nucleus while those from the lower quadrants end in the lateral portion. The macular area of the retina is represented by a relatively large central area of this nucleus. As noted in Figs. 9-5, 9-7, the lateral geniculate nucleus shows six fairly distinct layers. It has been established that those fibers arising in the contralateral retina end around cells in layers 1, 4, and 6 while the ipsilateral retina sends its impulses to layers 2, 3, and 5.

Neuron III. The cell bodies of these neurons lie in various portions of the lateral geniculate body. Their axons make up the *geniculocalcarine tract* (Figs. 9-3, 9-9). The most dorsal of these fibers pass almost directly backward to the cerebral cortex located along the calcarine fissure on the medial surface of the occipital lobe. The more ventrally placed fibers first run forward and downward into the temporal lobe, spread over the tip of the inferior horn of the lateral ventricle, and then loop backward, close to the lateral ventricular wall, to reach the calcarine cortex. Within the geniculocalcarine tract (optic radiations) which passes chiefly through the retrolenticular part of the internal capsule, the relation between retinal areas and tract fibers is also evident (Fig. 9-5). Diagramatically, the

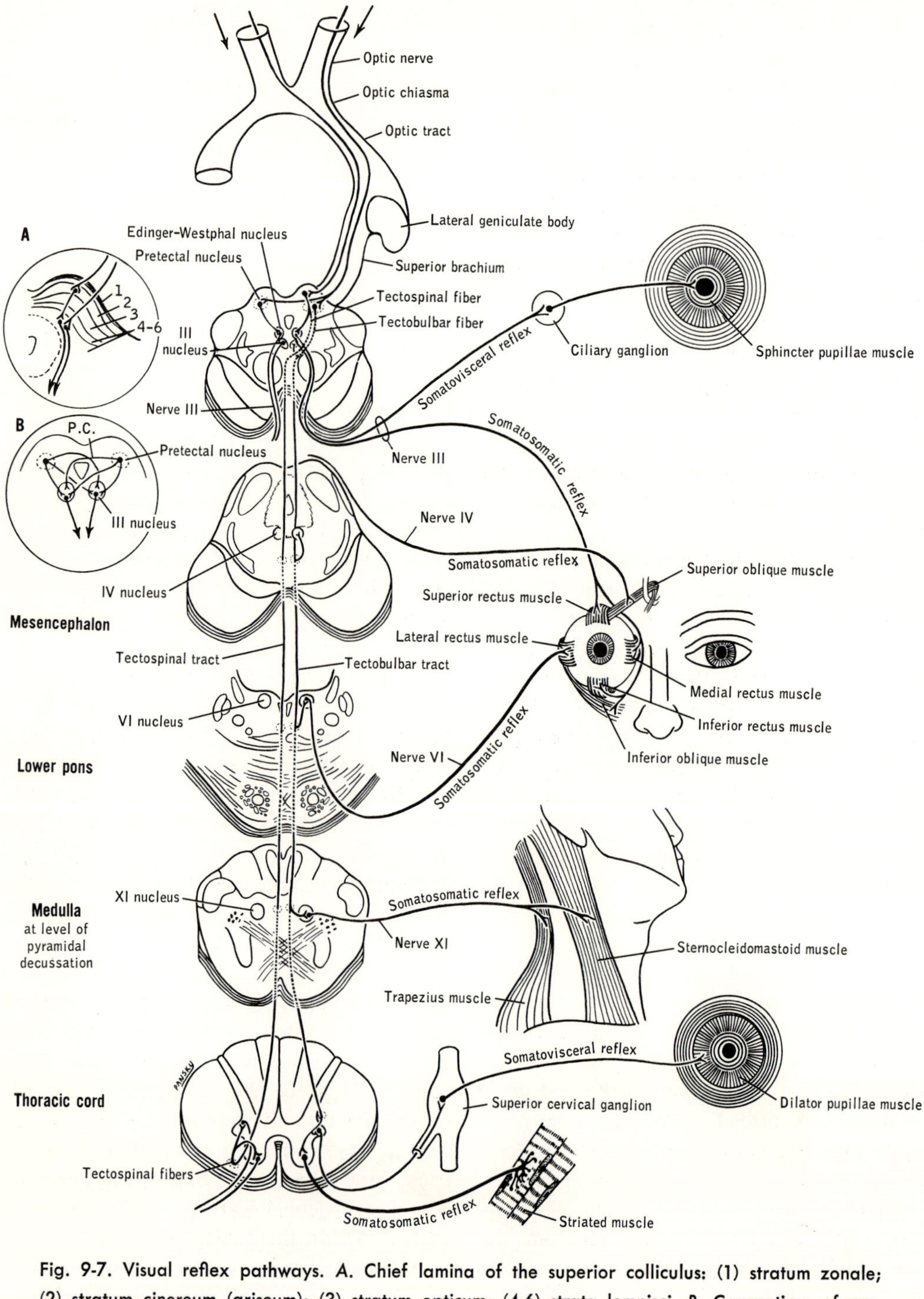

Fig. 9-7. Visual reflex pathways. A. Chief lamina of the superior colliculus: (1) stratum zonale; (2) stratum cinereum (griseum); (3) stratum opticum; (4-6) strata lemnisci. B. Connections of pretectal zone to oculomotor complex.

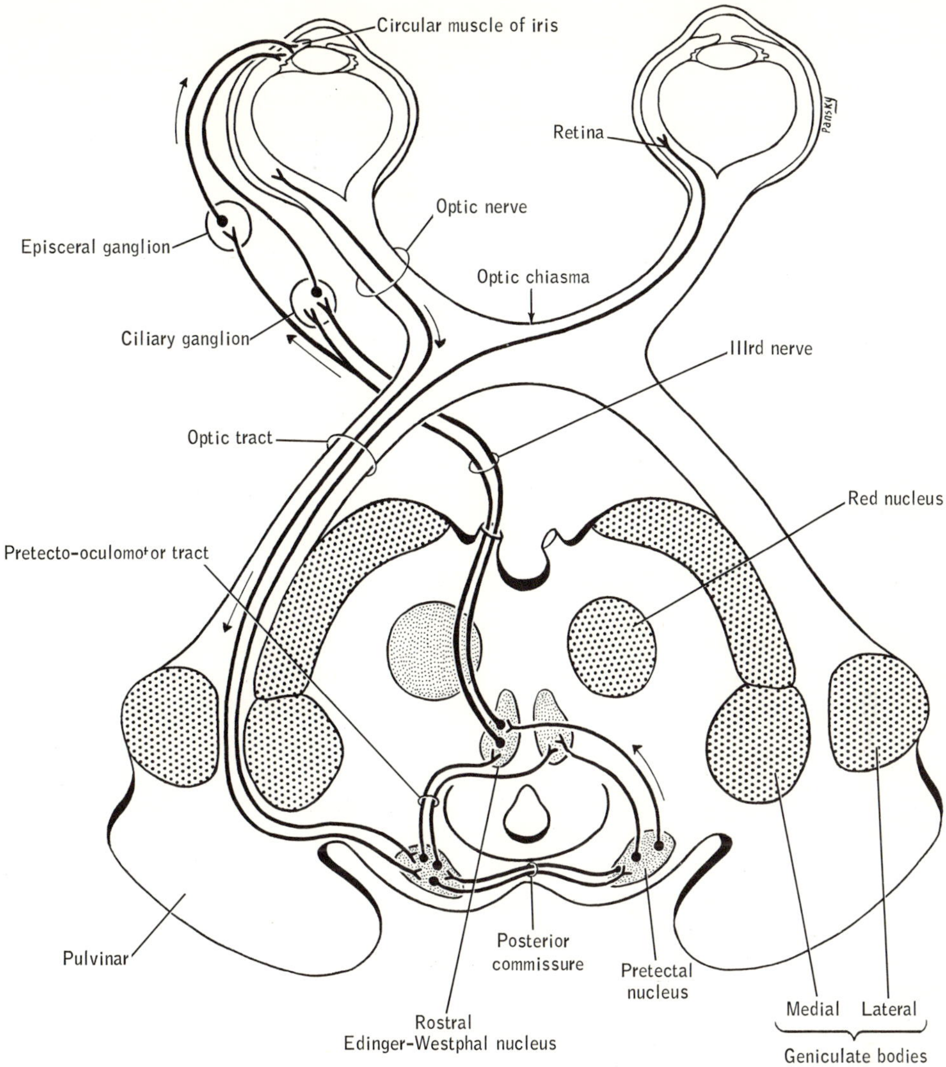

Fig. 9-8. Diagram of the light reflex pathway showing the left side only.

geniculocalcarine tract can be represented as being crescent-shaped with its concavity directed medially. The macular region of the retina occupies the entire body of the crescent and is most lateral in position. The fibers representing the upper quadrant of the retina lie along the superior arch while the inferior retinal quadrant pathway is on the inferior arch. The relationship between the areas of the lateral geniculate nucleus and the optic cortex is also very precise. From the medial half of the nucleus (upper retinal quadrants), third order neurons pass to the upper (superior) lip of the calcarine fissure while the lateral half of the nucleus (lower retinal quadrants) projects to the lower (inferior) lip of this fissure. The intermediate part of the nucleus, related to the macular retina, sending its fibers through the middle portion of

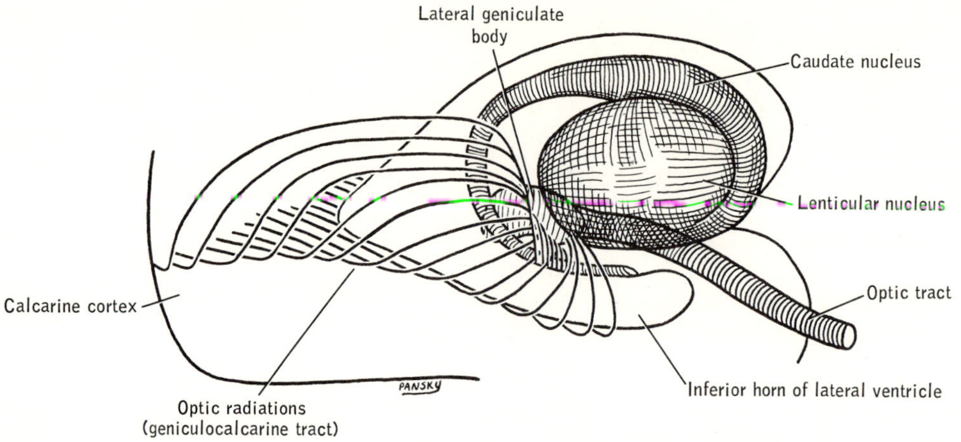

Fig. 9-9. Lateral view of the visual radiations showing the formation and course of the geniculocalcarine tract.

the optic radiations, is projected to a large cortical area along both sides of the posterior third of the calcarine fissure.[4]

Accommodation (Fig. 9-10.)

The process by which an image is kept in sharp focus when the gaze is shifted from a far object (beyond 16 in.) to a near object (less than 16 in.) is called *accommodation.* Several reflex activities are involved in this, including thickening of the lens, constriction of the pupil, and convergence of the eyes.

The reason for discussing this phenomenon at this point, rather than with other reflexes, lies in the fact that for the complete act of accommodation, it is necessary for the visual impulses to reach the cortex. This they do by way of the conscious pathways. Thus, when such impulses reach the cortical visual area, it is here that the reflex is initiated by associational neurons which pass forward to the motor centers of the frontal lobe. Secondary association neurons arising from such motor areas then descend through the internal capsule and diverge into the brachium of the superior colliculus to synapse there in the gray substance. From cells in the superior colliculus, fibers descend to the posterior portion of the Edinger-Westphal nucleus and the nucleus of Perlia (medial part of the third nucleus), where they synapse.

Efferent Limb. Some fibers from the Edinger-Westphal nucleus pass ventrally as preganglionic fibers to join the oculomotor nerve, with which they enter the orbit. They then diverge from the orbit to pass through the ciliary ganglion *without* synapse, terminating about the cells of the *episcleral ganglia* on the sclera of the eyeball. The short axons of the postganglionic fibers terminate in the ciliary muscle. Thus, this reflex results in an increase in thickness of the lens in its anteroposterior diameter.

Other fibers from the Edinger-Westphal nucleus pass by way of the third cranial nerve to the *ciliary ganglion,* where the preganglionic fibers terminate. From here, postganglionic fibers pass to the sphincter pupillae muscle of the iris, enabling *constriction of the pupil.*

From the *nucleus of Perlia,* fibers pass either directly to the medial recti muscles of the eyes or by way of short axons into the main third nucleus itself and then to the muscles. This reflex enables the eyes to *converge.*

[4] There is some controversy over the possibility that the maculae retinae have a bilateral cortical representation. If such pathways exist, they might account for the fact that, in large cortical lesions involving the occipital cortex, the macular region is often spared.

Clinical Considerations

Many clinical conditions, both congenital and acquired, lead to impairment of vision. Among them are coloboma, albinism, cataract, opaque cornea, and retinal separation. Furthermore, certain systemic conditions, not primarily concerned with vision but often affecting it adversely, such as severe diabetes, could be mentioned. However, these, together with the general ophthalmologic problems of astigmatism, myopia, and hyperopia, cannot be considered here (Fig. 9-11). Only the purely neurologic conditions will be discussed.

Further, visible signs about the eyes, such as drooping of the eyelids (ptosis) and constriction of the pupils (myosis), as seen in connection with Horner's syndrome, are closely associated with defects of the autonomic nervous system. Therefore, a discussion of this condition will be delayed until the study of the GVE system is undertaken (Chap. 15). Defects involving position and movement of the eye will also be considered under the GSE system (Chap. 14).

The terms *visual axis, visual fields, retinal fields,* and *macular vision,* discussed early in this chapter under General Definitions, should be reviewed. Other terms frequently encountered in reference to the visual system are *anopsia* (without vision); *hemianopsia* (blindness, unilateral or bilateral, in one-half of the visual field); *heteronymous hemianopsia* (bitemporal or binasal loss of vision); *homonymous hemianopsia* (loss of vision in the nasal half of one eye and the temporal half of the other).

Testing

Visual Fields. (Figs. 9-3, 9-5.) The examination of the visual fields is of great clinical importance in localizing lesions involving the visual

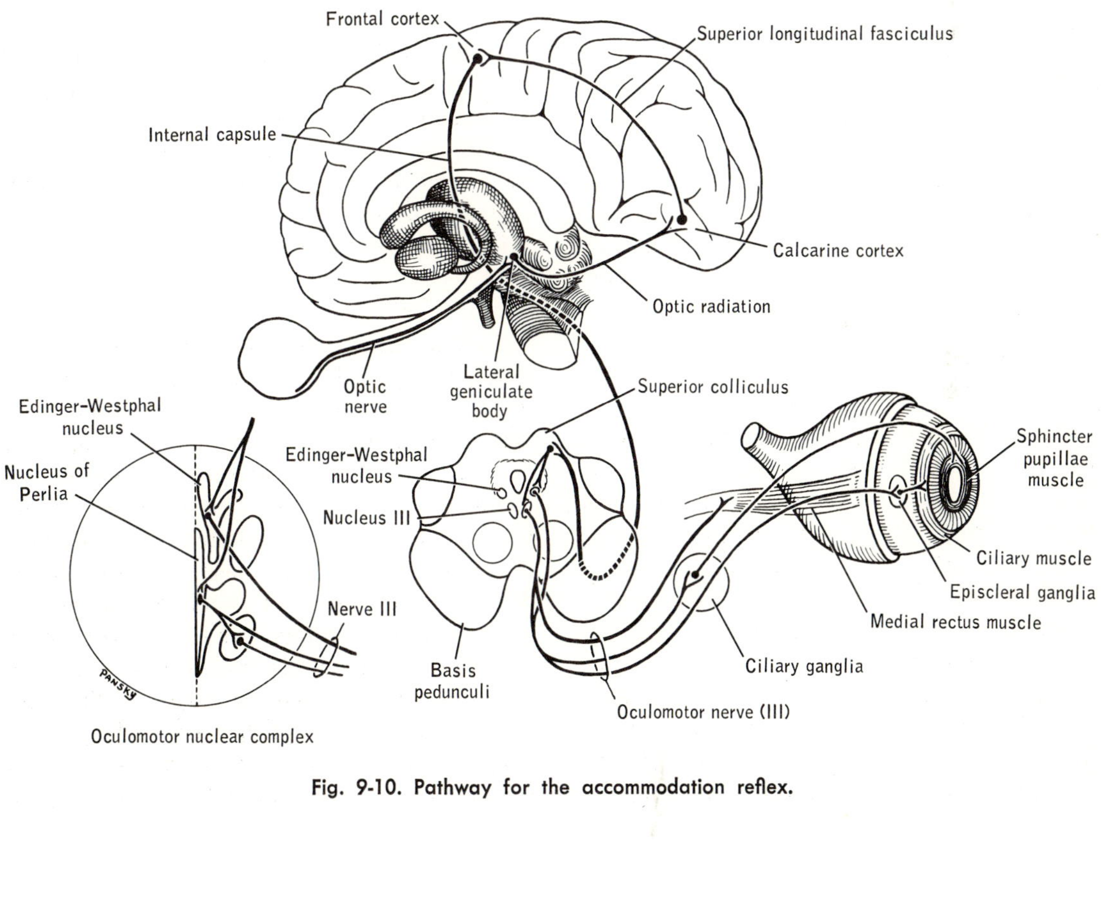

Fig. 9-10. Pathway for the accommodation reflex.

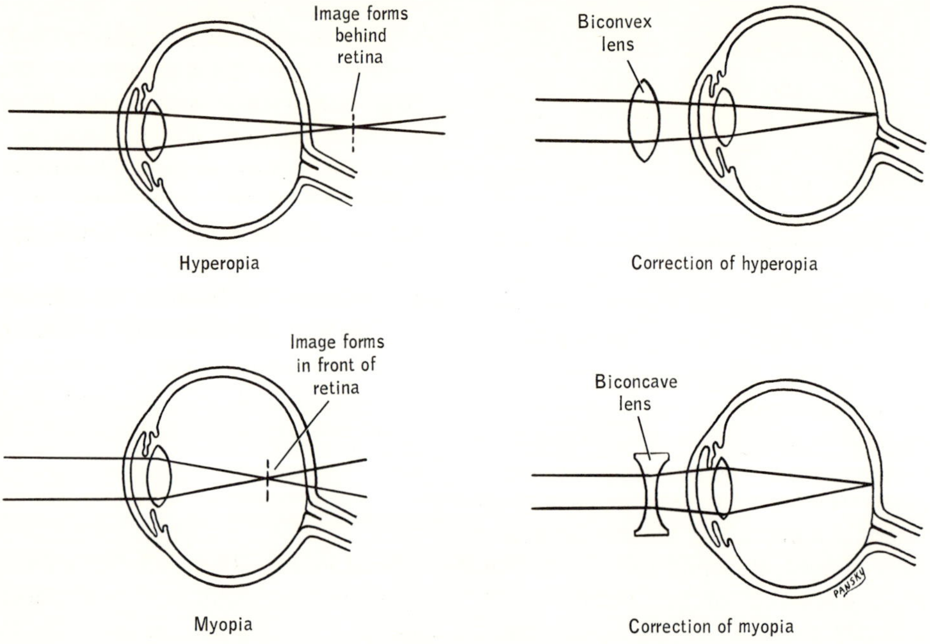

Fig. 9-11. Visual defects—myopia and hyperopia.

pathways. The fields may be mapped by the use of a perimeter or tangent screen. However, a fairly accurate picture may be produced by having the patient fix his gaze directly ahead, on a dark field several feet in front of him with one eye covered. The examiner then moves a small, silvered sphere on the end of a wand, from the periphery toward the central fixation zone. The patient is required to tell when he fails to see the sphere. This process is carried through to cover the four quadrants of the field, and is then repeated for the other eye.

Convergence and Reflex Pupillary Constriction. (Fig. 9-12.) With the examiner standing directly in front of the patient, the finger, wand, or comparable object is held some distance (more than 16 in.) from the patient's nose. It is then moved rapidly in toward the nose. It should be noted whether the eyes converge and the pupils constrict.

Light Reflex. A small beam of light is directed into one eye; it should be noted whether the pupil of the eye into which the light is shining shows constriction (*direct light response*), and then it should be noted whether the pupil in the other eye constricts simultaneously (*consensual light response*).

Ophthalmoscopic. In the sense used here, the examination of the retina through the ophthalmoscope is to search the retina for defects primarily located there.

Specific Pathology

Lesions Involving Optic Nerve, Optic Chiasma, or Optic Tract. (Fig. 9-13.) Figures indicate the location of possible lesions, fibers destroyed or damaged, and the resulting visual field defects. Thus, complete anopsia in one eye may result from loss of blood supply to the retina or optic nerve. Compression of the optic nerve in the orbit may also lead to variable degrees of blindness. Tumors, expanding forward from the pituitary gland or hypothalamus, may impinge upon the optic chiasma to such an extent that decussating fibers of the nasal retinae will be disrupted, thus leading to *bitemporal hemianopsia. Binasal hemianopsia,* in which the uncrossed fibers from the temporal retina of both eyes are interrupted with the consequent loss of both nasal visual fields, is theoretically possible, but rare. Bilateral aneurysms of the internal carotid arteries have been observed to cause binasal hemianopsia. Unilateral compression of one side of the chiasma due to this arterial defect, destroying the fibers from the temporal retina of the same side with the loss of the nasal visual field for that eye, is more common (*nasal hemianopsia*). Injuries or tumors may also involve the optic tracts, thus producing *homonymous hemianopsia.* However, the destruction of these tracts is often only partial. This is also true of the geniculocalcarine tract and the visual cortex. So many variations are possible that a complete description of all of them is too complex for this book.

Lesions of the Pretectal Zone. It has been pointed out that the reflex pathways for pupillary constriction and for accommodation are not

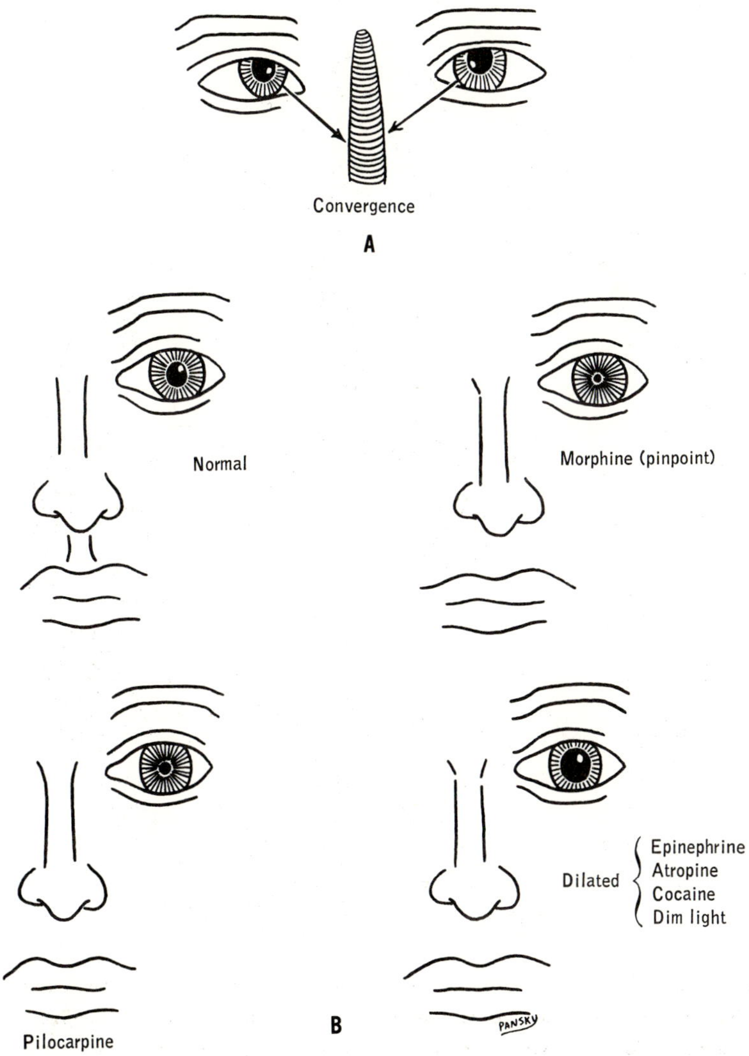

Fig. 9-12. Eye movement and pupil changes. *A.* Convergence. *B.* Variations in pupillary size due to various causes, especially the use of certain drugs.

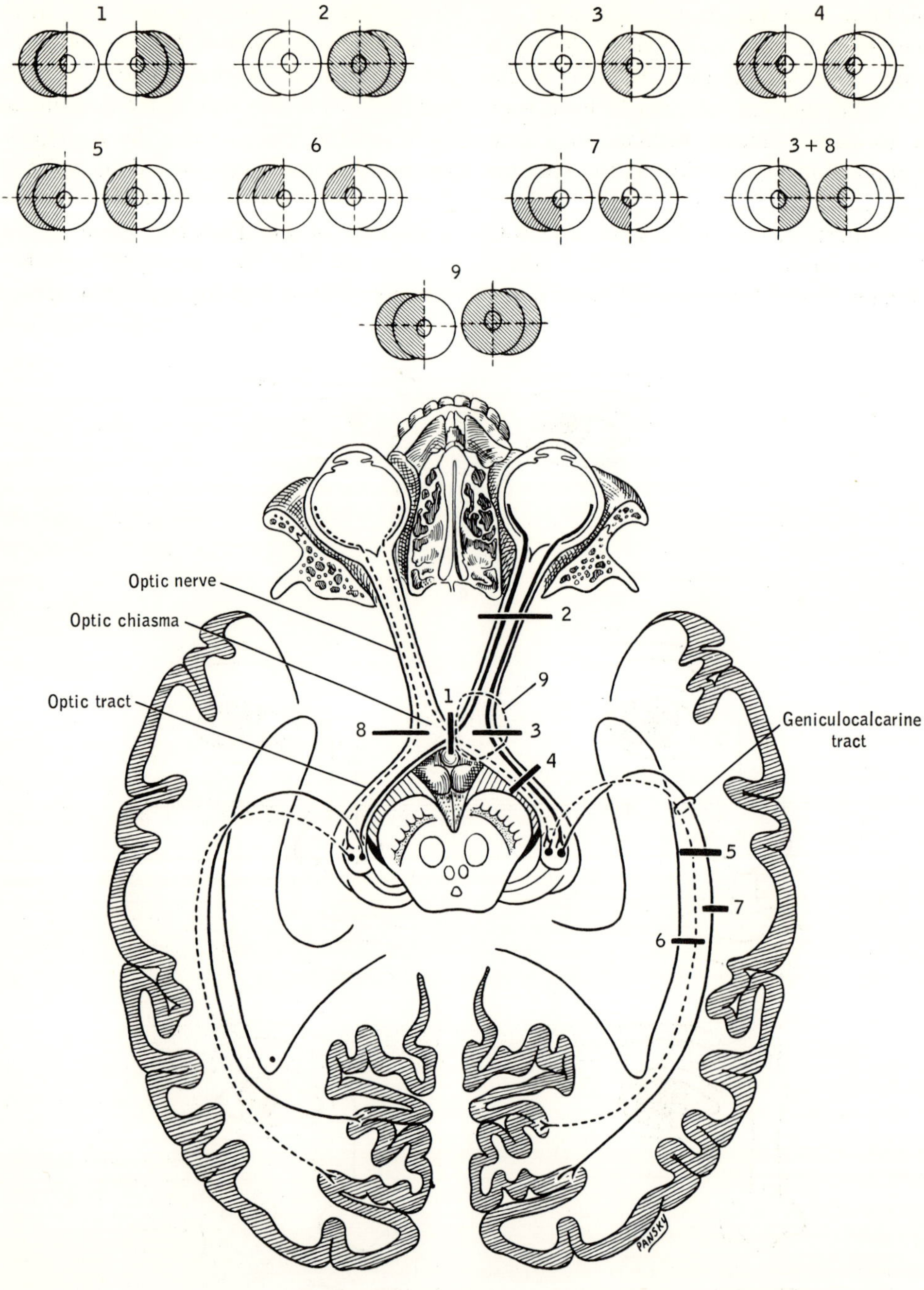

Fig. 9-13. Lesions in the visual pathways: (1) bitemporal heteronymous hemianopsia; (2) homolateral blindness; (3) right nasal hemianopsia; (4) lateral homonymous hemianopsia; (5) homonymous hemianopsia; (6) homonymous partial quadranticanopsia; (7) same as (6); (8) plus (3) nasal heteronymous hemianopsia; (9) homolateral blindness plus contralateral temporal hemianopsia. Note: Lesions shown at (6) and (7) would involve more than those fibers indicated, thus accounting for loss of visual fields for both eyes.

the same. Thus, if a disease such as tabes dorsalis spreads to the pretectal zone, an important link in the light reflex circuit is broken and *no pupillary constriction in response to light is elicited*. On the other hand, the *pupil does constrict for near vision*. This is the so-called *Argyll Robertson pupil*.

AUDITORY SYSTEM

Development (Figs. 9-14, 9-15.)

Unlike the eye, the essential structure for hearing, lying within the inner ear, develops from a thickening of the surface ectoderm along the dorsolateral aspect of the hindbrain. This essential structure first appears as a definite placode in embryos between 2.5 and 3.5 weeks. The series of changes which occurs during the next weeks of development is best described through illustration. The ear grossly approaches typical adult structure at 16 weeks, although hearing does not occur until some time after birth. The development of accessory structures important in the reception and transmission of sound waves, such as the tympanic membrane and auditory ossicles, etc., is shown in Fig. 9-15.

In order to understand how the energy of the sound waves in the air is transformed into nervous energy, it is necessary to visualize not only the inner ear but also the middle and external ears as well (Figs. 9-16, 9-17). With these gross relationships in mind, the orientation of the parts of the inner ear should next be studied by examining a section through the cochlea, including the endolymph and perilymph (Figs. 9-18, 9-19). Thus, sound waves pass through the external auditory meatus, where they impinge upon the tympanic membrane. The membrane is set into motion with the same frequency as the incident waves and in relatively the same amplitude. Since the ansa (handle) of the malleus, the first of the auditory ossicles, is fixed to the membrane, it transmits the motion to the incus and finally to the stapes. The foot plate of the stapes lies in an oval aperture, covered by a membrane, in the wall of the bony labyrinth (oval window, fenestra ovale). Thus, the motion of this membrane, initiated by the stapes, sets up waves in the perilymph. As the moving perilymph flows up through the scala vestibuli and down the scala tympani, certain portions of the thin membranous walls of the labyrinth begin to vibrate. This vibration initiates waves in the endolymph of the cochlear duct. These are the waves (endolymphatic) which initiate movement among the hairs of the cells in the organ of Corti, the sensory receptor of the cochlear mechanism (Fig. 9-19). The movement of the hairs in the receptor cells creates certain action currents in the neurons associated with them. It has been shown that cells in one part of the cochlea vibrate to waves of one frequency while those in another part are sympathetic to other frequencies.[5] Thus, tones of low pitch (frequency) are received in the apical coil of the cochlear duct, while those of high pitch are selected in the basal coil.

Pathways

Reflex (Fig. 9-20.)

Receptors. These are the *hair cells* which lie along the entire length of the organ of Corti, in the cochlear duct (Fig. 9-19).

Afferent Neurons. A network of neurofibril-like material surrounds each hair cell. These fibrils unite below the hair cells into a nonmyelinated nerve fiber. The nerve fibers pass down the cochlea in a small space just beneath the receptor cells, enter the basilar membrane, and turn medially in the latter toward the lip of the bony modiolus, which forms the core of the cochlea. Here, the fibers become myelinated. After a short course in this thin shelf of bone, the peripheral process joins its cell body. These bipolar cells lie in the bone, arranged along the inner edge of the spiral bony shelf. This aggregation of cells is the *spiral ganglion* (Fig. 9-23). From the ganglion cells, processes are directed

[5] It is not clearly understood whether selectivity of vibrations of various frequencies is an inherent function of the hair cells or whether this phenomenon is a function of the fibers in the basilar membrane upon which the hair cells rest.

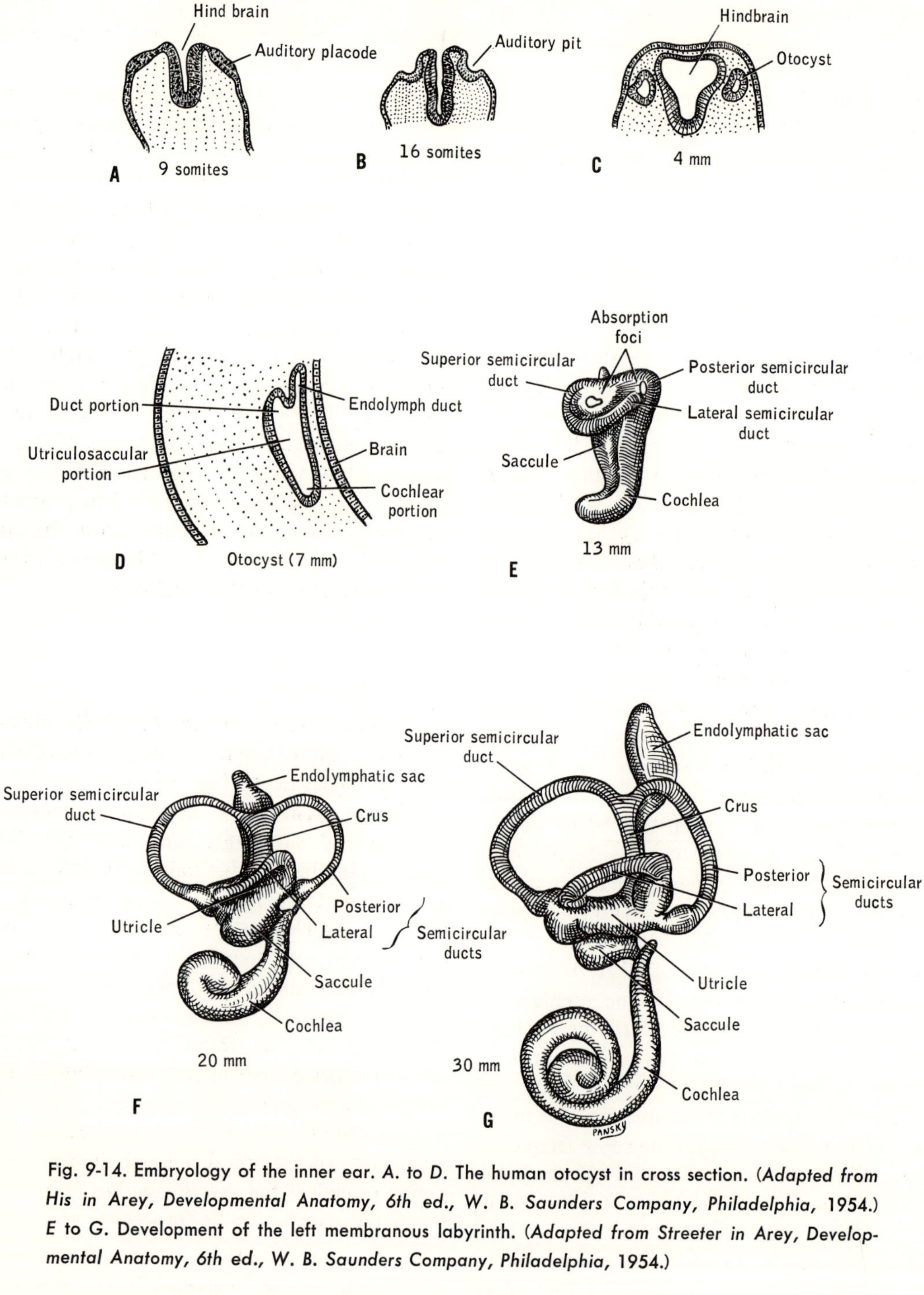

Fig. 9-14. Embryology of the inner ear. A. to D. The human otocyst in cross section. (*Adapted from His in Arey, Developmental Anatomy, 6th ed., W. B. Saunders Company, Philadelphia, 1954.*) E to G. Development of the left membranous labyrinth. (*Adapted from Streeter in Arey, Developmental Anatomy, 6th ed., W. B. Saunders Company, Philadelphia, 1954.*)

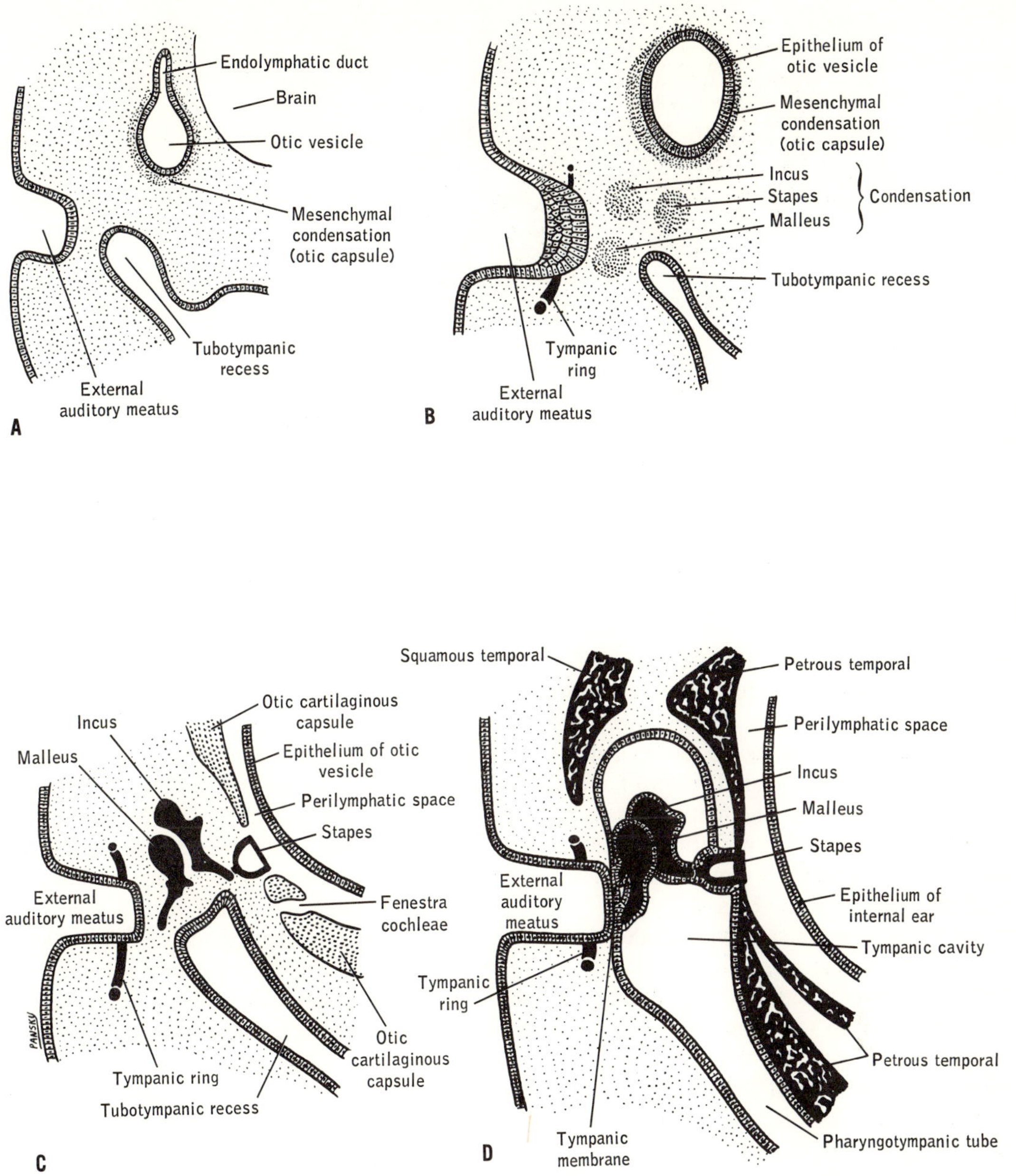

Fig. 9-15. Schematic representation showing four stages in the development of the auditory tube, the auditory ossicles, the middle ear, and the external auditory meatus. (*Adapted from Hamilton, Boyd, and Mossman, Human Embryology, 2d ed., The Williams & Wilkins Company, Baltimore, 1952.*)

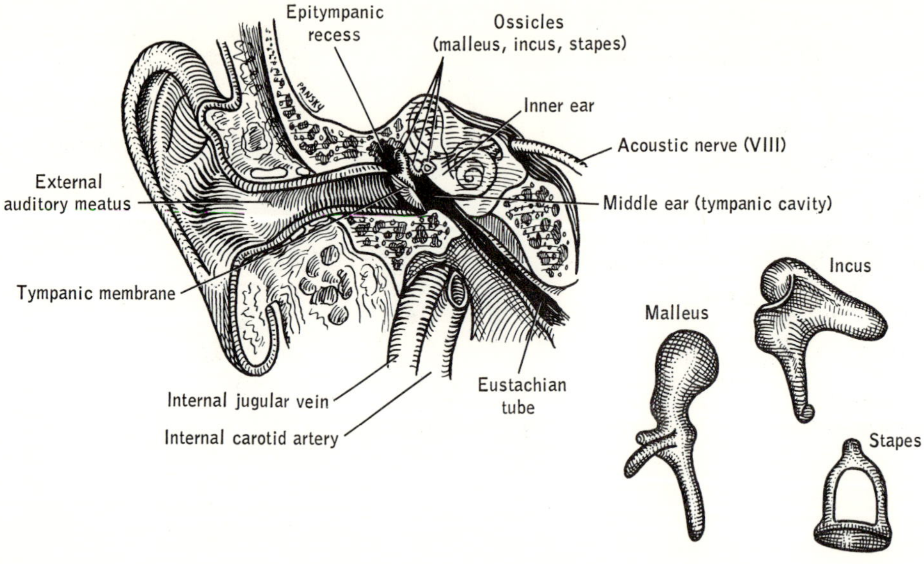

Fig. 9-16. Anatomy of the external, middle, and inner ear.

centrally, accumulated in the center of the modiolus. There, they turn downward toward the base of the cochlea, where they enter the internal acoustic meatus to be joined by the fibers from the vestibular division of the eighth nerve. They traverse the entire length of the meatus and enter the posterior cranial fossa, where they immediately enter the brain in the cerebellopontine angle (Figs. 2-7, 2-8).

After entering the substance of the brain, the cochlear fibers segregate into two main bundles. One group passes laterally and dorsally to the restiform body to terminate in the *dorsal cochlear nucleus* (Figs. 9-20, 9-21). The other group remains slightly ventral and medial to the restiform body and ends in the *ventral cochlear nucleus* (Figs. 9-20, 25-6).

First Association Neuron. The cell bodies of the first association neurons lie in either the dorsal or the ventral cochlear nuclei.

Fibers from the *ventral nucleus* pass medially with a slight rostral inclination and are collectively known as the *ventral trapezoid body* (Figs. 9-20, 9-21, 25-9). These fibers lie between the basilar and tegmental areas of the pons. The fibers of the trapezoid body cross the midline and, on reaching the level of the superior olivary nucleus, bend around the lateral side of this nucleus and turn rostrally, forming a band called the *lateral lemniscus* (Figs. 25-9 to 25-11). In its ascent, this becomes the most lateral part of the lemniscus system and can be traced into the caudal part of the mesencephalon. Some of the trapezoid fibers terminate in the nuclei of the trapezoid body, others in the superior olive, while still others merely give collaterals to these nuclei. Of the fibers in the lateral lemniscus, some terminate in the nucleus of the lateral lemniscus (Fig. 25-10) and others synapse in the inferior colliculus (Fig. 25-11). Collaterals from the fibers in the conscious pathway may also terminate in the nuclei of the lateral lemniscus and inferior colliculus (Figs. 2-39, 2-45, 9-20).

Fibers arising from the *dorsal cochlear nucleus* follow a variety of courses. Some remain on the same side, running rostrally to join the lateral lemniscus. Others travel medially, lying a little below the floor of the fourth ventricle. Reaching the raphé they cross to the opposite side and then run ventrolaterally to join the lateral lem-

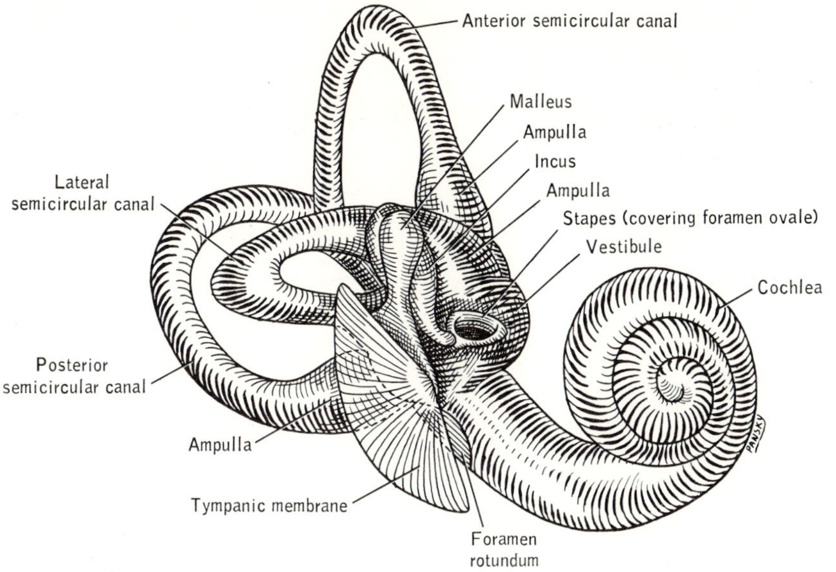

Fig. 9-17. Chain of transmission showing the tympanic membrane, the auditory ossicles, and the bony labyrinth.

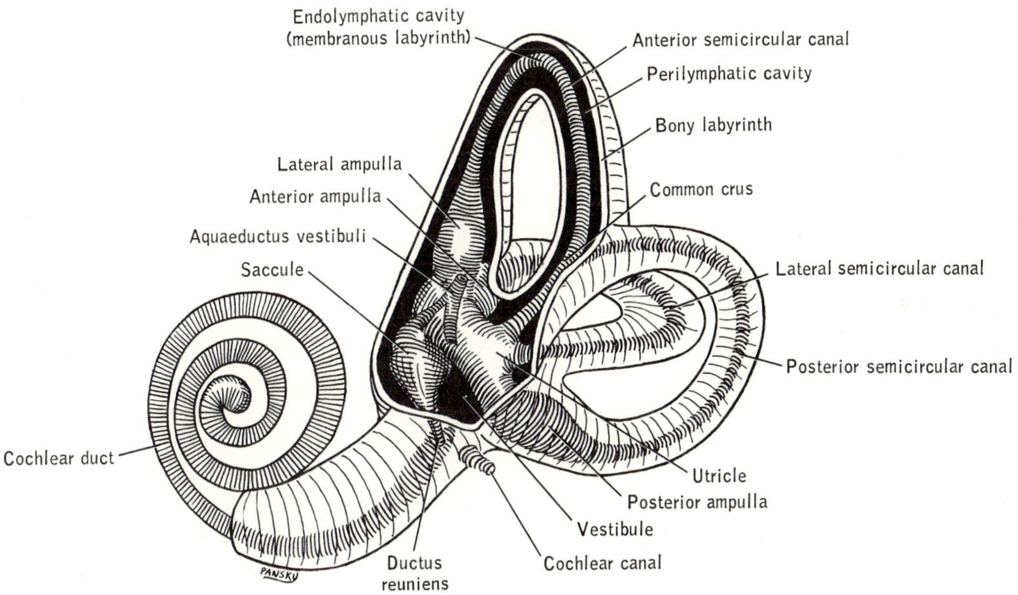

Fig. 9-18. Relationships of the parts of the inner ear with special emphasis on the endolymph and perilymph.

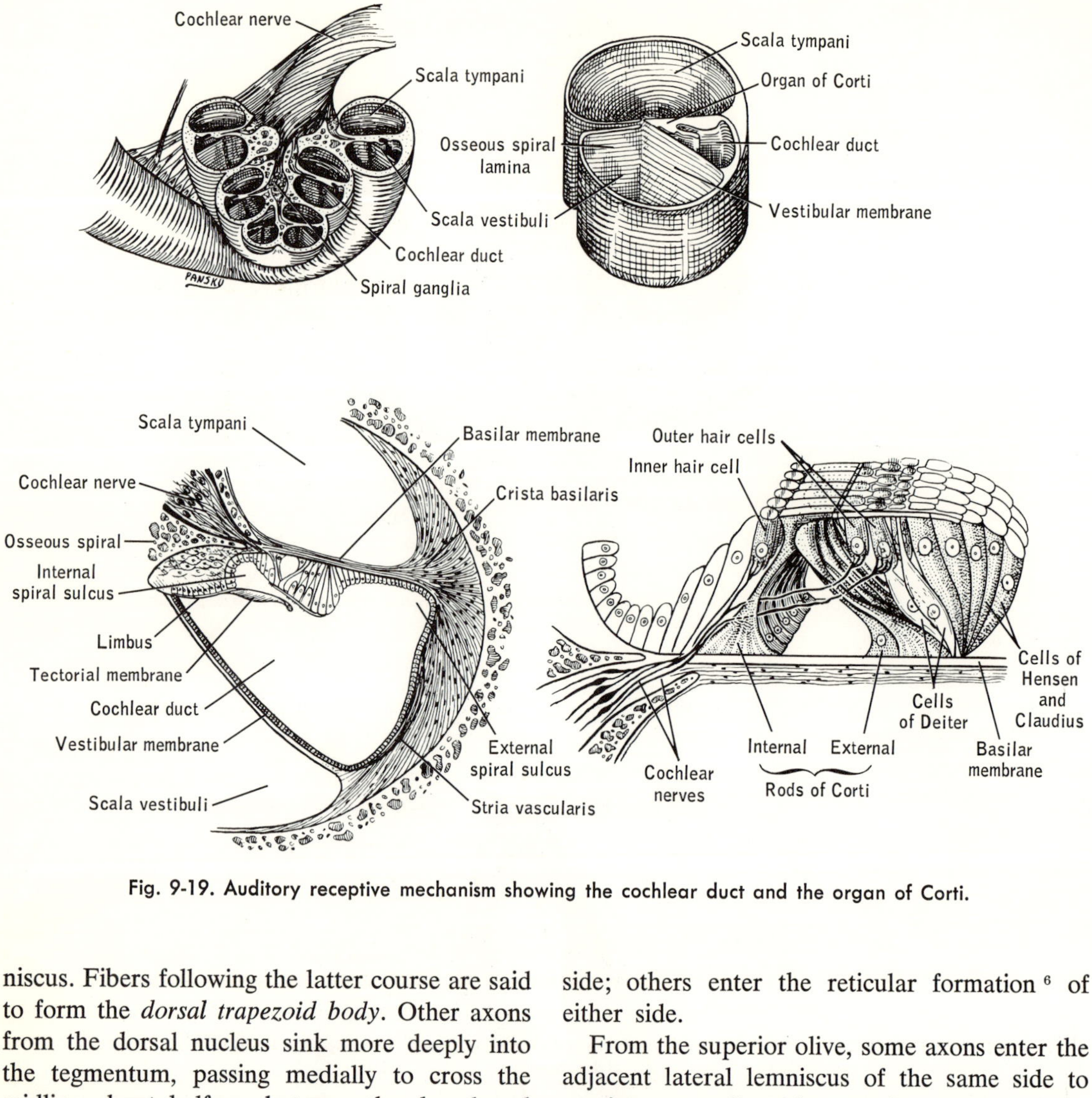

Fig. 9-19. Auditory receptive mechanism showing the cochlear duct and the organ of Corti.

niscus. Fibers following the latter course are said to form the *dorsal trapezoid body*. Other axons from the dorsal nucleus sink more deeply into the tegmentum, passing medially to cross the midline about halfway between the dorsal and ventral trapezoid bodies. After crossing, these fibers join the contralateral lateral lemniscus. These fibers comprise the *intermediate trapezoid body*.

Second Association Neuron. The cell bodies of such neurons are located in four nuclear masses: nucleus of the trapezoid body, nucleus of the superior olive, nucleus of the lateral lemniscus, and the inferior colliculus.

From the nucleus of the trapezoid body, some fibers cross to the superior olive of the opposite side; others enter the reticular formation [6] of either side.

From the superior olive, some axons enter the adjacent lateral lemniscus of the same side to continue rostrally either to the nucleus of the lateral lemniscus or to the inferior colliculus. Some fibers may enter the neighboring reticular formation,[6] still another group stream dorsomedially in the peduncle of the superior olive to join the medial longitudinal fasciculus (MLF) of either side. Among those fibers in the peduncle are some that arise either in the superior olive proper or in the medial accessory olive (or in

[6] Additional association neurons may be involved where fibers entering the tegmental reticular formation may make scattered synapses.

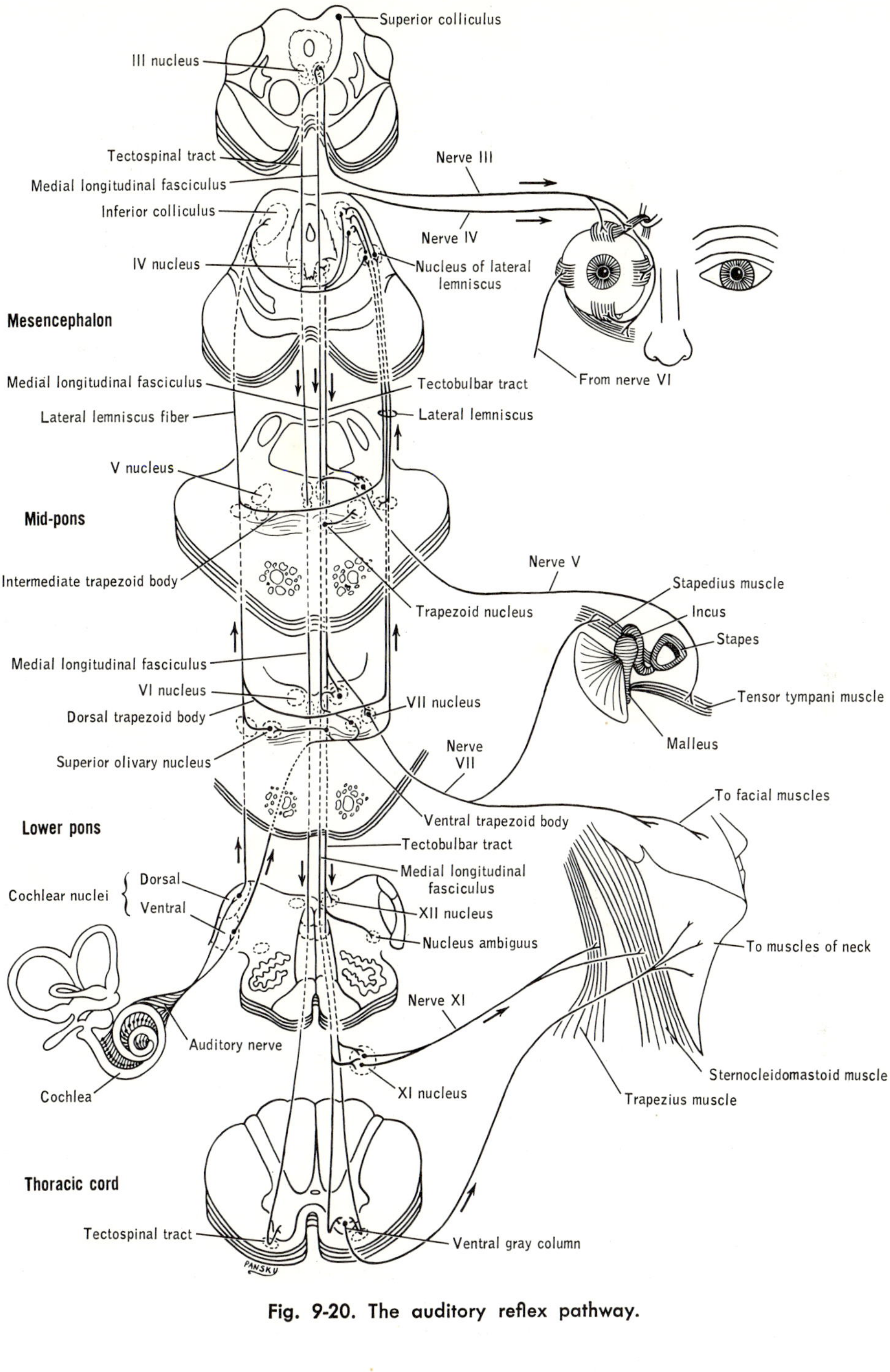

Fig. 9-20. The auditory reflex pathway.

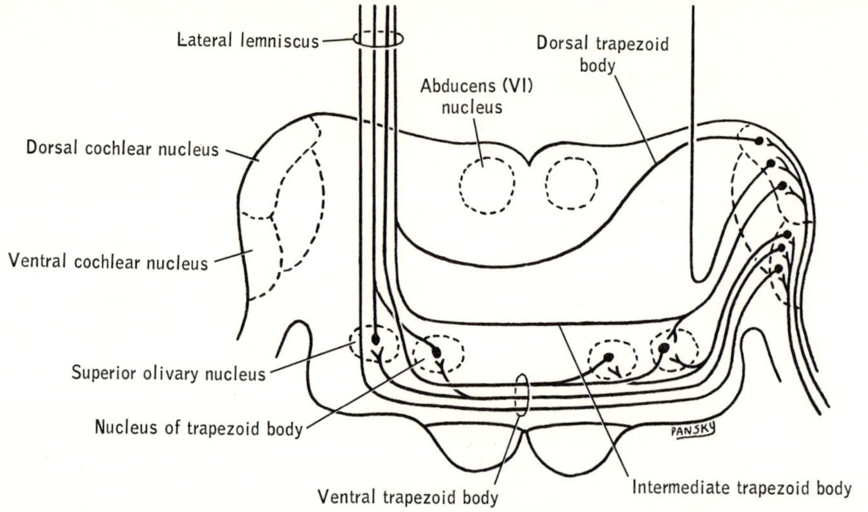

Fig. 9-21. Enlargement of the auditory pathway in the region of the medulla to illustrate the trapezoid bodies and the formation of the lateral lemniscus.

the adjoining tegmentum). This group is known as the *efferent cochlear bundle.* The latter cross inferior to the genu of the seventh nerve and leave the brain in company with the vestibular nerve of the opposite side. These may be joined by fibers originating in the principal cell mass of the superior olive of that side. Ultimately, both crossed and uncrossed fibers leave the vestibular nerve and join the cochlear with which they travel until they terminate on hair cells of the organ of Corti (Fig. 9-22). Stimulation of this bundle leads to suppression of activity in the cochlear nerve. This is basically a feedback mechanism from the primary auditory receptors. There is a possibility that other relay nuclei may also contribute to this system.

From the nucleus of the lateral lemniscus, some of the fibers merely continue upward in the lemniscus of the same side; others enter the tegmental reticular formation [6] of the opposite side; and a last group apparently reaches the lateral lemniscus of the opposite side to ascend to the inferior colliculus.

From the superior olive, axons may ascend or descend in the medial longitudinal fasciculus (Figs. 25-2 to 25-12) to reach cranial motor nuclei, particularly III, IV, VI (possibly V, VII, and XI), and the ventral columns of the cervical spinal cord. It is likely that the fibers from the superior olive, nucleus of the trapezoid body, and perhaps the lateral lemniscus reach these same motor regions through the reticular formation.

Third Association Neuron. Axons arising in the inferior colliculus pass ventromedially, cross the midline, and join fibers descending from the superior colliculus in the *tectospinal tract* (Figs. 25-1 to 25-11). In the higher mammals and man it is uncertain as to the number of descending fibers which actually take origin in the nucleus of the inferior colliculus. It appears that most of the fibers arising here ascend by way of the central gray or through capsular connections to the superior colliculus where they synapse. Cells in the latter then send their axons into the tectospinal and tectobulbar tracts. This tract sends its terminals into the ventral gray column of almost the entire cord. Some fibers apparently remain on the same side, traveling in the ipsilateral *tectobulbar tract,*[3] to terminate among the cranial motor nuclei. (Fig. 9-20.) Furthermore, connections from the inferior colliculus to the hypothalamus have been reported. Although the exact location is vague and their functions are not clear, it appears that sound does have effects upon visceral activity. The latter phenomenon might be explained on the basis of such connections.

Efferent Neuron. From cells in the anterior column of the cervical cord, fibers leave by way of the ventral roots of the cervical nerves to be distributed to muscles in the neck. Thus, a *somatosomatic reflex* enables the head to react to sound by turning toward the direction of the sound. This reflex is further augmented by fibers leaving the nucleus of cranial nerve XI to the sternocleidomastoid and trapezius muscles. Fibers leaving the nuclei of cranial nerves III, IV, and VI to the muscles of the eye also constitute a somatosomatic reflex, enabling the use of the eyes for sound locations. It should be understood that the reactions mentioned are in relation to ordinary sounds. However, the entire body may react to loud and unexpected sounds, since the tectospinal tract involves the entire extent of the cord.

Fibers arising from the motor nucleus of cranial nerves V and VII pass to the accessory muscles of the middle ear (tensor tympani and stapedius, respectively). This sets up a *special somatovisceral reflex* which increases the sensitivity to sounds and protects the delicate membranes of the middle ear against rupture. Incidental to loud and sudden noises, blinking of the eyelids and grimacing facial expression are produced by efferent neurons in these same two cranial nerves.

Conscious (Fig. 9-24.)

Receptors. These are the same as those given under Reflex, above.

Neuron I. These are identical with the afferent neurons of the reflex pathway. It has been found that fibers coming from the basal coils of the cochlea (for high pitch) terminate in the dorsal part of the dorsal cochlear nucleus. Those fibers arising in the apical coils (for low pitch) end in the ventral part of the dorsal cochlear nucleus and in the ventral nucleus.

Neuron II. The cell bodies of these neurons lie in the dorsal and ventral cochlear nuclei.

The course of the axons from these cells follows two alternate paths. It is perhaps best to describe first the more direct route to consciousness before the indirect (relay) circuit is attempted.

Direct Route. Some of the fibers from the ventral cochlear nucleus and perhaps most of the

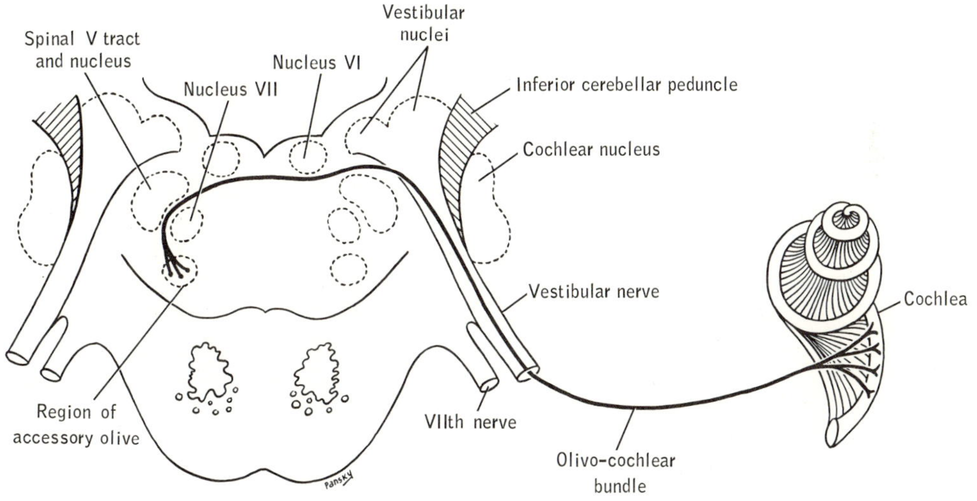

Fig. 9-22. Diagram showing the pathway by which activity of the auditory nerve is suppressed by the efferent fibers to the cochlea.

fibers from the dorsal nucleus that cross through the dorsal and intermediate trapezoid bodies bend rostrally and continue forward in the lateral lemniscus of the other side. When they reach the mesencephalon, near the caudal border of the inferior colliculus, they diverge more laterally, to bypass the colliculus (collaterals may be given off to the latter). This bundle is then known as the *brachium of the inferior colliculus* (Fig. 25-11). Its termination is the *medial geniculate nucleus* (*body*) (Fig. 25-12) of the thalamus. It is believed that the uncrossed fibers from the dorsal nucleus which travel in the ipsilateral lateral lemniscus also go directly to the medial geniculate body via the brachium of the inferior colliculus. (Figs. 2-35 to 2-37.)

Indirect (*Relay*) *Circuit*. The circuit begins in the ventral cochlear nucleus, the axons passing medially in the ventral trapezoid body, some of them terminating in the nucleus of that body, where another neuron arises. Almost certainly, the superior olive is an important relay station, receiving fibers both from the cochlear nucleus and from the nucleus of the trapezoid body. From the olive, fibers ascend in the lateral lemniscus, some synapsing in its nucleus, others continuing to the inferior colliculus. It is likely that some of the fibers in this chain, whose cells of origin lie

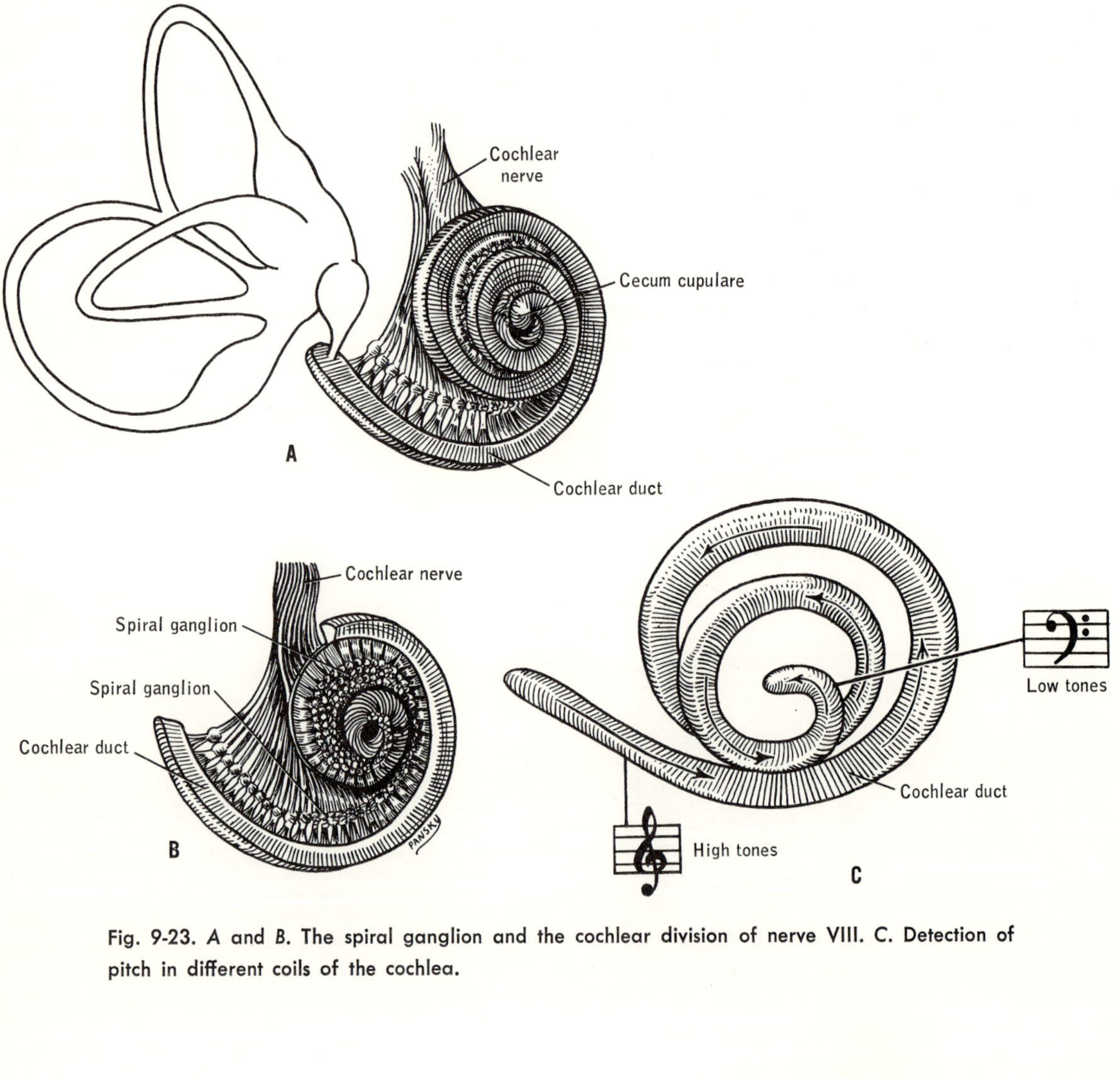

Fig. 9-23. *A* and *B*. The spiral ganglion and the cochlear division of nerve VIII. C. Detection of pitch in different coils of the cochlea.

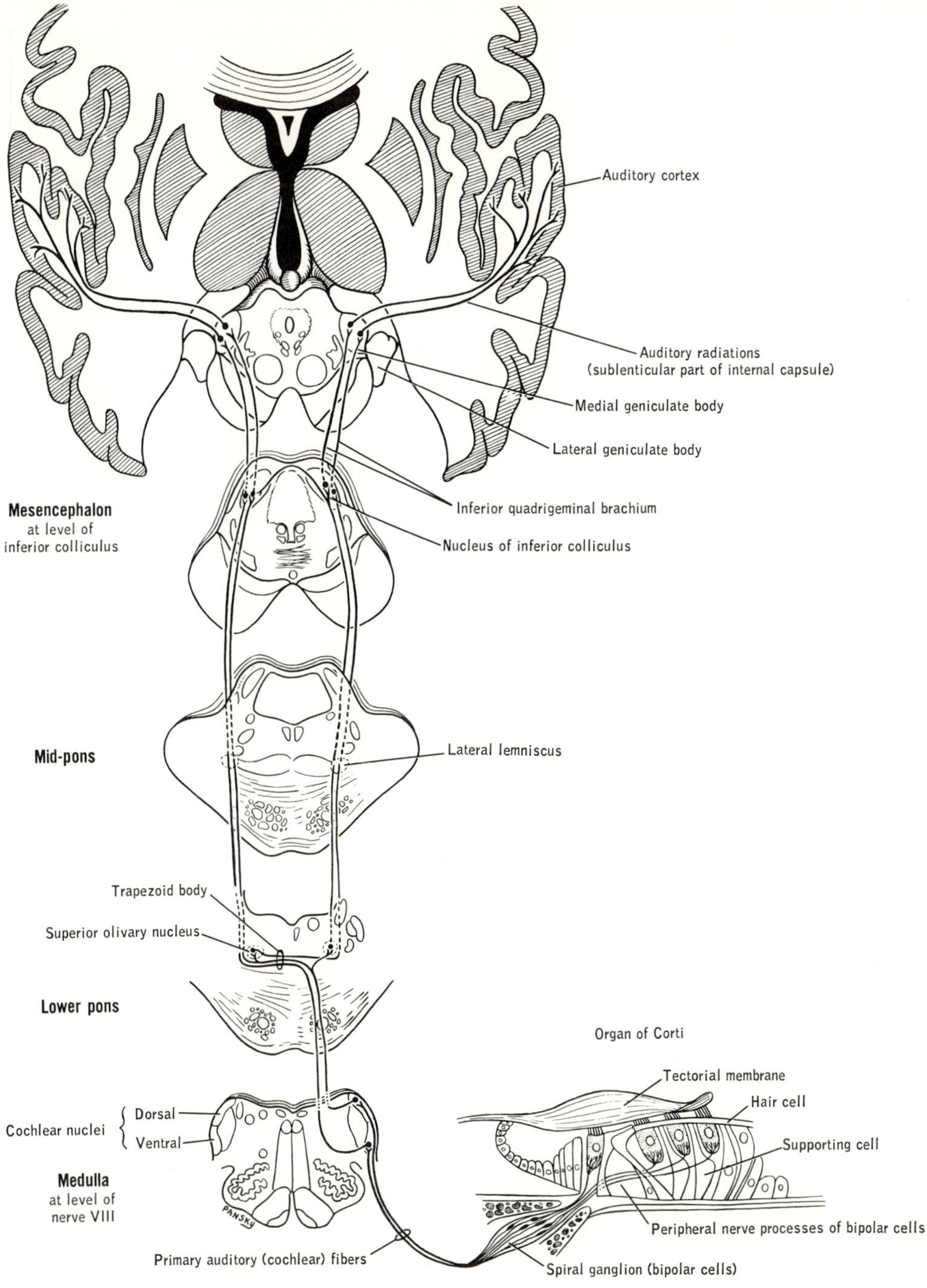

Fig. 9-24. Diagram of the conscious auditory pathway.

in such nuclei as the superior olive or the lateral lemniscus, enter the brachium of the inferior colliculus without entering the colliculus itself. The nucleus of the inferior colliculus is the largest of the relay centers. From the inferior colliculus, a large number of fibers originating there pass laterally and rostrally to form a major portion of the brachium of the inferior colliculus. Through this bundle, these, too, reach the medial geniculate body. Thus, it is apparent that all fibers, whether direct or relayed, eventually terminate in the medial geniculate nucleus of the thalamus. This nucleus is divided into a small ventral and large dorsal portion. It is the latter that receives most of the auditory impulses directed toward conscious levels.

Neuron III. The cell bodies of these neurons are located in the dorsal part of medial geniculate nucleus. Their axons, called *auditory radiations* or *the geniculotemporal tract,* pass laterally, mainly through the sublenticular part of the internal capsule, to terminate in the transverse temporal gyri. Tones of different frequencies have specific reception areas on the auditory cortex.[7] High tones are localized in the medial portion while low tones are perceived in the anterior and lateral portions.

Clinical Considerations

Testing

Two types of test are generally used, those designed to test auditory acuity and those used to differentiate between central and peripheral deafness.

Acuity. These are relatively simple and consist merely of noting the distance from either ear at which a patient can hear the ticking of an ordinary watch, one ear being tested at a time.

Differentiation. One of the more common tests used to differentiate between lesions of the nerve and disease in or around the transmitting mechanism (external meatus and middle ear, including ossicles) is the Rinné method. In it, a tuning fork is placed against the mastoid bone and the patient is instructed to state immediately when he no longer hears the sound. The interval is timed. Ordinarily, the patient can still hear the sound if the fork is removed and held behind the ear. The time at which he hears nothing is noted. The test result is said to be positive, or normal, when the tuning fork is heard about twice as long by air conduction as by bone conduction. An abnormal Rinné test result is a sign of middle ear or external meatus defect. When the nerve is involved, both air and bone conduction are reduced but the Rinné test result is normal. The Weber test is preferred by some examiners. In it, the base of a tuning fork is placed on the vertex of the skull. If hearing is normal, the sound will be heard by both ears. When there is disease of the middle ear or stoppage of the external meatus, the sound will be heard best on the diseased side. If the nerve is damaged, the sound will be stronger on the normal side.

Because some of the central auditory fibers cross, while others remain on the same side, a unilateral lesion within the CNS, unless large enough to destroy both cochlear nuclei or entering fibers of the acoustic nerve, would not cause total deafness. This holds true whether involvements include the lateral lemniscus, brachium of the inferior colliculus, geniculotemporal tract, or auditory cortex. Even total ablation of the auditory cortex will not cause deafness, although hearing in the opposite ear will be diminished.

Therefore, to localize exactly a lesion involving this system, it is often necessary to note how its parts are related to portions of other systems and to observe the various signs and symptoms of lesions in neighboring pathways. For example, a lesion along the course of the nerve may easily involve the vestibular portion of the nerve, whereas a lesion in the posterior part of the internal capsule might interfere with the visual system.

[7] There is also experimental evidence to indicate that there are descending fibers from the auditory cortex to the sensory receptors in the organ of Corti.

SUMMARY
Vision
REFLEX

Somatosomatic		*Somatovisceral* (special)
1. Rods and cones	Receptor	1. Same as somatosomatic
2. Bipolar cells with bodies in inner nuclear layer of retina, terminating with ganglion cells in retina	Afferent neuron	2. Same as somatosomatic
3. From ganglion cells in nasal half of retina, into optic nerve, across to opposite side through the optic chiasma, into the optic tract, then via brachium of superior colliculus to terminate in superior colliculus From ganglion cells in temporal half of retina, into optic nerve, through optic tract of the same side, terminating as above	Association neuron (1)	3. Same as somatosomatic
4. From cells in the superior colliculus, fibers descend via the tectobulbar tract to end in nuclei III, IV, and VI (also XII) From cells in superior colliculus, fibers descend in tectospinal tract to end in ventral gray columns of the cord	Association neuron (2)	4. Same as somatosomatic except that tectobulbar fibers terminate in nuclei of nerves V, VII, and XI (also IX and X) The SVE system is not represented in the cord
5. From nuclei III, IV, and VI through corresponding cranial nerves to extrinsic ocular muscles From nucleus XII through nerve XII to muscles of tongue	Efferent neuron	5. From nucleus V to muscles of mastication, etc. From nucleus of VII to facial muscles, etc. From nucleus XI to sternocleidomastoid and trapezius

Somatovisceral (general) for light		*Somatovisceral* (general) for accommodation
6. Same as somatosomatic	Receptor	6. A cortical reflex (see conscious pathway to cortex)
7. Same as somatosomatic	Afferent neuron	7. A cortical reflex (see conscious pathway to cortex)
8. In part, like somatosomatic except in this case fibers of brachium of superior colliculus terminate in the pretectal zone, while others terminate in the superior colliculus	Association neuron (1)	8. From cortex through internal capsule and brachium of the superior colliculus to terminate in the superior colliculus
9. From the superior colliculus through the tectospinal tract to end on cells in the intermediolateral cell column of the cord (dim light) From the pretectal zone to the EW nucleus (bright light)	Association neuron (2)	9. From the superior colliculus, fibers descend to synapse in EW nucleus and the nucleus of Perlia
10. From the intermediolateral column through preganglionic fibers ascending in the cervical sympathetic trunk to synapse in the superior cervical ganglion. Postganglionics ascend through the carotid plexus to reach dilator pupillae muscle From EW nucleus through preganglionics in nerve III to synapse in the ciliary ganglion from which postganglionics pass to sphincter pupillae muscle	Efferent neuron	10. From the EW nucleus, preganglionic fibers pass through nerve III, continue through the ciliary ganglion, without synapse, to end in the episcleral ganglion, from which postganglionics pass to the ciliary muscle From the EW nucleus, other fibers travel as above but terminate in the ciliary ganglion with postganglionics going to the sphincter pupillae muscle

CONSCIOUS

1. Same as in reflex	Receptors
2. Same as afferent neuron in reflex	Neuron I
3. Same as association neuron I in reflex except that here the fibers terminate in the lateral geniculate body	Neuron II
4. From cells in the lateral geniculate body through the geniculocalcarine fibers passing to the cortex along the calcarine fissure by way of the sub-and retrolenticular part of the internal capsule	Neuron III

SUMMARY
Hearing

REFLEX

Trunk		Head
Somatosomatic		*Somatovisceral* (special)
1. Hair cells in organ of Corti	Receptor	1. Same as somatosomatic
2. Through nerve VIII, with cells in spiral ganglion, ending in dorsal or ventral cochlear nuclei	Afferent neuron	2. Same as somatosomatic
3. From cells in ventral cochlear nucleus, across midline via ventral trapezoid body, turning rostrally in lateral lemniscus, terminating or giving collaterals to nucleus of trapezoid body; superior olive; nucleus of lateral lemniscus; inferior colliculus From cells of dorsal cochlear nucleus through either dorsal or intermediate trapezoid bodies into lateral lemniscus of the opposite side, having connections as above From cells of the dorsal cochlear nucleus, ascending in the lateral lemniscus of the same side, with connections similar to above	Association neuron (1)	3. Same as somatosomatic
4. From cells in nucleus of trapezoid body to superior olive or reticular formation From cells in superior olive through lateral lemniscus to end in nucleus of lateral lemniscus, in reticular formation, or in the inferior colliculus From cells in the superior olive through MLF to end in nuclei III, IV, or VI From cells in nucleus of lateral lemniscus to the lateral lemniscus of either side, ending in inferior colliculus	Association neuron (2)	4. Same as somatosomatic except that here MLF may terminate in nuclei V, VII, and XI (also IX and X)
5. From cells in reticular formation to any somatic motor nucleus of brain stem From cells in the inferior colliculus, descending through the tectobulbar tract to somatic motor nuclei of head From cells in the inferior colliculus, descending via the tectospinal tract to ventral gray columns of the cord	Association neuron (3)	5. Same as somatosomatic except terminations would be in nuclei V, VII, and XI (also IX and X) This system (SVE) has no representation in the cord.
6. From cells in nuclei III, IV, or VI through respective nerves to the extrinsic ocular muscles From cells of the ventral gray columns to skeletal muscle of neck, trunk, and extremities	Efferent neuron	6. From nucleus V via trigeminal nerve to muscles of mastication, tensor veli palatini, and tensor tympani From nucleus VII to muscles of facial expression, stapedius, and posterior belly of the digastric From nucleus XI to sternocleidomastoid and trapezius From nuclei IX and X (ambiguus) to muscles of pharynx and larynx

CONSCIOUS

Direct		Indirect
7. Same as in reflex	Receptor	7. Same as in the direct pathway
8. Same as afferent neuron in reflex	Neuron I	8. Same as in the direct pathway
9. Many fibers from cells in ventral cochlear nucleus and many from dorsal cochlear nucleus cross to the opposite side via the trapezoid bodies, enter the lateral lemniscus to mesencephalon, thence through the brachium of the inferior colliculus to end in medial geniculate body.	Neuron II	9. This is represented by a chain of neurons beginning in either of cochlear nuclei using nucleus of trapezoid body, superior olive, nucleus of the lateral lemniscus, and the inferior colliculus as relay stations, finally entering medial geniculate body via brachium of inferior colliculus
10. From cells in the medial geniculate body through geniculotemporal fibers in sublenticular part of internal capsule to superior temporal gyrus	Neuron III	10. Same as in direct pathway

10 GENERAL VISCERAL AFFERENT SYSTEM (GVA)

This system is predominantly concerned with the initiation of reflexes which control the activity of the viscera by way of the autonomic system. The sensations from the viscera at conscious levels are much less specific and are very poorly localized. They may, however, have great intensity, e.g., intestinal colic, labor pains, or injuries in the celiac plexus or testicles. Other forms of visceral sensibility include nausea, thirst, hunger, sexual feelings, and the sense of well-being or malaise. Since the question of visceral pain is often related to surface areas and is thus somatic in character, *referred pain* has been discussed in connection with the GSA system (Chap. 8).

TRUNK

Reflex Pathways (Fig. 10-1.)

Receptors

There are three major types of receptors: the many-branched *free* endings devoid of any coverings; the complex *tangle* of nerve fibers with or without a light capsule; and the heavily encapsulated and laminated *Pacinian corpuscles.* The free endings are usually found on mucous surfaces associated with the lining epithelial cells. The tangles are found both on serous surfaces and in the muscular coats of the viscera. They are adapted to register pressure changes. The Pacinian corpuscles are located in the mesenteries, in the supporting tissue of the viscera, and in the body wall.

Afferent Neuron

From the receptors in the walls of the viscera, the peripheral process of the afferent neurons accompanies efferent fibers to reach the cord. Thus, on the way to the cord, afferent fibers may pass through one or more autonomic ganglia, but they do not synapse in any of them. They enter the main spinal nerve trunk by way of the white rami communicantes and pass into either the lateral or medial division of the dorsal root, where their unipolar cells lie in the ganglia. The central process enters the cord along the dorsolateral sulcus in the thoracic, upper lumbar, and midsacral regions. Within the cord, these fibers undergo a typical bifurcation into long ascending and short descending branches. The collaterals and terminals of these branches end in the dorsal column of the cord.

Those fibers particularly concerned with *visceral pain* accompany the somatic pain fibers in the lateral division of the dorsal root to enter Lissauer's tract and terminate in the substantia gelatinosa. Those fibers particularly concerned with pressure go through the medial division of the dorsal root and end in the dorsal column just ventral to the substantia gelatinosa.

Association Neuron

Since the important part of this system lies in the reflexes which it initiates, it is of more than

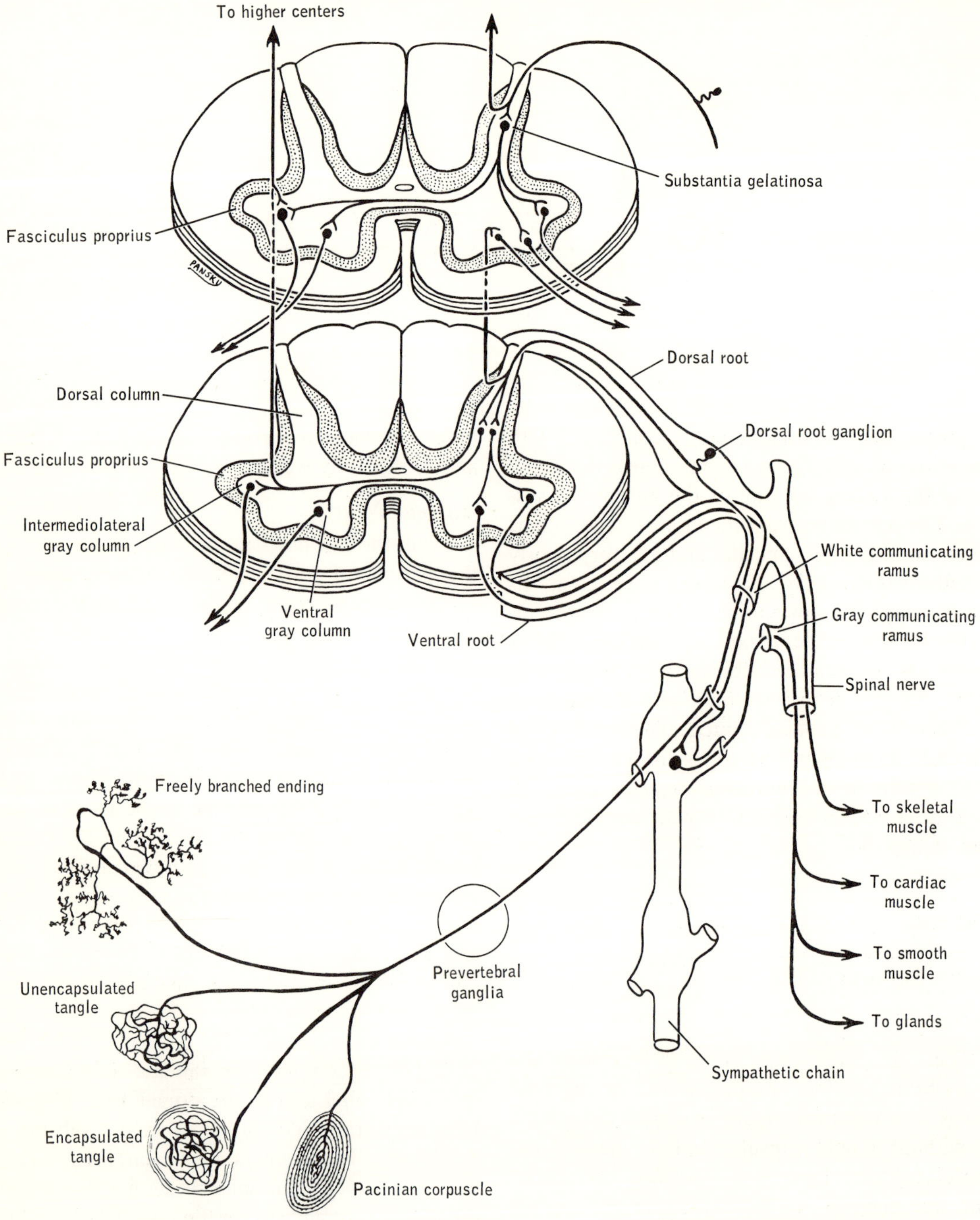

Fig. 10-1. General visceral afferent reflex pathway for impulses entering the CNS through spinal nerves.

passing interest to show how impulses entering via visceral afferents are distributed to the efferent limbs of the reflex arcs.

Associational neurons in the cord have their origins either in the substantia gelatinosa or in the more ventral portions of the dorsal column. Their distribution is variable. Some may run directly to the intermediolateral or ventral gray columns of the same side or may cross over to comparable regions of the other side through commissural fibers. Other associational fibers spread out through the fasciculus proprius of the same and opposite sides to reach the intermediolateral and ventral columns of other levels of the cord. It is likely that some of these fibers continue to ascend through either the fasciculus proprius or the reticular formation to influence the cranial motor mechanism.

Efferent Neuron

Reflexes of both the viscerosomatic and viscerovisceral types may occur. The efferent neurons innervating skeletal muscle will be discussed in Chap. 14. Those neurons involved with visceral reflexes, having their origin either in the intermediolateral cell column of the spinal cord or in certain brain stem nuclei and their terminations in smooth muscle, cardiac muscle or glands, comprise the autonomic nervous system (Chap. 15). Thus, through these efferents, the reflex mechanisms are completed which cause the secretion of glands and speed up peristalsis in response to the presence of food in the digestive tract; slow the heart and reduce blood pressure when pressure becomes too high in the vascular system; initiate exhalation when the air cells of the lungs are distended. Other examples will be cited in subsequent chapters (Chaps. 14, 15).

Conscious Pathways (Fig. 10-2.)

Receptors

These are the same as described under Reflex Pathways, above.

Neuron I

These are identical with the afferent neuron described under Reflex Pathways, above. However, some of the central processes may ascend in the dorsal funiculus (particularly in the fasciculus gracilis) to terminate in the nuclei of the dorsal funiculus.

Neuron II

These have their origins from cells of the substantia gelatinosa, cross the cord in the anterior white commissure, to join the lateral spinothalamic tract of the opposite side. Within this tract they bend rostrally and ascend to the posterolateral ventral nucleus of the thalamus, where they synapse. It has also been demonstrated that some of the fibers arising in the substantia gelatinosa do not ascend directly but do so through short, ascending relays in the fasciculus proprius, often remaining for some distance on the same side.

Neuron III

From cells in the posterolateral ventral nucleus of the thalamus, a small number of fibers ascends through the posterior limb of the internal capsule to be distributed to the postcentral gyrus according to the segmental arrangement of somatic afferent systems in which they run.

HEAD

Reflex Pathways (Fig. 10-3.)

Receptors

These are the same type as those described under the reflex pathways of the trunk, above. In addition however, special receptors are associated with cranial nerves IX and X. These are the carotid body and aortic bodies, respectively. They are small structures, somewhat glandlike in appearance, of the chemoreceptor type. They are sensitive to changes in concentration of carbon dioxide (and oxygen?) in the blood.

Afferent Neuron

From the receptors, the afferent neurons make up a portion of cranial nerves VII, IX, and X and pass with these nerves into the central nervous system.

Facial Nerve (VII). The distribution and course of the general visceral afferent system

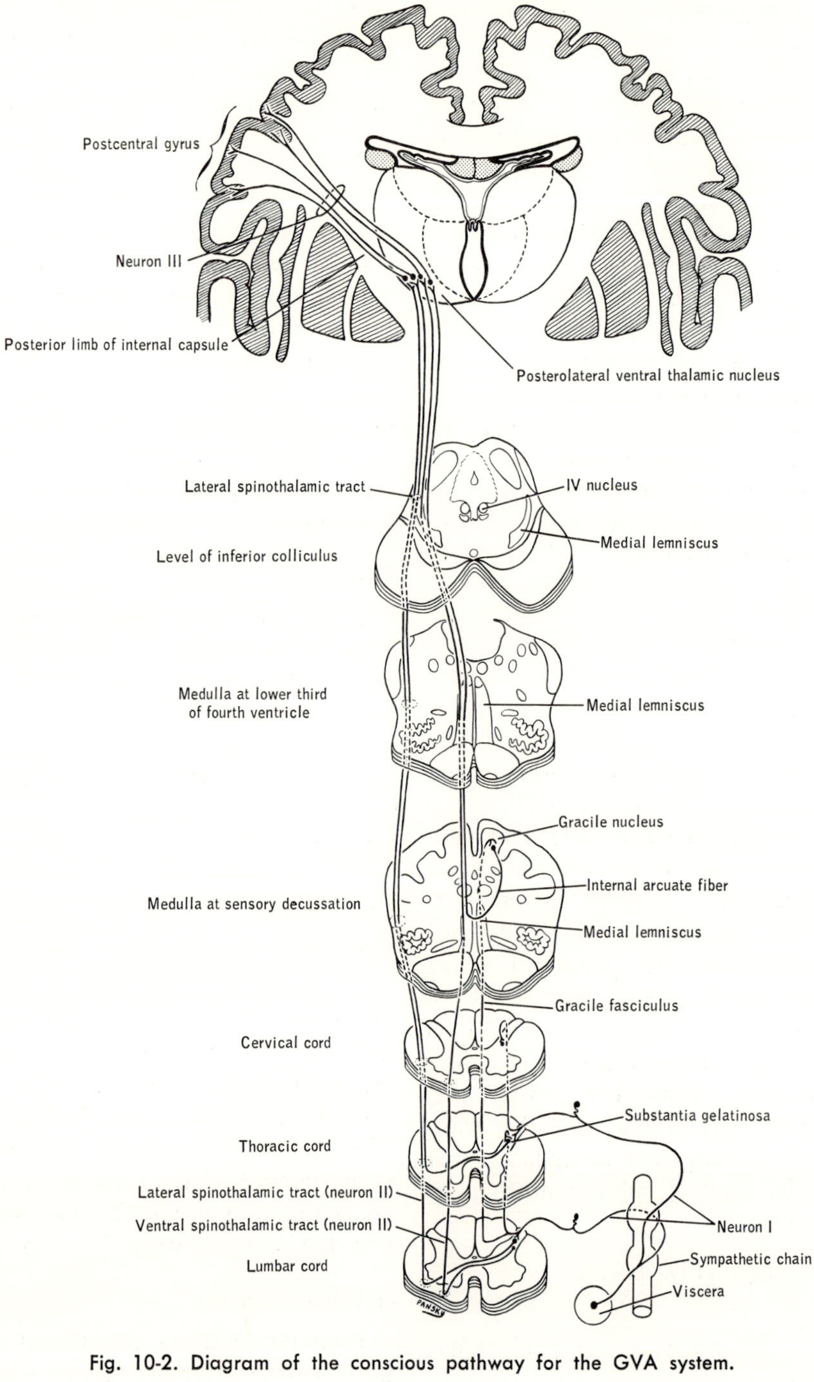

Fig. 10-2. Diagram of the conscious pathway for the GVA system.

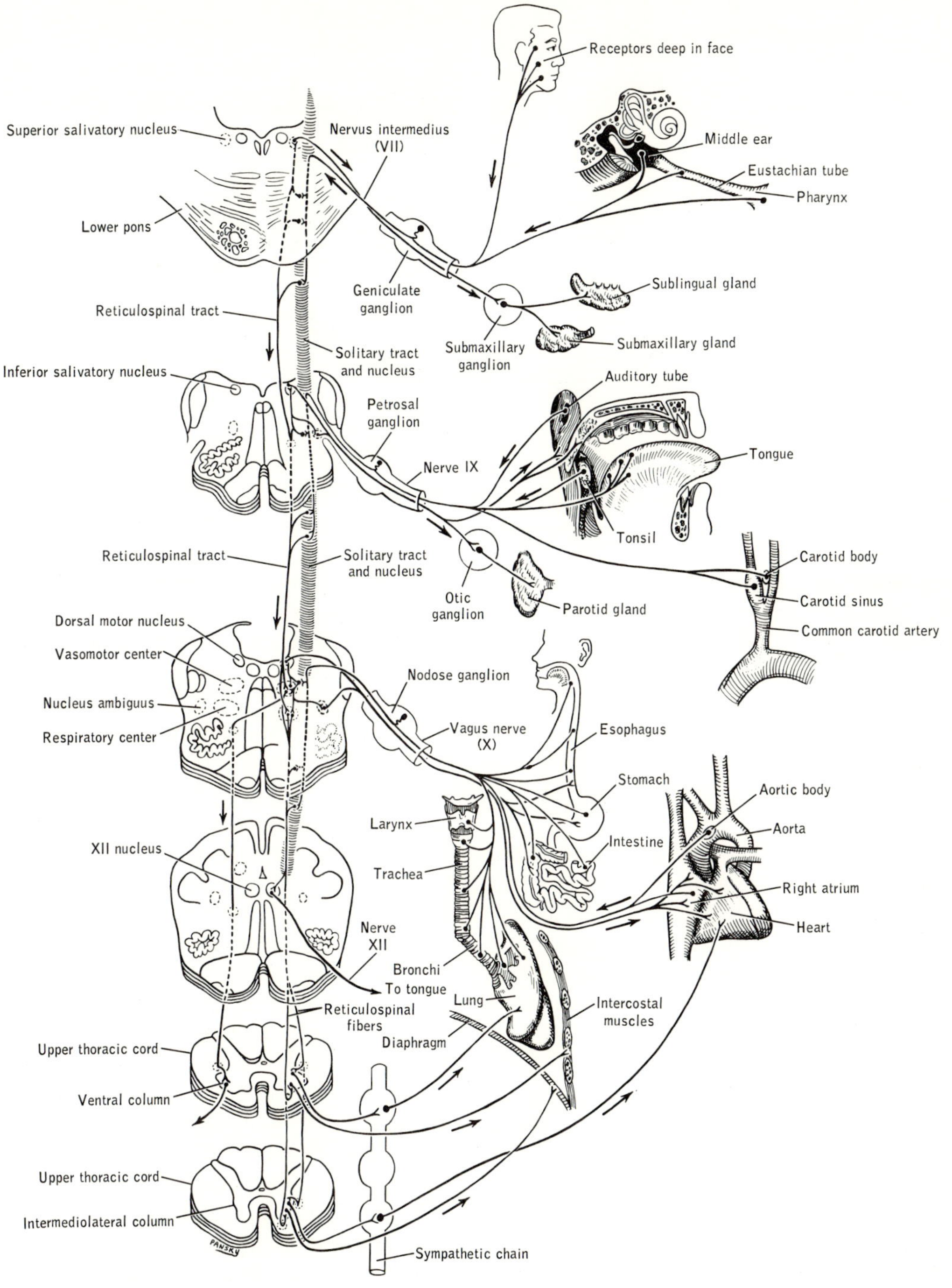

Fig. 10-3. The GVA reflex pathway for impulses entering the CNS through cranial nerves.

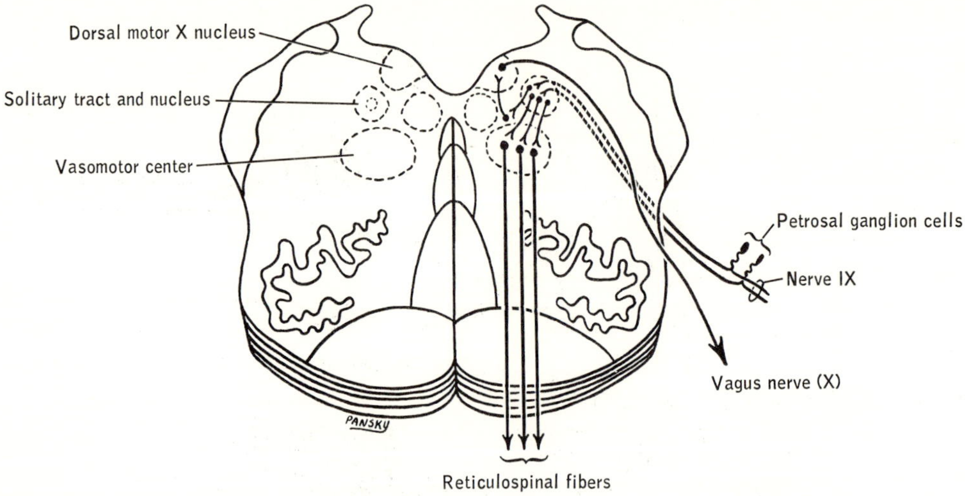

Fig. 10-4. Open part of the medulla with the vasomotor center enlarged.

in this nerve are controversial because so many of the impulses carried by this nerve remain below conscious levels. However, it is believed that the facial nerve is associated with receptors deep in the face, middle ear, auditory tube, and adjoining pharyngeal wall.

From these areas, the peripheral processes of all the afferent neurons become segregated in the sensory root of the facial nerve (VII), the *nervus intermedius*. The cell bodies for these neurons lie in the *geniculate ganglion* (Fig. 10-3). The central processes continue toward the brain, forming a distinct bundle which runs between the motor root of the facial nerve (VII) and the acoustic nerve (VIII) and joins the brain stem at the cerebellopontine angle (Figs. 2-7, 2-8, 25-7).

After entry into the brain, the central processes run dorsomedially and approach the lateral aspect of the fourth ventricle, where they turn caudally in a bundle called the *tractus solitarius* (Figs. 10-3 to 10-5 and Chap. 11). After running caudally for variable distances, all these fibers terminate in the *nucleus of the tractus solitarius,* which nearly completely surrounds the tract (Figs. 10-3 to 10-6, 25-2 to 25-5).

Glossopharyngeal Nerve (IX). From the receptors in the posterior tongue, tonsil, and auditory tube, the peripheral processes of the afferent neurons pass through the pharyngeal, lingual, and tympanic branches and enter the main trunk. Their cell bodies are found in the *inferior (petrosal) ganglion* (Figs. 10-3, 10-4). The central processes join the medulla along the posterolateral sulcus dorsal to the rostral end of the inferior olive (Figs. 2-7, 2-8, 25-5). After entry, the central processes course dorsomedially until they reach the *tractus solitarius* (Figs. 10-3 to 10-5). Here they bend caudally to become a part of that tract. They also synapse on the *nucleus of the tractus solitarius* (Figs. 10-3 to 10-6, 25-2 to 25-5).

Of special interest is the small *carotid sinus branch* of this nerve (Fig. 10-3). In this branch, afferent neurons run from the special chemoreceptors of the carotid body and from pressure receptors in the walls of the carotid sinus to join the main trunk nerve.[1] From here their course is similar to that just described.

Vagus Nerve (X). These afferent neurons originate in receptors in the walls of the viscera, including the entire digestive system, from the root of the tongue to the middle of the transverse

[1] There is some disagreement as to whether the pressure endings are associated with the sinus branch of nerve IX or with a small sinus branch of nerve X.

colon; the respiratory system, from the larynx to the pulmonary air sacs of the lung; and the arch of the aorta and the walls of the right atrium of the heart. The peripheral processes join the main trunk of the vagus at various points along its course. The cell bodies lie in the *nodose ganglion* (Figs. 10-3, 10-5). The central processes pass upward to join the medulla in the posterolateral sulcus just caudal to the rootlets of nerve IX (Figs. 2-7, 2-8, 25-4).

After entry, these fibers course dorsomedially to join the tractus solitarius (Figs. 10-3, 10-5) and descend as a part of the latter. They also terminate in the nucleus of the tractus solitarius (Figs. 10-3 to 10-6, 25-2 to 25-5).

First Association Neuron

The cell bodies for all associational neurons related to cranial nerves VII, IX, and X lie in the nucleus of the tractus solitarius. From here, some axons pass through the surrounding reticular formation to go directly to motor nuclei of the brain stem such as the *dorsal motor nucleus of the vagus* (Figs. 2-48, 25-4) or the *salivatory nuclei.* Others may descend into the cord via the reticulospinal tract to end about cells of the intermediolateral or ventral gray columns. The majority, however, probably synapse in various scattered groups of cells lying in the reticular formation of the medulla, some of which are referred to as *centers.* Thus, first associational neurons terminate in the *bulbar respiratory center,* the *vasomotor center,* or the *swallowing center* (Figs. 10-3 to 10-5).

Second Association Neuron

From cells in these and other centers of the medulla, secondary association neurons may pass to the dorsal motor nucleus of the vagus, the nucleus ambiguus, the hypoglossal nucleus of the brain stem, or may descend into the cord, probably by way of the reticulospinal tract. In the cord, these fibers terminate in the ventral gray columns of the cervical or thoracic regions or in the intermediolateral gray column in the thoracic cord.

Efferent Neuron

From cells in the dorsal motor nucleus of the vagus and from the intermediolateral column of the cord efferent neurons pass by way of the cardiac branches of the vagus and sympathetic

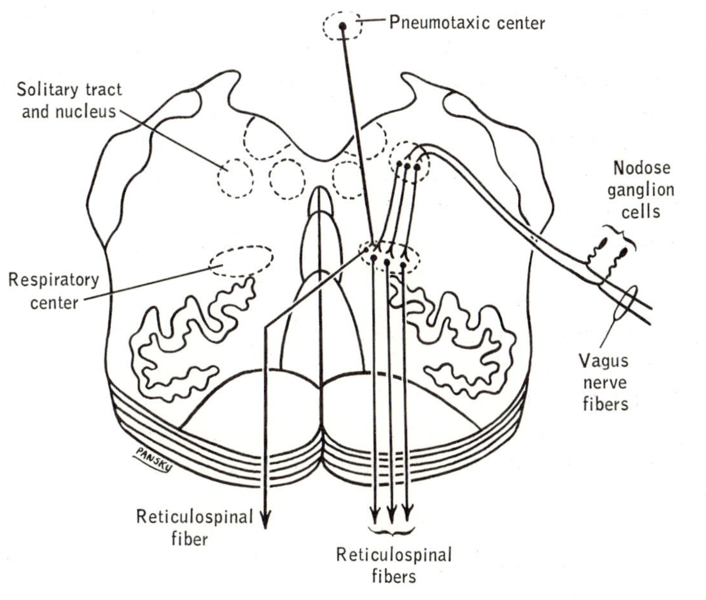

Fig. 10-5. Open part of medulla with the respiratory center enlarged.

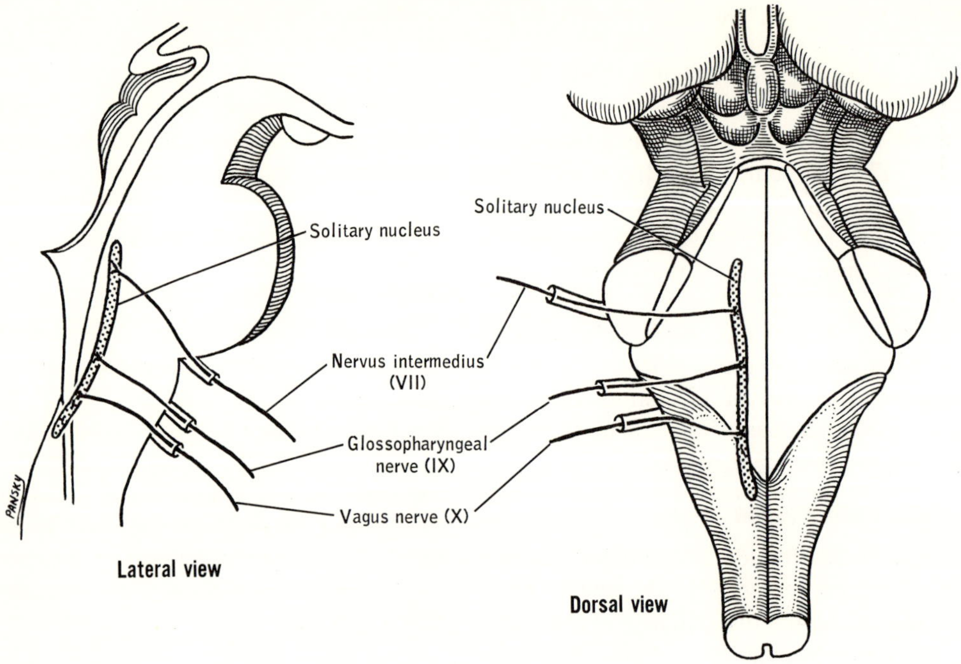

Fig. 10-6. Cranial nerves terminating in nucleus solitarius.

trunks, respectively. These reflexively control heart rate and blood pressure (Chap. 15).

From other cells in the dorsal motor nucleus of the vagus, streams of impulses are carried to glands of the digestive tract and to its smooth muscle to bring about secretion of enzymes and to speed up peristalsis.

From the cells of the salivatory nuclei, efferent neurons pass by way of the seventh and ninth cranial nerves to bring the salivary glands under reflex control (Chap. 15).

From the nucleus ambiguus, efferent fibers pass by way of the ninth and tenth cranial nerves to control reflexly the muscles of the pharynx and palate involved in swallowing.

Axons from cells in the hypoglossal nucleus are distributed by way of the twelfth nerve to muscles of the tongue, also concerned with the act of swallowing.

From the cells in the anterior gray column of the lower cervical and thoracic cord, axons pass by way of the phrenic, long thoracic, and intercostal nerves to the diaphragm, serratus anterior, and intercostal muscles, respectively. This pathway controls the rate and depth of respiration.

The first three reflexes cited above are of the *viscerovisceral* type; the fourth exemplifies a *special viscerovisceral* reflex; the last two are examples of the *viscerosomatic* type of reflex (Figs. 10-3, 10-7).

Conscious Pathways

The conscious pathways associated with the GVA system are not definitely known. It seems probable that the few fibers that do ascend to conscious levels accompany fibers of the somatic afferent system.

COMPARISON OF THE GSA AND GVA SYSTEMS

Structurally, the two systems are similar; they consist of neurons of the monopolar type, with cells located in ganglia outside the CNS. At cord levels, visceral and somatic fibers run in

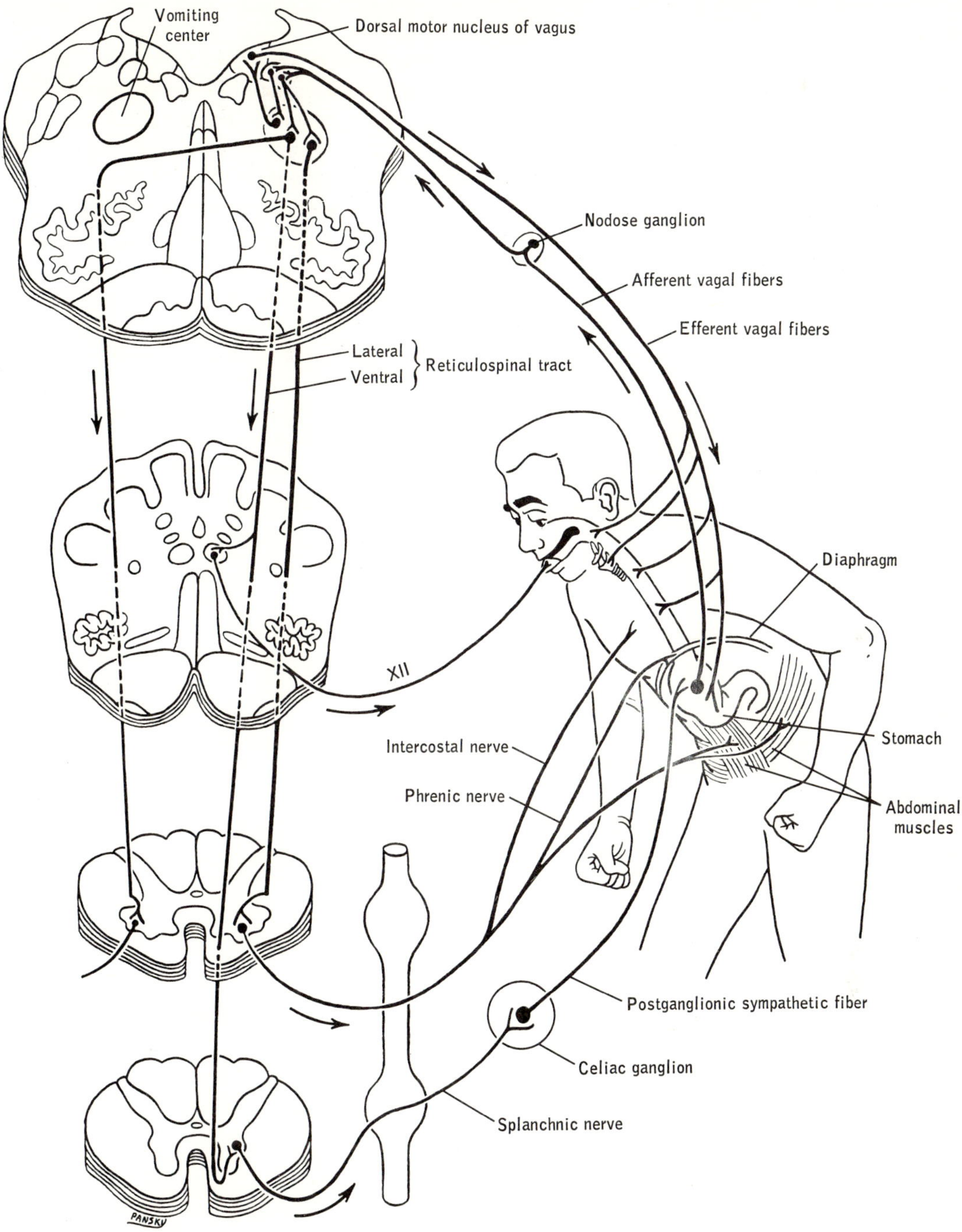

Fig. 10-7. Vomiting reflex. Diagram to show the viscerovisceral and viscerosomatic reflexes initiated from irritation of the stomach, the afferent impulses being carried by the GVA fibers in the vagus nerve (X). The actions involved are the following: (1) elevation of soft palate; (2) larynx and hyoid drawn forward; (3) salivation and opening of mouth; (4) closure of glottis; (5) relaxation of esophagus; (6) opening of cardia; (7) flaccid relaxation of stomach; (8) constriction of lower end of stomach; (9) inhibition of normal respiration; (10) forced inspiration; (11) sharp, spasmodic contraction of diaphragm and abdominal muscles; (12) characteristic posture—flexion at waist, clenched fists, etc.

the dorsal root and join the spinal cord in the same region.

On a structural basis, there are also several differences between the two systems. In the somatic system, sensory fibers are widespread and are contained in all the spinal nerves. Among the cranial nerves, the major portion of the somatic afferents are carried in the trigeminal nerve (V); a few somatic fibers are also present in the vagus nerve (X); some may run in the facial nerve (VII) and glossopharyngeal nerve (IX). Visceral afferents are found in only certain of the spinal nerves, those of the thoracic, upper lumbar, and midsacral levels.

In the spinal nerves, somatic sensations travel through the nerve trunks, following all branches. Visceral fibers of the cord leave the spinal nerve trunk by way of white rami communicantes and accompany the motor fibers of the autonomic system.

The majority of somatic receptors are sensitive to a great variety of environmental changes, whereas the majority of visceral receptors are of the stretch-pressure type, a few being sensitive to chemical changes.

Another difference lies in the fact that ascending secondary pathways within the CNS are well established for somatic sensation but poorly identified for visceral sensation.

CLINICAL CONSIDERATIONS

Since the physiology of this system is so intimately linked to motor activity, no attempt will be made to evaluate the integrity of the GVA system at this time.

SUMMARY
General Visceral Afferent

Trunk	REFLEX	Head
1. Free endings or complex tangles Pacinian corpuscles	Receptor	1. Many same as for trunk Chemoreceptors, sensitive to concentrations of O_2 and CO_2
2. Through fibers accompanying visceral efferents, to spinal nerves via white rami, with cells in dorsal root ganglia, entering the cord at thoracic, upper lumbar, and midsacral levels, to terminate in the dorsal gray column	Afferent neuron	2. From receptors deep in face, middle ear, and auditory tube through nerve VII with cells in the geniculate ganglion, into the brain stem, downward in tractus solitarius to end in the nucleus of the tractus solitarius From receptors in posterior tongue, tonsil, and pharyngeal wall through nerve IX with cells in the inferior petrosal ganglion, into the brain stem and downward in the tractus solitarius to end in the nucleus of the tractus solitarius From chemoreceptors of carotid body and pressure receptors of carotid sinus, through carotid sinus branch of nerve IX, thence as above From receptors in the walls of viscera, including heart, great vessels, lungs, and digestive system, through nerve X,with cells in the nodose ganglion, into the brain stem and downward in the tractus solitarius to end in the nucleus of the tractus solitarius
3. *Viscerosomatic* From cells in the dorsal gray column directly to ventral gray column at same level, same side; through the fasciculus proprius to the ventral gray at other levels of same side; through the anterior white commissure and fasciculus proprius to the ventral gray at same or other levels of opposite side *Visceroviscereal* Identical with above except for termination, which would be the intermediolateral cell column at any level on either side	Association neuron	3. *Visceroviscereal* (general) From cells in the nucleus of the tractus solitarius directly, or through relays in the reticular formation, to superior and inferior salivatory nuclei; dorsal motor nucleus of the vagus; intermediolateral cell column of the cord by way of reticulospinal tract From cells in the nucleus of the tractus solitarius to the bulbar respiratory and vasomotor centers, which relay to the dorsal motor nucleus of the vagus and, through the reticulospinal tract, to the intermediolateral cell column of the cord *Visceroviscereal* (special) From cells in the nucleus of the tractus solitarius to the bulbar swallowing center, which relays to the nucleus ambiguus *Viscerosomatic* From the cells in the nucleus of the tractus solitarius to the bulbar respiratory and swallowing centers, which relay to the nucleus of nerve XII and, through the reticulospinal tract, to the ventral gray columns of the cord
4. *Viscerosomatic* From the ventral gray column to skeletal muscle of neck, trunk and extremities *Visceroviscereal* From the intermediolateral cell column by way of preganglionics to synapse in autonomic ganglia, thence by postganglionics to heart, smooth muscle, and glands	Efferent neuron	4. *Visceroviscereal* (general) From the superior and inferior salivatory nuclei through nerves VII and IX, respectively, to autonomic ganglia and by postganglionics to major salivary glands From dorsal motor nucleus of vagus through preganglionics of nerve X to autonomic ganglia and thence, through postganglionics to heart and other viscera From the intermediolateral cell column of the cord, through preganglionics, to autonomic ganglia, thence through postganglionics to heart, blood vessels, and other viscera *Visceroviscereal* (special) From cells in nucleus ambiguus through nerves IX and X to the muscles of the pharynx and larynx *Viscerosomatic* From nucleus XII to muscles of the tongue; from ventral gray columns to diaphragm and other respiratory muscles

CONSCIOUS

Trunk	CONSCIOUS	Head
5. Same as for reflex	Receptor	5,6,7,8. Indefinite; probably similar to course and distribution of the trigeminal nerve
6. Same as for reflex except that some fibers ascend in dorsal funiculus to end in nuclei of dorsal funiculus	Neuron I	
7. From cells in the dorsal gray column, through the anterior white commissure, to lateral spinothalamic tract of opposite side, ascending in the latter to terminate in the posterolateral ventral nucleus of the thalamus From the nuclei of the dorsal funiculus (gracilis and cuneatus), through internal arcuate fibers, across the midline to the opposite medial lemniscus, in which they ascend to the posterolateral ventral nucleus of the thalamus	Neuron II	
8. From the posterolateral ventral nucleus of the thalamus, through the posterior limb of the internal capsule, to be distributed to the postcentral gyrus according to the segmental arrangement of neuron I	Neuron III	

11 SPECIAL VISCERAL AFFERENT SYSTEM (SVA)

OLFACTION

In man, smell may not be so important as other special senses. However, the reflex relationships of olfactory impulses are of such fundamental significance in relation to visceral control that their importance should not be overlooked.

Many neuroanatomists describe this system merely as a part of the functional activity of the ancient rhinencephalon. Others describe it as a completely separate system. However, since it is so intimately tied up, either directly or indirectly, with visceral function (location, ingestion, and preparation for digestion of food, or the location and recognition of the opposite sex), it seems logical to place it within the visceral afferent system.

Because of the widespread distribution and separation of parts of the olfactory system, a thorough review of the gross aspects of the brain is essential (Chap. 2). However, certain features of this apparatus require further elucidation.

That portion of the basal region of the hemispheres which extends forward from the anterior commissure and the lamina terminalis to the caudal end of the olfactory tracts is the septal (paraterminal) area. This area includes the subcallosal gyrus, the anterior continuation of the hippocampus, and the parolfactory area (Figs. 11-1, 11-2).

The cortex around the lateral olfactory stria is known as the *lateral olfactory gyrus* (*prepyriform area*). The gyrus curves laterally along the border of the anterior perforated substance and, under cover of the temporal lobe, bends caudomedially toward the inner surface of the temporal lobe. The region where the bend occurs is the *limen insulae*. The gray matter of this gyrus then spreads out to become continuous with the head of the hippocampal gyrus. Where this cortical substance spreads out, it forms the *ambient* and *semilunar gyri,* which directly overlie the *amygdaloid complex* (Figs. 5-14, 11-1 to 11-3, 25-17, 25-18).

The *amygdaloid complex* is a large nuclear mass located near the rostral end of the inferior horn of the lateral ventricle, buried in the substance of the temporal lobe (Figs. 11-1 to 11-3). Medially, it is continuous with the cortex of the uncus. Above it lies the lenticular nucleus. Dorsally and rostrally is the anterior perforated substance, and caudally it appears to be continuous with the tail of the caudate nucleus.

The *hippocampal formation,* located in the temporal lobe, consists of the *hippocampus,* the *dentate gyrus,* and *subiculum* (Figs. 2-19, 2-33, 11-2, 11-4, 25-14 to 25-17). The rostral end of the hippocampus spreads out in the rostral end of the inferior horn of the lateral ventricle. Caudally, the hippocampus curves upward and around the splenium of the corpus callosum to become continuous with the *supracallosal gyrus,* the latter terminating in the septal area. Although not easily seen, the supracallosal

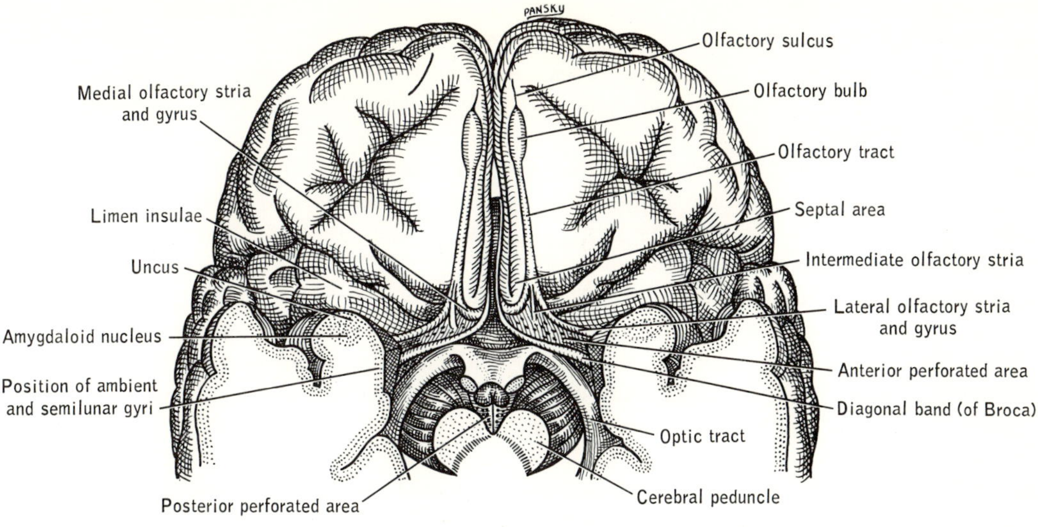

Fig. 11-1. Basal aspect of the brain showing the olfactory cortex and adjoining structures.

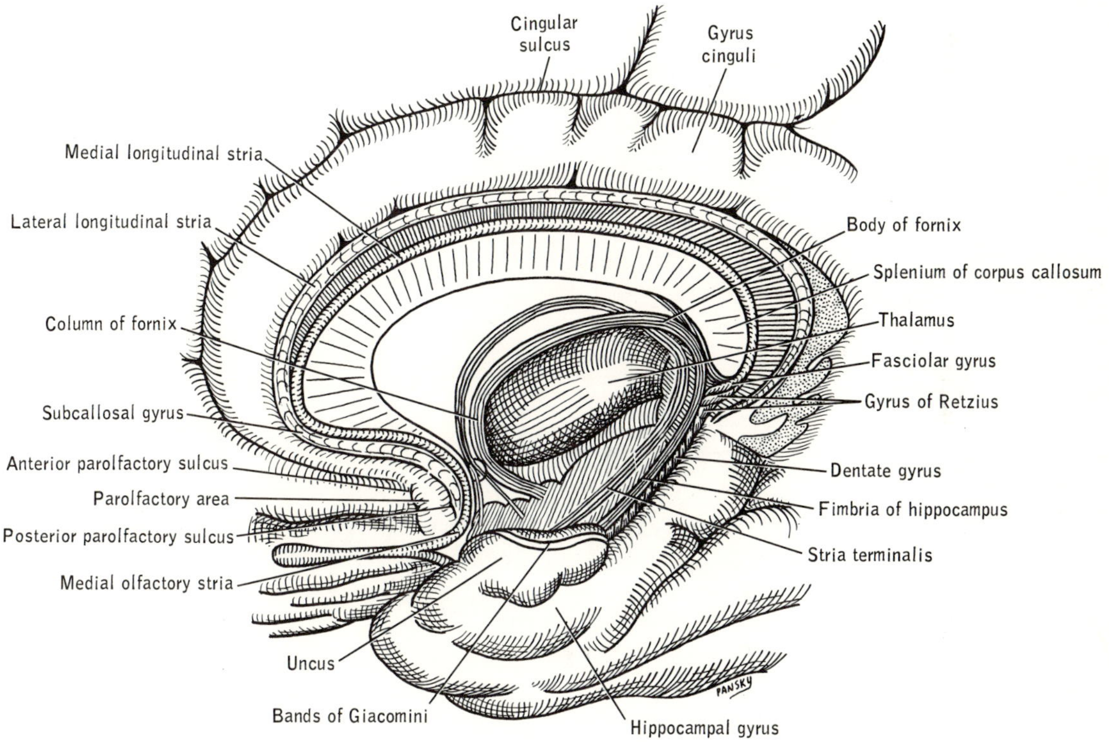

Fig. 11-2. Sagittal section of the brain showing the olfactory cortex and associated structures.

gyrus contains the medial and lateral longitudinal striae. Rostrally, these striae join to form a single fascicle which passes beyond the subcallosal gyrus to enter the *diagonal band of Broca* (Fig. 11-1). The *dentate gyrus* (Fig. 25-14) is a much-grooved, narrow band of cortex which lies across the hippocampal fissure from the hippocampal gyrus (Figs. 2-19, 2-33, 11-2). It is surrounded by the hippocampus, except on its medial side, where it lies in the depths of the *hippocampal fissure* (Figs. 2-33, 11-4, 25-15). Rostrally, the dentate gyrus extends to the notch of the uncus. There, it turns, continuing across the inferior surface of the uncus to spread over its medial surface as the *bands of Giacomini* (Fig. 11-2). Posteriorly, the dentate gyrus can be traced into the *fasciolar gyrus* (Fig. 11-2), which runs beneath the splenium of the corpus callosum to join the supracallosal gyrus (indusium griseum). The *subiculum,* together with the *presubiculum,* is an area of transition between the hippocampus and the hippocampal gyrus and may be seen along the lower border of the hippocampal fissure (Fig. 11-4).

Besides the longitudinal striae mentioned above, there are two other sets of bands. The first of these is the *stria terminalis,* which runs in a groove separating the dorsal thalamus from the body and tail of the caudate nucleus (Fig. 11-2). These striae connect the hypothalamus and the amygdaloid nuclei. The second set, the *stria medullaris thalami* (Figs. 11-7, 25-14), runs rostrally from the habenula along the lateral margin of the roof of the third ventricle and can be traced toward the region of the medial olfactory stria and gyrus.

The major portion of the fornix has already been observed (Chap. 2). However, it should be

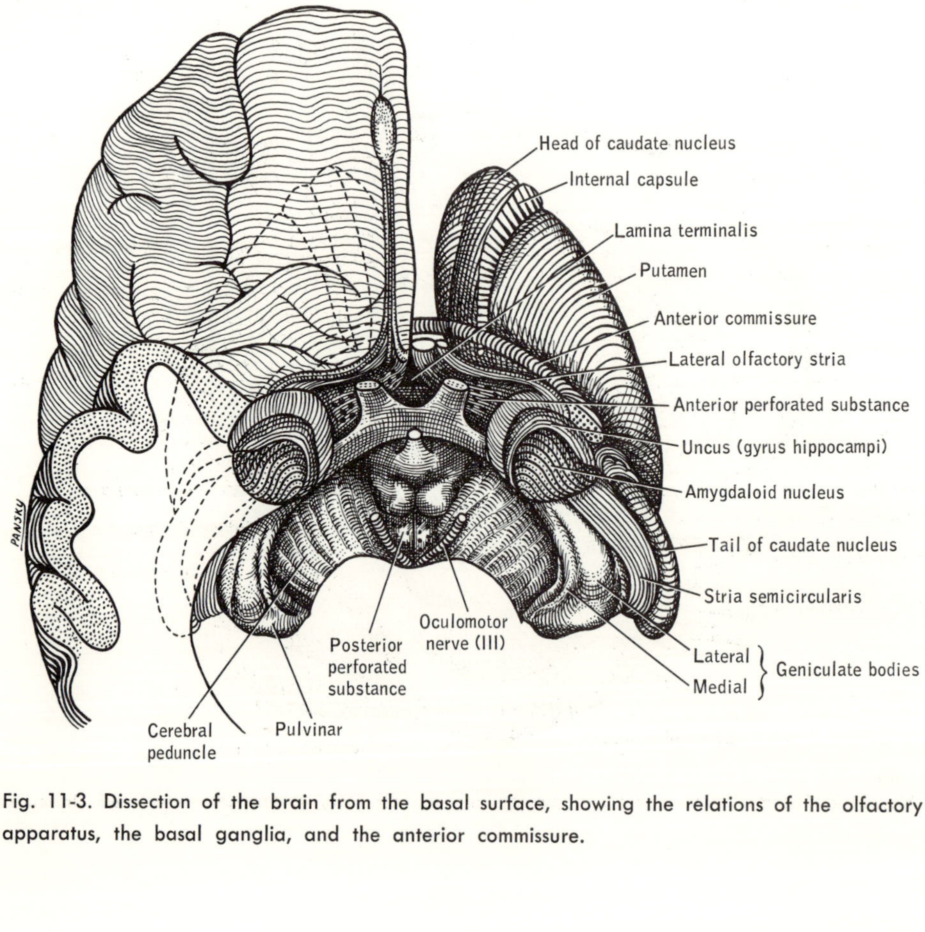

Fig. 11-3. Dissection of the brain from the basal surface, showing the relations of the olfactory apparatus, the basal ganglia, and the anterior commissure.

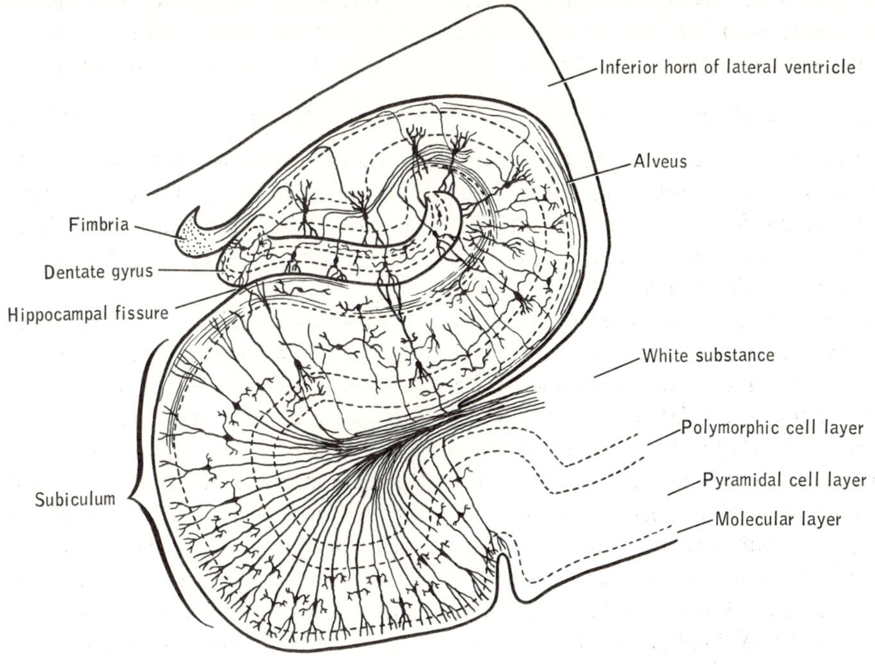

Fig. 11-4. Diagrammatic representation of a transsection through the hippocampus, showing its layers as well as the origin of the fornix.

made clear that the fimbria of the fornix originates in the hippocampal formation. Its fibers curve upward through the *alveus* (Fig. 11-4), a zone of white matter lying along the lateral periphery of the hippocampus. The fibers of the alveus pass medially in the floor of the inferior horn of the lateral ventricle to join the fimbria (Fig. 11-4).

Reflex Pathways

Receptors (Fig. 11-5.)

The olfactory receptors lie in a specialized portion of the nasal epithelium occupying the upper part of the nasal chamber, extending about one-third of the way down the nasal septum medially, and over the superior nasal concha, laterally. The olfactory membrane is composed of two types of cells. The first are purely supporting and are of a modified simple columnar type. At the surface, these cells join to form a cuticle which is penetrated by the sensory cells. The latter are very slender cells, the nuclei of which lie at a deeper lever in the membrane than those of the supporting cells. Extending toward the surface from the region of the nucleus is a cytoplasmic process which penetrates the cuticle of the supporting cells. Ten to twelve short hairs arise from the end of the process. These hairs become embedded in the mucus overlying the olfactory surface. The central process of this receptor cell is very fine and pierces the basement membrane of the epithelium. The central processes of adjoining cells combine to form fascicles of nonmyelinated neural elements. The fascicles pierce the bony roof of the nasal cavity through the cribriform plate of the ethmoid and enter the overlying olfactory bulb, where a synapse is made.

Afferent Neuron (Fig. 11-5.)

The bipolar cell described as the receptor also serves as the afferent neuron of the reflex pathways. These pathways terminate in the olfactory bulb by synapsing with the dendrites of mitral cells lying in a glomerular net (Fig. 11-5).

Association Neuron (Figs. 11-5, 11-6.)

From the mitral cells, axons pass caudally in the central portion of the olfactory tract. Some of these association fibers terminate in the anterior olfactory nucleus, which at least partially surrounds the tract. From this nucleus, secondary association fibers arise which accompany the primary neurons in their caudal course.

Near its caudal end, each olfactory tract shows a divergence of fibers, the *lateral and medial olfactory striae* (Fig. 11-1). Each of the striae is accompanied by gray substance, the *lateral and the medial olfactory gyri,* respectively (Figs. 11-1 to 11-3, 11-6). Both primary and secondary association fibers enter the medial and lateral striae. Those in the lateral stria may terminate in either the nucleus of the lateral olfactory tract which lies along the stria or in some of the nuclei of the amygdaloid complex. Those running in the medial stria enter either the olfactory tubercle, to pass to the nuclei of the septal area (Fig. 25-20) or the anterior continuation of the hippocampus, or the anterior commissure, to terminate in the contralateral amygdaloid nuclei associated with the stria terminalis.

Further Association Neurons (Fig. 11-7.)

From the lateral olfactory nucleus, short fibers may pass into the amygdaloid complex. There are also association connections from the amygdaloid complex to the septal nuclei by way of the diagonal band of Broca.

From the septal nuclei, fibers descend through the *medial forebrain bundle.* Some of the fibers of this bundle terminate in the *preoptic nuclei,* the *lateral hypothalamic nuclei,* and the *mammillary nuclei* (Figs. 21-1, 21-2). Others from this bundle continue caudally into the tegmentum of the mesencephalon and traverse the brain stem through the reticular formation to synapse around autonomic motor centers of both brain and cord. However, it should be emphasized that the fibers associated with the hypothalamus are probably more important than those continuing directly through the brain stem (Chap. 21).

From the amygdaloid complex, fibers pass by way of the *striae terminalis,* which pass caudally along the tail of the caudate nucleus, arch over

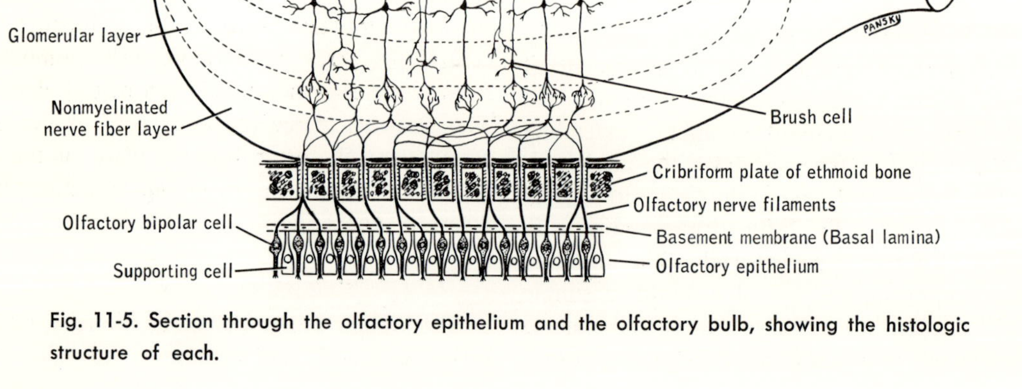

Fig. 11-5. Section through the olfactory epithelium and the olfactory bulb, showing the histologic structure of each.

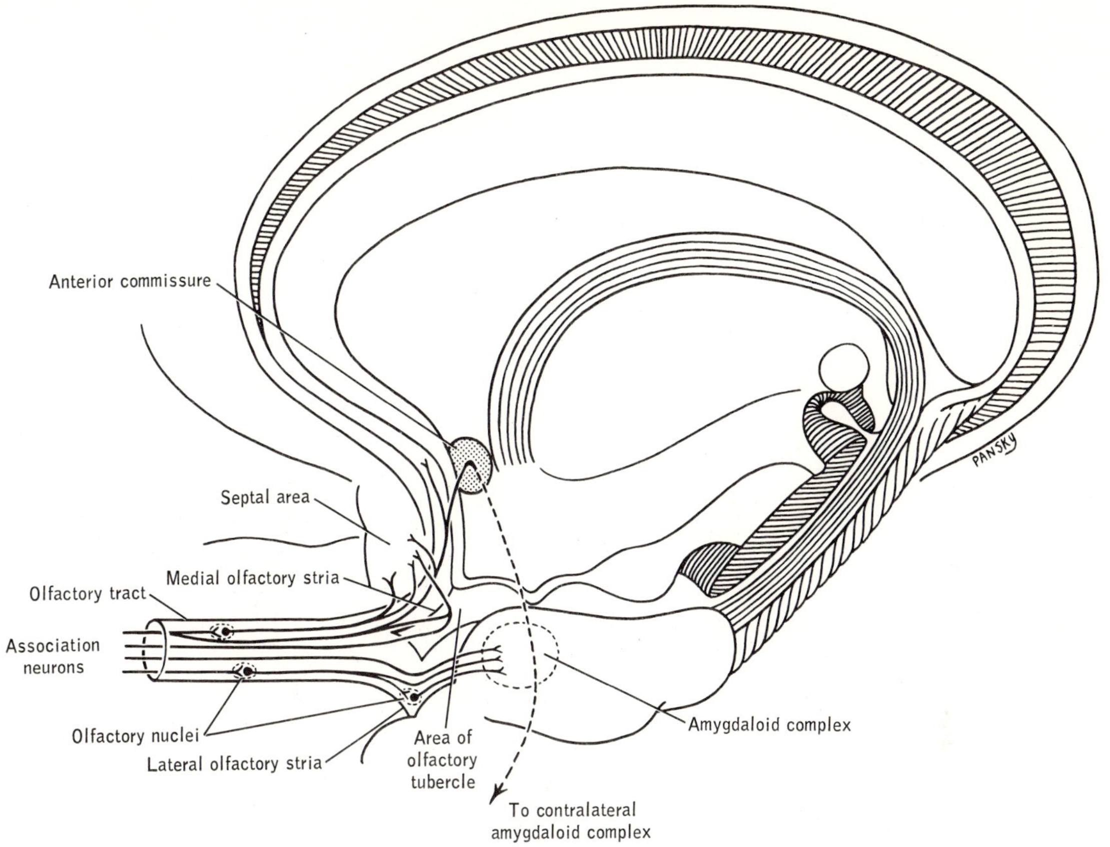

Fig. 11-6. First series of association neurons in the olfactory system.

the dorsal aspect of the thalamus in a sulcus between the latter and the caudate nucleus, to terminate in the *septal nuclei,* the *preoptic region,* and the *paraventricular nuclei* of the hypothalamus (Chap. 21). From the preoptic nuclei additional association fibers descend by way of the *medial forebrain bundle* to autonomic centers of brain stem and cord to reinforce the fibers from the septal nuclei mentioned above.

From the septal nuclei, amygdaloid complex, and hypothalamic nuclei, fibers pass by way of the *stria medullaris thalami.* This bundle passes along the lateral edge of the roof of the third ventricle. Most of its fibers end in the habenula (Fig. 25-13) of the same side, while the remainder cross in the habenular commissure to terminate in the habenula of the opposite side. From the habenula still other association fibers pass ventrocaudally by way of the *habenulopeduncular tract* to terminate in the *interpeduncular nucleus.* This nucleus extends along the interpeduncular fossa from the level of the oculomotor nucleus of the mesencephalon to the pons. From this nucleus still other association fibers run into the reticular nuclei, especially the *dorsal tegmental nucleus.* From this nucleus, fibers pass by way of the *dorsal longitudinal fasciculus* (of Schütz) (Figs. 25-8 to 25-10), to terminate in both somatic and visceral motor nuclei of the brain stem and cord.

Efferent Neuron

From the cranial motor nuclei of the brain stem (III, IV, VI, and XII) and the ventral col-

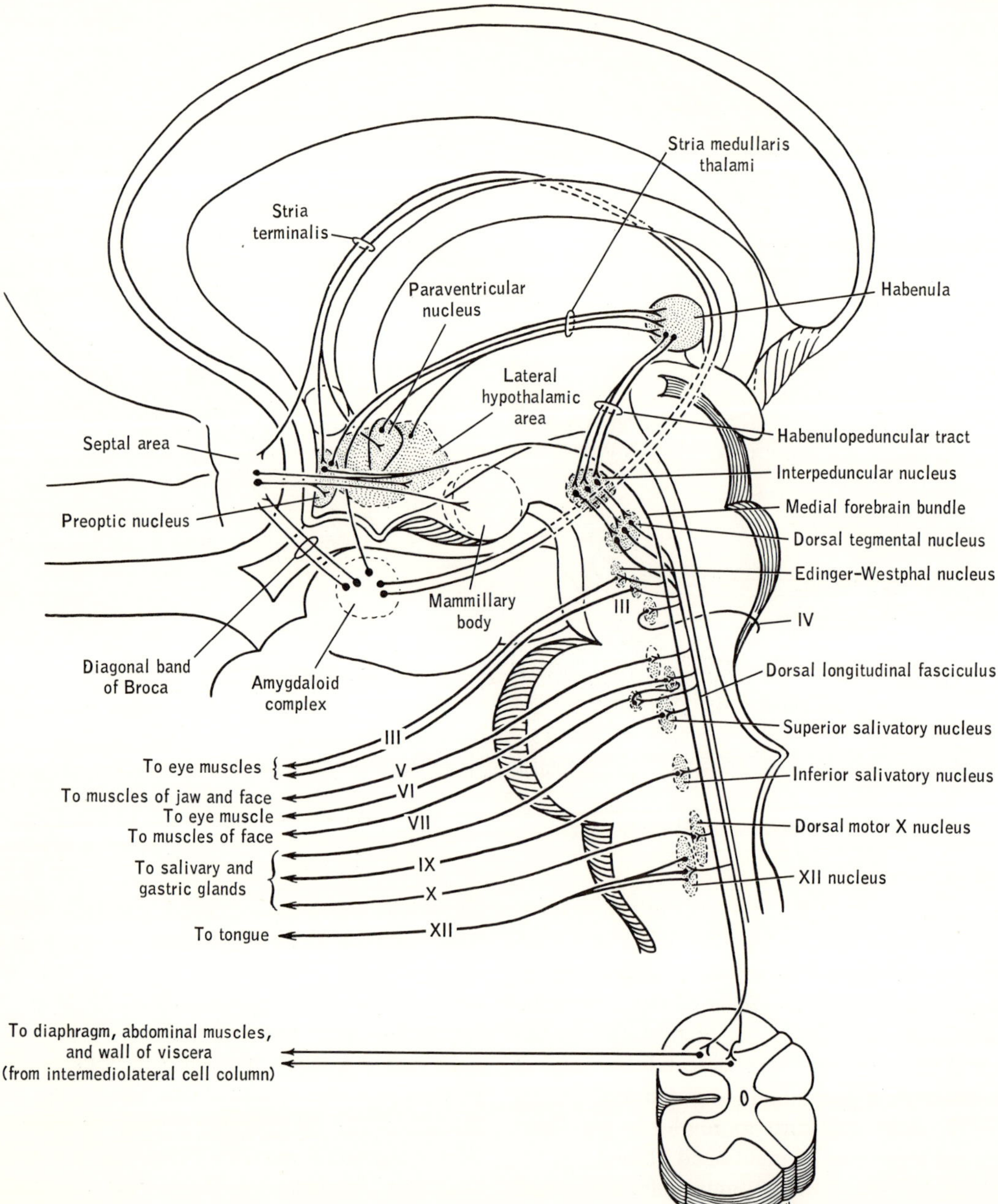

Fig. 11-7. Further association neurons of the olfactory system.

umns of the spinal cord, axons pass by way of certain cranial and any of the spinal nerves to initiate viscerosomatic reflexes (olfactosomatic). These reflexes consist of movements of the eyes, tongue, and neck, as well as of the trunk and extremities, in relation to both pleasant and unpleasant odors. Other reflexes of this type involve the nerves to the diaphragm and abdominal musculature used in retching or vomiting in response to highly disagreeable odors.

From the general visceral efferent column of the brain stem, including the superior and inferior salivatory nuclei, together with the dorsal motor nucleus of the vagus, fibers pass by way of nerves VII, IX, and X to initiate the general viscerovisceral (olfactovisceral) reflexes. These consist of the secretion of salivary and gastric glands in response to odors. From the intermediolateral cell column of the cord, as well as others supplied by the vagus, fibers pass through the autonomic system (Chap. 15) to the walls of the viscera, which play a part in the vomiting and retching reflexes. These, too, are *viscerovisceral* in nature.

From nuclei of the special visceral efferent column in the brain stem, fibers pass by way of certain cranial nerves to muscles of the jaws, face, and pharynx to initiate *special viscerovisceral reflexes*. These are especially important in vomiting and retching.

Conscious Pathways (Fig. 11-8.)

Receptors

These are the same as described under Reflex Pathways, above.

Neuron I

This is identical with the afferent neuron described under Reflex Pathways, above.

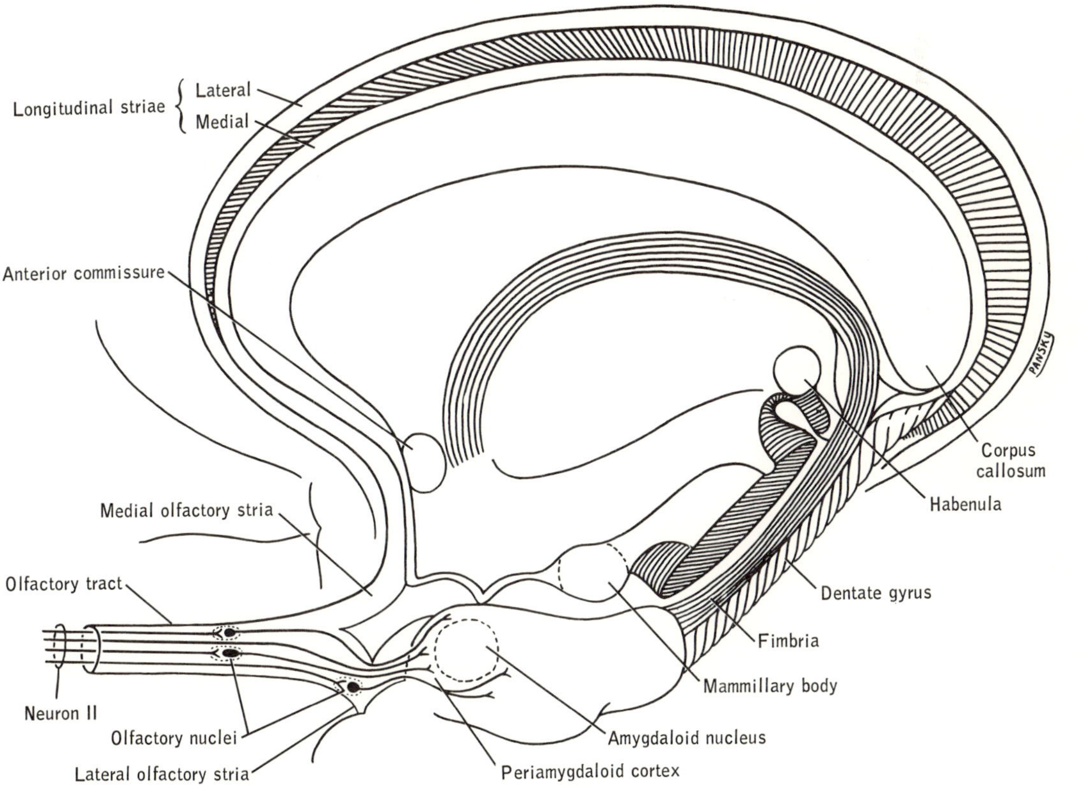

Fig. 11-8. The conscious olfactory pathway.

Neuron II

These neurons arise from mitral cells in the olfactory bulb. The axons of some of these neurons may go directly to the cortex,[1] whereas others may synapse along their course toward the cortex [1] in the anterior or lateral olfactory nuclei.

Both the direct and indirect fibers from the bulb or olfactory nuclei, respectively, terminate in the *prepyriform* or *periamygdaloid* (*semilunar* and anterior part of the *ambient gyrus*) cortex.

Clinical Considerations

Testing

In the average examination, the measurement of olfactory ability is not considered. Generally, it is enough to test the ability of the patient to recognize test odors when introduced one at a time, into each nostril separately. In addition, quantitative tests have been devised in which a measured amount of test odor is used in one nostril at a time, the patient holding his breath for a moment. The least amount of odor necessary for recognition is called the *minimal identifiable odor* (MIO). When this is determined, a steady stream of test odor is passed through the nostril until fatigue occurs, at which time the patient no longer is aware of the odor. Then each nostril is tested at 30-second intervals with the minimal identifiable odor in order to determine the duration of fatigue.[2]

Pathology

Anosmia (Loss of Smell). Loss of the sense of smell, especially if bilateral, is ordinarily not of great significance and may be a manifestation of a peripheral defect rather than of one involving the nuclei or tracts of the central nervous system. Local conditions, such as catarrhal or atrophic rhinitis and polyps, impair the olfactory sense. There are some people who suffer from congenital anosmia. Unilateral anosmia has considerably more significance.

[1] It should be understood that since this pathway does not involve the thalamus, there are no true tertiary neurons (neuron III) in the sense used in describing other afferent systems.

[2] It should be remembered that head colds or local nasal disorders will adversely affect such test results.

Brain tumors, for example *meningiomas,* in the floor of the anterior cranial fossa may compress the olfactory tract and lead to varying degrees of anosmia. The pressure on the tract will cause an increase in minimal identifiable odor on the diseased side. If the tumor is *intracerebral,* in such a position that no pressure is put upon the olfactory tract, an increase in the duration of fatigue but not in minimal identifiable odor is observed. If the intracerebral tumor lies in the frontal lobe in such a position that compression of the olfactory tract also occurs, there is an increase in minimal identifiable odor as well as an increase in duration of fatigue.

Aneurysms of the internal carotid artery may compress the tracts and lead to anosmia.

Basal skull fractures involving the anterior cranial fossa may also cause anosmia.

Uncinate Fits. Sometimes these are a manifestation of irritations of the medial, basal part of the temporal lobe, possibly involving the uncus or hippocampal gyrus. The patient usually describes a disagreeable, though often unfamiliar odor.

Olfactory Hallucinations. These may result from the irritation of either the primary olfactory or entorhinal (associative) cortex. Sometimes a tumor may be present. In some cases olfactory hallucinations represent epileptic aura. They may occur in the insane.

GUSTATION

Reflex Pathways

Receptors (Fig. 11-9.)

For the sense of taste, the receptors are *taste buds,* actually a type of chemoreceptor, located in the stratified squamous epithelium lining the mouth and oral pharynx. By far the majority are found on the dorsal surface of the tongue; they are particularly numerous on the sides of the *circumvallate papillae* and, to a lesser degree, on the *fungiform papillae.* Taste buds are round or

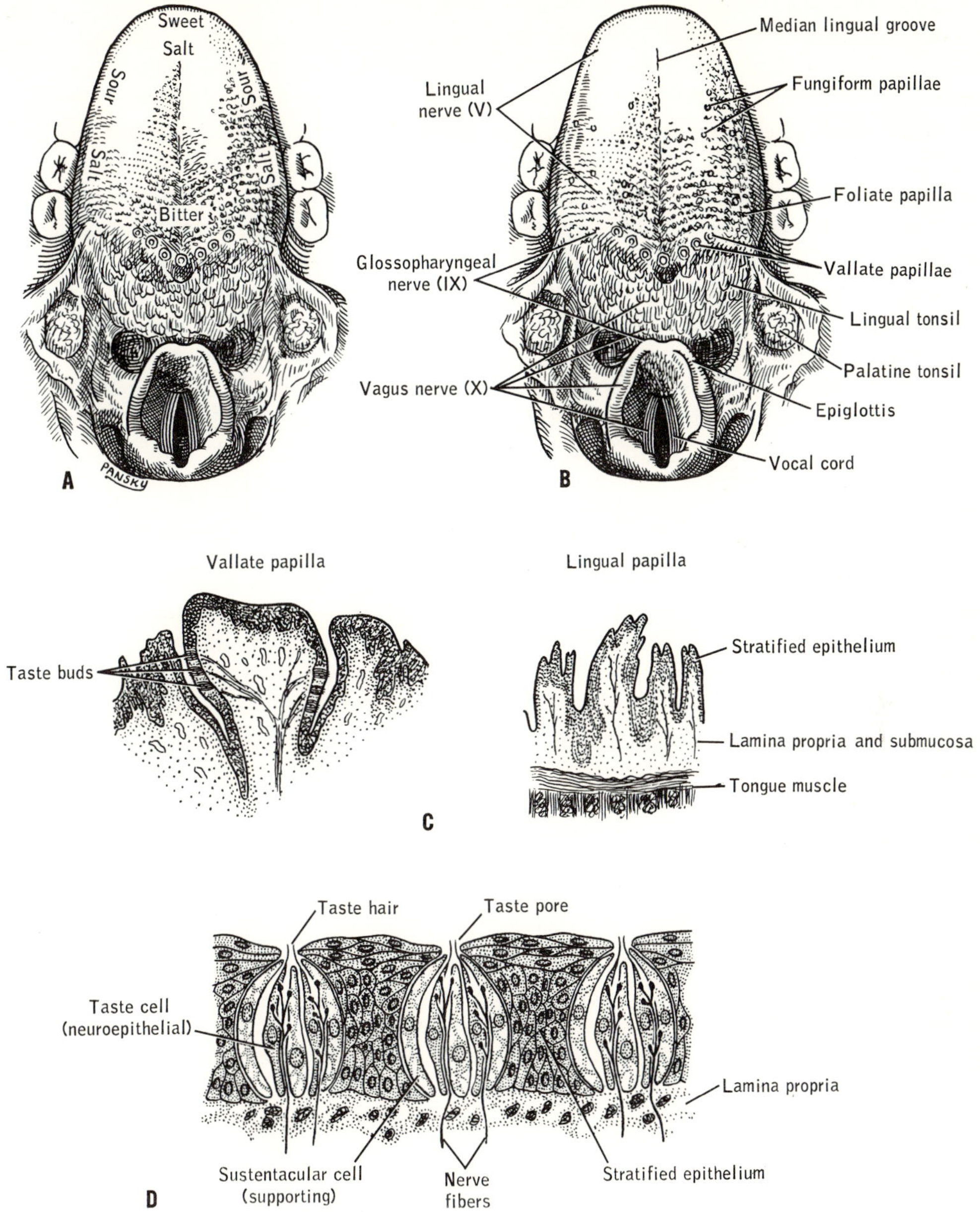

Fig. 11-9. The gustatory apparatus. *A*. Dorsal view of the tongue indicating the areas of sensibility to the various modalities of taste. *B*. Dorsal view of the tongue showing the distribution of the different kinds of papillae and the areas supplied by various cranial nerves. C. Histologic picture of two types of papillae. *D*. Finer structure of the taste buds.

oval in shape, with supporting cells (sustentacular) arched parallel to the outer curvature of the bud. Near the surface, the tips of the sustentacular cells surround a very small opening, the inner taste pore. The latter coincides with a small hiatus in the overlying epithelium, the outer taste pore. From 4 to 20 sensory cells are interspersed in this framework. The sensory cells are slender and rodlike, with a darker nucleus near the middle. The superficial process extends toward a pitlike excavation located in the center of the bud beneath the inner pore. At the end of the process is a small taste hair which projects into the pit. Thus, substances ingested, when in a liquid form, easily enter through the taste pores, to stimulate these cells.

Unlike other special senses, taste receptors are not concentrated in one relatively small area. On the contrary, they have a fairly wide distribution and are associated with cranial nerves VII, IX, and X. For this reason, it is helpful to localize the taste buds into definite zones: anterior two-thirds of the tongue; posterior third of the tongue; inner surface of the lips; lining of the cheeks; soft palate; glossopalatine arch; pharynx; posterior wall of the larynx and epiglottis.

Afferent Neuron. (Fig. 11-10.) All the peripheral processes of the afferent neurons, regardless of the cranial nerve eventually followed, penetrate the basement membrane of the epithelium in the form of nonmyelinated fibrils which end in the taste bud, either diffusely or in some form of intimate contact with the receptor cells.

It is generally easier to describe this circuit by starting with the cranial nerves which are associated with the taste buds in zones previously described.

Facial Nerve (VII). (Fig. 11-10.) From receptors on the anterior two-thirds of the tongue, peripheral processes of the neurons join the branches of the *lingual nerve,* a major branch of the mandibular division of the trigeminal nerve. After following the lingual nerve for some distance, taste fibers diverge to enter the *chorda tympani nerve.* This nerve passes obliquely backward to the petrotympanic fissure, enters the petrous temporal bone and crosses the lateral wall of the tympanic cavity to join the main trunk of the facial nerve in the facial canal. As an alternate route, some taste fibers from this same portion of the tongue traverse about half the length of the chorda tympani, leave the latter to pass through one of the roots of the *otic ganglion,* which they cross *without* synapse, and enter the *greater superficial petrosal nerve.* They follow the latter to the facial trunk, which they join just below the geniculate ganglion.

From the taste buds of the palate, the peripheral processes of the neurons ascend through the *palatine nerves* into the sphenopalatine ganglion. They pass through this ganglion *without* synapse and leave its dorsal side with the *Vidian nerve,* to become a part of the *greater superficial petrosal nerve.* Through this they join the facial nerve just below the geniculate ganglion.

The cell bodies of all the SVA neurons from the anterior tongue or palate are of the monopolar type and lie in the *geniculate ganglion of the facial nerve* (VII). From here the central processes accumulate in the *nervus intermedius* and continue through this nerve to the brain stem (Figs. 2-7, 2-8). From here they travel dorsomedially through the substance of the medulla, approach the lateral wall of the fourth ventricle, and turn caudally in the *tractus solitarius* (Figs. 11-10, 25-5). The taste fibers in this tract then terminate in the *nucleus of the tractus solitarius* [3] (Figs. 25-2 to 25-5).

Glossopharyngeal Nerve (IX). (Fig. 11-10.) From the taste buds on the posterior one-third of the tongue and the anterior pharyngeal wall, the peripheral processes of the afferent neurons run in the *lingual* and *pharyngeal branches,*

[3] There is a difference of opinion among neuroanatomists as to the termination of the primary taste neurons. The majority favor the belief that the principal synapses are in the nucleus of the tractus solitarius, particularly in the rostral end of it. Others have suggested the presence of a specific cell group called the *gustatory nucleus,* said to lie just medial to the nucleus of the tractus solitarius. In many cases, a definite nuclear mass may be seen, at first squeezed between the dorsal motor nucleus of the vagus and the hypoglosal nucleus. Actually, it may even extend to the medial side of the latter (Fig. 25-4). When it is in this location, the term *nucleus intercalatus* is often applied.

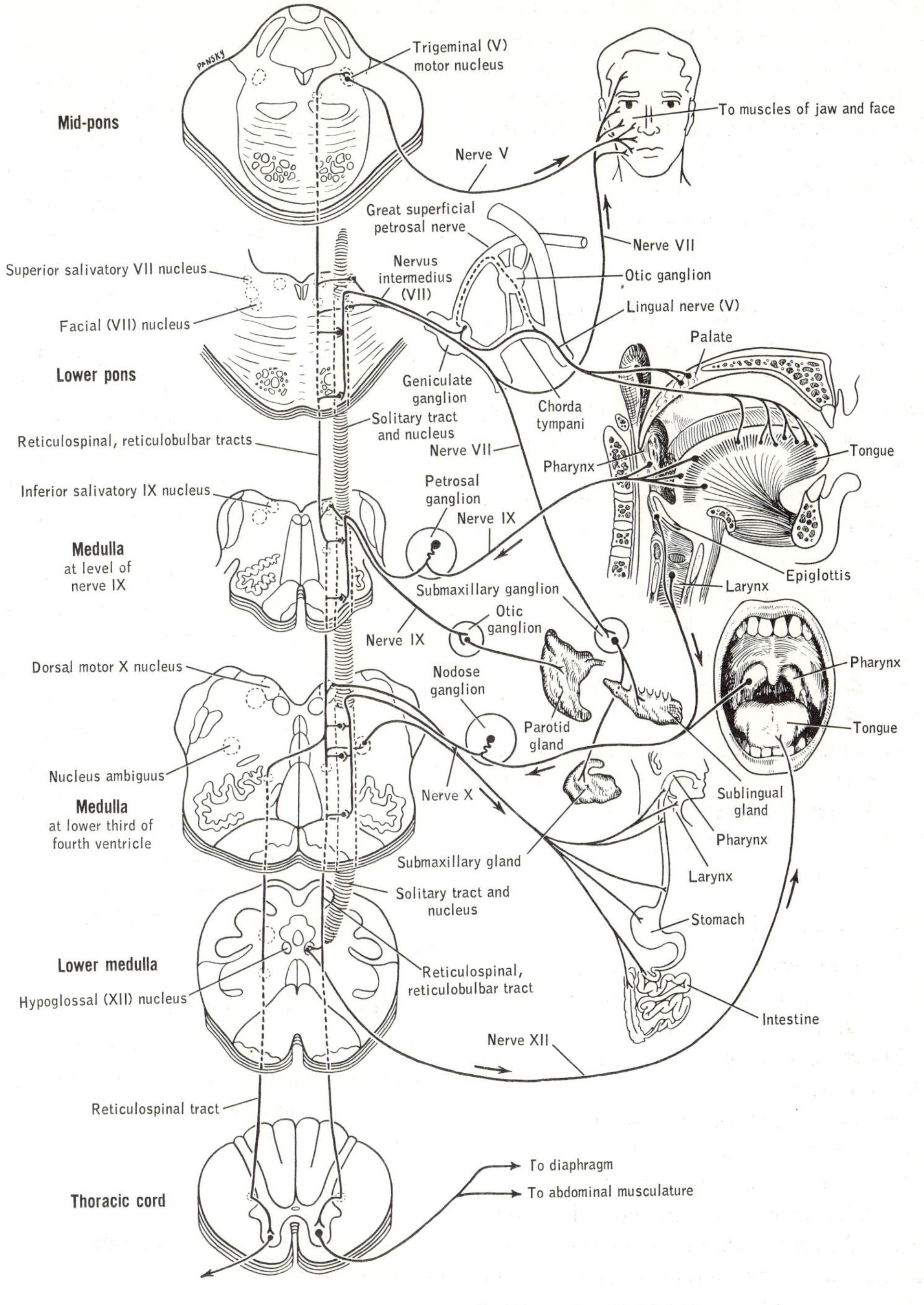

Fig. 11-10. Gustatory reflexes, especially those elicited by pleasant tastes.

respectively, of the glossopharyngeal nerve, through which they ascend to the main trunk of that nerve to reach their cell bodies, which lie in the *petrosal ganglion.* The central processes continue their ascent to the superficial attachment of nerve IX (Figs. 2-7, 2-8, 25-5). The intramedullary course is similar to that of nerve VII, in that taste fibers turn caudally in the *tractus solitarius* (Fig. 25-2 to 25-5) to end in the nucleus of that tract.[3]

Vagus Nerve (X). (Rig. 11-10.) The peripheral processes of afferent neurons whose receptors lie in the posterior pharynx run through the *pharyngeal branch of the vagus nerve,* passing through the pharyngeal plexus, to join the vagus nerve (X) below its nodose ganglion. Fibers from the epiglottis and larynx travel through the *superior laryngeal branch of the vagus,* which joins the main trunk of nerve X. In either case, the monopolar cell bodies for all taste fibers traveling in the vagus lie in the *nodose ganglion.* The central processes ascend with the vagus to its superficial attachment to the brain stem (Figs. 2-7, 2-8, 25-4).

The intramedullary course of these afferent neurons is essentially the same as that described in nerves VII and IX, all eventually bending caudally in the *tractus solitarius* to end in the nucleus of that tract.[3]

Association Neuron (Fig. 11-10.)

The direct observation and tracing of such neurons has not been possible. However, reflex reactions which occur in response to taste are so well established that there can be little doubt that such fibers do exist.

The cell bodies for these neurons lie in either the *nucleus of the tractus solitarius* or in the *gustatory nucleus.*[3] Their axons immediately enter the reticular formation, through which they are distributed to the superior and inferior salivatory nuclei; the dorsal motor nucleus of the vagus; the nucleus of the trigeminal and facial nerves; the nucleus ambiguus; and the cells of the ventral gray columns in the cord by way of the reticulospinal tract.

Efferent Neuron (Fig. 11-10.)

From cells in the superior and inferior salivatory nuclei and the dorsal motor nucleus of the vagus nerve, efferent neurons, by way of cranial nerves VII, IX, and X, are distributed to the major salivary glands (parotid, submaxillary, and sublingual), the gastric glands, and the muscularis of the alimentary canal. These initiate *viscerovisceral* reflexes which produce secretion in the glands and peristalsis in the digestive tract in response to food in the mouth.

From cells in the motor nuclei of the trigeminal and facial nerves, axons are distributed to the muscles of the jaws and face. This initiates a *special viscerovisceral* reflex which causes changes in facial expression and movements in the jaws in response to food in the mouth.

All the reflexes thus far mentioned are associated predominantly with pleasant tastes. There are also others related to tastes of an unpleasant nature. Among these are reflexes initiated by axons from the dorsal motor nucleus of the vagus (viscerovisceral); from the nucleus ambiguus (special viscerovisceral); from the hypoglossal nucleus (viscerosomatic); from the ventral gray column of the cervical cord and from the ventral gray column of the thoracic cord (viscerosomatic). These fibers, distributed to the musculature of the digestive tract, pharynx, tongue, diaphragm, and abdomen, are all necessary in the vomiting-retching reflex.

Conscious Pathways (Fig. 11-11.)

The pathways followed to cerebral levels have not been definitely established. However, since man does become conscious of many tastes, such pathways must exist.

Receptors

These are the same as described under Reflex Pathways, above.

Neuron I

These are identical with the afferent neuron described under Reflex Pathways, above.

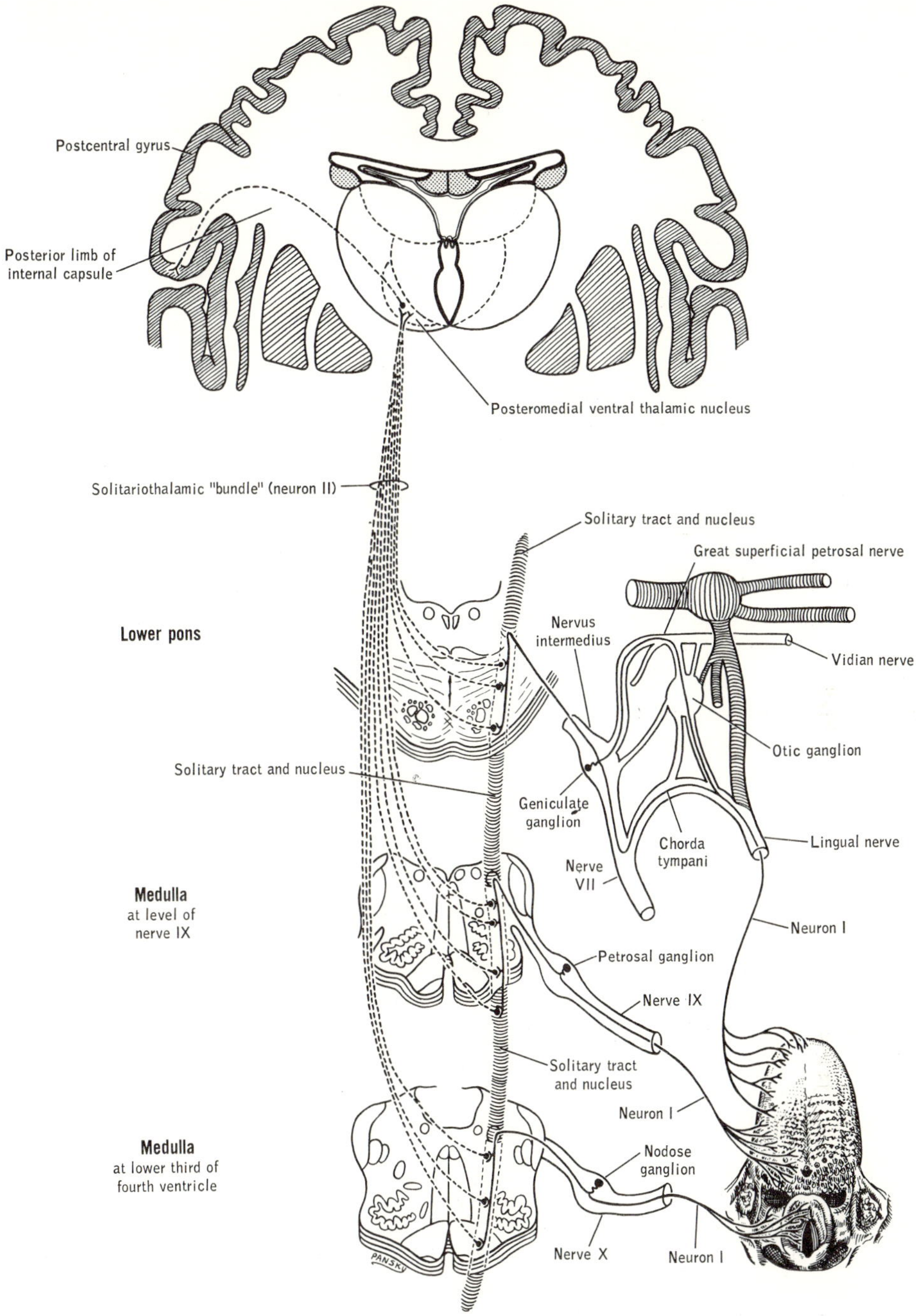

Fig. 11-11. Conscious gustatory pathway.

Neuron II

The cell bodies for these neurons lie either in the rostral end of the *nucleus of the tractus solitarius* or in the *gustatory nucleus.*[3] Most of the axons of these neurons may cross the midline before ascending as the so-called *solitariothalamic bundle* (visceral lemniscus). The course of these fibers is uncertain. However, it appears safe to assume that they would accompany other bundles ascending toward the thalamus, such as the spinothalamic tracts, or the medial lemniscus, or the trigeminothalamic lemnisci. Since the trigeminothalamic bundles are already carrying general somatic impulses arising from receptors of the head, including the mucous membrane of the tongue and mouth, it certainly would not be illogical for the secondary neurons of taste to lie close to them.

There is likewise disagreement as to the exact thalamic nucleus which serves as a terminus for these secondary neurons. Evidence seems to favor the *medial* part of the *posteromedial ventral nucleus,* or an *accessory semilunar nucleus* which adjoins the latter on its medial side.

Neuron III

The cells of origin of the third neuron lie in either the posteromedial ventral nucleus or an accessory semilunar nucleus. Their axons travel through the posterior limb of the internal capsule. From this point there is further disagreement as to the terminations of these fibers in the cortex. More recent information favors the most ventral part of the postcentral gyrus (opercular part), with extensions deep into the lateral fissure, as the primary gustatory cortex. Since this area is so close to the general sensory cortex for the tongue and also is near the motor areas for movement of the tongue and jaws, such a conclusion seems logical. The older concepts favored either the uncus or the anterior part of the insula as the primary gustatory cortex.

Since the hypothalamus is the highest direct effector center for the visceral efferent mechanism, it would be strange if taste, a special visceral sense, were not connected to some part of the hypothalamus. At least one possibility is suggested by the fact that secondary taste fibers are running in the tegmental reticular formation. These fibers may be carried rostrally to make connections in the reticular formation of the upper pons or lower mesencephalon. From the latter, another set of neurons enters the mammillary peduncle (Chap. 21) to be carried into the mammillary nuclei of the hypothalamus.

Clinical Considerations

Qualities of Taste (Fig. 11-9*A*.)

There is some tendency to consider four kinds of taste, namely: sour, sweet, bitter, and salt. These may be thought of as modalities of sensation, just as cold, hot, pain, and temperature are modalities of somatic sensation. This idea is supported by some evidence. First, certain regions of the tongue are more sensitive to one taste than another, and even individual papillae have a fair degree of specificity. Next, the application or use of certain drugs causes a loss of one kind of taste but not of others. Lastly, one kind of taste elicits one type of response while another initiates another type, as diametrically opposed as swallowing and vomiting. Thus, the tongue is regionally divided on the basis of the taste modality to which it is most sensitive. The tip apparently can distinguish all four modalities, although even here there is a greater sensitivity to sweet and salt. The edges of the tongue are more responsive to sour, while the base is more sensitive to bitter.

Taste sensibilities are described as *ageusia,* a complete absence of taste; *hypogeusia,* diminished taste; and *parageusia,* hallucination or the misinterpretation of taste.

Testing

Since olfaction and gustation are functionally and subjectively so closely allied, an apparent ageusia or hypogeusia may, to a major extent, be due to local conditions of the nose (congestions due to a cold or an obstruction of the passageway). Therefore, as a first step, the examination should begin with an investigation of the nasal chambers.

When the examination of the nose is completed, the various regions of the tongue should be tested with substances possessing the four basic qualities of taste. It is particularly important to note whether a loss of taste is over the entire tongue or over either the right or left halves only. If the anterior two-thirds or the posterior third of the tongue is tested, it could be determined whether the pathologic condition is in the peripheral course of the glossopharyngeal nerve or involves the chorda tympani and facial nerves.

Pathology

Since pathologic conditions involving taste almost inevitably produce far more striking symptoms which can be related directly to other functional components of nerves VII, IX, or X, no attempt will be made to describe specific pathologic alterations. Some of these alterations will be considered in the section dealing with cranial nerves (Chap. 17). Centrally located lesions will also give more striking symptoms referable to other pathways.

SUMMARY
Smell

REFLEX

Viscerovisceral (general)		*Viscerovisceral* (special)
1. Hair cells in upper nasal chamber	Receptor	1. Same as viscerovisceral (general)
2. Part of receptor cell, whose central process terminates in the olfactory bulb	Afferent neuron	2. Same as viscerovisceral (general)
3. From olfactory bulb, through olfactory tract, some terminating in anterior olfactory nucleus, others continuing caudally From olfactory bulb and from anterior olfactory nucleus, through either medial or lateral olfactory stria Fibers of medial stria either end in nuclei of septal area or cross to opposite amygdala Fibers of lateral stria either end in nucleus of lateral stria or in amygdala of same side From lateral olfactory nucleus to amygdala	Association neuron to brain centers	3. Same as viscerovisceral (general)
4. From amygdala, via diagonal band of Broca, to septal nuclei From amygdala, through terminal stria to septal nuclei, preoptic region, and paraventricular nuclei of hypothalamus From septal nuclei, through medial forebrain bundle, to preoptic nuclei, lateral hypothalamic area, and mammillary nuclei From septal nuclei, amygdala, and hypothalamus through stria medullaris thalami to the habenula From habenula through habenulopeduncular tract to the interpeduncular nucleus From the interpeduncular nucleus to the dorsal tegmental nucleus From septal nuclei through medial forebrain bundle directly to the tegmental reticular nuclei	Association neuron between centers	4. Same as viscerovisceral (general)
5. From septal nuclei and preoptic nuclei through medial forebrain bundle to autonomic nuclei of brain stem and intermediolateral column of cord From tegmental reticular nuclei through the reticular formation and reticulospinal tract to autonomic nuclei of brain stem and intermediolateral column of the cord From dorsal tegmental nucleus via the dorsal longitudinal fasciculus to autonomic nuclei of the brain stem and the intermediolateral column of the cord	Descending fiber to lower motor nuclei	5. Same as viscerovisceral (general) except for the terminations, the reticular formation, medial forebrain bundle, and dorsal longitudinal fasciculus terminating in nuclei V, VII, IX, and X
6. From the autonomic nuclei of the brain stem (superior and inferior salivatory and dorsal motor nucleus of the vagus) through preganglionics running in nerves VII, IX, and X, to synapse in autonomic ganglia, thence through postganglionics to salivary glands and the muscles and glands of the digestive system From the intermediolateral cell column of the cord through preganglionics in the ventral roots of spinal nerves and by white rami, to autonomic ganglia, thence by postganglionics to smooth muscle and glands	Efferent neuron	6. From nucleus V through trigeminal nerve to muscles of mastication From nucleus VII through facial nerve to muscles of face From nucleus IX and X (ambiguus) through glossopharyngeal and vagus nerves to muscles of pharynx and larynx
Viscerosomatic		
1-4. Same as above	1-4 Same as above	
5. Same as above except the reticular formation, reticulospinal tract, and dorsal longitudinal fasciculus end around cranial somatic nuclei III, IV, VI, and XII and the ventral gray column of the cord	Descending fiber to lower motor nuclei	
6. Efferent neurons from III, IV, and VI pass through their respective nerves to extrinsic ocular muscles From nucleus XII, fibers pass to the tongue From the ventral column, fibers innervate muscles of neck, trunk and extremities	Efferent neuron	

CONSCIOUS

Direct		*Indirect*
7. Same as in reflex	Receptor	7. Same as in reflex
8. Same as afferent neuron in reflex	Neuron I	8. Same as afferent neuron in reflex
9. From cells in olfactory bulb through the lateral olfactory stria to end in the prepyriform area, the periamygdaloid area, and the anterior ambient gyrus N.B. Since the thalamus is not involved in this system directly, there is no true neuron III as seen in other afferent systems	Neuron II	9. From cells in the olfactory bulb, ending in anterior or lateral olfactory nuclei From olfactory nuclei to same areas of cortex as in direct pathway

SUMMARY
Taste

REFLEX

Viscerosomatic		*Viscerovisceral* (general)
1. Taste buds	Reflex	1. Same as viscerosomatic
2. From receptors on anterior two-thirds of tongue via lingual, chorda tympani, and facial nerves, with cell bodies in the geniculate ganglion, into the brain stem bending caudally in the tractus solitarius and ending in the nucleus of that tract (or gustatory nucleus) From receptors on posterior third of tongue via glossopharyngeal nerve, with cell bodies in the petrosal ganglion, into the brain stem, bending caudally in the tractus solitarius and terminating in the nucleus of that tract (or gustatory nucleus) From receptors near epiglottis and the posterior pharynx via the vagus nerve with cell bodies in the nodose ganglion, into the brain stem, bending caudally in the tractus solitarius and terminating the nucleus of that tract (or gustatory nucleus)	Afferent neuron	2. Same as viscerosomatic
3. From cells in the nucleus of the tractus solitarius (or gustatory) to the nucleus of the hypoglossal nerve From cells in the nucleus of the tractus solitarius (or gustatory) through the reticular formation and reticulospinal tract to the ventral gray column of the cord	Association neuron	3. From cells in the nucleus of the tractus solitarius (or gustatory), through the reticular formation to salivatory nuclei; dorsal motor nucleus of vagus; through reticulospinal tract to intermediolateral column of the cord
4. From the hypoglossal nucleus through nerve XII to muscles of tongue From the ventral gray columns of the cord through spinal nerves to muscles of neck, trunk, and extremities	Efferent neuron	4. From salivatory nuclei by preganglionics in nerves VII and IX to autonomic ganglia, thence, through postganglionics, to the salivary glands From the dorsal motor nucleus of the vagus by preganglionics in nerve X, to terminal autonomic ganglia, thence by short postganglionics to muscles and glands of digestive system From the intermediolateral cell column, through preganglionics in the ventral roots of spinal nerves and by white rami to autonomic ganglia, thence by postganglionics to muscles and glands of digestive system

Viscerovisceral (special)	
5. Same as viscerosomatic	Receptor
6. Same as viscerosomatic	Afferent neuron
7. From cells in the nucleus of the tractus solitarius (or gustatory) through the reticular formation to nuclei V, VII, IX, X, and XI	Association neuron
8. From nucleus V to muscles of mastication through trigeminal nerve From nucleus VII to muscles of face via facial nerve From nucleus ambiguus through nerves IX and X (glossopharyngeal and vagus) to muscles of pharynx and larynx From nucleus of XI through accessory nerve to sternocleidomastoid and trapezius muscles	Efferent neuron

CONSCIOUS

1. Same as in reflex	Receptor
2. Same as afferent neuron in reflex	Neuron I
3. From the nucleus of the tractus solitarius (or gustatory), probably traveling with the trigeminothalamic tracts, to terminate in the medial side of the posteromedial ventral nucleus of the thalamus (sometimes called the accessory arcuate or semilunar nucleus)	Neuron II
4. From the accessory arcuate nucleus through the posterior limb of the internal capsule to reach the extreme ventral end of the postcentral gyrus (area 43)	Neuron III

12 GENERAL PROPRIOCEPTION (GP)

By definition, proprioception means receiving stimuli originating in the muscles, tendons, and joints. It is the mechanism involved in the self-regulation of posture and movement. Thus, both position and posture are maintained by a continuous flow of impulses from the musculoskeletal apparatus.

Although the proprioceptive system is of prime importance wherever a complex musculature exists, its activity passes almost unnoticed, for its conscious aspects are less highly developed than those of the exteroceptive senses. However, it does express itself primarily in terms of reflexes.

TRUNK

Simple Reflex Pathways (Figs. 12-1, 12-2.)

Receptors

The receptors, located in and among muscles, tendons, and joints, are of several types.

The intramuscular variety are known as *muscle spindles*. Each spindle is composed of a variable, but usually small number of atypical, slender skeletal muscle fibers. These are the *intrafusal fibers* and are enclosed in a connective tissue sheath. The latter tissue is attached at the ends of the spindle with the endomysium of the normal skeletal muscle fibers—*the extrafusal fiber*. Toward their ends, the intrafusal fiber is striated and is contractile. The central portion of these fibers is expanded and contains an abnormally large number of nuclei for which reason it is referred to as the *nuclear bag region*. Between the connective tissue and the sarcolemma of the bag there is a considerable fluid-filled space crossed by connective tissue fibers and nerves. The intrafusal fiber is related to three kinds of neurons: (1) small efferents, the *gamma efferents,* which have motor end plates in the polar region of the fiber; (2) primary afferents (A-afferents), the largest of the three, which wind around the nuclear bag region as the *annulospiral ending;* (3) secondary afferents (B-afferents) which terminate in a group at the periphery of the bag region as the *flower spray endings*. Because the intra- and extrafusal fibers are parallel, they are both stretched when the entire muscle is stretched. The act of stretching stimulates the annulospiral endings. A similar effect is obtained when the polar region of the intrafusal fiber contracts in response to activity in the gamma efferents for, in such a contraction, the bag region is put under tension.[1]

The flower spray endings are thought to be activated by a maximum contraction of the muscle fiber.

Within the tendons are *tendon spindles,* similar in basic structure to the muscle spindle ex-

[1] The importance of these activities will be further considered with the Somatic Efferent System (Chap. 14 and the suprasegmental control mechanisms (Chaps. 18, 19, 20) are discussed.

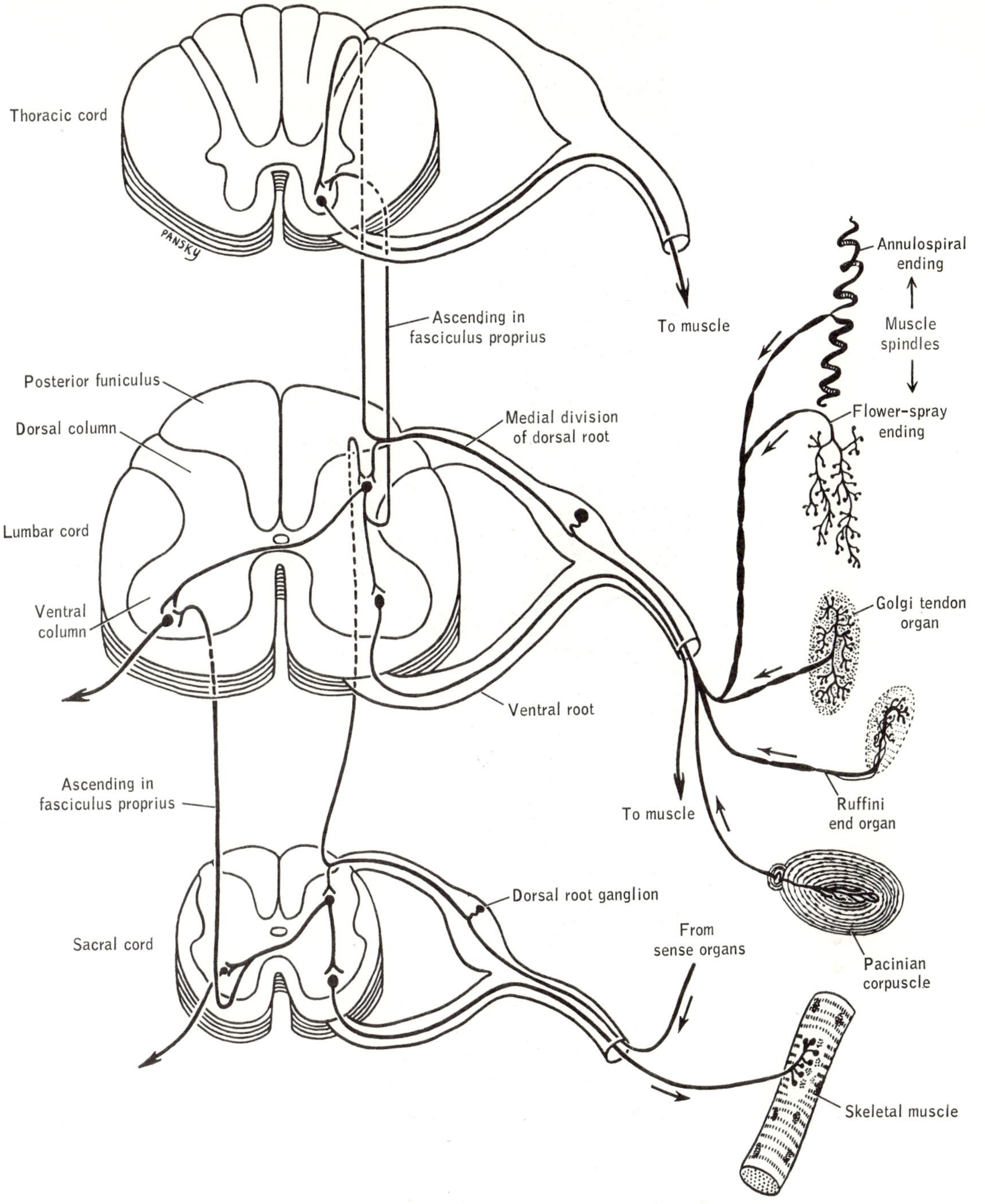

Fig. 12-1. Diagram of the general proprioceptive (GP) reflex paths for afferent impulses reaching the CNS through spinal nerves.

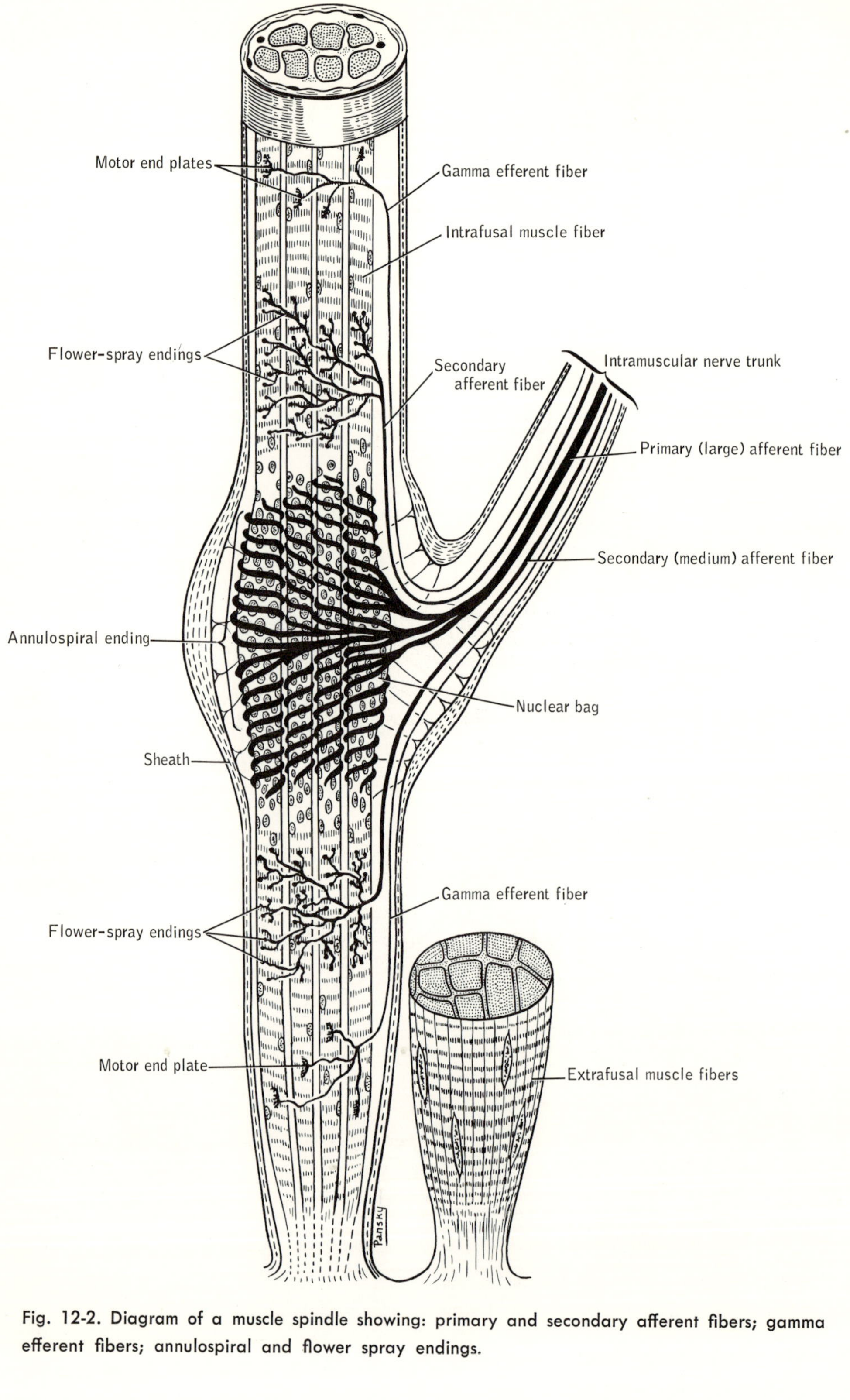

Fig. 12-2. Diagram of a muscle spindle showing: primary and secondary afferent fibers; gamma efferent fibers; annulospiral and flower spray endings.

cept that the modified fibers are collagenous, rather than muscular. Between tendon fibers are *corpuscles,* similar to those of Ruffini (Chap. 8), which are believed to react to stretching of the tendon. In addition, there are also the *neurotendinous organs of Golgi,* which are adapted to register submaximal muscular contractions.

Pacinian corpuscles are found in fascia and intermuscular septums and about joint capsules. In the two former locations, they are activated by the swelling of the entire muscle or its larger subdivisions (as in contraction), while those situated within articular capsules record movements at joints.

Corpuscular structures, not named specifically, have also been observed near joints.

Afferent Neuron

The neuron related to the annulospiral ending is large and heavily myelinated. It is referred to as an A-afferent. Its monopolar cell in the dorsal root ganglion is also large. The fiber associated with the flower spray and tendon endings is intermediate in size with a moderately large monopolar cell in the dorsal root ganglion. These are the so-called B-afferents. All central processes are collected in bundles comprising the *medial division* of the dorsal root. As soon as entry into the cord is made through the dorsolateral sulcus, these fibers join the posterior funiculus, those coming in at lower spinal levels lying more medially in the funiculus (Chap. 8). Each individual fiber then bifurcates into long ascending and short descending branches both of which give off collaterals that end either around cells in the dorsal column or directly around cells in the ventral column. In addition, branches of the same A-afferent fibers also make synapses on both sides of the cord with small, multipolar neurons of the intercalated type which are located among the motor cells of the ventral column. The axons of the latter synapse with other efferent neurons.

The B-afferents carrying impulses from the flower spray and tendon endings also send collaterals into the ventral column to terminate on the same motor cells that received the terminations of the A-afferents.

As pointed out, collaterals of both A and B afferents terminate in the body of the dorsal column. Fibers arising there are distributed, like other associational neurons, to a number of places as part of typical polysynaptic reflex arcs.

Association Neuron

The central processes of the dorsal root ganglion cell related to the afferent neuron of the annulospiral receptor passes directly to synapse with the motor cells in the ventral columns on both sides of the spinal cord without the interposition of an association neuron. This is a monosynaptic (two neuron) reflex arc and is the anatomical basis of the *stretch* or *myotatic reflex.*

The ganglion cells which transmit impulses from the flower spray endings send their central processes into the gray substance of the cord. Some of these also terminate directly on motor cells of the ventral column. The others end in the proper nucleus of the dorsal column. Fibers arising in that nucleus are distributed widely as part of typical polysynaptic reflex arcs. Some pass to the ventral column on the same side. Many travel up or down the cord through the fasciculus proprius to reach the ventral column at other levels. Still others cross to the opposite side of the cord through the anterior white commissure to terminate either directly upon motor cells of the ventral column in the same spinal segment or upon segments at other levels, through the fasciculus proprius.

Efferent Neuron

Like the efferent limbs of all spinal reflexes, these, too, have their cells of origin in the ventral columns. Their axons cross through the anterior funiculus, exit from the cord along the ventrolateral sulcus, and form the ventral root of each spinal nerve, subsequently passing to all skeletal muscle.[1]

Coordination (Cerebellar) Reflex Pathway (Fig. 12-3.)

So many of man's activities are carried out subconsciously that there is little conception of

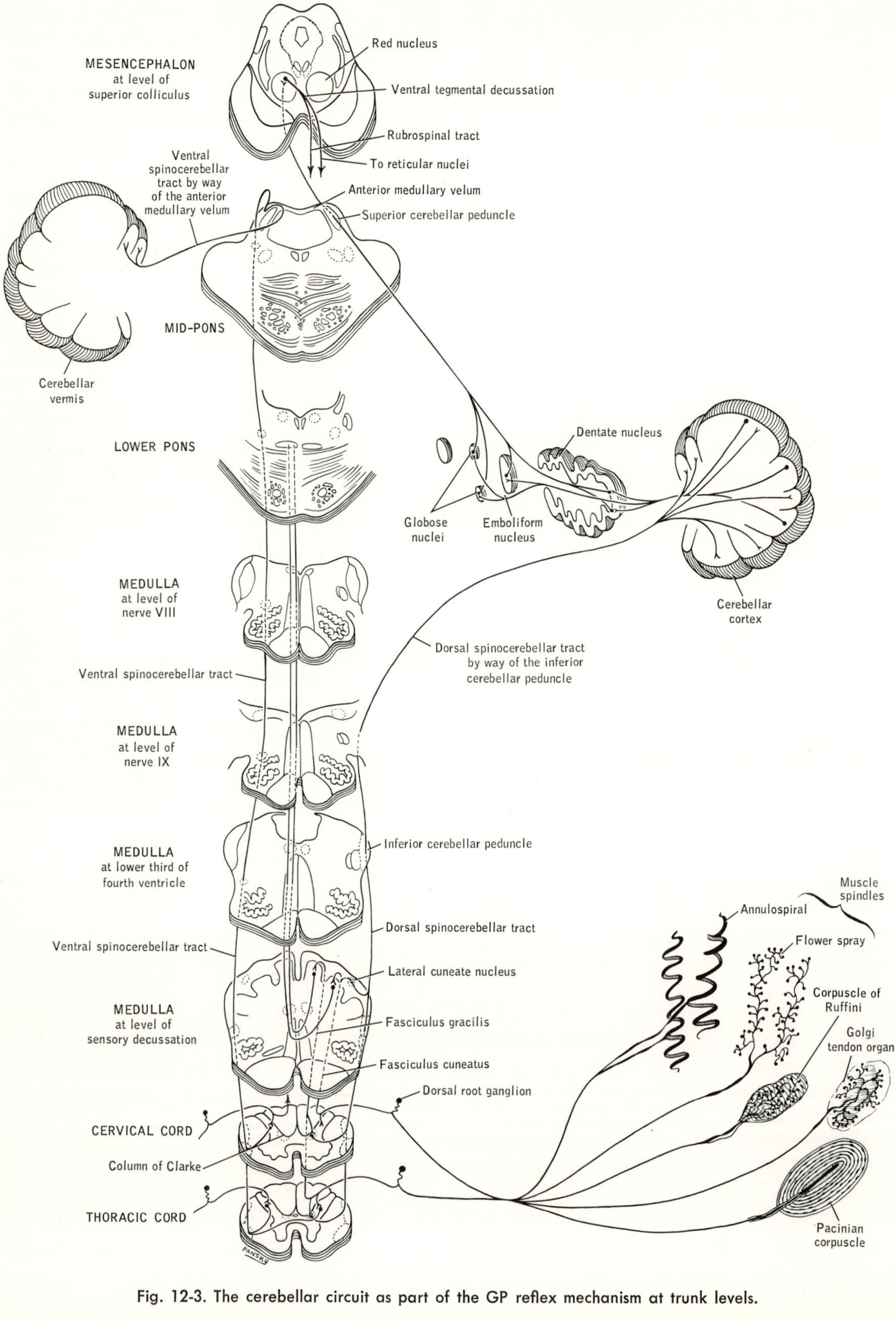

Fig. 12-3. The cerebellar circuit as part of the GP reflex mechanism at trunk levels.

the tremendous amount of adjustment necessary for proper function. Not only must a set of muscles contract, but the contraction must be to the correct extent while, at the same time, an opposing group must relax to the appropriate degree. Whether in the retention of normal posture or during increased activity due to emergency reactions, a constant flow of impulses from receptors in the trunk musculature must reach the central nervous system in order to keep the entire body in the proper state of tonus. Consider, for example, the reflex reactions which occur when an attempt is made to regain the normal position after having stumbled or turned an ankle. This requires the rapid contraction of many muscles over a wide area of the body, all demanding regulation and coordination. For both of these processes, the cerebellum plays an important role. However, only a brief account of the descending chains through which the cerebellum mediates its influence upon muscular action will be given here. The details will be added in the chapter on the cerebellum (Chap. 18).

Receptors

These are the same as those described under Simple Reflex Pathways, above.

Afferent Neuron

The first neuron in the cerebellar circuit is the same as the afferent limb of the simple reflex arc. However, there is one difference, namely, collaterals from the primary fibers synapse not only in the body of the dorsal column but also in the column of Clarke (nucleus of Clarke), which extends from the eighth cervical through the second lumbar segments (Fig. 3-5).

Association Neuron—Ascending

Axons originating from the dorsal column proper may cross to the opposite side of the cord through the anterior white commissure, pass to the periphery of the cord in the ventral portion of the lateral funiculus, and there turn rostrally as the *ventral spinocerebellar tract*. Fibers in this tract carry impulses from all regions of the body, including the upper extremity and neck. In its upward path, the ventral spinocerebellar tract remains lateral and superficial throughout the cord (Fig. 3-7). It takes a position dorsal to the inferior olive and medial to the lateral spinothalamic tract in the medulla (Figs. 25-1 to 25-3). In the pons, it shifts gradually more laterally (Figs. 25-6, 25-7) and then courses dorsally around the external surface of the superior cerebellar peduncle to reach the anterior medullary velum (Fig. 25-9). Through the latter, this tract enters the rostral end of the cerebellar vermis. Other axons having similar origin in the body of the dorsal column pass laterally to the *ventral spinocerebellar tract* on the same side. Thus, this tract contains both crossed and uncrossed fibers.

From Clarke's column most of the axons turn almost directly laterally on the same side of the cord, where they extend almost to the periphery of the most dorsal portion of the lateral funiculus. Here, they turn rostrally as the *dorsal spinocerebellar tract* (Fig. 3-7). Impulses traveling in this tract originate primarily in the trunk and lower extremity.[2] Throughout the cord, the dorsal spinocerebellar tract maintains its superficial, dorsolateral position. In the medulla it lies just beneath the surface, overlying the spinal V tract (Figs. 25-1 to 25-3). Gradually it shifts dorsally and joins the inferior cerebellar peduncle (restiform body), through which it enters the cerebellum to spray out to the cerebellar cortex at both its rostral and caudal ends.

Association Neuron—Descending

Axons leave the cerebellar cortex, passing through the white cores of the folia to reach the central cerebellar nuclei (Chap. 18). Arising from these nuclei, fibers leave the cerebellum through its superior peduncle, decussate, and terminate in the red nucleus of the midbrain. The *rubrospinal tract* [3] arises from large cells in

[2] Since Clarke's column does not appear below the second lumbar segment, this tract is not found caudal to that level.

[3] In man the rubrospinal tract is very small, its existence being denied by some authorities. It is more generally agreed, however, that it can be traced as an entity at least as far as the upper thoracic cord.

this nucleus. It crosses the midline in the ventral tegmental decussation and descends through the reticular formation of the brain stem into the lateral funiculus of the spinal cord to terminate about the cells of the ventral columns.

From small cells of the red nucleus, other axons descend in the reticular formation, most of them terminating in the reticular nuclei (Chap. 19). From the latter nuclei, fibers continue downward into the lateral funiculus of the spinal cord by way of the *reticulospinal tract* to terminate about the cells of the ventral columns. This pathway is probably of greater significance than the rubrospinal tract in transmitting cerebellar influence to muscular activity.

Efferent Neuron

These are the same neurons as described under Simple Reflex Pathways, above.

Conscious Pathway

Receptors

These are the same as described under Simple Reflex Pathways, above.

Neuron I

This is identical with the afferent neuron described above for simple reflexes.

Neuron II and Neuron III

In so far as proprioceptive impulses are carried to conscious levels, it is believed that the secondary and tertiary neurons follow the same course as indicated for tactile discrimination (Chap. 8).

HEAD

Simple Reflex Pathways

Receptors

These are similar to those of the trunk and are found among the muscles of mastication and facial expression, around the temporomandibular joint, and in the sockets of the teeth.[4]

[4] Mastication, the adjustment of strength of bite, and at least the first part of deglutition all require some degree of self-regulation.

Afferent Neuron

The peripheral processes from each receptor travel in all three divisions of the trigeminal nerve. A few are in the ophthalmic branch. From the hard palate and sockets of the upper teeth, some pass via the maxillary branch. However, the vast majority, from the sockets of the lower teeth, the muscles of mastication, and the temporomandibular joint, are found in the mandibular division. Unlike other sensory systems, there is no cell body for these afferent fibers either in the semilunar ganglion or anywhere else outside the central nervous system. The peripheral processes merely pass through the ganglion to join the motor root (portio minor), traveling in that root to the lateral aspect of the pons where it enters the brain. Its fibers run obliquely dorsomedially and pass between the motor and chief sensory nuclei of the trigeminal nerve (Fig. 25-9). As these fibers approach the ventrolateral aspect of the fourth ventricle, their course becomes rostral, continuing along the superior portion of the ventricle and into the mesencephalon along the cerebral aqueduct. Thus, the term *mesencephalic root* has been given to this group of proprioceptive fibers belonging to the trigeminal nerve (Figs. 2-45, 2-46). From the point where these fibers begin their rostral course until they finally play out in the midbrain, typical monopolar ganglion cells are associated with each neuron. These collectively are known as the *mesencephalic nucleus* (Figs. 25-9, 25-10). The central process from these cells is difficult to follow. Undoubtedly some of these processes make direct synapse with cells in the motor nucleus of the trigeminal nerve, thus forming a *two-neuron reflex arc*. It is probable that others of the central processes make synapses among cells in the reticular formation.

Peculiarly enough, there is no certainty about the course of proprioceptive impulses arising in the extrinsic muscles of the eye, the tongue, or pharynx. Therefore, these impulses will be considered in a very general way.

There is some evidence to indicate the presence of proprioceptive fibers associated with typical receptors in the muscles of the orbit. Some investigators feel that such fibers eventually join the ophthalmic division of the trigeminal nerve and make their way to its mesencephalic nucleus. However, since the mesencephalic nucleus traverses the same midbrain levels which contain the motor nuclei of both cranial nerves III and IV, it is possible that proprioceptive fibers accompany the motor roots of these nerves into the tegmentum, where they diverge dorsally to enter the mesencephalic nucleus.

The muscles of facial expression are also supplied with proprioceptive afferents. Because of numerous connections between nerves V and VII, some investigators have suggested that the mesencephalic nucleus contains the cell bodies of these neurons as well. The evidence supporting this contention is poor. Others have suggested that proprioceptive fibers pass through the nervus intermedius, have their cell bodies in the geniculate ganglion of nerve VII, and terminate in the nucleus solitarius. This same group have also suggested that fibers from the palate and nose travel by way of the greater superficial petrosal nerve, with cells in the geniculate ganglion and endings in the nucleus solitarius.

Because speech requires delicate controls, it must be assumed that proprioceptive fibers, coming from the pharynx and larynx, play a vital role in this process. Since the motor nerves of these areas are carried by way of the glossopharyngeal and vagus nerves, each of these nerves possessing ganglia for other sensory components, it is possible that the cell bodies of afferent proprioceptive neurons are also located there. One can only speculate upon the course and connections of such fibers beyond the borders of the medulla, but the nucleus solitarius is a possible terminus.

It is evident that the movements of the tongue are finely controlled. Furthermore, histologic evidence indicates the presence of numerous proprioceptive receptors in the tongue. These facts notwithstanding, there are no ganglia associated with nerve XII. Although the hypoglossal nerve communicates with both nerve V and nerve IX, there is no good evidence that proprioceptive fibers from the tongue enter either of these nerves. Thus, the peripheral course, as well as the central pathways, is open to debate.

Another school of thought suggests that proprioceptive nuclei may lie in or closely adjacent to the motor nuclei which supply the orbital, facial, lingual, pharyngeal, and laryngeal muscles. However, decisions on this matter must be reserved pending future investigation.

Association Neuron [5]

From cells in the reticular formation of the brain stem, axons spread to all the general somatic and special visceral motor nuclei.

Efferent Neuron

From the motor nucleus of the trigeminal nerve, axons pass through the portio minor to the muscles of mastication by way of the mandibular division.

From the facial nucleus, axons are distributed to the muscles of facial expression.

From the nucleus ambiguus, fibers are carried to the muscles of the pharynx and larynx by way of the glossopharyngeal and vagus nerves.

From the nuclei of the oculomotor, trochlear, and abducens nerves, axons bring the extrinsic muscles of the eye under reflex control.

Efferent fibers from the hypoglossal nucleus, via nerve XII, bring the muscles of the tongue under reflex control.

Conscious Pathway

Receptors

These are the same as described under Trunk, Simple Reflex Pathways.

Neuron I

This is identical with the afferent neuron described above under Head, Simple Reflex Path-

[5] It should be recalled that certain reflexes, such as some of those involving mastication, are of the two-neuron type, in which the central process of the afferent neuron from the mesencephalic nucleus of the trigeminal nerve substitutes for the association neuron of the typical three-neuron arc.

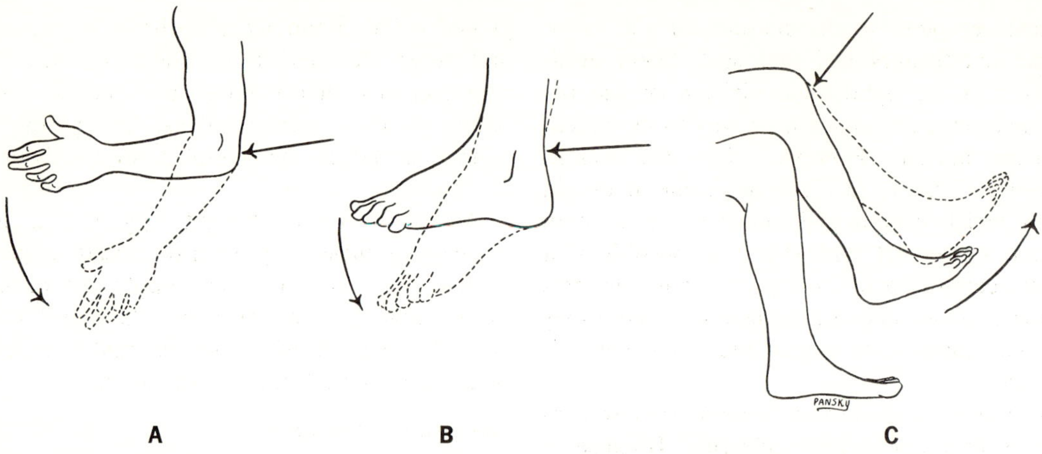

Fig. 12-4. Reflex tests. *A.* Extension of the forearm; *B.* Plantar flexion of the foot; C. Extension of the leg.

ways, except that in this case, it is believed that the short central process from the mesencephalic nucleus terminates in the main sensory nucleus of the trigeminal nerve.

Neuron II and Neuron III

As far as is known, these neurons may follow the course described for the tactile system of the head (Chap. 8).

CLINICAL CONSIDERATIONS

Testing

A sharp tap is applied to any of several extensor tendons (Fig. 12-4), for example: the triceps, just above the olecranon: the quadriceps tendon, just below the patella; the Achilles tendon, above the calcaneus. If the parts—forearm, leg, or foot as the case may be—are in a state of at least partial flexion at the time the stimulus is applied, the normal response is an extension of the part. By using a variety of testing sites it is possible to more nearly localize a lesion, thus: triceps—C6, C7, (C8?); quadriceps—L2, L3, and L4; ankle—S1 and S2.

With the eyes closed, the patient is asked to identify or to describe objects placed in his hands. This is a continuation of the same tests applied for tactile discrimination (Chap. 8).

With the patient in bed and his muscles as much relaxed as possible, the different parts of his limbs are moved by the examiner. First, the patient is asked to tell in what position the limbs have been placed and then to tell in what direction the movement has occurred.

The patient is asked to stand with his feet together and his eyes closed. Is it necessary for him to move his feet to keep his balance?

Ask the patient to walk and observe his gait. Can he walk with his eyes closed?

Additional information concerning coordination can be obtained by asking the patient, with his eyes closed, to touch one finger to the tip of his nose or to place the heel of one foot to the opposite knee, then push it down along the shin.

On examination, lesions involving this system, yield the following findings: *areflexia,* in which no reflexes are elicitable; *astereognosis,*[6] in which the patient, with eyes covered, fails to identify familiar objects placed in his hand; *ataxia,*[7] in which the patient has difficulty in standing without moving his feet, or in walking

[6] It should be recalled that stereognosis is actually a cortical function which depends upon the blending of two or more basic modalities. Thus, loss of proprioception would contribute to the inability to recognize objects.

[7] Since ataxia is also a finding in cases of lesions in other parts of the nervous system, further tests are necessary before a lesion can actually be localized.

without using his eyes; *incoordination,* or *asynergia,* in which the various muscles fail to work together or in normal sequence.

Generally destruction of nerve roots begins near the caudal end of the cord and progresses cranially. Usually the medial division of the dorsal roots of the spinal nerves is attacked and destroyed. Since this is the part carrying the afferent neurons of the proprioceptive reflex arcs, no tendon reflexes in the area of the lesion can be elicited. Likewise, the patient cannot tell in which position his limbs have been placed or in what direction they have been moved. In order to walk without falling, he must use his eyes to determine where his feet must be placed because he does not receive the normal impulses from his muscles and joints. He is unable to identify objects placed in his hands, if the disease has spread as far as the lower cervical levels.

Trauma

Any injury which leads to a destruction of the posterior funiculi will result in a loss of the sense of position and movement below the site of the lesion on the same side of the cord.

SUMMARY
General Proprioception

SIMPLE REFLEX

Trunk		Head
1. Neuromuscular endings (annulospiral and flower spray) Neurotendinous spindle Tendon-joint corpuscular endings	Receptor	1. Same as for trunk, plus endings in sockets of teeth
2. Through dorsal roots of all spinal nerves, with cell bodies in dorsal root ganglia, into dorsal funiculus (fasciculus gracilis and cuneatus) of the cord to terminate in the dorsal gray columns	Afferent neuron	2. Through the trigeminal nerve and into the brain stem with cell bodies in the mesencephalic nucleus of V, the central processes ending either in reticular formation or directly in the motor nucleus of V
3. From cells in the dorsal gray columns to ventral gray column on same side at same level; through the fasciculus proprius to the ventral gray column at other levels on the same side; through the anterior white commissure and fasciculus proprius to the ventral gray column at the same and other levels on the opposite side of the cord	Association neuron	3. From the reticular formation to other cranial nuclei, especially nuclei VII and XII
4. From the ventral gray columns to skeletal muscle of the neck, trunk, and extremities	Efferent neuron	4. From nucleus V through trigeminal nerve to muscles of mastication From nucleus VII through facial nerve to muscle of face From nucleus XII through the hypoglossal nerve to muscles of the tongue

CONSCIOUS

Trunk		Head
5-8. See conscious pathway for Tactile Discrimination (Chap. 8)	Receptor Neuron I Neuron II Neuron III	5-8. See conscious pathway for Tactile Discrimination (Chap. 8)

CEREBELLAR CIRCUIT

Trunk		Head
1. Same as simple reflex, trunk	Receptor	1. Same as simple reflex, head
2. Same as afferent neuron, simple reflex, trunk terminating in the column of Clarke	Afferent neuron	2. Same as afferent neuron, simple reflex, head, except, in this case, fibers end either in the reticular formation or the chief sensory nucleus of the trigeminal
3. From dorsal gray column to ventral spinocerebellar tract on same side, thence rostrally through the cord and brain stem, through the anterior medullary velum to terminate in the rostral vermis From dorsal gray column, across the cord in the anterior white commissure to ventral spinocerebellar tract of the opposite side, then as above From Clarke's column, into the dorsal spinocerebellar tract of same side, rostrally through the cord, entering the restiform body and terminating in both rostral and caudal portions of the cerebellar cortex	Afferent cerebellar neuron	3. From the reticular formation through reticulocerebellar fibers which enter the cerebellum through the restiform body to end in posterior semilunar lobule From chief sensory nucleus through trigeminocerebellar fibers which enter the cerebellum with the ventral spinocerebellar tract through the anterior medullary velum to terminate as above
4. From Purkinje cells of cerebellar cortex through the cerebellar medullary core to the central cerebellar nuclei	Corticonuclear neuron	4. From Purkinje cells of the cortex through the white core to reach the central cerebellar nuclei
5. From central nuclei, through the brachium conjunctivum to end in the red nucleus	Efferent cerebellar neuron	5. From central nuclei, through the brachium conjunctivum, to end in the red nucleus
6. From the red nucleus, some fibers decussate in the ventral tegmental decussation and descend through the rubrospinal tract to terminate in the ventral gray column of the cord From the red nucleus, fibers terminate in the reticular nuclei and from the latter, fibers pass through the reticulospinal tract to terminate in the ventral gray columns of the cord	Descending neuron	6. From the red nucleus, terminating in the reticular formation and passing through this to reach the motor nucleus of V
7. Same as in simple reflex, trunk	Efferent neuron	7. From nucleus V through the trigeminal nerve to muscles of mastication

13 SPECIAL PROPRIOCEPTION (SP)

The special proprioceptive system involves the maintenance of the position of the eyes and body in relation to changes in the orientation of the head. This requires the presence of special receptors located in the *membranous labyrinth* of the vestibular portion of the inner ear.

The membranous labyrinth consists of several parts (Figs. 9-16, 13-1*A*): the saccule, the utricle, and three semicircular canals, are filled with a fluid called *endolymph*. The semicircular canals are set at right angles to each other and represent all planes of space. They are named according to orientation and their relations, namely: horizontal, anterior, and posterior. The adjoining segments of the anterior and posterior canals fuse to form a single channel to the utricle called the *common crus*. The ends of all others empty separately into the utricle. Each of the canals has an enlargement, called the *ampulla,* near the opening.

SIMPLE REFLEX PATHWAYS (Fig. 13-2.)

Receptors (Fig. 13-1.)

The receptors lie in both the ampullae of the canals and in the utricle and saccule. In the latter two locations they are composed of hair cells surrounded by supporting elements. Cilia project from the free surface of the sensory cells, while the terminal filaments of the vestibular division of the eighth cranial nerve entwine about their bases. The area of ciliated cells is covered with a cap of jellylike substance in which are embedded small crystals of calcium carbonate, the otoliths (otoconia). For this reason the entire cap may be spoken of as the otolithic membrane.

The patch of hair cells in both the utricle and saccule is called the *macula*. In the saccule, the macula is oriented in the sagittal plane, the cilia are directed laterally. In the utricle, the macula lies in the horizontal plane (Fig. 13-1) with the cilia directed upward. In both locations, the maculae are prolonged slightly onto the curved surfaces of their respective receptacles, both prolongations being predominantly directed in the frontal plane. Thus, macular surfaces are provided for each of the three planes of space.

Both maculae are thought to be related to posture.[1] In the normal, erect position, the receptors in the utricle are least stimulated. When the head changes position, the maculae are tilted and the otoliths, falling with gravity, exert their influence on the gelatinous cap. This results in a bending or pulling of the cilia, an action sufficient to stimulate the nerve. For example, the right macula of the saccule is maximally stimulated when the individual lies on his right side, while that in the left saccule is least affected.

[1] It has been suggested that the macula sacculi is also sensitive to vibrations (vibroreceptor) and that the macula utriculi responds, at least to some extent, to linear acceleration.

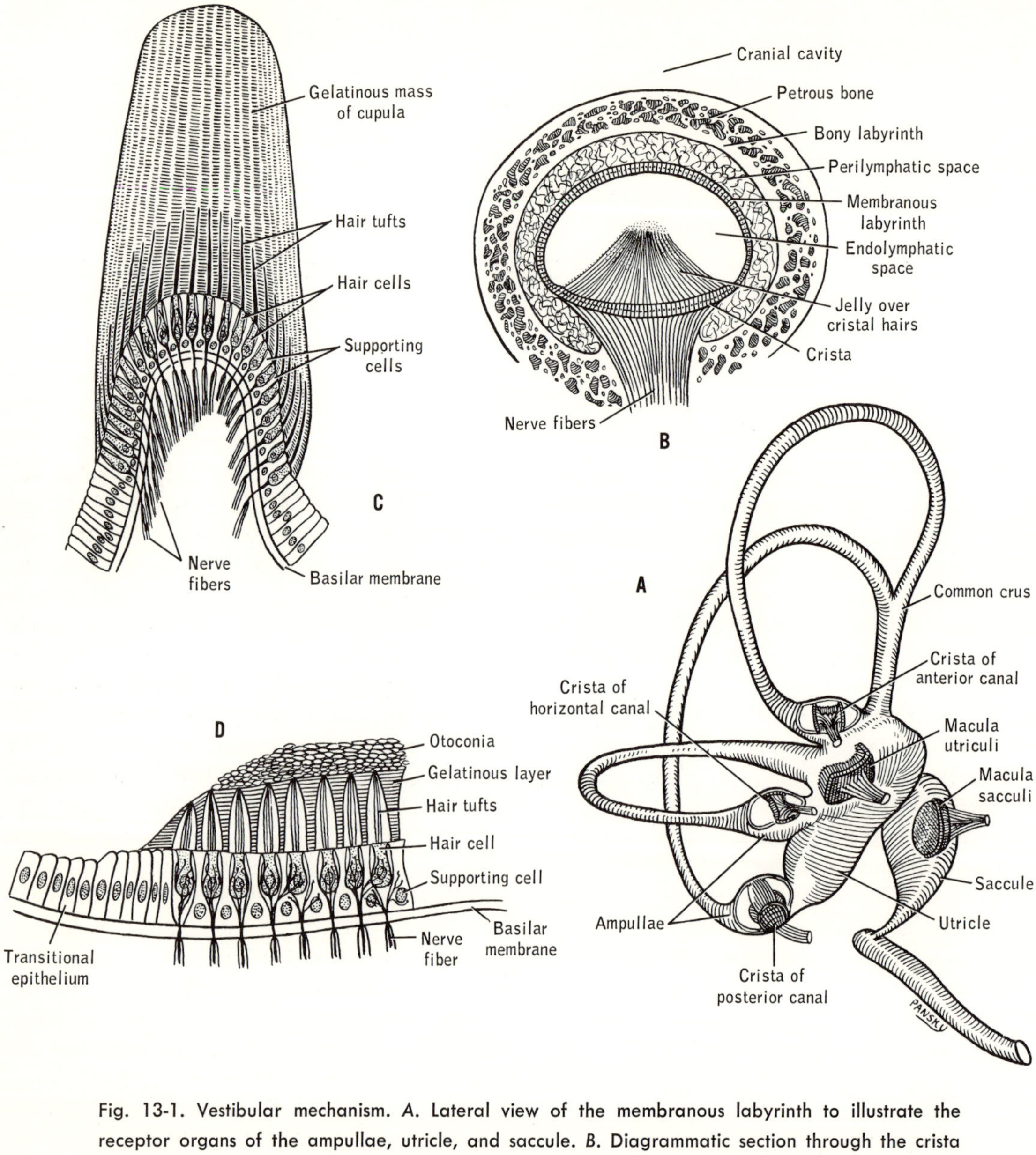

Fig. 13-1. Vestibular mechanism. *A.* Lateral view of the membranous labyrinth to illustrate the receptor organs of the ampullae, utricle, and saccule. *B.* Diagrammatic section through the crista of a semicircular canal. (*Adapted from Krieg, Functional Neuroanatomy, 2d ed., McGraw-Hill Book Company, Inc., Blakiston Division, New York, 1953.*) C. Schematic representation (enlarged) of a crista ampullaris as seen in longitudinal section. *D.* Schematic enlargement of a macula.

The groups of hair cells in the ampullae of the semicircular canals are called cristae (Fig. 13-1). Here, too, there appears to be a gelatinous cap into which the cilia protrude. The latter are displaced by movements of the endolymph contained in the canals, the greatest amount of stimulation arising during rotation, acceleration, and deceleration, all three planes of space being represented. For example, if the head moves clockwise (to the right) pressure is exerted maximally at the anterior end of the right horizontal canal due to the inertia of the endolymph. Thus, the crista in this location will be activated. However, when rotation to the right stops, the pressure of the moving fluid would be maximal against the crista in the anterior end of the left horizontal canal. Thus, it is evident that these receptors are best adapted to record movement.

Afferent Neuron (Figs. 13-2, 13-3, 13-4.)

The myelinated peripheral processes from the cristae and maculae combine to form the *vestibular portion of the eighth nerve.* They enter the internal auditory meatus, at the base of which is located the *vestibular ganglion.* The cells of this ganglion are of the *bipolar type.* The central processes continue into the cranium to enter the brain at the cerebellopontine angle (Figs. 2-7, 2-8, 25-7). Within the medula they run dorsomedially until they have traversed about two-thirds of the distance to the lateral angle of the fourth ventricle. Here each bifurcates into ascending and descending branches.

These branches terminate in four vestibular nuclei (Figs. 13-3, 13-5, 25-4 to 25-7): *the superior, medial, lateral, and spinal (descending).* The superior (nucleus of Bechterew) is triangular in shape, extending rostrally from near the level of nerve entry, along the floor and lateral aspects of the superior recess of the fourth ventricle. The lateral (nucleus of Deiters) is a relatively small, irregular area, containing particularly large cells, lying just ventral to the region where the primary afferent neurons bifurcate. The medial (dorsal or principal nucleus) is the largest of the four and is also triangular in shape, its broadest portion lying at the level of entry of the eighth nerve, tapering to an apex far down the medulla. The spinal, or descending, nucleus is a long column of cells extending caudally to the level of the nucleus gracilis, the cells being distributed among the fibers of the spinal, or descending, vestibular tract. All these nuclei occupy a field in the rhomboid fossa of the fourth ventricle called the *area acoustica* (Figs. 2-38, 13-5).

The ascending branches of the primary fibers pass mainly to the rostral end of the medial nucleus and to the entire superior nucleus. The descending branches unite, forming the *descending,* or *spinal, vestibular tract.* The latter terminates in the lateral, descending, and possibly the caudal part of the medial nuclei.

Association Neuron

These have their cell bodies in any of the vestibular nuclei.

Fibers from the superior nucleus enter the *medial longitudinal fasciculus* (MLF) (Figs. 13-2, 13-3, 25-1 to 25-11) of the same side and turn rostrally to terminate among the cells of cranial nerves III, IV, and VI.

From the lateral nucleus, the vast majority of fibers descend on the same side through the brain stem and down the length of the cord in the anterior funiculus as the *vestibulospinal tract* (Fig. 13-2), which terminates among the cells of the ventral columns of the cord.

From the descending nucleus, fibers pass medially, cross the midline, and descend in the medial longitudinal fasciculus, to terminate in the nucleus of the accessory nerve and the ventral columns of the cervical cord.

From the medial nucleus, axons cross the midline, enter the opposite medial longitudinal fasciculus, and bifurcate into fibers which ascend or descend within that fascicle to terminate as indicated for other fibers traveling in it. Some fibers from this nucleus enter the reticular formation of both sides to be distributed to the motor nuclei belonging to the autonomic system in the brain stem and the intermediolateral

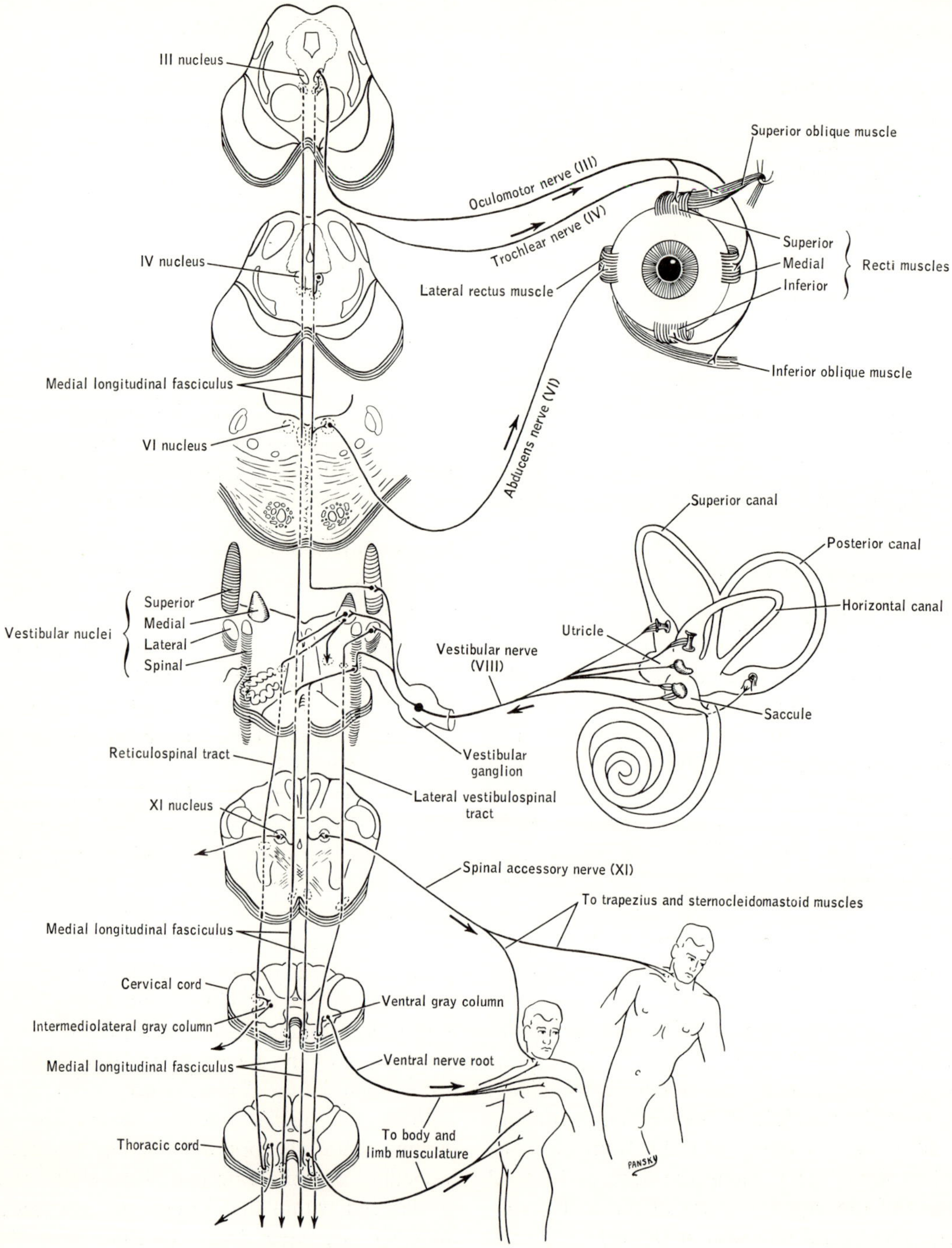

Fig. 13-2. Simple vestibular reflex pathways.

column of the cord, by way of the reticulospinal tract.

Efferent Neuron

Axons from the ventral columns of the cord, extending from the lower cervical to the lower sacral levels, are distributed to the skeletal muscles of the trunk and extremities, thus completing a typical somatic reflex. This is very important in relating movements of the body with those of the head and is definitely significant in maintaining balance.

Fibers from the ventral columns of the cord in the cervical region and from the nucleus of the spinal portion of the accessory nerve are distributed to the muscles of the neck, the sternocleidomastoid and trapezius. These muscles are particularly important in maintaining the normal position of the head. (Fig. 13-2.)

Axons from the somatic efferent columns of the brain stem, particularly the nuclei of the oculomotor, trochlear, and abducens nerves, supply the extrinsic muscles of the eyes, thus coordinating movements of the eyes with those of the head. There is some indication that a definite pattern of afferent limb, association neuron, and efferent limb exists, i.e., from specific semicircular canals to specific eye muscles. The following scheme has been given (Fig. 13-6): from the anterior canal to the homolateral superior rectus and contralateral inferior oblique muscles; from the posterior canal to the homolateral medial rectus and the contralateral lateral rectus muscles.

Fibers arising from the autonomic centers, especially the dorsal motor nucleus of the vagus and the intermediolateral cell column of the cord, account for the nausea, vomiting, and pallor manifested after overstimulation of the vestibular system.

COORDINATION (CEREBELLAR) PATHWAY (Fig. 13-7.)

Although the details of cerebellar connections will be given later, it should be emphasized at this point that the cerebellum does exert control over activities initiated by the stimulation of vestibular receptors.

Direct Route

Receptors

These are the same as described under Simple Reflex Pathways, above.

Afferent Neuron

These are also the same as those indicated under Simple Reflex Pathways. However, cerebellar impulses travel through the ascending branches, only, and terminate in the nodulus and flocculus of the cerebellum (Chap. 18).

Descending Association Neuron

From cells in the cortex of the nodulus and flocculus, fibers descend to terminate in the fastigial nucleus. From this nucleus some axons descend by way of the medial segment of the inferior cerebellar peduncle body to end in the vestibular nuclei. Other axons from the fastigial nucleus cross the midline and descend to the vestibular nuclei of the opposite side by way of the *uncinate bundle* (of Russell). Thus, the cerebellum is able to exert influence directly upon the vestibular nuclei. Additional association fibers from these nuclei are then carried by the pathways already described (vestibulospinal tract, medial longitudinal fasciculus, and reticular formation) to the same terminations. It is quite possible that large numbers of these additional neurons are unnecessary, since vestibular reflexes have, to some extent, already been modified or regulated by fibers descending from the cerebellum to the vestibular nuclei.

Efferent Neuron

These are the same as described under Simple Reflex Pathways, above.

Indirect Route

Receptors

These are the same as for the direct route, described above.

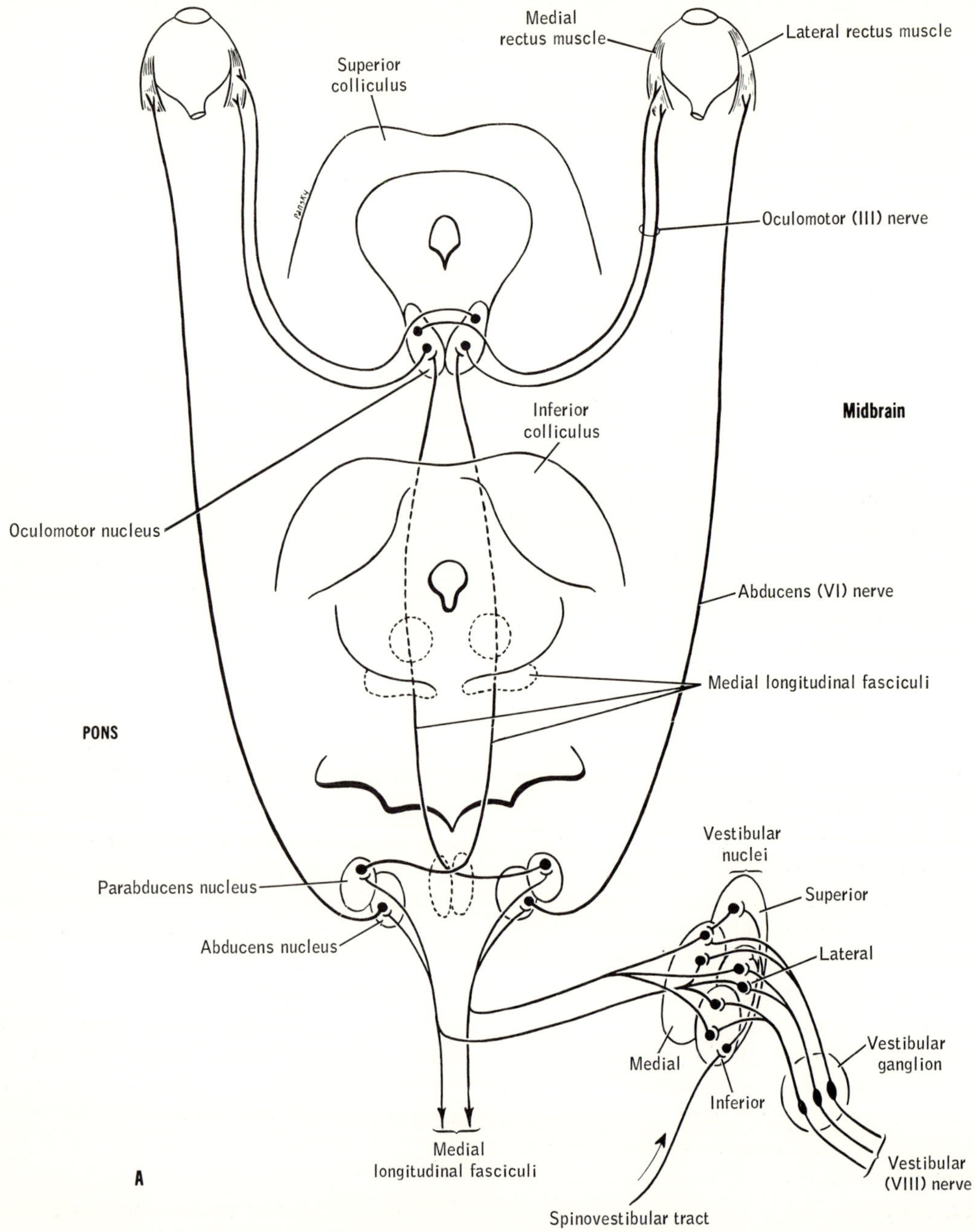

Fig. 13-3. *A*. Relations of the vestibular connections to eye movements in the horizontal plane. *B*. Relations of vestibular connections to eye movements in the vertical plane.

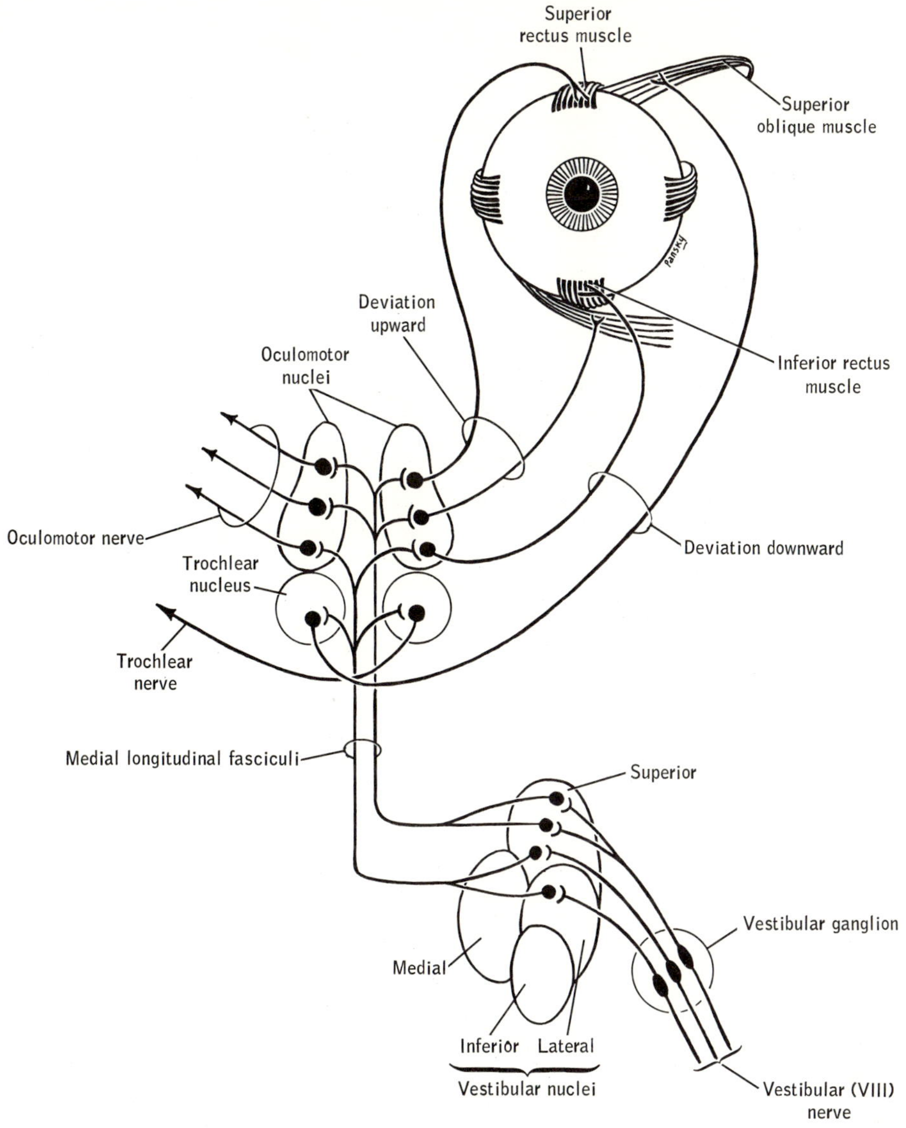

B

Afferent Neuron

These are the same as those indicated for the direct route except that they terminate in the superior and lateral vestibular nuclei.

Association Neuron—Ascending

From cells mainly in the superior nucleus but also from the lateral nucleus, fibers ascend in the medial segment of the inferior cerebellar peduncle (the juxtarestiform body). They terminate both in the flocculonodular lobe and in the lingula and uvula of the cerebellum (Chap. 18).

Association Neuron—Descending (Fig. 13-7.)

From cells in the cerebellar cortex of the regions mentioned above, fibers descend both to

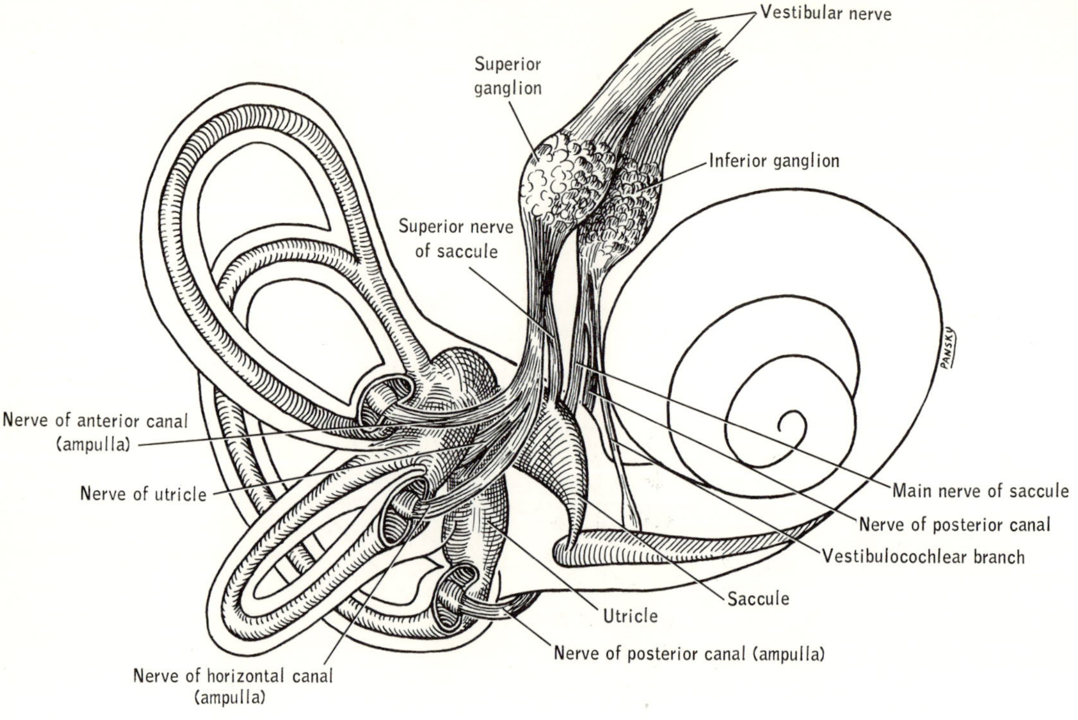

Fig. 13-4. Divisions of the vestibular portion of nerve VIII and the vestibular ganglion.

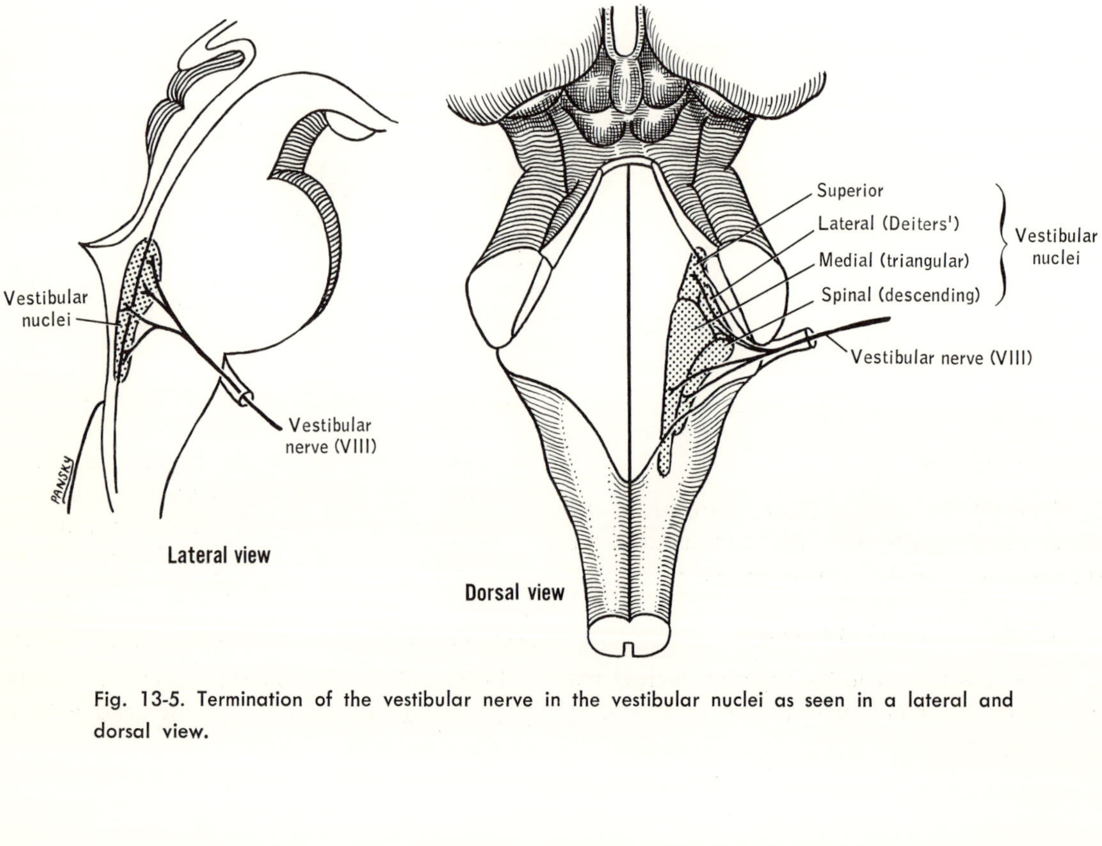

Fig. 13-5. Termination of the vestibular nerve in the vestibular nuclei as seen in a lateral and dorsal view.

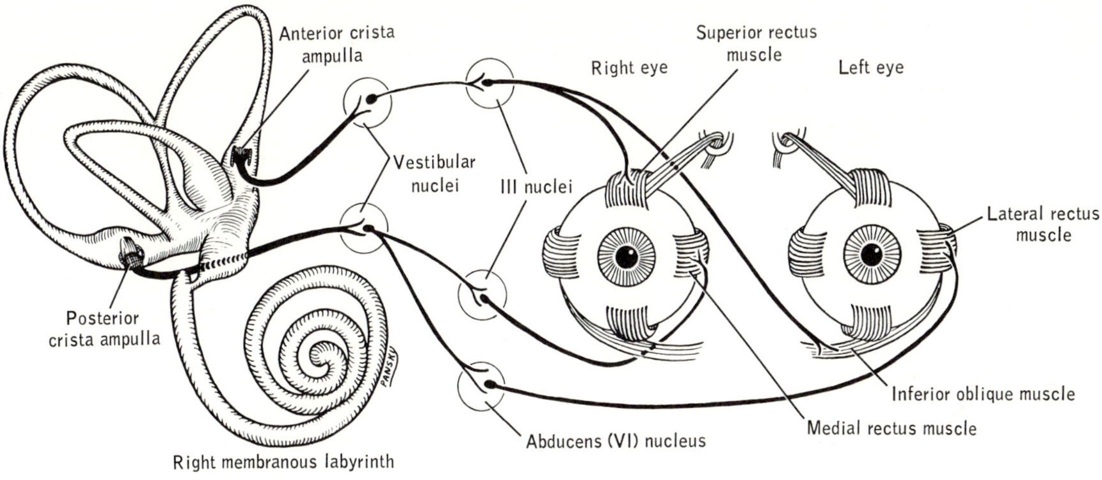

Fig. 13-6. Relation of the semicircular canals to specific muscles and movements of the eye.

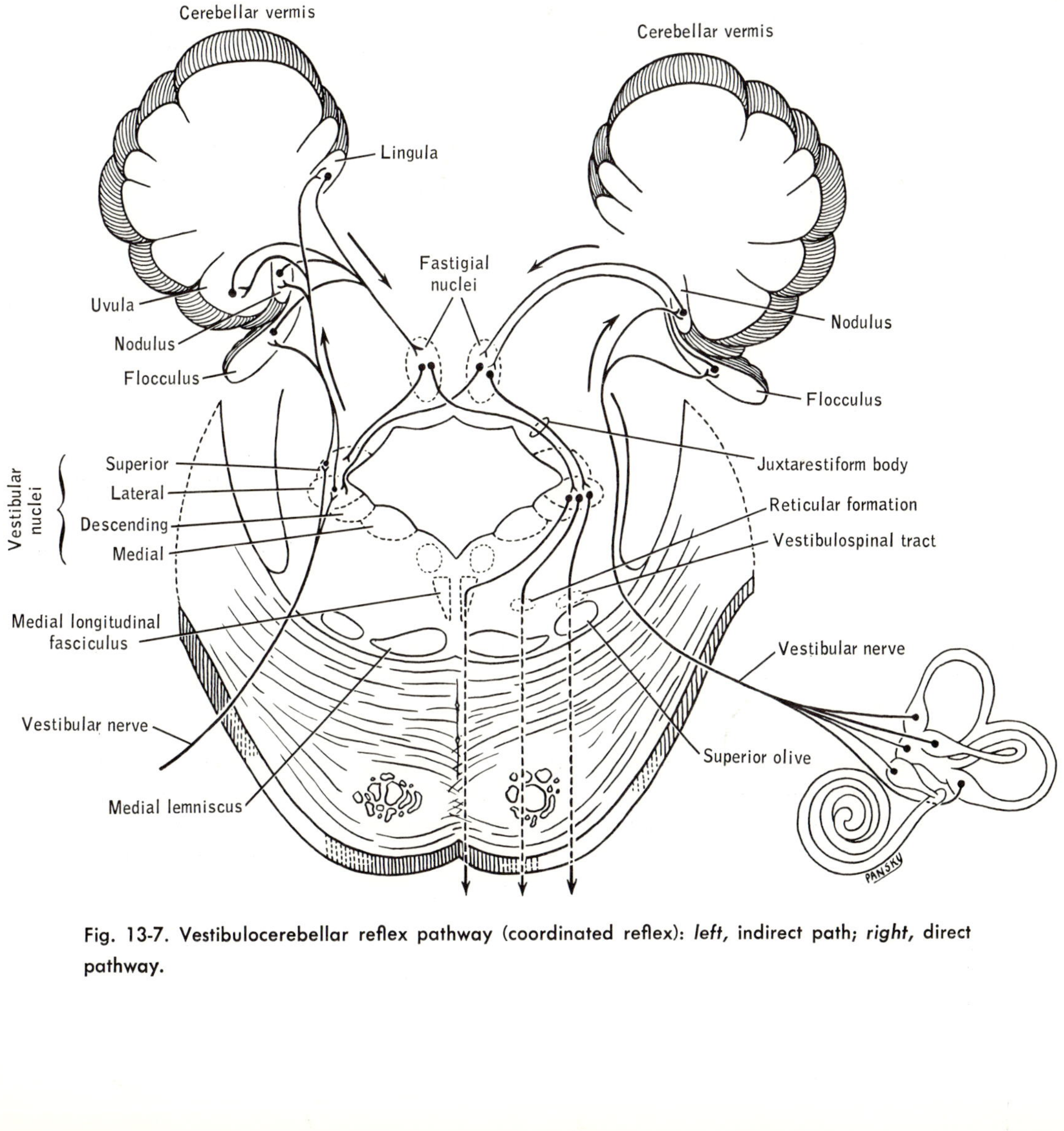

Fig. 13-7. Vestibulocerebellar reflex pathway (coordinated reflex): *left,* indirect path; *right,* direct pathway.

the fastigial and to the globose nuclei. Arising from both fastigial and globose nuclei, axons descend by the same pathways and have the same terminations as those described for the descending association fibers of the direct route.

Efferent Neuron

These are also the same as given under Simple Reflex Pathways and explained under the direct cerebellar pathway.

CONSCIOUS PATHWAY

Little is known about such connections. The receptors certainly would be the same as described for reflexes. The major portion of the primary neuron would also be the same as the afferent neurons of the reflex arcs. However, one group of investigators has suggested that some of these afferent neurons end in the ventral cochlear nucleus and from there follow the auditory pathways to consciousness (Chap. 9).

CLINICAL CONSIDERATIONS

Disease in the vestibular mechanism expresses itself in disturbances of equilibrium, balance, and coordination. Therefore, the simple observation of the patient standing or walking becomes an integral part of the examination. Furthermore, since this system is so intimately tied up with reflex movements of the eyes, such reflexes are important in trying to localize a lesion.

Testing

Tests which apply chiefly to the cerebellar circuits are discussed in Chap. 18.

Before taking up any of the special testing

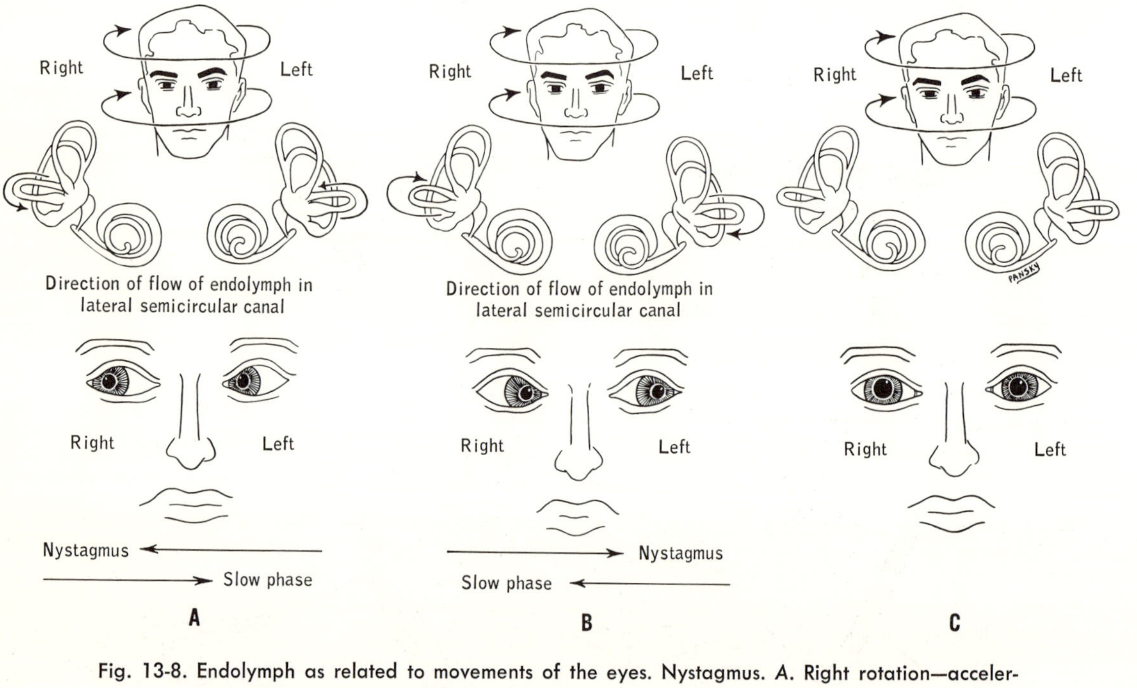

Fig. 13-8. Endolymph as related to movements of the eyes. Nystagmus. *A*. Right rotation—acceleration. The endolymph moves from right to left; thus nystagmus is to the right, and the slow phase is to the left. *B*. Right rotation—deceleration. The endolymph moves from left to right; thus nystagmus is to the left, and the slow phase is to the right. C. Right rotation—constant velocity. There is no movement of the endolymph and thus no eye movement.

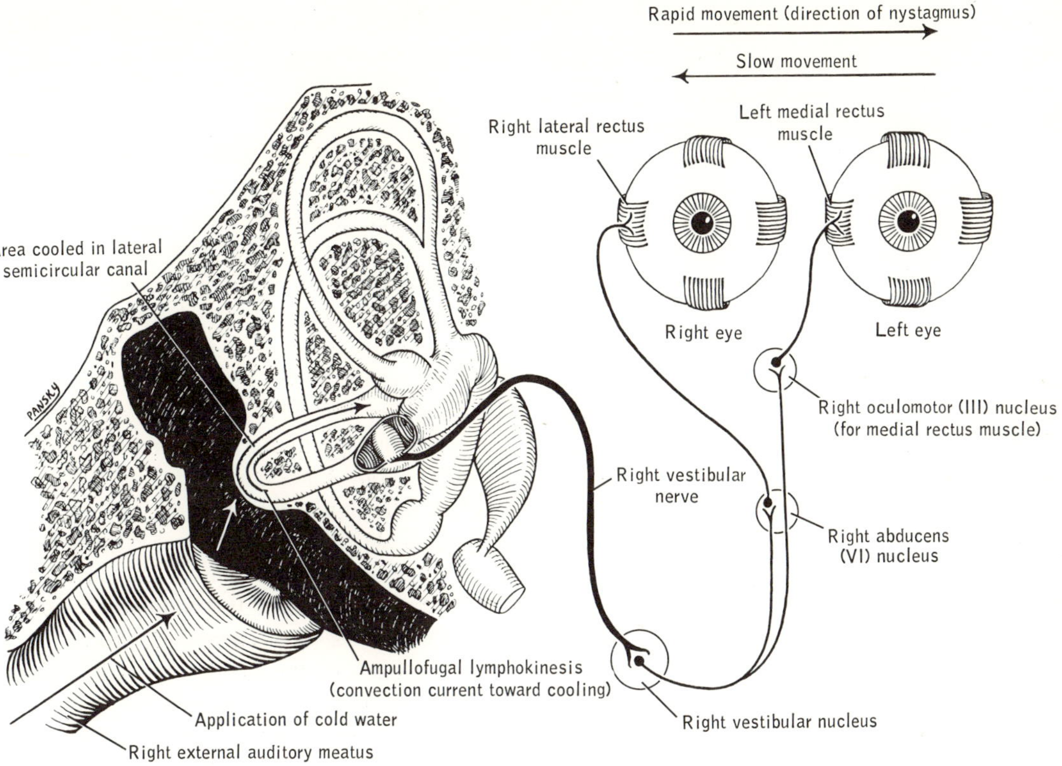

Fig. 13-9. Caloric test. Cold water introduced into right external meatus showing effects opposite to that produced by introduction of hot water.

procedures, it is necessary to discuss the relationships between the vestibular system and the maintenance of position of the eyes during positional changes of the head. In general, when the head moves slowly in any plane, the eyes do not follow but tend to retain their fixation on the original field. This, in effect, is the same as though they deviated in an opposite direction to that in which the head is turned. (This is true whether the motion is from side to side or up and down.) When the eyes, after a slow movement, reach the limit of deviation in one direction, they move quickly back toward the other extreme. This is called *nystagmus*. The slow movement is a manifestation of activation of the ocular muscle centers through irritation of the vestibular system, whereas the quick movement is regarded as a cerebral reflex, returning the eyeballs to their former position. The *direction of the nystagmus is named in accordance with the direction of the quick, reflex movement*.

Currents in the semicircular canals cause motion of the eyes away from the direction of the movement of the head. Thus, when the head stops moving, the resultant reversal in direction of the flow of the current, due to the inertia of motion, will reverse the direction of the eye movements. This accounts for the dizziness, or vertigo, which is the subjective sensation that the world is revolving. It should be noted, however, that this vertigo occurs only after excessive rotation, which definitely cannot be considered a normal stimulation, since the vestibular system is not adapted to compensate for such excesses.

Rotation (*Bárány*) (Fig. 13-8.)

The patient is placed in a rotary chair with a headrest which enables the head to be fixed in the desired position to bring one particular pair of semicircular canals into play. In order to produce pure horizontal nystagmus, the head is tilted forward about 30°. The chair is then rotated about ten times quickly in succession. This rotation produces *lymphokinesis,* or motion of the endolymph, in the horizontal canals. At first, the endolymph is displaced in a direction opposite to that in which the canal is moving. This has the effect of causing the eyes to move slowly in a direction opposite to the direction of rotation. When the eyes have reached the limit of movement in this direction, they are quickly snapped back by the cortical fixation reaction. Thus the quick motion, or nystagmus, is in the direction of the rotation. Because the patient is being turned so rapidly, this escapes notice. Gradually, with each successive revolution, the endolymph gathers momentum and begins to move in the direction of the rotation. However, when the chair is suddenly stopped, the momentum of the endolymph causes it to continue to move in the direction of the original movement. Thus, what is seen by the examiner is a horizontal nystagmus in the *direction opposite to the rotation.*

Besides observing nystagmus, one should ask the patient to stand erect, with the eyes closed and the feet together (Romberg position), to note any postural deviations which take the form of falling to one side or the other. Normally, the deviations observed consist of a tendency to fall in a direction opposite to that of the nystagmus. In other words, in *a direction towards the rotation.*

Directional movements of the limbs may also be carried out after the chair has been stopped. The patient is asked to point to the observer's finger, which is held up in front of the patient at such a distance that he just reaches it with his forefinger with the elbow locked in full extension. He is then asked to shut his eyes, let his arm fall at his side, and then raise the arm to point at the observer's finger. Deviation *opposite to that of the nystagmus,* in the direction of the rotation, is seen.

Caloric (Fig. 13-9.)

In this test, the external auditory meatus is douched with hot (50 to 55°C) or cold (18 to 25°C) water, whereby convection currents are set up in the endolymph. For this purpose, an ordinary ear syringe of 100-cc capacity is sufficient. Three or four syringes in quick succession will generally suffice to elicit a reaction. The great advantage of this test is that it is unilateral, that is, either vestibule can be tested separately, and even one particular semicircular canal can be singled out for examination by placing the head in different positions.

When cold water is introduced into the external meatus, it cools the prominence of the lateral canal, condenses the endolymphatic fluid, and thereby sets up a current downward or toward the back of the head when the patient is lying in the dorsal position (on the back). This flow is thus away from the ampulla of the horizontal canal (ampullofugal), and the eyes are then turned slowly toward the side of the irrigated ear, the movement being alternately interrupted by a quick return movement toward the *contralateral side.* For example, if the cold water is introduced into the right ear, left nystagmus results. With hot water, the prominence is warmed. Thus, the expanding endolymph produces a current toward the ampulla (ampullopetal), which gives rise to a slow turning of the eyes toward the opposite side with a subsequent quick reflex return to the *homolateral side* (Fig. 13-9). For example, with the patient lying on his back, hot water introduced into the right ear causes right nystagmus.[2] It should be noted that the optimal position for eliciting this reaction is the vertical for whatever canal is to be tested. Thus, in order to place the horizontal canal in this plane, the head is inclined backwards about 60°, which position the head usually assumes

[2] This is according to Ewald's law, which states that the direction of the ocular movements corresponds to the direction of the convection current set up in the semicircular canals.

when the patient lies on the bed with a small pillow under the back of the head.

If the caloric test is performed in the upright position, the horizontal canal is far removed from the optimal position. For this reason one sees only a faint horizontal nystagmus mixed with a stronger rotatory nystagmus as a result of stimulation of the other two canals, which are now nearly vertical. By changing the position of the head, one can elicit a number of different responses: (1) by introducing cold water into the right ear when the patient is recumbent, one will observe a horizontal nystagmus to the left with past pointing to the right and a slight tendency to fall to the right; (2) by repeating the test with the patient in the sitting position, one will observe a slight nystagmus to the left with much rotatory motion of the eyes (rotatory nystagmus), a past pointing to the right, and a strong tendency to fall toward the right, due mainly to lymphokinesis in the anterior canal.

Before either of the above-described tests can be applied and before their results can be interpreted, it is necessary to determine whether there is evidence of spontaneous nystagmus, past pointing, or postural deviations. For example, in irritative lesions in the inner ear, along the vestibular nerve, or in certain parts of the cerebellum, all these phenomena may occur, usually with the nystagmus away from the diseased side and the past pointing and tendency to fall toward it. On the other hand, total destruction of the labyrinth on one side may cause the head to decline toward the destroyed vestibule. Furthermore, associated with the spontaneous signs, there may be vertigo, nausea, pallor, and perspiration.

If any of the signs (nystagmus, etc.) appears, it should be ascertained whether any condition exists which could increase the pressure in the middle ear, since vertigo can be caused by such pressure. It is also necessary to be sure that the external auditory meatus is free from obstruction. This is particularly important if the caloric tests are to be used.[3]

[3] Air should be substituted for water if there is evidence of perforated tympanic membranes.

It should be obvious that in the rotation tests, both horizontal canals are irritated. However, the canal opposite the side toward which rotation is taking place is being subjected to a more intensive irritation than the other, since it moves through a greater arc. But if one canal is diseased and rotation is set up in the direction toward the diseased side, this side will give a more marked reaction than will the normal side. For example, a spontaneous tendency to fall to the right will be changed to a tendency to fall backward if rotation is toward the right. Of course, in cases where there is a bilateral destruction of the vestibule or its nerve, none of the typical signs appears after rotation.

If the caloric test fails to elicit nystagmus, past pointing, or postural deviations, it can be assumed that a destructive lesion exists on the side being tested.

As a last consideration, an attempt should be made to determine whether the lesion is located peripherally, either in the membranous labyrinth or in the extramedullary course of the vestibular nerve; centrally, within the brain stem; or in the cerebellum.

Concerning the cerebellum, only one point will be made here. The spontaneous nystagmus of cerebellar origin is not altered by changes in position of the head. That of vestibular origin *is* altered by changes in head position.

There are certain definite indications of peripheral lesions. First, because of the close anatomic relations of the auditory and vestibular receptors, together with their afferent neurons, lesions frequently involve hearing, either in the form of such sounds as buzzing, roaring, or clicking (tinnitus) or by varying degrees of deafness. If the caloric test fails to elicit any response, the lesion is definitely peripheral in location. Lastly, as pointed out previously, peripheral irritative lesions usually produce nystagmus away from the diseased side, together with past pointing and postural deviations toward it. This may be accompanied by episodes of variable length of vertigo, nausea, etc.

In case of central lesions, the caloric test elicits past pointing and postural deviations but *no nystagmus.* Further, there is a tendency for the subjective signs, such as vertigo, to be more continuous. However, certain central lesions cause no vertigo and the nystagmus may be coarser and slower, with a tendency to fall toward the normal side. Central disease may also involve other sensory mechanisms or motor apparatus which could not easily be affected by a peripheral lesion.

Specific Pathology

Vertigo is the most characteristic symptom of vestibular disease. Vestibular manifestations may be caused by disease of the labyrinths themselves, the vestibular nerve, the vestibular nuclei, or the supranuclear connections. Vertigo may also, however, be a symptom of general, rather than focal, disease. The labyrinths may be affected by inflammation (Voltolini's disease), hemorrhage, edema, pressure changes, etc. The so-called *Ménière's syndrome* is characterized by paroxysmal attacks of vertigo, usually associated with unilateral tinnitus and deafness. It is believed to be due to edema of the labyrinth. Some investigators consider it an inflammatory process or a type of neuralgia affecting the eighth nerve. Other lesions, such as basal or pontine tumors or hemorrhages, can involve either the extra- or intramedullary course of the afferent fibers of the vestibular nerve.

SUMMARY
Special Proprioception

SIMPLE REFLEX

1. Hair cells in macula of saccule; macula of utricle; cristae of the ampullary region of semicircular canals of inner ear	Receptor
2. Through fibers of vestibular portion of nerve VIII with cells in the vestibular ganglion, into the brain stem to terminate in medial, spinal (descending), superior, or lateral vestibular nuclei	Afferent neuron
3. From medial, spinal, and superior nuclei, fibers ascending and descending on both sides of the brain stem in the MLF, from which terminals are given to cranial nuclei III, IV, and VI and to the ventral gray columns of the spinal cord, in the cervical region From the lateral vestibular nucleus, fibers descending via the vestibulospinal tract to the ventral gray columns throughout the cord	Association neuron
4. From cranial nuclei III, IV, and VI, fibers passing through their respective nerves to the extrinsic muscles of the eye From the ventral columns of the cord to skeletal muscles of the neck, trunk, and extremities	Efferent neuron

CEREBELLAR CIRCUIT

Direct		*Indirect*
1. Same as in simple reflex	Receptor	1. Same as in simple reflex
2. Same as in simple reflex except that these fibers pass directly to the flocculus and nodulus of the cerebellum (instead of vestibular nuclei)	Afferent neuron	2. Same as in simple reflex except that the termination is in the superior and lateral vestibular nuclei only
3. In this case, the same as above	Afferent cerebellar neuron	3. From the superior and lateral vestibular nuclei, fibers ascending in the juxtarestiform body to end in the flocculus, nodulus, lingula, and uvula
4. From Purkinje cells of the flocculus and nodulus to the fastigial nucleus	Corticonuclear neuron	4. From the cortex (above) to both the fastigial and globose nuclei
5. From the fastigial nucleus, through the juxtarestiform body, descending as the fastigiobulbar tract to end in the vestibular nuclei on the same side From the fastigial nucleus, across the midline, to descend in the uncinate fasciculus, terminating in the vestibular nuclei of the opposite side	Efferent cerebellar neuron	5. Same as efferent cerebellar neuron in the direct cerebellar circuit
6. Same as for simple reflex	Descending neuron	6. Same as descending neuron in the direct cerebellar circuit
7. Same as for simple reflex	Efferent neuron	7. Same as in simple reflex

14 GENERAL SOMATIC EFFERENT SYSTEM (GSE)

Early in development, an intimate relationship between the primitive nervous system and the mesodermal tissue from which muscles are derived is established (Chap. 5). This relationship is maintained throughout development regardless of how far the muscle tissue may migrate (Fig. 5-17). This is well exemplified by the muscles of the abdominal wall, the forearm and hand, or the leg and foot, all of which, in adult man, are innervated by fibers whose origin (from the cord) is far removed from the muscle innervated. Although it has proved impossible in higher animals to follow the actual course of development, it is fairly clear that the muscles of the eye, supplied by nerves III, IV, and VI, as well as those of the tongue, supplied by nerve XII, likewise trace their origins to somites and that, therefore, these nerves can likewise be classified as GSE.

The neurons of this system are all of the multipolar type (Chap. 6). The cell bodies are large, possessing many dendrites which ramify within the gray substance in which the cells are located. The wide distribution of dendrites makes contact possible with a variety of other neurons. The single axon is large and leaves the CNS to terminate in *motor end-plates* on skeletal muscle fibers, to form what is referred to as a *myoneural junction* (Fig. 14-1).

As a motor nerve bundle approaches a muscle, it begins to separate into its individual fibers. These, in turn, branch repeatedly, so that a single nerve fiber may supply many muscle fibers. As each branch nears the muscle fiber which it is to innervate, the endoneurium becomes very fine and delicate, spreading out over the sarcolemma, perhaps becoming continuous with the endomysium. The myelin sheath disappears completely, while the neurilemma ends at, or becomes confluent with, the sarcolemma. At the point of contact, which lies near the middle of the muscle fiber, the sarcoplasm of the muscle forms a mass of variable size and shape. The naked axis cylinder enters this mass, called the *motor end-plate,* and breaks up into a number of terminal twigs which ramify in the plate and end in small, club-shaped enlargements (Figs. 6-16, 14-1).

The muscle fibers, which are ultimately supplied by a single nerve fiber through its branchings (plus the nerve itself), are called a *motor unit*. There is a considerable difference in the size of these units, depending upon the size of the entire muscle and upon the precision of action of that muscle. Thus, in some of the largest, most powerful muscles, one nerve fiber may supply 200 muscle fibers, while in some of the more delicate muscles, the extrinsic ocular group for example, ratios of 1:1 or 1:2 have been reported.

The complete dependence of skeletal muscle upon the integrity of its motor nerve is one of the most striking relationships encountered in the entire human body. Almost immediately upon the loss of its nerve, histologic changes are noted in the muscle. At first, these changes are in the nature of shrinkage, a process which can be reversed when and if new nerve fibers are supplied. Eventually, however, complete atrophy occurs [1] and the muscle is replaced by connective tissue.

Those neurons arising from cells in the brain stem and cord directly supplying the muscles are also known as *lower motor neurons* (for upper motor neuron, see Chap. 20). Since constant allusion has been made to the synapsing of association neurons from sensory systems with the cell bodies or dendrites of these lower motor or efferent neurons, it should now be clear that impulses arising from many sources can activate this fiber (Fig. 14.2). However, though many systems intiate or modify muscular action in some way, the pathway through which this is accomplished constitutes what is spoken of as a *final common path.*

SPINAL PATHWAYS

Cell Body

These cells are located in the ventral gray columns of the spinal cord. They tend to be grouped into two major nuclear masses (Fig. 3-5), a *medial mass,* found throughout the length of the cord and thought to supply fibers that go to muscles of the trunk; and a *lateral mass,* found only at the levels of the brachial and lumbosacral plexuses, thus contributing to the girdle musculature and the muscles of the extremities. The medial group is usually subdivided into ventral and dorsal nuclei. The ventromedial group sends its fibers to the muscles of the back, while the dorsomedial distributes its anxons to the intercostal and abdominal muscles. The lateral cell territory is likewise subdivided, the ventrolateral group sending its fibers to the arm or thigh and the dorsolateral to the forearm or leg. At the lower level of each of the plexus enlargements, a third group of cells, called the retrodorsal lateral, is added for the muscles of the hand or foot.

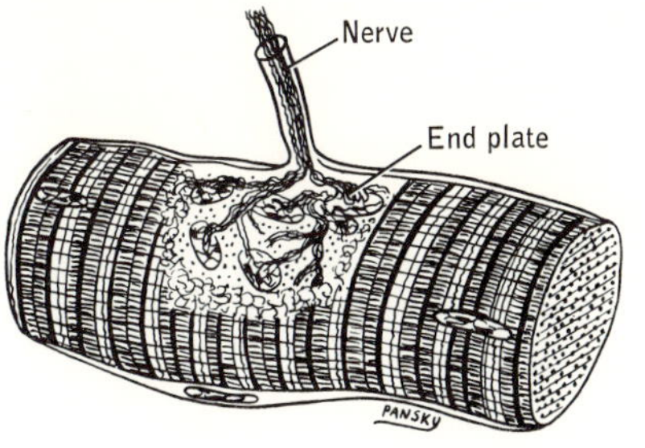

Fig. 14-1. Structure of motor end-plate.

In general, within each of the cell groups of the ventral column at all levels, there is a functional and regional division. The cells in the more ventral portions of the group supply axons to the extensor muscles while the more dorsally placed cells supply the flexors. Scattered among the large multipolar neurons in the ventral column are other, much smaller cells. Some of these give rise to the small gamma efferent fibers. Others are the so-called Renshaw cells which lie very close to the motor cells. Still others are the cell bodies of small intercalated neurons whose axons remain within the ventral column of the same side of the cord but synapse with cells in the opposing region of the same cell group—that is, from the extensor region to the flexor or vice versa.

Axon

The single axon of the large multipolar motor cells passes in a ventrolateral direction. Before leaving the gray substance of the ventral column, it gives off at least one recurrent collateral which makes a synapse with a neighboring Renshaw cell whose axon, in turn, synapses with the same motor cell which gave origin to the motor axon. The main (chief) axon streams out into the white matter where it becomes myelinated and emerges from the spinal cord along the ventrolateral sulcus forming a part of the *ventral root* (Fig. 3-3A).

The fine axons from the small motor cells

[1] Apparently the rate of atrophy varies in different muscles and it is thought that the entire process can be reversed at any time up to the point of complete replacement.

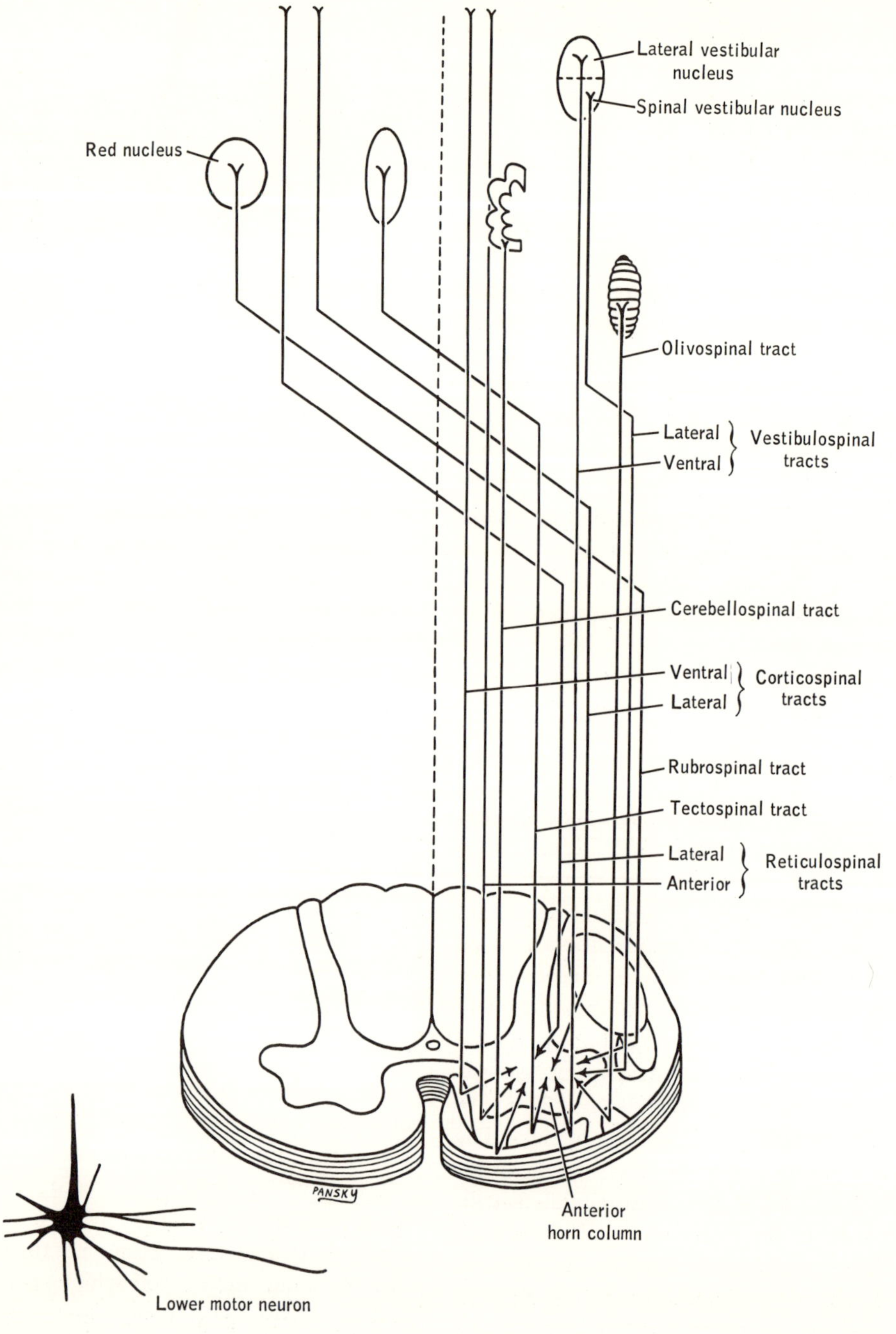

Fig. 14-2. Neurons from numerous sources which terminate around and thus influence the lower motor neurons of the ventral column of the spinal cord. Illustration of the principle of the "final common path."

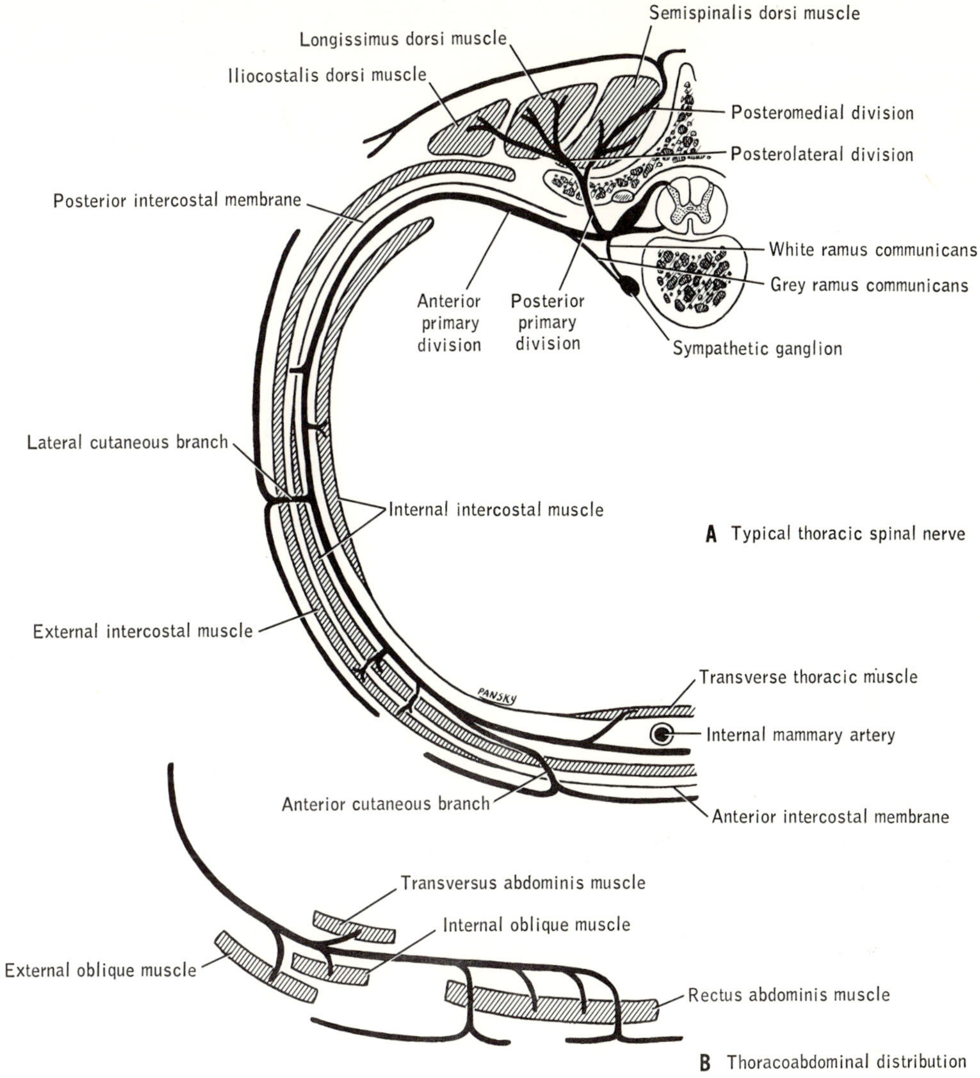

Fig. 14-3. Diagram of a typical spinal nerve as demonstrated by a cross section of the body at a midthoracic level.

follow the same course but have no collaterals. These are the gamma efferents which terminate on the intrafusal fibers of the muscle spindle (Chap. 12). At variable distances from the cord, they join the dorsal root, forming the nerve trunk. These, at appropriate levels, leave the vertebral column through the intervertebral foramina. The subsequent ramifications of a typical spinal nerve are indicated diagrammatically (Fig. 14-3). All the motor fibers terminate in motor end-plates. Thus, impulses traveling along any of the spinal motor fibers of the general somatic efferent (GSE) system can produce contraction on the part of the skeletal musculature of the neck, trunk, and extremities.

CRANIAL PATHWAYS

In the brain stem, there is also representation of the GSE system. Here, however, the linear continuity of the column is interrupted, the cells being grouped together in four nuclear masses, the axons of which contribute to four different cranial nerves. For this reason, the description which follows will be based upon this division.

Hypoglossal Nerve (XII)

Cell Body

These are aggregated in a nucleus of considerable length which lies just beneath the floor of the fourth ventricle on either side of the midline. Grossly, location of the nucleus can be distinguished as it lies beneath the hypoglossal trigone (Figs. 2-35, 14-4, 25-2 to 25-4). Although the nucleus is slender, it is nearly 2 cm in length, extending rostrally from some distance below the olive, nearly to the lower edge of the cochlear nuclei. Its typical relations are best demonstrated through illustration (Figs. 2-48, 2-49). The cells are similar in size and morphology to those in the ventral gray of the cord.

Axon

The large, single axons of each cell at first stream ventrally through the reticular formation. There is just enough lateral drift so that they bypass the medial lemniscus (Figs. 2-48, 2-49, 25-2 to 25-4). When they reach the dorsal border of the pyramids, they turn to pass between the latter and the inferior olive, emerging from the side of the medulla in a groove marking the interval between the bulges made by the inferior olivary nucleus and the pyramid (Figs. 2-7, 2-8, 2-48, 2-49, 25-2 to 25-4). The rootlets of the hypoglossal nerve converge to form the main trunk, the terminations of which lie either in the extrinsic (styloglossus, hyoglossus, and genioglossus) or in the intrinsic muscles of the tongue (Fig. 14-4). Through the action of these muscles, the tongue can be protruded, retracted, or moved from side to side. Such activity and extreme mobility make the tongue of inestimable importance in mastication, deglutition, and phonation.

Abducens Nerve (VI)

Cell Body (Figs. 2-47, 25-7, 25-8.)

These are grouped in a small, spherical nucleus located close to the midline in the pons. Because fibers of the facial nerve bend around the nucleus, making a bulge in the floor of the fourth ventricle—the facial colliculus—this nucleus is easily located (Figs. 2-35, 2-36).

Axon (Figs. 2-7, 2-8, 25-8.)

The single axons from each cell pass almost directly ventrally near the lateral border of the medial longitudinal fasciculus. At the same time, there is a considerable caudal drift, the

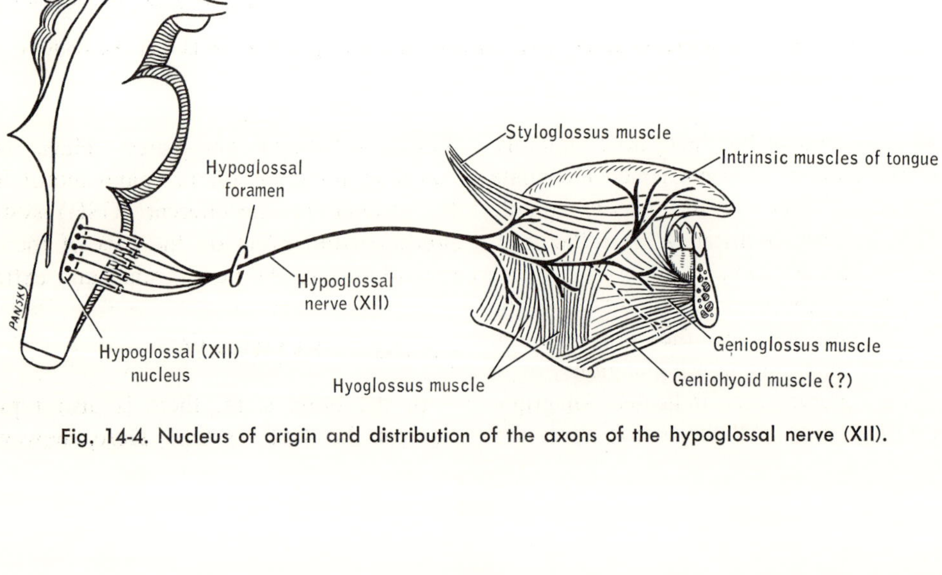

Fig. 14-4. Nucleus of origin and distribution of the axons of the hypoglossal nerve (XII).

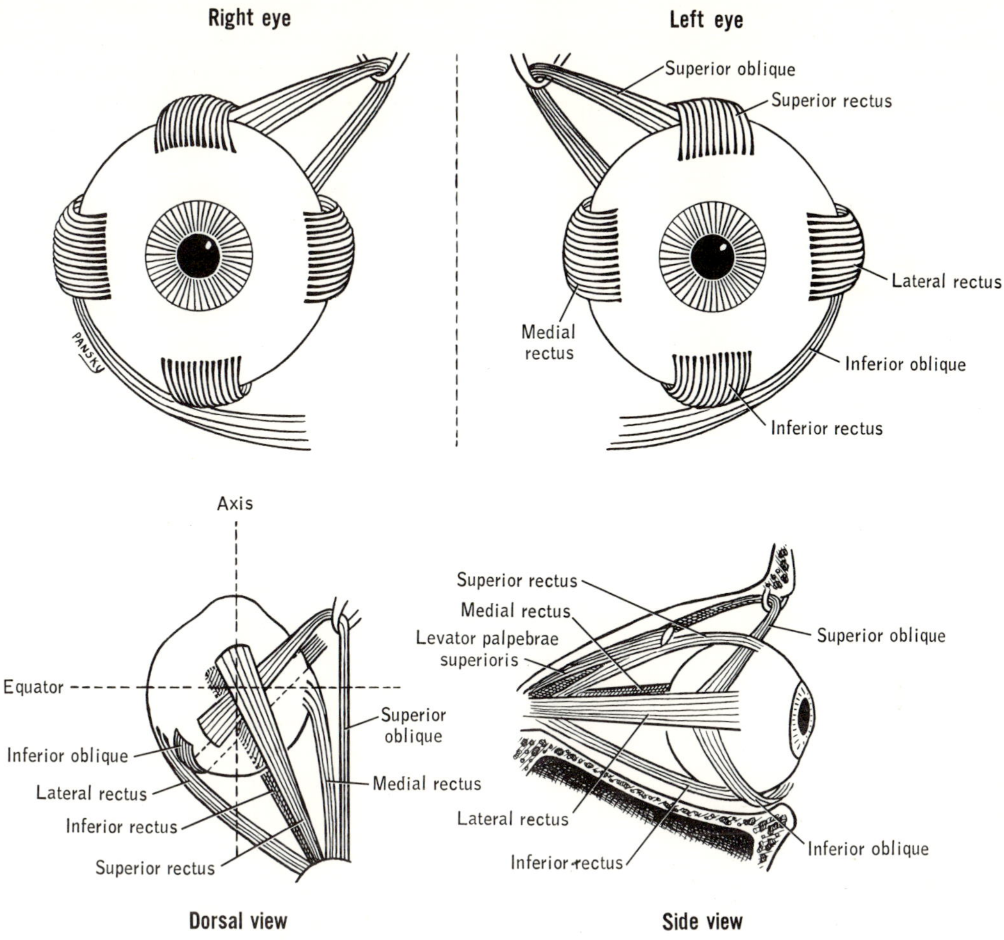

Fig. 14-5. The extrinsic ocular muscles seen from various angles.

fibers emerging from the base of the brain stem in a groove between the caudal border of the pons and the medulla to terminate in the lateral rectus muscle of the eye (Fig. 14-5). A contraction of the lateral rectus muscle produces a horizontal turning of the eye toward the side of the head (abduction) and to some extent a retraction of the eyeball (along with the other recti muscles (Fig. 14-5).

Trochlear Nerve (IV)

Cell Body (Figs. 2-39, 25-11.)

These cells lie in a small, oval nuclear mass adjoining the midline in the region of the lower mesencephalon, just below the cerebral aqueduct at the level of the rostral portion of the inferior colliculus.

Axon (Figs. 25-10, 25-11.)

The large single axons from the cells of the nucleus emerge from the latter along its dorsolateral aspect and curve dorsally along the border of the central gray substance surrounding the cerebral aqueduct. At the same time, there is considerable caudal drift, so that these fibers reach the dorsal side of the brain stem caudal to the inferior colliculus. Here, they enter the anterior medullary velum, decussate, and thus leave the brain stem through its roof (Fig. 2-35). These axons, now grouped together as the trochlear nerve (IV), curve ventrally around the lateral aspect of the brain stem and appear at the basal aspect of the brain at the side of the pons, just rostral to the superficial attachment of the trigeminal nerve (Figs. 2-7, 2-8). The trochlear nerve terminates in the superior oblique muscle of the eye (Figs. 14-5, 14-7).

Unlike the lateral rectus muscle, which produced movement of the eye in one plane, the superior oblique muscle produces action in more than one plane. It rotates the eyeball on its dorsoventral axis and turns it laterally on its vertical axis (abducts) and downward on its horizontal axis. Because of its action from a medially placed trochlea near the anterior aspect of the eye socket, the muscle also protrudes the eyeball.

Oculomotor Nerve (III)

Cell Body (Figs. 2-38, 14-8, 25-12, 25-13.)

These lie in a large nucleus which represents the highest level attained by the general somatic efferent (GSE) column. Since this nerve, unlike nerves IV and VI, supplies five muscles rather than one, its nucleus is considerably larger than the nuclei of either nerve IV or VI. The oculo-

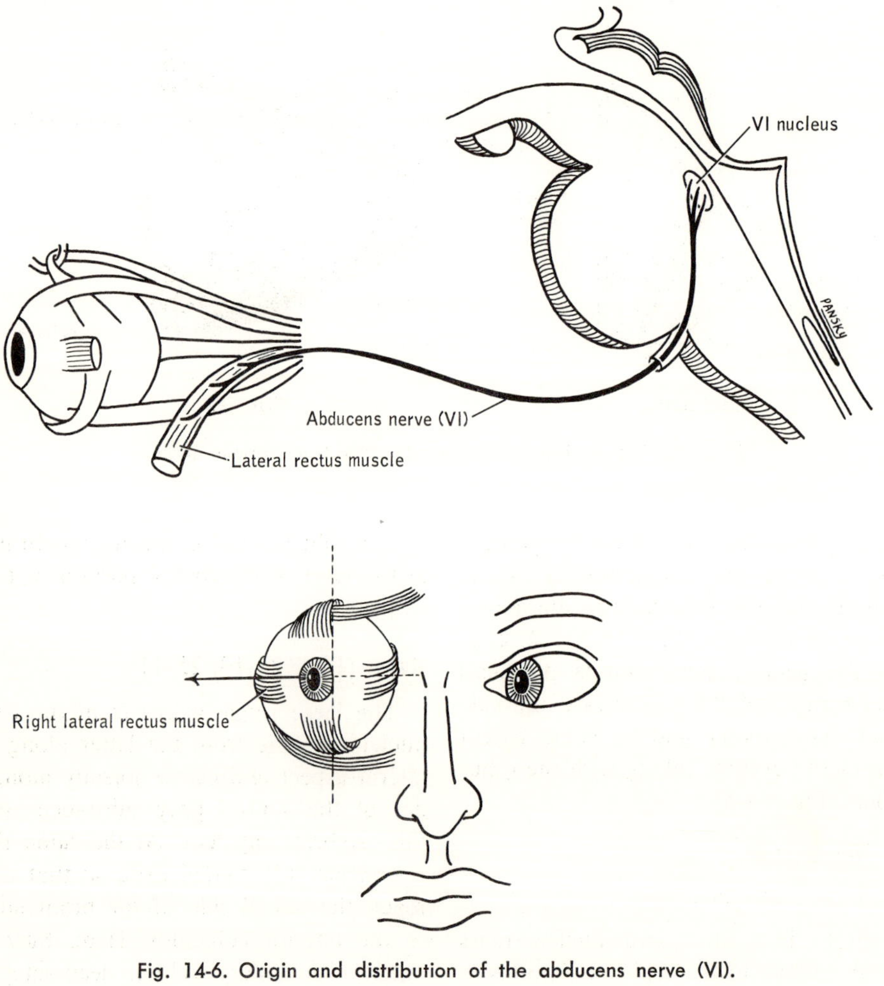

Fig. 14-6. Origin and distribution of the abducens nerve (VI).

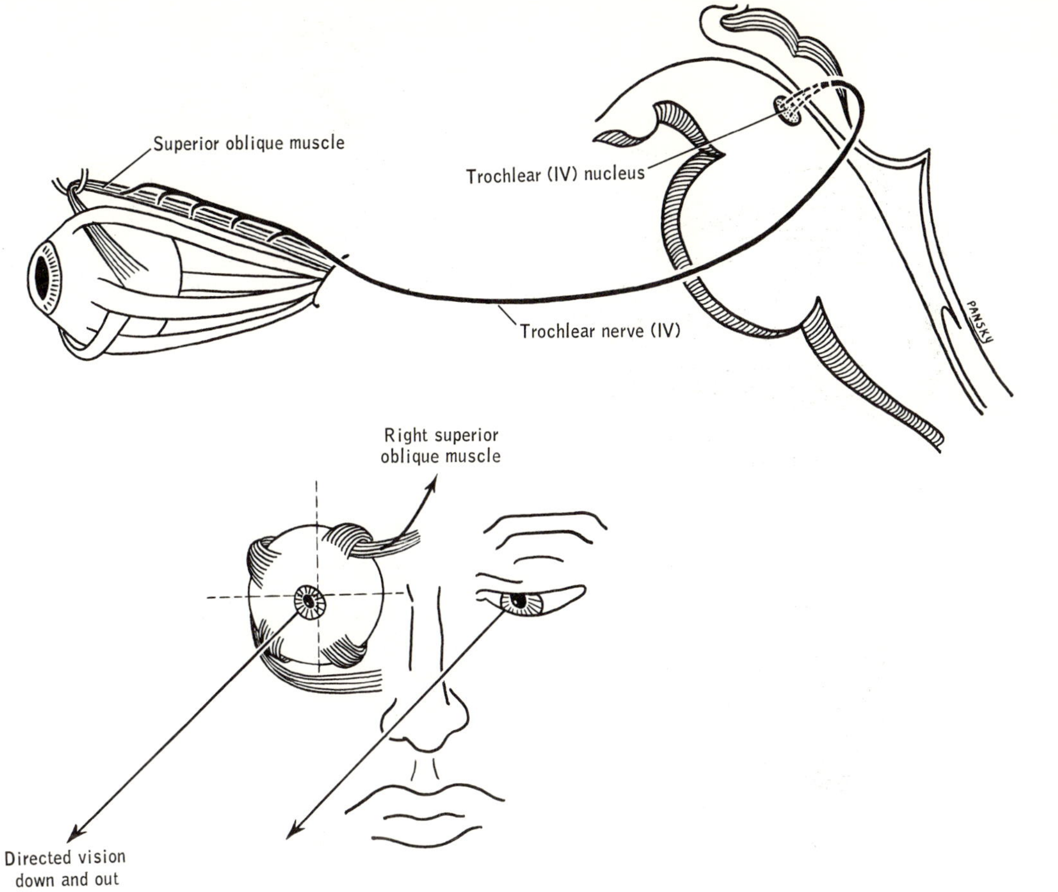

Fig. 14-7. Origin and distribution of the trochlear nerve (IV).

motor cell groups lie adjoining the midline and beneath the central gray substance around the cerebral aqueduct in the rostral portion of the mesencephalon. Their lower limits actually lie near the rostral end of the inferior colliculus, while the rostral limit lies ventral to the most rostral part of the superior colliculus. Because of its size and the different muscles it supplies, attempts have been made to divide the nucleus into parts (Fig. 14-9). Roughly, it may be said that the more dorsal cell groups send fibers to the muscles in the superior part of the orbit, the inferior groups innervate the muscles in the floor of the orbit, while the more medial group is concerned with the medial rectus muscle. A group of cells lying in the most medial portion of the latter group may represent the nucleus of convergence (nucleus of Perlia).

Axon (Figs. 2-7, 2-8, 2-38, 25-12.)

They leave the cell bodies in the nucleus and stream almost directly ventral, cutting through the dorsal tegmental decussation and along the medial border of the red nucleus, to emerge from the brain stem along the oculomotor sulcus, into the interpeduncular fossa. Some fibers to the medial rectus muscle apparently cross before leaving the brain just dorsomedial to the substantia nigra. Just before reaching the superior orbital fissure through which entry into the orbit is attained, the nerve breaks up into two major branches, a superior to supply the

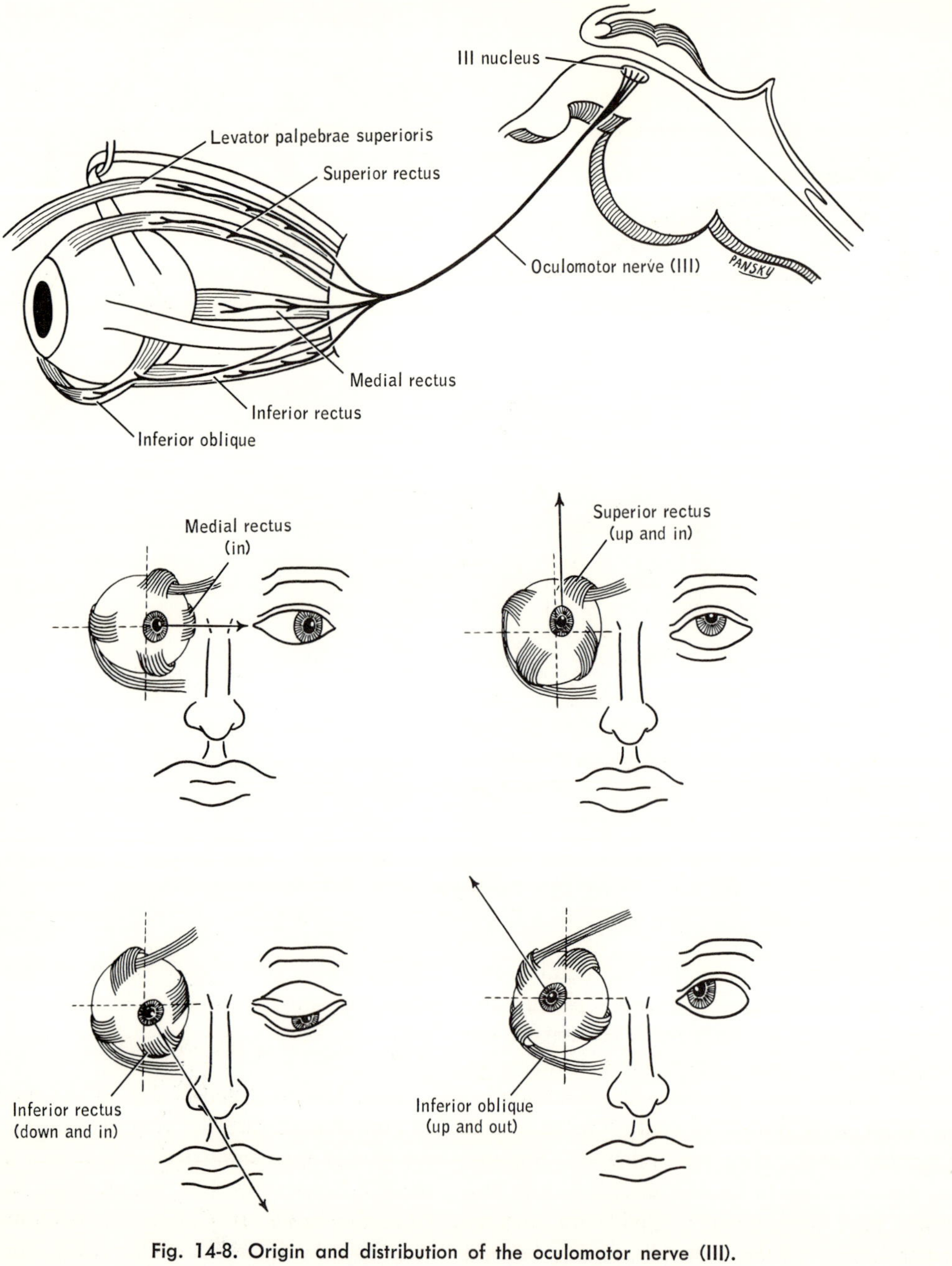

Fig. 14-8. Origin and distribution of the oculomotor nerve (III).

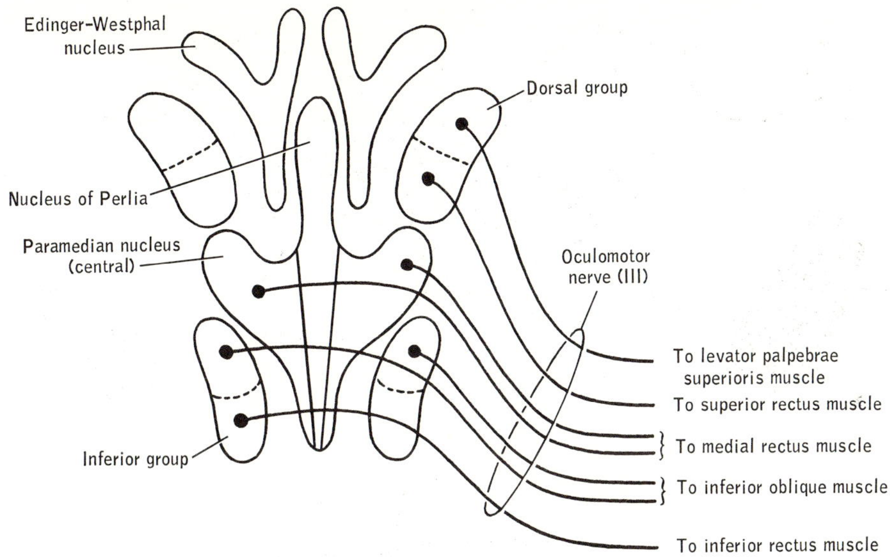

Fig. 14-9. Divisions of the oculomotor nucleus.

levator palpebrae superioris and the superior rectus muscles; an inferior, sending its terminals into the medial rectus, the inferior rectus, and the inferior oblique muscles (Figs. 14-5, 14-8).

As the name implies, the levator palpebrae muscle raises the upper lid and is not concerned with movements of the eyeball. Because of the direction of muscle fibers and their attachments, the superior and inferior recti muscles not only rotate the eye around its horizontal axis, raising or lowering the bulb, respectively, but also produce some rotation around the vertical axis, turning the eyeball somewhat inward (adduction). The medial rectus muscle produces a pure medial rotation (adduction) around the vertical axis, swinging the eyeball inward toward the nose. The recti muscles, because of their origin, also help retract the eyeball to some degree. The inferior oblique muscle also produces complex movements, as did the superior oblique. It first swings the eyeball on its vertical axis, turning it outward (abduction), and then turns the eye around its horizontal axis, directing it upward. There is also a rotation around the dorsoventral axis. Like the superior oblique muscle, the inferior, because of its origin, also tends to protract the eyeball.

STRETCH (MYOTATIC) REFLEX (Figs. 12-2, 14-10.)

This reflex is basic, not only for the maintenance of posture but also as a background for much of muscular activity. Furthermore, all or parts of the mechanism involved in this reflex are utilized when movement is initiated, controlled or modified by suprasegmental centers. Thus, a detailed account is essential at this point.

Before considering the actual circuit, several fundamental concepts must be reviewed. First, the maintenance of posture is opposed to gravity. Were it not for a large mass of skeletal muscle often referred to as "antigravity," the body would fall. Second, muscles are arranged around articulations in opposing groups (flexors-extensors; abductors-adductors). When one set of muscles contracts, its opposing set (on the other side of the joint) must relax, otherwise no movement would occur. Third, an afferent neuron from the stretch receptor can directly

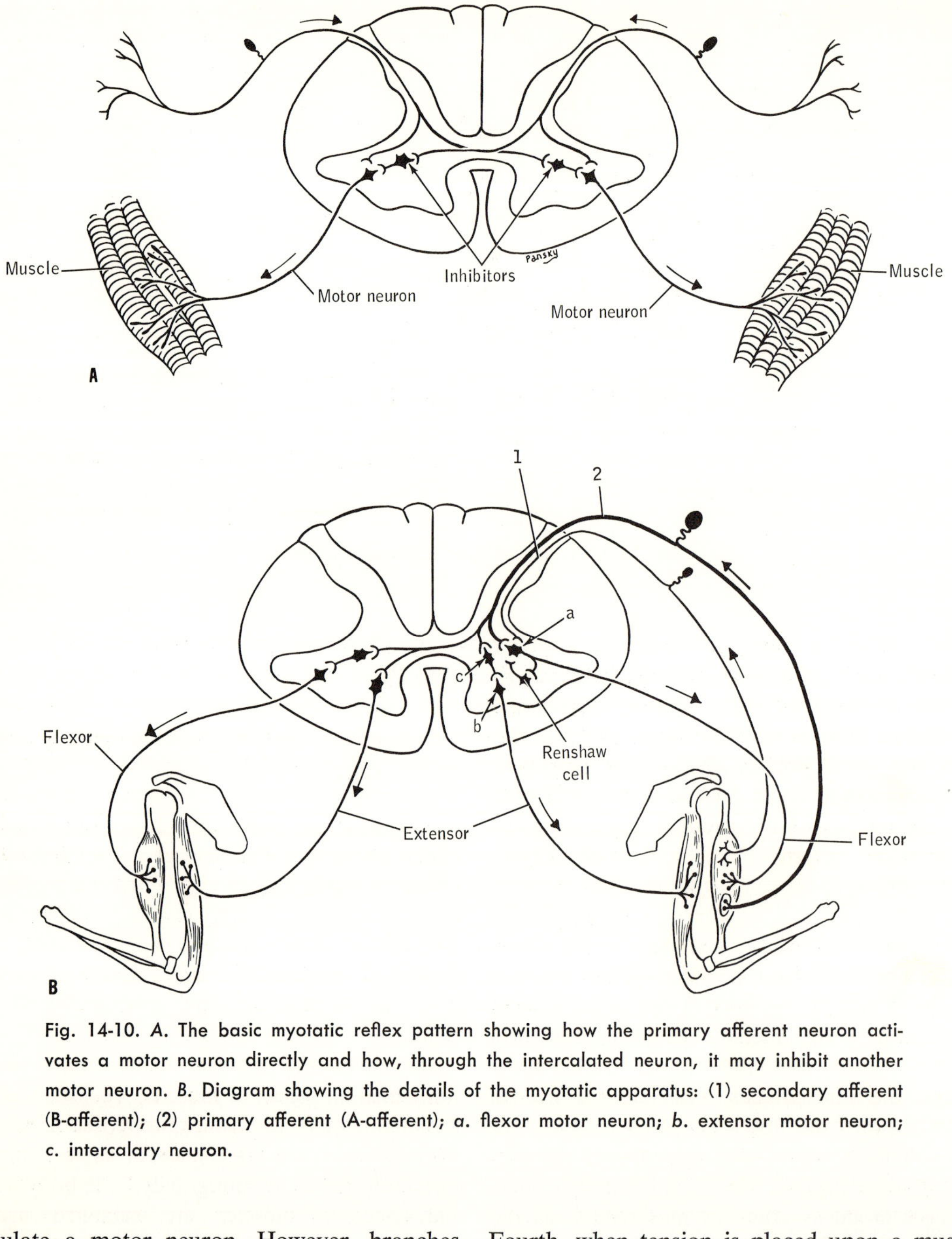

Fig. 14-10. *A.* The basic myotatic reflex pattern showing how the primary afferent neuron activates a motor neuron directly and how, through the intercalated neuron, it may inhibit another motor neuron. *B.* Diagram showing the details of the myotatic apparatus: (1) secondary afferent (B-afferent); (2) primary afferent (A-afferent); *a.* flexor motor neuron; *b.* extensor motor neuron; *c.* intercalary neuron.

stimulate a motor neuron. However, branches of this same afferent fiber can not directly inhibit the neuron of the opposing group since no afferent neuron can be a stimulator and inhibitor at the same time. This activity must be carried out through a short, intercalated neuron. Fourth, when tension is placed upon a muscle, all of the stretch receptors are not usually fired at the same time. And, fifth, there must be built-in safe-guards to prevent the overcontraction of the muscle, as a protection against rupture or evulsion.

With the above facts in mind, let us examine the myotatic reflex as it concerns posture. With the body in the erect position, the force of gravity is trying to pull the body down. Thus, to varying degrees depending upon the location of the antigravity muscle, body weight puts muscle fibers on the stretch. Actually, the pull of but a fraction of an ounce is sufficient to stimulate the annulospiral endings which are especially numerous in antigravity muscles. Thus, a volley of impulses passes over the A-afferent fibers. Since these make direct synapses on motor cells, a contraction of muscle fibers in the area of the stimulated spindle occurs. When the muscle fiber has contracted, its spindle is no longer stimulated, impulses along the afferent fiber are diminished and thus the muscle in this area relaxes. Since the set of muscle fibers which has just reacted is refractory, momentarily, to another stimulus, a group of adjoining muscle fibers goes through the same cycle. Thus, an endless series of small group reactions sweeps through the entire muscle. So, in effect, the muscle is in a state of continuous activity and posture is maintained. However, there is more to it than this since the opposing muscles must relax. Although the A-afferent can not in itself be activator and suppressor at the same time, it has been shown that some of its telodendria synapse with cells of small intercalated neurons. The axons of the latter travel a short distance within the cell group where they synapse on cells whose axons innervate the flexors. Thus, it is the intercalated neuron which acts as the inhibitor. As a part of this same mechanism, the same afferent neuron sends some of its branches across the cord to come into synaptic relations either directly with motor cells for stimulation or with intercalated neurons for the inhibition of muscular activity on the other side of the body.

It seems obvious that, with an extremely powerful stretch, a muscle might be stimulated into such a powerful contraction that it could be damaged. Theoretically, when a muscle contracts, the annulospiral receptors are no longer activated (stretched) and the muscle should relax from want of an action current. However, there are two other circuits which are involved in the inhibitory mechanism and make possible better control of the extent of muscular contraction. The first of these utilizes the B-afferents. These are associated with both the flower spray endings in the muscle spindle and the tendon endings. The flower sprays are stimulated by a thickening of the intrafusal fiber as the muscle contracts, the tendon receptors are stimulated by the pull of the contracting muscle on its tendon. The central processes of the B-afferents terminate directly upon the motor cells responsible for the contraction, thus inhibiting them and leading to relaxation. The second pathway involves the axon collaterals. These arise from the axons responsible for the muscle contraction. The collaterals synapse with Renshaw cells whose axons, by terminating upon the same cell which gave rise to the original axon, depress activity of the mother cell.

Using these same basic patterns, suprasegmental influences can be brought to bear upon the lower motor system. For example, consider the act of picking up some object. This requires the action of the flexors of the forearm (biceps, brachialis, etc.). The descending pathway from the voluntary motor cortex sends terminals into the anterior column to synapse with the cells of the gamma efferents causing a contraction of the polar region of the intrafusal fibers. This, in effect, stretches the bag region of the intrafusal fiber just as though the muscle were being stretched by an extrinsic force. Thus, a stretch reflex is initiated and the flexors contract. However, it is equally important that the extensors (triceps brachii) relax. Therefore, the A-afferent neuron not only synapses with the neurons for the flexor group but also has connections with intercalated neurons which synapse with the neurons of the extensor group, thus inhibiting the activity of the triceps. The recurrents of the motor axons through the Renshaw cell circuit and the B-afferents make possible a modicum of control over the extent of muscular contraction. Perhaps more important from the point of view of purposeful movement, is the fact that the great pool of efferent and intercalated neurons in the ventral column is open not only to activation initiated by the voluntary cortex but also to other suprasegmental influences which can transform the basic reflex muscle "twitch" into a prolonged action, reinforced, facilitated, or suppressed as the need demands (Chaps. 18, 19, 20).

CONJUGATE MOVEMENT

For all animals whose eyes are set in the front of the head, facing forward, it is essential that both eyes move together so that objects under observation can be kept in focus on both retinae at the same time (Fig. 14-11). This is called *conjugate movement.* Such movements are, of course, controlled or influenced by association neurons from many sources in the CNS, at both reflex and voluntary levels. However, the majority of impulses which set off movements of the eye pass to the GSE motor nuclei indirectly through intercalary neurons, the cells of which lie in either the tectum or tegmental reticular formation. Such cell groups are referred to as "centers for conjugate movement," and it has been suggested that the superior colliculus is concerned with vertical movement; the parabducens nucleus with horizontal movements; and the nucleus of Perlia with convergence.

CLINICAL CONSIDERATIONS

Before one can reasonably expect to understand the clinical investigation of this motor system, certain fundamental definitions must be understood.

Definitions

Atrophy

Generally, this means a diminution in size or a wasting away of muscle.

Areflexia

This is a complete absence of all reflexes.

Tone

All muscle, even when in an essentially resting stage, has a certain amount of normal tension, which is actually an extremely low-grade contraction.

Atonia

A condition in which muscle tone is absent.

Spasm

This is almost the exact opposite of atonia, for here there is a strong, involuntary contraction of a muscle or group of muscles. This may be persistent, in which case it is a *tonic spasm,*

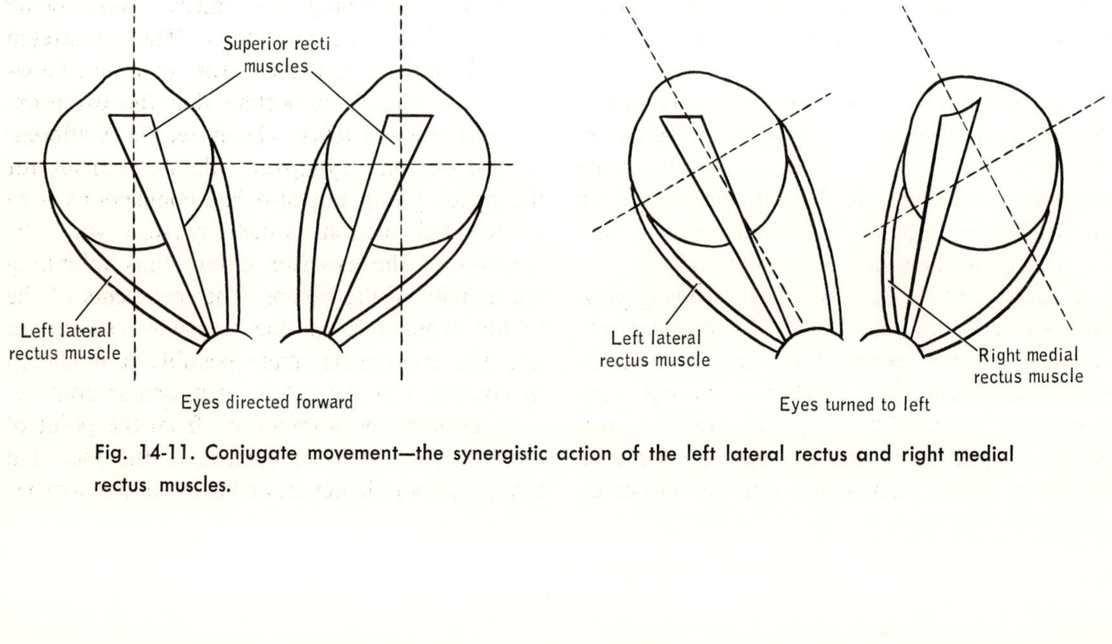

Fig. 14-11. Conjugate movement—the synergistic action of the left lateral rectus and right medial rectus muscles.

or it may alternate with periods of relaxation, in which case it is called a *clonic spasm.*

Contracture

This also means a contraction, particularly in the sense of a shortening or distortion, and frequently implies a condition of some permanency, as from the shrinkage of a muscle or from scar formation.

Paralysis

In general, this merely means loss or impairment of motor function because of lesions in the neural or muscular mechanism. This chapter is concerned primarily with the neural part. Usually, two types are dealt with. The first is a *flaccid* paralysis, characterized by atonia, areflexia and, later, atrophy. The second type is a *spastic* paralysis, characterized by increased tone (*hypertonia*), increased deep-tendon reflexes (*hyperreflexia*), and absent superficial (cremasteric and abdominal) reflexes.

Strabismus

This is the uncontrolled deviation of the eye.

Diplopia

This is double vision, in which a single object appears to be two.

Testing

As in all other diagnoses, it is important to check the case history carefully for evidence of disease or injury. Frequently, important clues are furnished through careful questioning.

A general superficial inspection is made for physical evidence of trauma, either recent, as indicated by a fresh wound, or old, as evidenced by scars. Wasted or shrunken areas should be looked for, since damage to or interruption of lower motor neurons leads to the atrophy of the muscles supplied.

The extremities are bent by the examiner to determine muscle tone and resistance to passive movement (Chap. 18). Tendons are also tapped at certain points to see if reflexes occur (Chap. 12). Both atonia and areflexia are evidence of lower motor neuron defects (flaccid paralysis) and may be apparent long before muscle atrophy is evident. The patient is asked to protrude the tongue. If it deviates toward one side, there is a lesion of the hypoglossal mechanism on the side *toward* which the deviation occurs (Fig. 14-12). This is because of the action of the unopposed muscles, such as the genioglossus, which is normally contracting and which, being the muscle of protrusion, pushes the tongue to the weakened side. If the lesion is of long standing, the tongue will also show atrophic changes on that side.

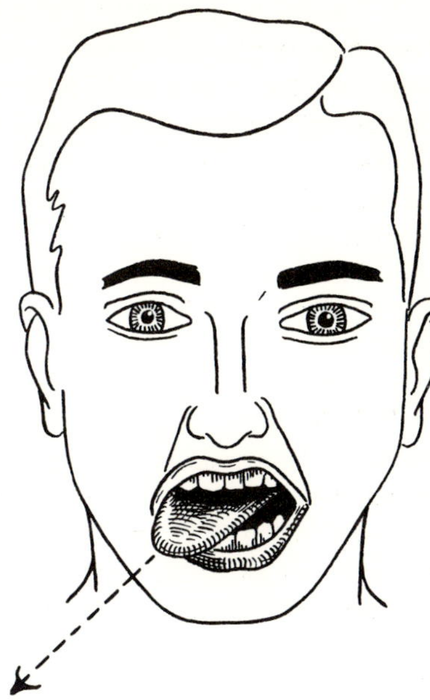

Fig. 14-12. Lesion in the right hypoglossal nerve, or its nucleus, showing the deviation of the tongue toward the side of the lesion.

The eye movements must be checked, first by observing the eyes when the patient is directed to look straight ahead, and then by having the patient attempt to follow a slowly moving object, with both eyes open and the head stationary (Fig. 14-13). The eyes should be watched for evidence of strabismus, and the patient should be asked whether he experiences diplopia. If strabismus is encountered, certain general rules for diagnosis may be noted. First, the eye on the affected side cannot be turned in the direction the paralyzed muscle normally turns it; and next, the opposing muscles exert a tonic pull, causing the eye at rest to tend to look in a direction opposite to the paralyzed muscle. Usually, when the patient attempts to look toward the affected side, he experiences diplopia. Lastly, the face tends to be turned to the affected side to try to compensate for the lack of function of the ocular muscles affected.

General Pathology

The pathology can usually be classified according to the place where the neuron is affected, i.e., whether within the CNS, where it is classed as *intramedullary,* or along the peripheral course, where it is classified as *extramedullary.*

Intramedullary

Tumors. These may do any of several things, all of serious consequence to the neuron. They may destroy the nucleus by direct encroachment upon its cells; they may interrupt the emergent axons from the nucleus; or they may interfere with the blood supply of either nucleus or fibers.

Infectious Agents. These may be either bacteria or viruses, which usually attack the cell bodies.

Trauma. This could be of several sorts, either from a direct penetrating agent or from penetrations of bone or bone fragments of vertebrae or skull. This damage can cause direct destruction of the nucleus or of the emergent axons. Interruption of blood supply may also occur.

Vascular Accident. These spontaneous ruptures of arterial vessels can lead to motor involvement in two ways, either through pressure of the clot, or through the direct interruption of vital blood supply to the nucleus or fibers.

Extramedullary

Tumors. These may develop either in the meninges or bony structure near the superficial attachment of a nerve to the CNS or in any tissue along the course of the nerve where it can impinge upon the efferent fibers.

Infections. These may involve the meninges and may involve the nerves while they are still

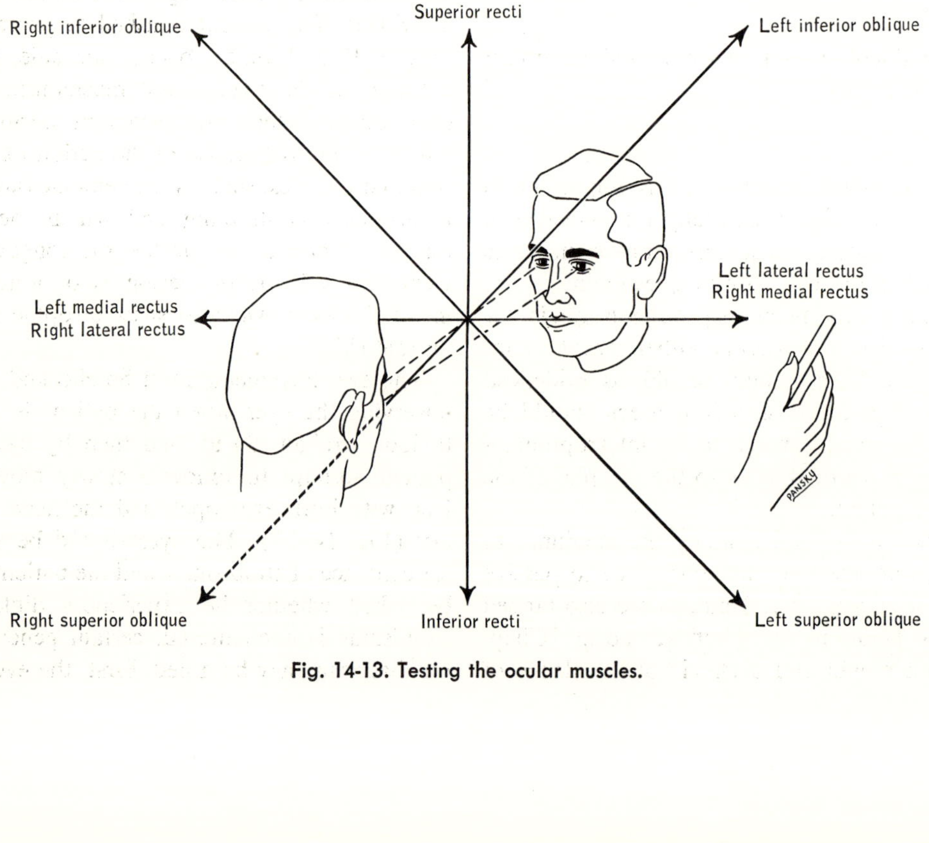

Fig. 14-13. Testing the ocular muscles.

within the bony skull or vertebral canal. Infections may also involve nerve sheaths in the more distal parts of the course of the nerve.

Trauma. In this case, nerve fibers may be severed by the direct act of a penetrating agent or through secondary involvement of surrounding traumatized tissue.

Pressure. This may be applied to nerves in various ways. First, a rise in intracranial pressure for any reason. Clots from hemorrhage in the meninges may exert pressure. Displaced parts, such as herniated intervertebral disks, may encroach on neighboring nerves. Aneurysms (abnormal regional dilatation of arteries) may also disrupt fibers in nerves which adjoin them.

Specific Pathology

Poliomyelitis

This is a condition in which a virus attacks nerve cell bodies. A variable number of cells are killed and this leads to the complete atrophy of all muscle fibers (100 to 200) supplied by the axon of the dead cell. At the onset, however, spasticity of the muscles or increased resistance to passive movement is observed. This is probably because of irritation of the anterior gray column cells. However, as the toxic effect of the virus finally overwhelms these cells, flaccidity appears. At this time, many cells are attacked and their axons become nonfunctional. Eventually, some of the cells do recover. Thus, muscles which at first appear to be completely paralyzed may return to partial function.

In the bulbar type of poliomyelitis, the gray matter of the medulla is affected, with the result that vital functions, including respiration, are interfered with.

Myasthenia Gravis

This is a syndrome of fatigue and exhaustion of the muscular system marked by progressive paralysis without sensory disturbance. It can affect any muscle(s) of the body, but the muscles of the face, lips, tongue, throat, and neck are especially selected by this condition.

To understand myasthenia gravis, it is necessary to understand how a nerve stimulates a muscle. On the humoral basis, acetylcholine is produced at the myoneural junction when current passes through the nerve. Usually, enough of this substance is formed to produce an adequate response. Any residue or excess remaining is destroyed by cholinesterase. In myasthenia, there is inadequate acetylcholine formation, a too-rapid destruction of acetylcholine by cholinesterase, or interference with the process in which acetylcholine reaches, and in some way acts upon, the muscle. This is similar in some ways to the process in which curare, a toxic drug, causes the complete paralysis of muscle by its interference with the action of acetylcholine. Since Prostigmine and neostigmine apparently protect acetylcholine, these drugs are used in such cases. In fact, Prostigmine may be used in the diagnosis of myasthenia. When employed for this purpose, 2 or 3 ml of a 1:2,000 solution (with $\frac{1}{150}$ grain atropine) is injected intramuscularly. If the muscular weakness improves in $\frac{1}{2}$ to $\frac{3}{4}$ hour and actually disappears altogether in 2 hours, the indications are that myasthenia gravis is present.

Erb's Palsy

It is sometimes called *upper-trunk palsy* and is usually due to injury incurred at birth in which

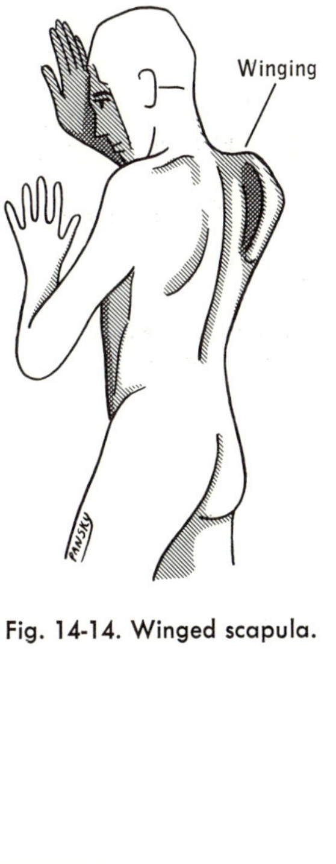

Fig. 14-14. Winged scapula.

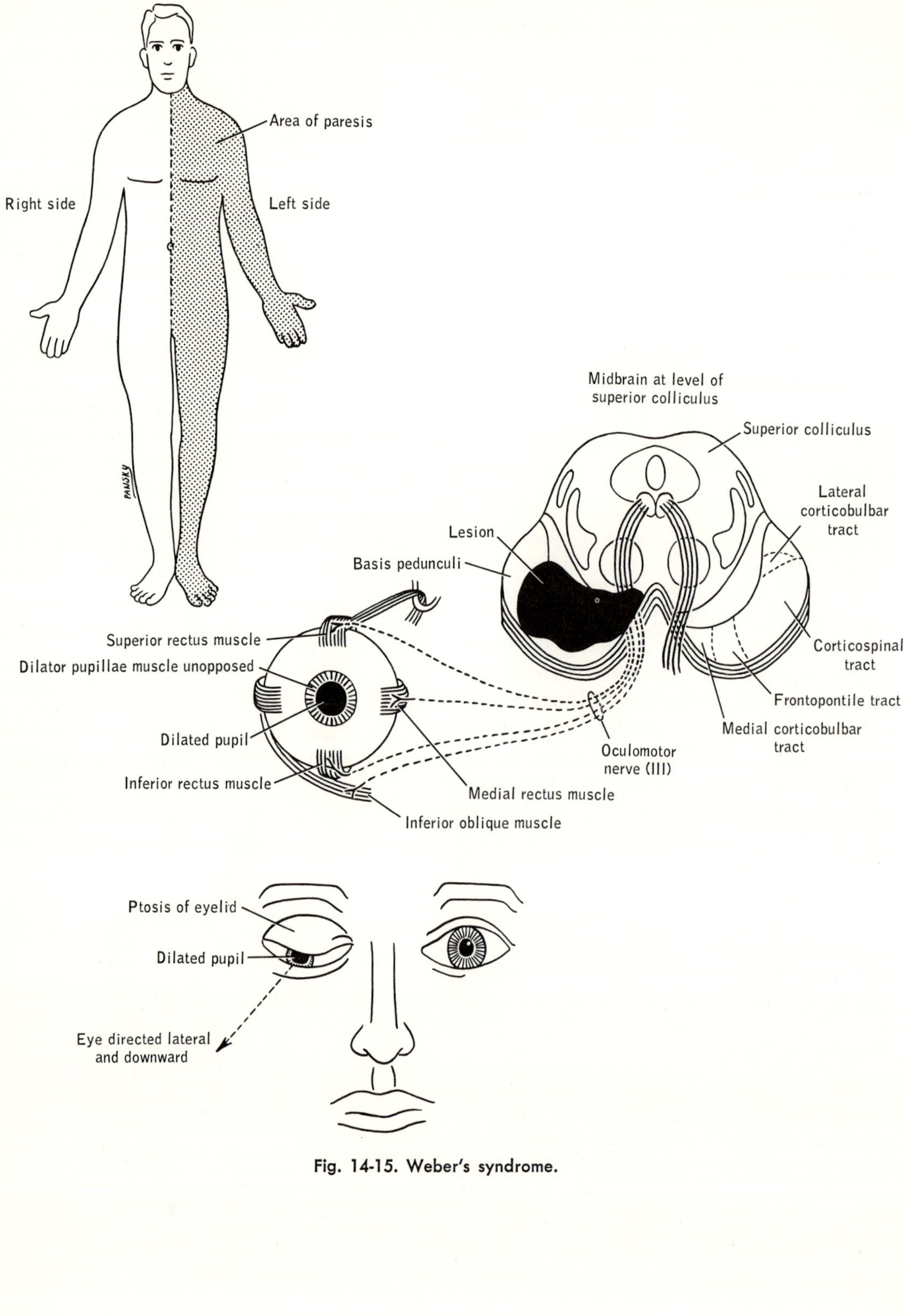

Fig. 14-15. Weber's syndrome.

the fifth and usually the sixth cervical nerves are broken as their ventral roots emerge from the cord. This leads to flaccid paralysis and atrophy of all the muscles supplied by these nerves. The condition is particularly evident in muscles like the upper part of the serratus anterior, innervated by the long thoracic nerve [atrophy results in *winged scapula* (Fig. 14-14)]; the deltoid, supplied by the axillary nerve (with atrophy causing *loss of roundness* of the shoulder); and in the anterior arm, where the musculocutaneous nerve supplies the biceps brachii.

Syringomyelia

This condition, described in connection with other systems (Chap. 8), involves the breakdown of portions of certain sensory pathways. However, since it involves a gross enlargement of the spinal canal, it can increase in diameter to such an extent that it encroaches upon the ventral columns, destroying motor cells locally in the region of the enlargement. This will lead to bilateral flaccid paralysis of the corresponding muscles. However, the sensory mechanism will give an even more accurate location for the lesion.

Weber's Syndrome (Crossed Oculomotor Paralysis) (Fig. 14-15.)

In this case, the lesion occurs along the side of the interpeduncular fossa. Recalling the anatomy of this region, it will be seen that the emergent fibers of the oculomotor nerve (III), together with the medial portion of the basis pedunculi, will be destroyed. This will lead to complete paralysis of all muscles supplied by the oculomotor nerve, leaving the superior oblique and lateral rectus muscles (nerves IV and VI) unopposed. Thus, the eye on the affected side will be directed laterally and downward. Since the motor fibers for pupillary constriction, both to light and accommodation, travel in this nerve, there will be failure of closure of the pupil. Because of involvement of the basis pedunculi there is also a contralateral paresis of the lower face, tongue, and extremities.

Oculomotor Ophthalmoplegia

In this condition there is complete block of nerve III. Its symptoms, as far as the eye is concerned, are the same as those for Weber's syndrome (see above), but no other systems appear to be involved.

Hemiplegia Alternans Hypoglossica

This condition results from a lesion either at the surface of the medulla, involving the emerging fibers of nerve XII and the pyramids, or within the medulla, catching the hypoglossal fibers in their intramedullary course and the pyramids as well. A paralysis of the tongue occurs on the affected side, since the tongue musculature is deprived of its innervation. When protruded, the tongue points toward the side of the lesion, and in time this side of the tongue will appear shrunken because of muscular atrophy. Because of the inclusion of the pyramid in the lesion, above the decussation, spastic paralysis will occur in the muscles of the opposite side of the body. The extent, again, may be variable, depending upon whether all or only part of the pyramid is disrupted.

SUMMARY
General Somatic Efferent

Spinal		Cranial
1. In the somatic efferent column of the spinal cord Ventral gray column throughout the length of the cord Medial group - throughout the length of the cord Dorsal division Ventral division Lateral group - only in region of brachial and lumbosacral plexuses Retrodorsal division Dorsal division Ventral division Central group - midcervical and sacral levels	Cell body	1. In somatic efferent column of the brain stem Oculomotor nucleus in middle and upper mesencephalon: Dorsal group Ventral group Medial group Trochlear nucleus (IV) in lower mesencephalon Abducens nucleus (VI) in pons Hypoglossal nucleus (XII) in medulla
2. Through the somatic efferent components of all spinal nerves From medial group: Dorsal division--to intercostal and abdominal muscles Ventral division--to axial muscles From lateral group: Retrodorsal division--to muscles of hand and foot Dorsal division--to muscles of forearm and leg Ventral division--to muscles of arm and thigh From central group--to muscles of diaphragms	Efferent fiber	2. Through somatic efferent components of corresponding cranial nerves Through oculomotor nerve (III): From dorsal group to superior rectus muscle of the eye and the levator palpebrae of the upper lid From the ventral group to the inferior rectus and inferior oblique muscles of the eye From the medial group to the medial rectus muscle of the eye Through the trochlear nerve (IV) to the superior oblique muscle of the eye Through the abducens nerve (VI) to the lateral rectus muscle of the eye Through the hypoglossal nerve (XII) to the muscles of the tongue
3. All motor end-plates of the muscles of neck, trunk, and extremities derived from somites	Termination	3. All in motor end-plates of skeletal muscles, indicated above, derived from somites

15 GENERAL VISCERAL EFFERENT SYSTEM (GVE) (AUTONOMIC SYSTEM)[1]

This is the motor system which regulates the organs (viscera) of the body. It includes the control of all smooth (involuntary) muscle, cardiac muscle, and glands.

Certain fundamental features concerning its structure and function must be pointed out. (1) In general, most viscera are supplied by two opposing sets of fibers, one stimulating, the other inhibiting activity. (2) Both the stimulating and inhibiting mechanisms require a two-neuron chain between the nucleus of origin in the CNS and the peripheral organ which is innervated (Fig. 15-1). This necessitates a synapse between the two neurons which occurs in ganglia outside the CNS. Using the ganglion as a point of reference, the fiber lying closest to the brain or cord is called *preganglionic* (presynaptic might be more appropriate). The second fiber, the cell of origin of which lies in one of the ganglia and which carries impulses to an organ, is called *postganglionic* (or postsynaptic). (3) The cells are of the multipolar type, but they are small. Within the CNS, the cells are located either in the *intermediolateral cell column of the cord* or in nuclei in the brain stem. (4) The termination of the visceral fibers is peculiar. In the organs, fine nerve terminals end in small knobs in contact with a muscle fiber or gland cell, but not all the cells or fibers receive such endings. In fact, the vast majority do not receive any direct nerve terminals. It has already been suggested (Chap. 6) that a substance, acetylcholine, is formed at the terminals of somatic efferent fibers and that this substance initiates muscle activity. In the visceral system, such a mechanism is especially necessary, since relatively few cells or fibers actually receive a nerve ending. Thus, large amounts of chemical substances form at the nerve terminals. These pass through the tissue fluids and even through the blood stream to reach and thus stimulate other cells. Since this is a liquid substance which spreads out from its source, the term *humoral mediation* has been applied to the mechanism. There are apparently two basic humors: one, similar to epinephrine, is called *sympathin;* the other is acetylcholine. Sympathin is apparently of two sorts: *excitatory,* sympathin E; *inhibitory,* or sympathin I. Those nerve terminals liberating sympathin are called *adrenergic;* those liberating *acetylcholine* are called *cholinergic*.

It is usual to divide the general visceral efferent system into two major portions, based upon the origin of the preganglionic fibers from the CNS. The preganglionic fibers arising from the thoracic and lumbar spinal cord are referred to as the *thoracolumbar* division, or "sympathetic." The preganglionic fibers originating either in certain cranial nerve nuclei or the sacral cord are referred to as the *craniosacral* division, frequently called "parasympathetic."

[1] The term *autonomic,* freely interpreted, means autonomous—having independent functions, or self-controlling. In other words, it regulates visceral function automatically, without cerebral control, or independent of it.

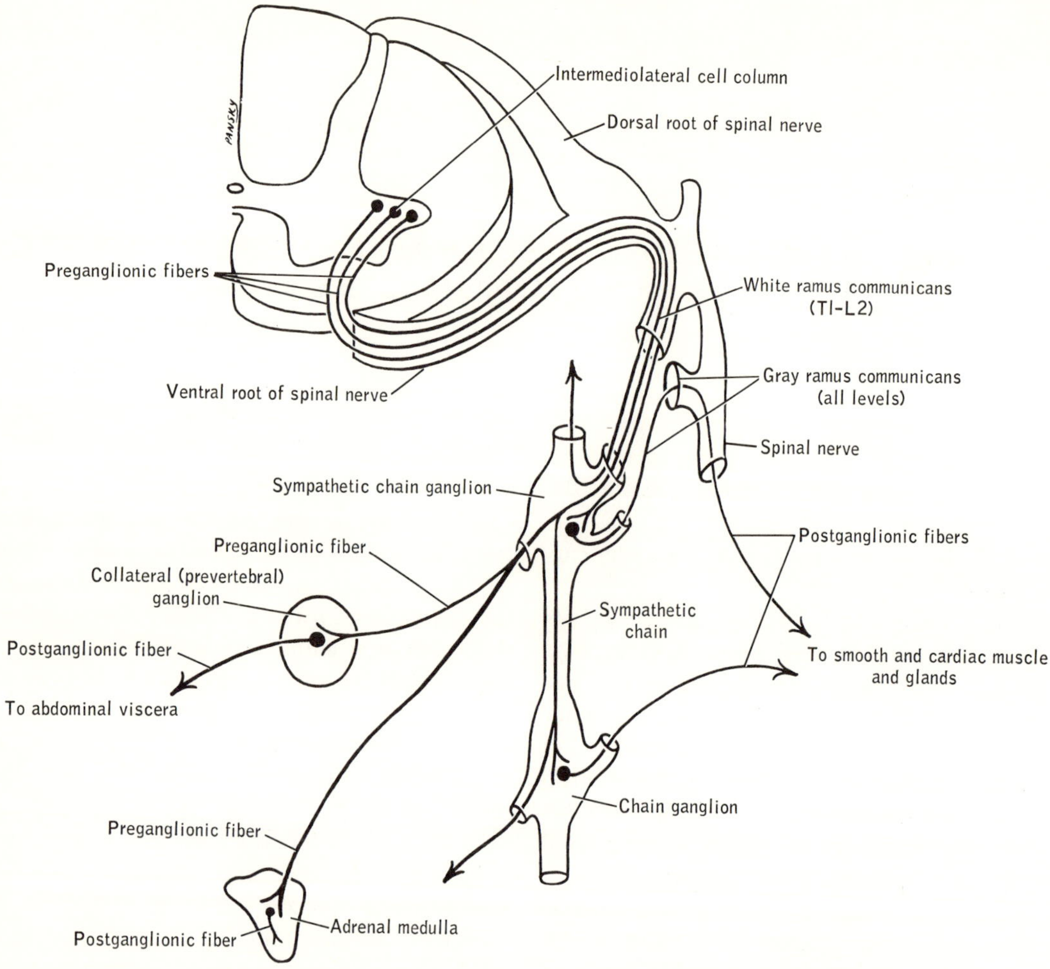

Fig. 15-1. Diagram of a section of the spinal cord, two sympathetic chain ganglia, a collateral ganglion, a terminal ganglion, and the connecting nerves to show the distribution of pre- and postganglionic fibers.

The ganglia of the thoracolumbar (sympathetic) outflow are located opposite each spinal segment, lying adjacent to the lateral side of the bodies of the vertebrae (Fig. 15-2). These ganglia are all interconnected by longitudinal fibers, thus forming a continuous chain. The ganglia are termed *chain* or *paravertebral ganglia.* The thoracic portion of the chain is continued rostrally into the neck as the cervical sympathetic trunk. Only three ganglia are associated with the latter: the *superior, middle,* and *inferior cervical* ganglia. The lumbar portion of the trunk is continued caudally as far as the coccyx.

THORACOLUMBAR DIVISION

Structure

Cells of the Preganglionic Neuron

These cells are of the multipolar type and are aggregated in the intermediolateral gray column of the thoracic and upper lumbar cord (Fig. 3-5).

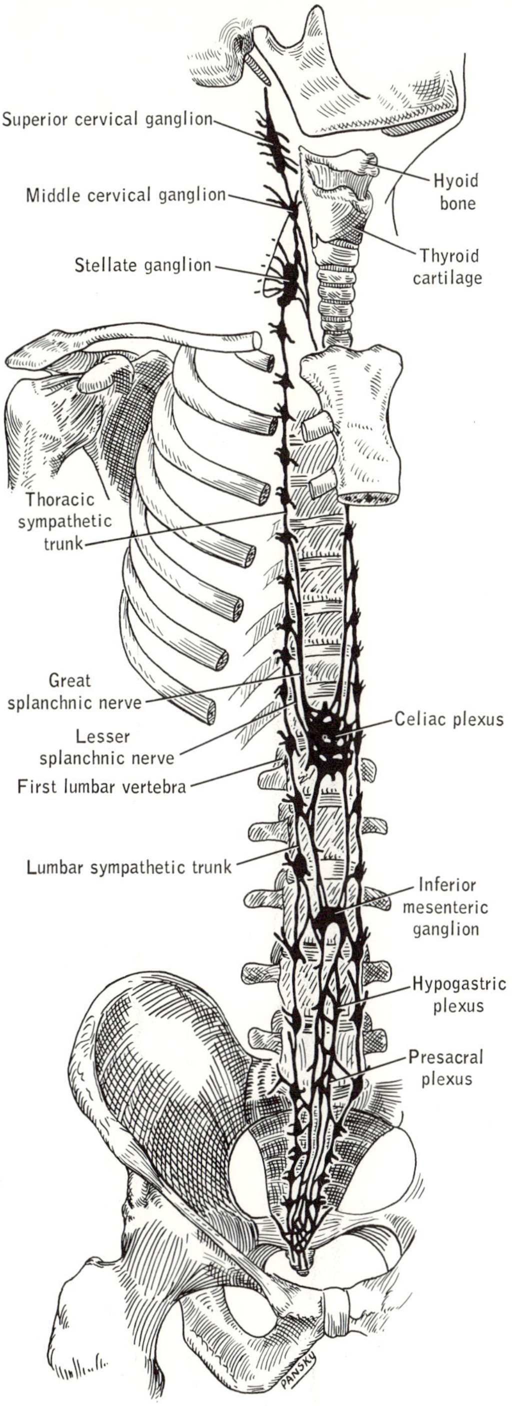

Fig. 15-2. Sympathetic ganglionated chain, the communicating rami, and the splanchnic nerves of the human adult.

Axons of the Preganglionic Neurons
(Figs. 15-1, 15-3, 15-4.)

These axons leave the cell column and pass ventrally through the ventral gray column, leaving the latter to cross the anterior funiculus (white matter), where they pick up myelin. They emerge from the anterolateral sulcus of the cord in company with the somatic efferents, to enter the ventral root of all thoracic and upper lumbar nerves. They travel in the latter to just beyond the point where the dorsal and ventral roots join to form the spinal nerve trunk. There, the visceral efferents leave the trunk as *white rami communicantes*. After a short distance, the white rami enter the thoracic or lumbar sympathetic trunk. On reaching the sympathetic trunk in the region of the nearest chain ganglion, the white ramus may do one of several things: terminate by synapse with a cell or cells in the chain ganglion at the level of entry; pass up or down in the trunk to synapse in one of the chain ganglia above or below the point of entry; pass rostrally through the chain into the cervical sympathetic trunk, many traveling all the way to the superior ganglion before terminating; or pass transversely through the thoracic trunk, forming special nerves which run caudally and ventrally to terminate in ganglia which lie in front of the vertebral column. The latter fibers form the *splanchnic nerves* (Figs. 15-2 to 15-4), and the ganglia in which they terminate belong to the class of *prevertebral ganglia* (Figs. 15-1, 15-3, 15-4). Some of the fibers running in the splanchnic nerves pass on through the ganglia to end in the adrenal medulla. It should be emphasized that a fiber may pass through many ganglia but will synapse in only one. Thus, regardless of how many ganglia are traversed, a fiber must not be considered postganglionic until a synapse has actually been made.

Cells of the Postganglionic Fibers
(Figs. 15-1, 15-3, 15-4.)

These multipolar cells are located in any one of the ganglia listed above which serve as synaptic stations for preganglionic fibers: the paravertebrals (including three cervical ganglia); the thoracic or lumbar chain ganglia; or the prevertebral (including the celiac ganglia and its subdivisions).

Axons of the Postganglionic Fibers
(Figs. 15-1, 15-3, 15-4.)

Most axons arising from the chain ganglia reenter the spinal nerve trunk by way of *gray rami communicantes*. Such rami leave the sympathetic trunk at all levels to join spinal nerves regardless of whether or not a white ramus is present. These postganglionic fibers then travel with the nerve and follow all its branchings and ramifications to terminate in the walls of peripheral blood vessels, in sweat glands, and in the erector muscles of the hair.

In the upper thorax, some of the postganglionic fibers pass medially to supply the bronchi and lungs.

From the cervical ganglia (Fig. 15-5) many descend, especially from the inferior and middle ganglia, to form the cardiac nerves to the heart.

From the superior cervical ganglion, most of the postganglionic fibers ascend along the branches of the carotid artery to reach the walls of the vessels of the head, sweat glands of the face, the erector muscles of the hair, the salivary glands, and the dilator muscles of the pupil (Figs. 15-6 to 15-8).

From the celiac or other prevertebral ganglia, the axons follow the branching of the mesenteric blood vessels, sending fibers into their walls and into the muscular coats of all the viscera.

General Function

No hard-and-fast rule can be made regarding the manner in which this division of the autonomic system will act. Its activity is often determined by the individuality of the organ supplied. However, two general concepts help in predicting what the reaction is to be. First, the discharge of impulses over this system is associated with expenditure of energy. The second point, closely related to the first, concerns the idea that thoracolumbar outflow is an emergency mechanism.

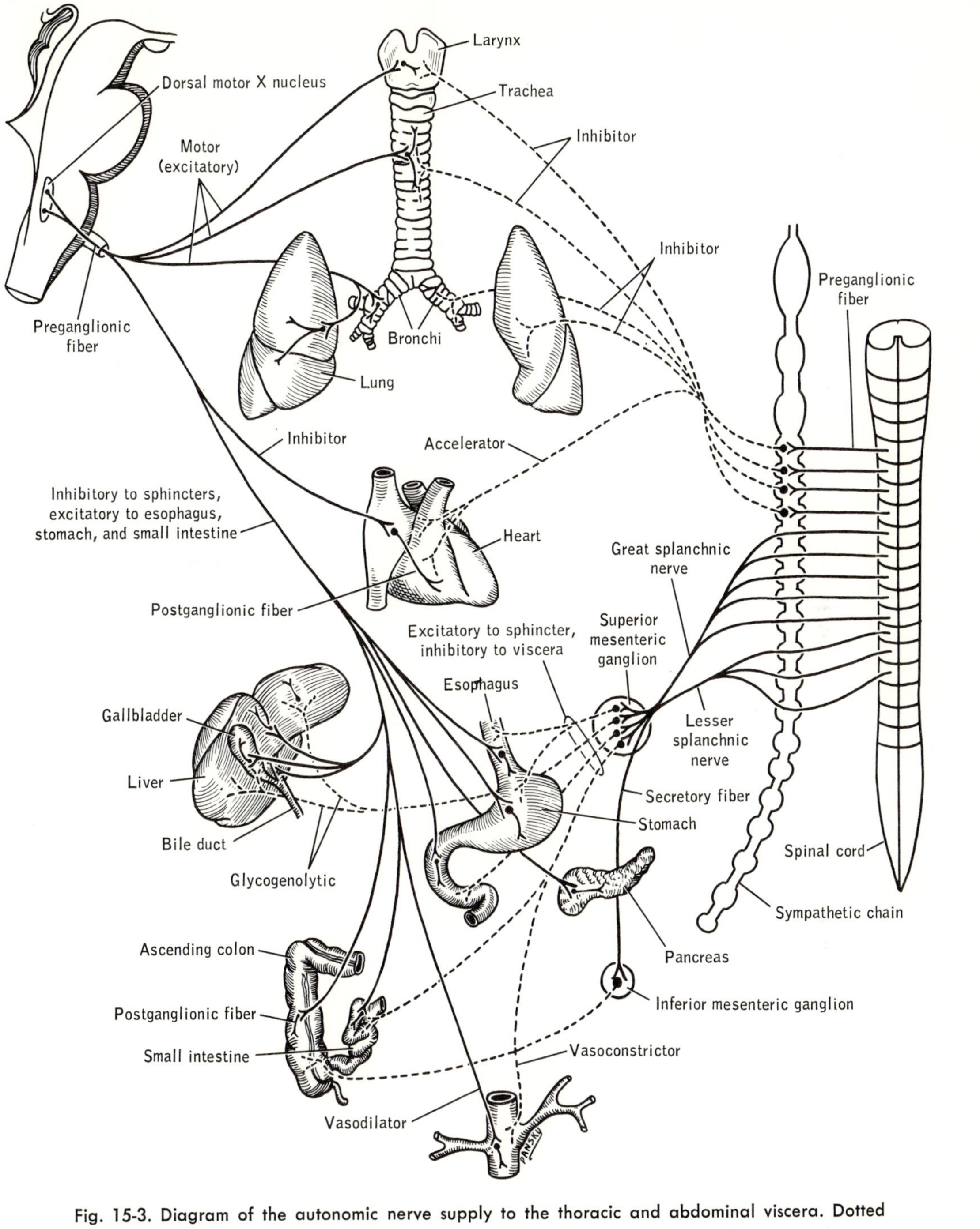

Fig. 15-3. Diagram of the autonomic nerve supply to the thoracic and abdominal viscera. Dotted lines—postganglionic fibers of the thoracolumbar outflow. The postganglionic fibers of the craniosacral outflow are represented by short solid lines, usually in or on the walls of the structures innervated. Some functional values have also been assigned to some of the fibers shown on the figure.

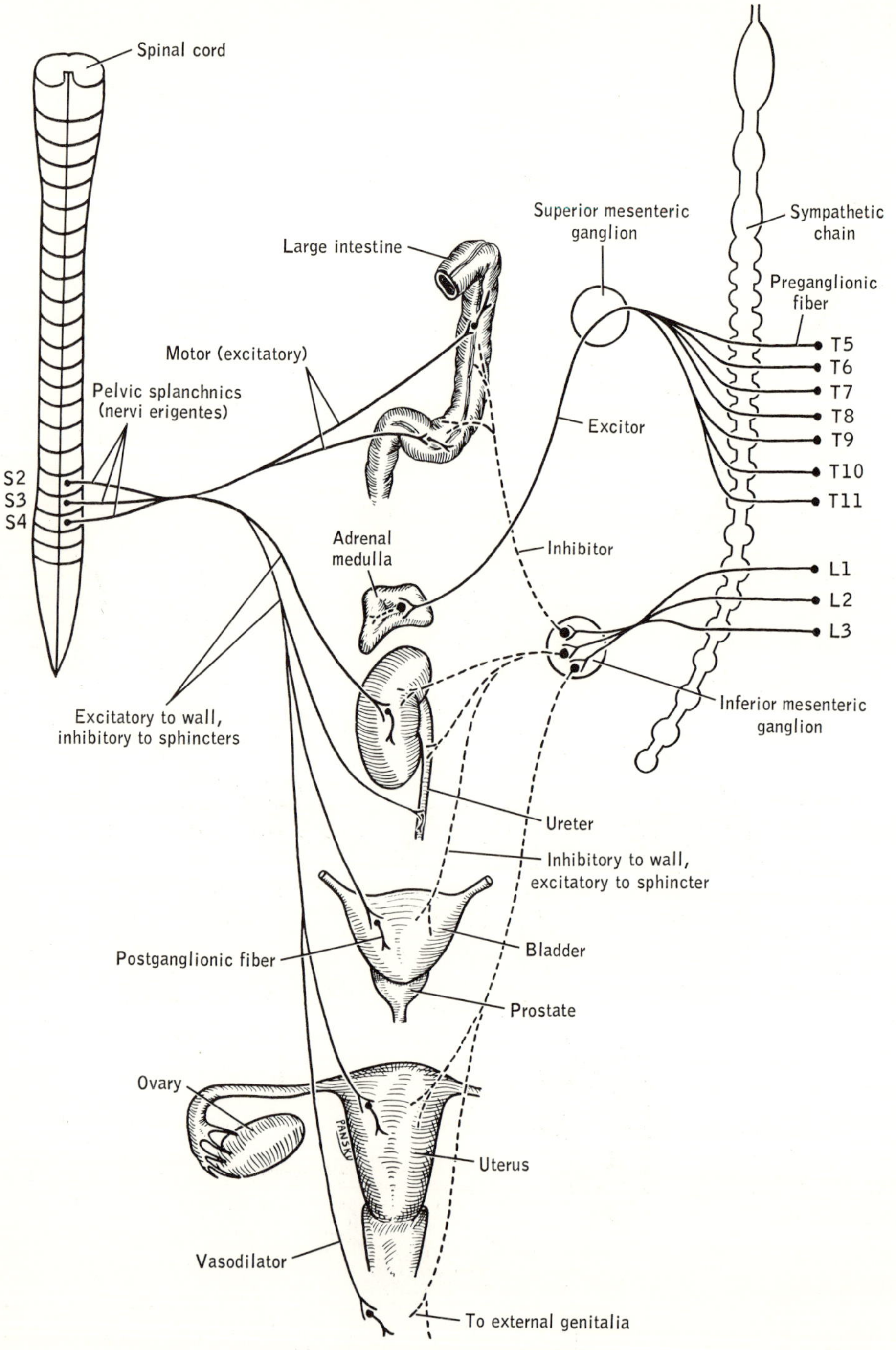

Fig. 15-4. Diagram of the autonomic nerve supply to the viscera of the lower abdomen and pelvis. Dotted lines—postganglionic fibers of the thoracolumbar outflow. The postganglionic fibers of the craniosacral outflow are indicated by short solid lines, usually in or on the walls of the structures innervated. Some functional values have been assigned to some of the fibers shown on the figure.

Since most crises are physical in nature, it is necessary to marshal all possible reactions of the body which would help to meet these forces. First, there must be a release of energy-supplying substances into the blood stream. This is accomplished by glycogenolysis in the liver. Second, there must then be an increase in blood supply to carry energy materials and oxygen to skeletal muscles and to carry away the increased waste resulting from their activity. The stepped-up circulation is accomplished by heart rate acceleration with accompanying constriction of peripheral and mesenteric blood vessels. Third, an increase in circulating oxygen and a means of disposing of excess carbon dioxide from the blood are necessary; these changes are aided by an increase in the diameter of the air passages.

Concomitant with the above-mentioned reactions it is important to suppress any energy-consuming activity during the time of emergency. Thus, secretion of glands and the contraction of visceral muscles are inhibited.

It is obvious from the foregoing that since the entire body economy is involved, the effects of this system must be widespread. This far-reaching influence is effected in several ways. First, the cells of origin of the system cover a large and physically continuous column. Next, it is regulated by a higher center, the hypothalamus (Chap. 21), the descending fibers of which can fire off the entire thoracolumbar column. Further, the humors at its axon terminals are readily transmitted through the tissues and even the blood stream without destruction by enzymatic action. Lastly, impulses flowing through some preganglionic fibers enter the adrenal medulla, which secretes a hormone, *epinephrine,* in response to stimulation.

Specific Reactions

In the light of the foregoing discussion of general functions, it seems appropriate to enumerate some of the specific reactions which occur as a result of the activation of the thoracolumbar mechanism.

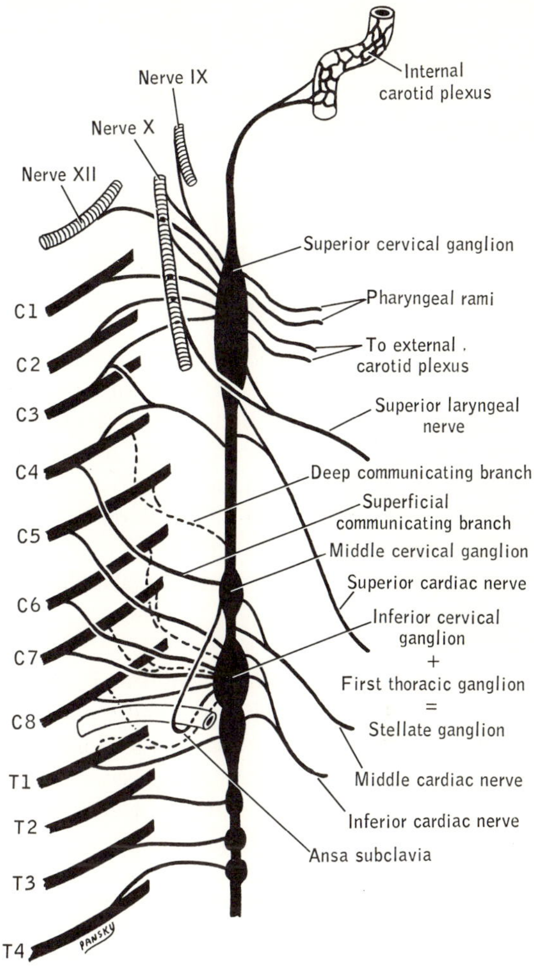

Fig. 15-5. The cervical sympathetic trunk and its ganglia. (*Adapted from Woerdeman, Atlas of Human Anatomy, McGraw-Hill Book Company, Inc., Blakiston Division, New York, 1950.*)

Pupil of the Eye

The pupils widen because of excitation of the dilator pupillae muscle (Fig. 15-8).

Blood Pressure

This is elevated through two methods: (1) constriction of the peripheral (skin) and visceral arteries; (2) cardiac acceleration.

Cardiac Rate

This is greatly *increased* (Fig. 15-3).

Visceral Musculature

Its activity is inhibited, accounting in part for "sour stomach" if a crisis occurs immediately after eating (Fig. 15-3).

External Sphincters

Their function is *activated*. Thus, the sphincters are closed more tightly (Figs. 15-3, 15-4).

Salivary and Digestive Glands

Their activity is *inhibited*. This accounts for dryness of the mouth, so often encountered, and also, in part, for indigestion when emergencies arise after eating (Figs. 15-6, 15-7). It is likely that the inhibition of glandular activity is not brought about by a direct influence on the cells themselves but through the constriction of blood vessels which supply the glandular alveoli.

Adrenal Medulla

Its function is *activated*. Epinephrine is poured into the blood stream, enhancing and reinforcing all the activities just mentioned. In addition, it is responsible for the release of glycogen from the liver, the material necessary to furnish energy for muscle contractions (Fig. 15-4).

Reflex Circuits Involving the Thoracolumbar Outflow

It is now possible to trace certain specific reflexes, the afferent limbs of which have been discussed elsewhere in a general way (Chaps. 8, 9, 10, 11).

Somatovisceral Type

A stimulus is applied in a somatic area, and afferent impulses travel over the GSA system. The efferent limb is the thoracolumbar part of the autonomic system. Such reflexes are dilation of the pupil caused by severe pain owing to injury to any part of the body or to sweating as a result of pain.

Viscerovisceral Type

Stimuli produced by changes within the viscera lead to reflex action. The afferent limb belongs to the GVA system, the efferent limb again being the thoracolumbar outflow. This action includes such reflexes as a rise of blood pressure when internal pressure in the great vessels falls too low, and an increase in cardiac rate due to low oxygen or high carbon dioxide concentration in the blood.

CRANIOSACRAL DIVISION

Although the cells of this division occupy a portion typical for the visceral efferent system in the CNS, the column is interrupted in many places. Even in the brain stem, where much of the division's concentration occurs, there are considerable gaps between cell groups (Fig. 15-9). For example, the distance between the nucleus of the vagus, the most caudal portion of the cranial outflow, and the second sacral segment of the cord, is enormous. Because of the discontinuity of both nuclei and the nerves in which the fibers run, it is necessary to describe the cranial and sacral parts individually.

Cranial Outflow

Cells of the Preganglionic Fibers

Edinger-Westphal Nucleus. (Figs. 15-8, 15-9.) The small cells belonging to this nucleus are located at the upper level of the mesencephalon, where they make a cap for the rostral end of the oculomotor nucleus, some cells being medial, others dorsal and somewhat lateral to the latter.

Superior Salivatory Nucleus. (Figs. 15-7, 15-9.) This is a group of small cells the exact position of which is in some doubt. It apparently lies in the junctional zone between medulla and pons,[2] in line (longitudinally) with the dorsal motor nucleus of the vagus and just a short distance rostral to the latter.

Inferior Salivatory Nucleus. (Figs. 15-6, 15-9.) This actually represents the caudal end of the superior salivatory nucleus.

[2] According to some investigators, it lies in the lateral reticular formation close to the rostral end of the nucleus ambiguus. This, however, would seem to be too far lateral.

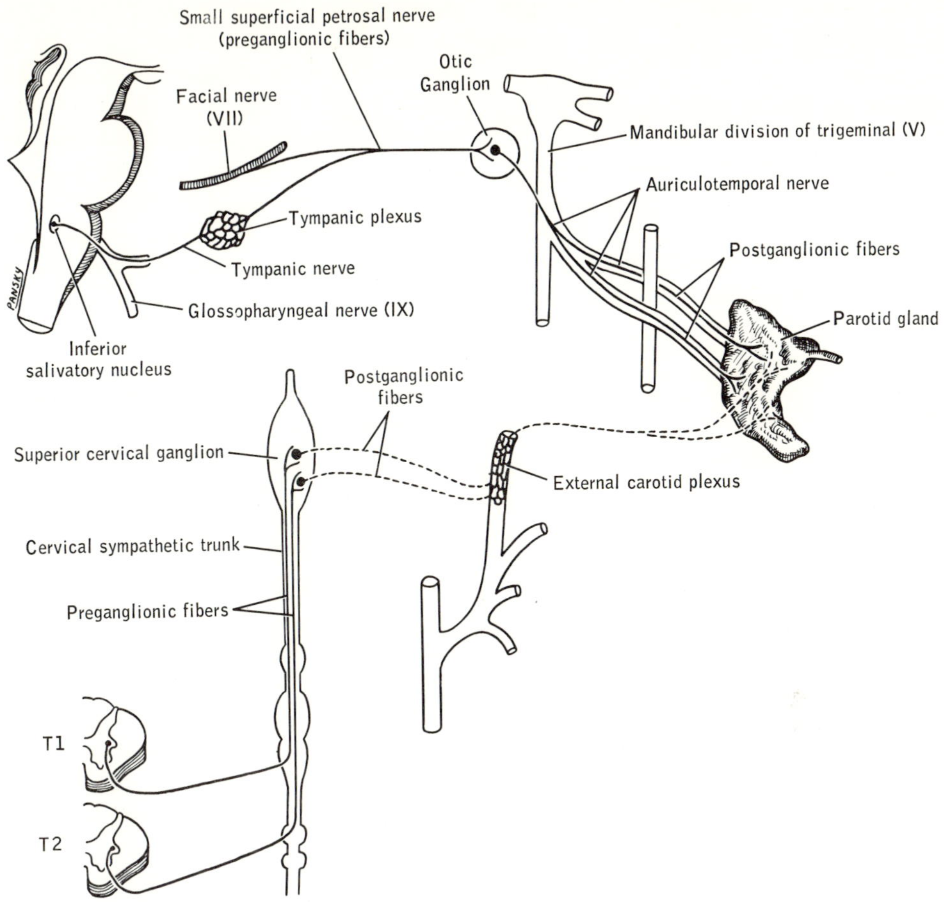

Fig. 15-6. Cranial autonomic nerves, with special emphasis on the connections of the otic ganglion, chiefly through nerve IX and the superior cervical sympathetic ganglion. Dotted lines—postganglionic fibers of the thoracolumbar outflow.

Lacrimal Nucleus. (Figs. 15-7, 15-9.) Although its presence has not been definitely established, some of the cells lying in the same region or at the rostral end of the superior salivatory nucleus may be especially concerned with the secretion of the lacrimal gland.

Dorsal Motor Nucleus of the Vagus. (Figs. 15-3, 15-9, 25-2 to 25-4.) This fairly large group of cells extends from near the pons-medulla junction to the level of the pyramidal decussation. It lies parallel and just lateral to the nucleus of the hypoglossal nerve, just below the floor of the fourth ventricle, in the area called the *ala cinerea.*

Axons of Preganglionic Fibers

Edinger-Westphal Nucleus. (Fig. 15-8.) Axons pass ventrally from the nucleus and join those fibers arising in the oculomotor (III) nucleus. The intramedullary and peripheral course to the orbit is the same as already described for nerve III. On entering the orbit, the oculomotor nerve divides into superior and inferior rami. The visceral efferents run in the larger, inferior ramus. They follow this a short distance and then diverge to form the *short root* of the *ciliary ganglion,* in which the preganglionic fibers terminate. There is now some evidence that certain of these preganglionic fibers continue through the ciliary ganglion without synapse and, passing through the short ciliary nerves, reach the ocular bulb, where they terminate among cells in or on the sclera, the *episcleral ganglion.*

Superior Salivatory Nucleus (and Lacrimal). (Fig. 15-7.) From this nucleus, the axons pass ventrolaterally to join the second part of the facial nerve, the fibers of which they accompany to the periphery, where they join the incoming sensory fibers. Together with the latter, these autonomic preganglionic fibers form the *nervus intermedius,* which lies at the medial side of the large motor root of nerve VII. From the brain stem, the autonomic fibers accompany the facial nerve to just beyond the geniculate ganglion. As the facial nerve bends sharply to enter the facial canal, a large number of autonomic fibers continues forward as the *greater superficial petrosal nerve.* As this nerve emerges from the cranial cavity through the hiatus of the facial canal, it passes over the foramen lacerum, where it is joined by the *deep petrosal nerve* (autonomic sympathetic) to form the *nerve of the pterygoid canal* (vidian). This nerve runs through the pterygoid canal at the base of the medial pterygoid plate to enter the pterygopalatine fossa, where it joins the sphenopalatine ganglion. The parasympathetic preganglionic fibers of the facial nerve terminate in this ganglion.

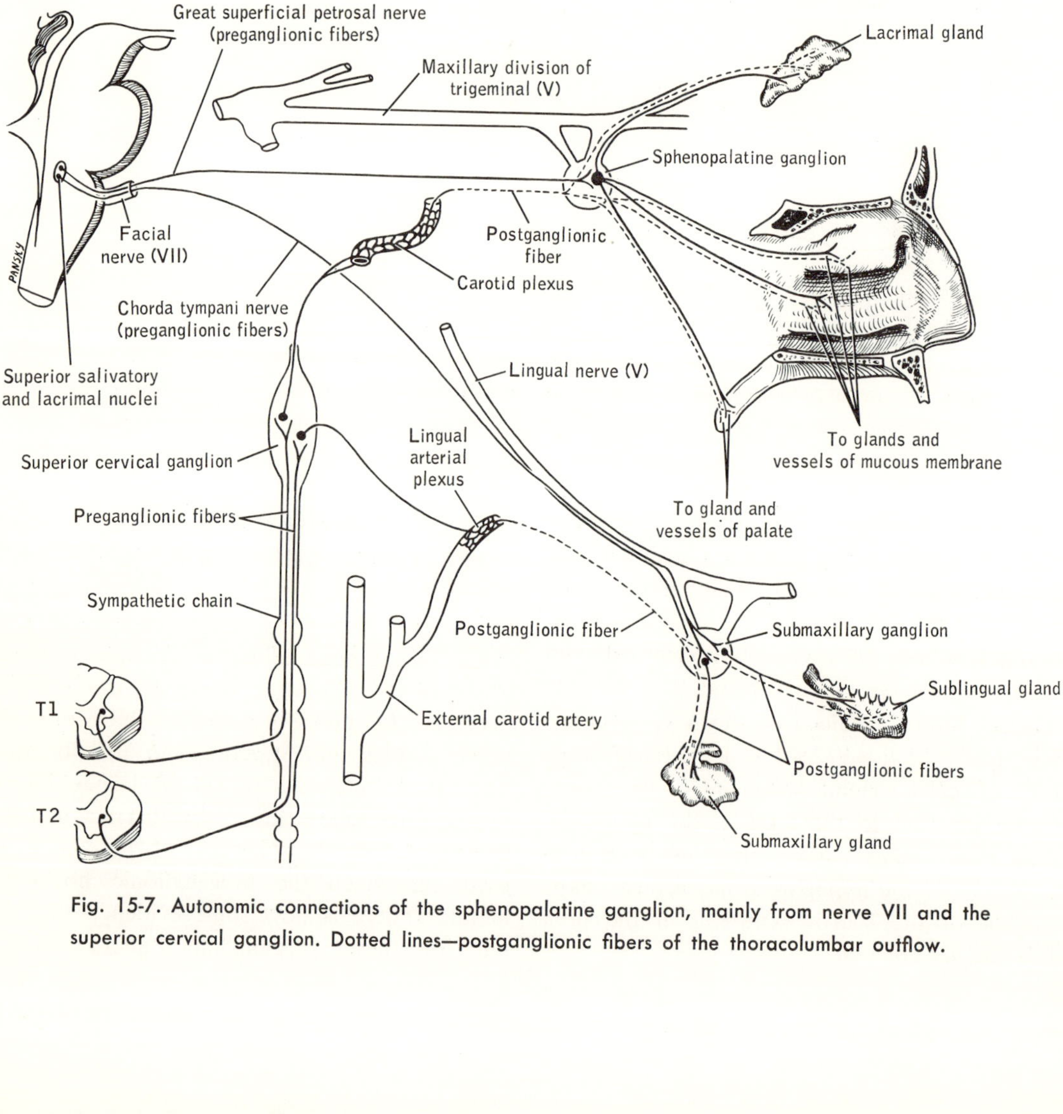

Fig. 15-7. Autonomic connections of the sphenopalatine ganglion, mainly from nerve VII and the superior cervical ganglion. Dotted lines—postganglionic fibers of the thoracolumbar outflow.

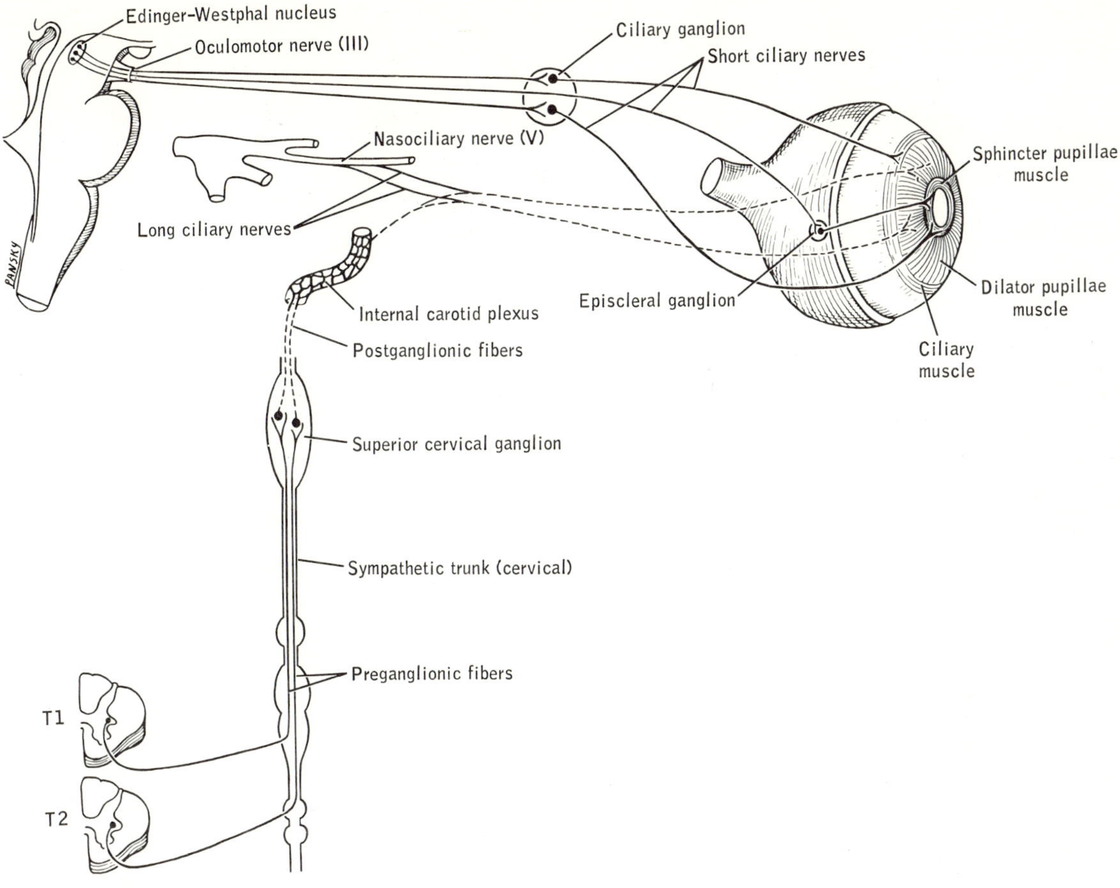

Fig. 15-8. Autonomic connections of the ciliary and episcleral ganglia through the oculomotor nerve (III) and the superior cervical ganglion. Dotted lines—postganglion fibers of the thoracolumbar outflow.

Some of the fibers arising in the *superior salivatory nucleus* continue for some distance through the facial canal behind the tympanic cavity. Above the stylomastoid foramen, the autonomic fibers diverge, running upward and forward to enter the tympanic cavity. The fibers cross the lateral side of this cavity, between the malleus and the incus, as the *chorda tympani* nerve. This nerve now leaves the tympanic cavity through the petrotympanic fissure and descends to join the posterior border of the lingual branch of the mandibular division of the trigeminal nerve (V). As the latter swings above the submandibular gland, the preganglionic autonomic fibers leave the lingual nerve to enter the *submandibular ganglion,* where they terminate.

Inferior Salivatory Nucleus. (Fig. 15-6.) Axons from this nucleus pass ventrocaudally, join the SVE fibers of the glossopharyngeal nerve (IX), which they accompany to the point at which this nerve leaves the skull through the jugular foramen. Just below this foramen, the autonomic fibers leave the main trunk and pass upward as the *tympanic nerve* (Jacobson) into the middle ear cavity, where the nerve forms a plexus (tympanic) on the medial wall of the tympanic cavity. From the plexus, the *lesser*

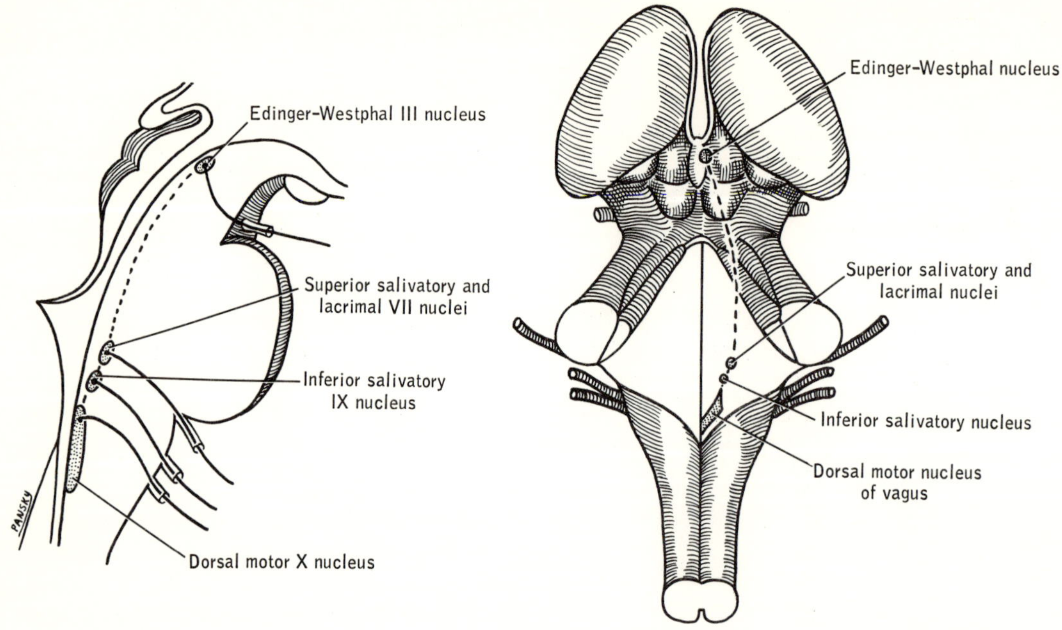

Fig. 15-9. Diagram of the cranial nuclear column of the GVE system. *Left,* lateral view; *right,* dorsal view.

superficial petrosal nerve runs forward to join the *otic ganglion.*

Dorsal Motor Nucleus of the Vagus Nerve. (Figs. 15-3, 25-4.) Axons from this nucleus pass ventrolaterally to join the SVE fibers, which they accompany in their intramedullary course. They continue downward through the neck, into the thorax and abdomen, synapsing in the *terminal ganglia* located in or near the walls of the viscera which are to be innervated.

Cells of the Postganglionic Fibers

These lie in the ganglia indicated above, namely: the ciliary, sphenopalatine, submandibular, otic, and terminal.

Axons of Postganglionic Fibers (Figs. 17-18, 17-22.)

Ciliary Ganglion. (Fig. 15-8.) Several groups of fibers, the *short ciliary nerves,* pass forward from this ganglion. They pierce the sclera of the eye and run forward to reach the ciliary and the sphincter pupillae muscles. Those fibers arising in the ciliary ganglion and passing to the sphincter are said to function mainly in reflex reactions involving light. Recent studies of the nerve terminals in the muscles of the iris using electronmicrography have demonstrated that there are two types of endings. The first contains numerous small, agranular vesicles 200–500 Å in diameter (synaptic vesicles). In addition, there are a few large vesicles 800–1000 Å in diameter containing central cores of variable size and density. These are found in the sphincter pupillae and are cholinergic. The second type also shows the same small nongranular vesicles but contains a large number possessing a central granule of high density. These are found in the dilator papillae and are adrenergic.

Sphenopalatine Ganglion. (Fig. 15-7.) From this ganglion, some postganglionic fibers join the maxillary division of the trigeminal nerve. They travel in its zygomatic branch, then diverge to join the *lacrimal branch of* the *ophthalmic division of nerve V,* and pass with this nerve to innervate the *lacrimal gland.* Other postganglionic fibers accompany the *nasal* and *palatine nerves* to supply the *glands* in the *mucous membranes of the nose and palate.*

Submandibular Ganglion. The postganglionic fibers here are short and almost immediately enter the substance of the submandibular and sublingual glands where they terminate especially around some of the serous cells.

Otic Ganglion. (Fig. 15-6.) The postganglionic fibers leave the ganglion by two small twigs which join both roots of the *auriculotemporal branch of the mandibular division of nerve V.* This nerve then carries the autonomic fibers in its upward course. As it passes the parotid gland, the autonomic postganglionic fibers leave the main nerve trunk and enter the parotid gland among the serous acinar cells. It should be recalled that the sympathetic postganglionic fibers terminate around the smooth muscle of the blood vessels and thus inhibit secretion of the gland by vasoconstriction.

Terminal Ganglia. From these, the postganglionic fibers tend to be very short. To the sphincter pupillae, they represent axons from the cells lying upon the sclera in the so-called *episcleral ganglion* (Fig. 15-8). These are the fibers said to subserve the reflex constriction of the pupil in near vision (accommodation). For the heart and lungs, fibers arise from ganglion cells lying upon the heart wall and bronchi (the cardiac and pulmonary plexuses, respectively) (Fig. 15-3). In the viscera of the alimentary tract, they lie entirely within the walls of the viscera (Fig. 15-3). One group of ganglion cells lies in the connective tissue between the smooth muscle coats. This is called *Auerbach's* (*myenteric*) plexus. The postganglionic fibers arising here supply the smooth muscles. Another group of ganglion cells lies in the submucous coat. This is *Meissner's* (*submucosal*) *plexus.* Its fibers (postganglionic) supply the glands of the tract.

Sacral Outflow

Structure

Cells of the Preganglionic Fibers. (Fig. 15-4.) The cells of this portion of the system lie in the intermediolateral cell column of the spinal cord at the second, third, and fourth sacral segments.

Axons of the Preganglionic Fibers. These fibers pass ventrally to leave the cord with the ventral roots of the second, third, and fourth sacral nerves by *white rami communicantes,* which together are considered pelvic splanchnic or pelvic nerves. These nerves pass ventrally across the pelvis to end in terminal ganglia about the pelvic viscera and in the wall of the colon, from the region of the splenic flexure downward.

Cells of the Postganglionic Fibers. (Fig. 15-4.) These cells lie in terminal ganglia in the connective tissue coverings of the pelvic viscera and the lower half of the colon.

Axons of the Postganglionic Fibers. (Fig. 15-4.) These are relatively short, arising from cells lying in or on the wall of the viscera and passing to the smooth muscle and glands of the pelvic viscera and colon.

General Function

As with the thoracolumbar outflow, there is no set pattern of reaction. This, too, is determined by the individuality of the organ supplied. However, when the underlying function of this division as a whole is understood, many of its specific reactions can be predicted.

Unlike the sympathetic portion, the craniosacral outflow is a *conservative mechanism*—to save wear and tear and to conserve energy. On this basis, its effects are directly opposed to that of the sympathetic system. It brings visceral function back to a normal level of activity after sympathetic activation. In accomplishing this, there are certain striking differences between these two parts of the autonomic system. In the first place, the parasympathetic system is not anatomically adapted to work as a unit, its regions of origin in the CNS often being widely separated. Furthermore, there is no gland (adrenal medulla) whose hormones act upon the tissues of the entire body. This division of the autonomic systems appears to be somewhat less influenced by higher control centers. In other words, this system can work upon individual organs or organ groups one at a time, as circumstances in those organs demand at a given time. This latter condition is made more certain by the fact that any excess acetylcholine produced at the axon terminals of this division is immediately destroyed by cholinesterase before it can spread through the tissues or into the blood stream.

Specific Reactions

Pupil. The pupil is constricted, thus exhibiting a form of conservation. First, by cutting down the light, visual purple is not broken down so rapidly. Second, it makes the effort put out by the ciliary muscle to accommodate for near vision more efficient by letting in just the correct amount of light.

Blood Pressure. Since high blood pressure is more wearing on the walls of the vessels and upon other tissues and organs, as well as on the heart, it is reasonable that the parasympathetic system should *reduce blood pressure*.

Cardiac Rate. Logically, the faster the heart works, the more energy must be expended and the greater will be the strain put upon the cardiac muscle fibers. Therefore, the parasympathetic system *slows the heart rate*.

Bronchial Smooth Muscle. This is *activated* to constrict the bronchioles. This constriction may occur to protect the delicate pulmonary air sacs from exposure to substances in the inhaled air.

Visceral Smooth Muscle. This is *activated*. Intestinal motility is essential for the digestion and absorption of ingested food and is, therefore, conservative.

Glands of the Alimentary Canal. These are *stimulated to secrete* enzymes, an action necessary for the utilization of ingested materials.

Certain Sphincters. When one understands that the elimination of waste substances is essential for better function of the body and is, therefore, conservative, the *relaxation of certain sphincters* (internal) about the *urethra* and *anal canal,* together with the *contraction of the smooth muscle of the bladder and rectum,* seems perfectly reasonable.

Reflex Circuits Involving the Craniosacral Outflow

It is now possible to complete some of the reflexes the afferent limbs of which were described under the sensory systems (Chaps. 8 to 11).

Somatovisceral

Several reflexes of this type are well-known; among them are lacrimation, due to corneal or conjunctival irritation; and engorgement of the penis, resulting from stimulation of the genital region. Both require the GSA system for the afferent limb. Constriction of the pupil in bright light belongs to this group, except that in this case the SSA system acts as the afferent portion.

Viscerovisceral

Among the more common of these reflexes is the reflex secretion of the salivary glands in response to either taste or smell. In either case, the SVA system is the afferent limb. Slowing of the heart when blood pressure becomes too high, and the activation of glands of the digestive system in response to the presence of material in the lumen of the viscera are also reflexes of this general class. In such instances the GVA system acts as the afferent limb.

CLINICAL CONSIDERATIONS

Thoracolumbar (Sympathetic) System

Testing

There may be many observations which involve parts of this system, but it becomes a problem whether the essential pathologic condition lies in this part of the autonomic system or whether it lies elsewhere but is manifested through this system. Some of the necessary observations include (1) the size and reactions of the pupil; (2) the color and temperature of the skin, especially the distal portions of the upper and lower extremities; (3) cardiac rate and blood pressure under various conditions of rest and exercise; (4) roentgenologic visualization of the blood vessels (angiography). In addition, information should be sought concerning the digestive processes, including salivation and the activities of the lower bowel; lacrimation; temperature control, especially sweating; and the function of the bladder.

Specific Pathology

Horner's Syndrome.[3] This syndrome is characterized by miosis, due to paralysis of the dilator of the pupil; a partial ptosis, due to paralysis of the upper tarsal muscle; and enophthalmos, due to paralysis of the orbital or retrobulbar muscle of Müller. In addition, in complete Horner's syndrome, there are ipsilateral dilatation of vessels of the face, hand, neck, and conjunctiva, plus ipsilateral anhidrosis. This syndrome may be the result of the interruption of the descending sympathetic pathways in the brain stem or spinal cord, of lesions in the cord at the level of the ciliospinal center, of lesions of the preganglionic fibers in or after they leave the cord, of injury to the cervical sympathetic ganglia, or of involvement of postganglionic fibers.

Raynaud's Disease. This is characterized by pallor or cyanosis of the distal extremities, especially the fingers. Sometimes the nose and ears are involved. This is usually brought on by cold or emotion. When of long standing, cutaneous gangrene, due to lack of adequate circulation, may occur. This condition may be the result of overactivity of the vasoconstrictor fibers of the thoracolumbar outflow.

Buerger's Disease (Thromboangiitis Obliterans). This is said to be an inflammatory and obliterative disease of the blood vessels, particularly of the lower extremities. Reduced circulation here may also lead to gangrene. This condition may have had its inception in, or may be aggravated by, overactivity of the vasoconstrictor fibers.

[3] Some of the terms used to describe this syndrome are defined as follows: miosis, an excessive contraction of the pupil; ptosis, drooping of the upper eyelid; enophthalmos, abnormal retraction of the eye into the orbit; and anhidrosis, an abnormal deficiency of sweat.

Erythromelalgia. This disease affects the vessels of the extremities, most frequently the hands, in which there is paroxysmal, bilateral vasodilatation, with burning pain and increased skin temperature. It may possibly be due to a lack of activity on the part of the vasoconstrictor fibers.

Hirschsprung's Disease. This is characterized by hypertrophic dilatation of the colon. It may have had its basis in overactive inhibitor fibers acting upon the colon, allowing dilatation to occur because of the accumulation of fecal material. It may also be due to congenital autonomic aplasia.

Hypertension. This term is used here to denote generalized high blood pressure. Because of the importance of this part of the autonomic system in raising blood pressure, it becomes suspect in the hypertensive patient.

Craniosacral (Parasympathetic) System

Testing

It should be realized that because of the intimate relations of the fibers of this system with others, both motor and sensory, there is little chance that only general visceral efferents will be involved. Therefore, symptoms due to damage of the parasympathetic nerves will be brought out when examination of individual cranial nerves is made. In general, the following items should be kept in mind: (1) the pupils should be checked for constriction in response to light and near objects; (2) the eye can be examined for evidence of the lack of lacrimation; (3) the use of such substances as lemon juice is adequate to test salivary secretion; (4) the usual check of cardiac rate and blood pressure, particularly the time required for both to return to normal, after exercise, may give some clue to the integrity of the system; (5) the digestive processes and the condition of the alimentary canal may give evidence about the parasympathetic nerves; (6) information concerning sexual activity, particularly the ability to erect the penis, should be sought, since engorgement of the genital vessels is a part of the parasympathetic function.

SUMMARY
General Visceral Efferent

Thoracolumbar Division		Craniosacral Division
1. Intermediolateral gray column of the thoracic and upper lumbar cord	Cell body	1. Edinger-Westphal (EW) nucleus, in upper mesencephalon Superior salivatory nucleus at pons-medulla junction Inferior salivatory nucleus, just caudal to the above nucleus Dorsal motor nucleus of the vagus, in medulla Intermediolateral cell column of the sacral cord at levels S2, S3, and S4
2. Through the ventral roots of thoracic and upper lumbar spinal nerves and by white rami communicantes to: Synapse in chain (paravertebral) ganglion at level of entry Ascend or descend in thoracic and lumbar sympathetic trunk to synapse in chain ganglia above or below level of entry Ascend in the cervical sympathetic trunk to synapse in the inferior, middle, or superior cervical ganglia Continue transversely through the sympathetic chain, still as preganglionics, especially at levels T6 through T12 (the splanchnic nerves), to synapse in the prevertebral ganglia (i.e., celiac) or the adrenal medulla	Preganglionic fiber and synapse	2. From the EW nucleus via nerve III to terminate by synapse either in ciliary ganglion or episcleral ganglion From superior salivatory ganglion via nervus intermedius, facial nerve (VII), great superficial petrosal nerve, and nerve of the pterygoid canal to terminate in the sphenopalatine ganglion From the superior salivatory ganglion via nervus intermedius, facial (VII), chorda tympani, and lingual nerves to the submaxillary ganglion From the inferior salivatory nucleus through the glossopharyngeal nerve (IX), tympanic nerve, tympanic plexus, and lesser superficial petrosal nerve to synapse in the otic ganglion From the dorsal motor nucleus of the vagus via the vagus nerve (X) to terminal ganglia lying near, in, or on the walls of the viscera Through the ventral roots of the corresponding sacral nerves (S2, S3, and S4), as the pelvic splanchnic nerves, to terminate in the terminal ganglia in or on the walls of the lower colon and pelvic viscera
3. From chain ganglia, through gray rami communicantes to spinal nerves for distribution to peripheral blood vessels; smooth muscle (arrector pili); and glands of the skin From certain chain ganglia, especially upper thoracic, to bronchi and lungs From inferior and middle cervical ganglia as cardiac nerves to the heart From the superior cervical ganglion, mainly through the carotid plexus and by fibers along the branches of the carotid, to the blood vessels of the head; the glands of the head; the smooth muscles and glands in the skin of the head; and the dilator pupillae, together with the smooth muscle of the lids and orbit, of the eye	Postganglionic fiber and termination	3. From ciliary ganglion to ciliary muscle and sphincter pupillae muscles, for light From the episcleral ganglion to muscles as above, for accomodation From sphenopalatine ganglion, to maxillary division of trigeminal (V), through zygomatic branch, to the lacrimal branch of the ophthalmic division of the trigeminal (V), to the lacrimal gland From the sphenopalatine ganglion, through nasal and palatine nerves, to glands of nose and palate From submaxillary ganglion to submaxillary and sublingual glands From otic ganglion through the auriculotemporal branch of the mandibular division of the trigeminal nerve (V) to the parotid gland From terminal ganglia of: Cardiac plexus--to heart Pulmonary plexus--to bronchi Auerbach's plexus--to smooth muscle of viscera (digestive system) Meissner's plexus--to glands of viscera (digestive system) From terminal ganglia of pelvis to smooth muscles and glands of pelvic viscera including lower colon

INNERVATION OF THE VISCERA

ORGAN	SYMPATHETIC PREGANGLIONIC	SYMPATHETIC POSTGANGLIONIC	SYMPATHETIC ACTION	PARASYMPATHETIC PREGANGLIONIC	PARASYMPATHETIC POSTGANGLIONIC	PARASYMPATHETIC ACTION
Arrector pili	All levels	All ganglia of trunk and chain	Erects hair	Not proved to be present		
Bladder muscle	TII-L2	Hypogastric gang. and plexus	Relaxes	S2-S4	Intrinsic ganglia	Contracts
Cavernous tissue	L2	Hypogastric gang. and plexus	Deturgescence	S2-S4	Vesical plexus	Turgescence
Ciliary muscle	C8-T3	Sup. Cervical gang.	Relaxes	E.-W. nucieus	Episcleral gang.	Contracts
Colon	T6-T10	Sup. and Inf. Mesenteric Gang. and Plexi	Inhibits Peristalsis	Dorsal Motor X	Myenteric and Submucosal Plexi	Excites peristalsis
Coronary vessels	T1-T5	Cervical and Thoracic gang.	Dilates	Dorsal Motor X	Cardiac plexus and ganglia	Constricts
Heart Muscle	T1-T5	Cervical and Thoracic gang.	Accelerates rate	Dorsal Motor X R. Vagus..SA node L. Vagus..AV node	Cardiac plexus and ganglia	Decelerates rate
Iris of eye	C8-T3	Sup. Cervical gang.	Dilates pupil	E.-W. nucleus	Ciliary gang.	Constricts pupil
Kidney	T10-T11	Renal Gang. and plexus	Constricts pelvis and vessels	Not proved to be present		
Lacrimal gland	T1-T3	Sup. Cervical gang.	Vasoconstricts to reduce secretion	Lacrimal or Superior salivatory	Sphenopalatine gang.	Stimulates secretion
Liver	T5-T6	Celiac gang. and plexus	Glycogenolysis	Dorsal Motor X	Unknown	Contracts Gall Bladder
Lung	T2-T5	Thoracic gang.	Relaxes bronchial mm.	Dorsal Motor X	Pulmonary plexus	Constricts bronchi
Mammary gland	T2-T6	Thoracic gang.	Constricts ducts	Not proved to be present		
Nasal and oral glands	T1-T3	Sup. Cervical gang.	Vasoconstr. to reduce secretion	Lacrimal or sup. salivatory nuclei	Sphenopalatine gang.	Stimulates secretion
Pancreas	T5-T6	Celiac gang. and plexus	Vasoconstr. to reduce secretion	Dorsal Motor X	Intrinsic ganglia	Increases secretion
Parotid Gland	T1-T3	Sup. Cervical gang.	Vasoconstr. to reduce secretion	Inf. Salivat. nucleus	Otic ganglion	Stimulates secretion
Stomach	T6-T10	Celiac gang. and plexus	Inhibits peristalsis, Vasoconstr., Inhibits secretion	Dorsal Motor X	Myenteric and submucosal plexi	Stimulates peristalsis and secretions
Small Intestine	T6-T10	Celiac and Sup. mesenteric gang. and Plexus	Inhibits peristalsis, Inhibits secretion, Vasoconstr.	Dorsal Motor X	Myenteric and submucosal plexi	Stimulates peristalsis and secretion
Sphincters						
Anal	L2	Hypogastric gang. and Plexus	Constricts	S2-S4	Intrinsic gang.	Relaxes
Pyloric	T6-T10	Celiac gang. and plexus	Constricts	Dorsal Motor X	Myenteric gang.	Relaxes
Urethral	L2	Hypogastric gang. and plexus	Constricts	S2-S4	Intrinsic gang. and plexus	Relaxes
Sublingual and Submaxillary glands	T1-T3	Sup. Cervical gang.	Vasoconstr. to reduce secretion	Inf. Salivat. nucleus	Sphenopalatine and Submandibular ganglia	Stimulates secretion
Sweat glands	All levels	All trunk and chain ganglia	Stimulates secretion	Not proved to be present		

16 SPECIAL VISCERAL EFFERENT SYSTEM (SVE)

This is the motor system which supplies striated, skeletal muscle derived from the embryonic branchial arches. In the latter respect, it is different from the somatic efferent system which innervates muscle derived from somites (Chap. 14).

Early in development, the mesoderm surrounding the foregut becomes divided into four complete segments and one incomplete segment by the appearance of pharyngeal pouches and clefts (Figs. 5-16, 5-17). These divisions are called *branchial arches* and are usually designated by numbers arranged consecutively from rostral to caudal. One cranial nerve enters each of the first three arches: the trigeminal (V) into the first; the facial (VII) into the second; and the glossopharyngeal (IX) into the third. Branches from the vagus nerve (X) supply both the complete fourth and partial fifth arches.

Almost from the beginning, the nerves in each arch establish a close relationship with the premuscle masses which differentiate in the arch. This relationship persists throughout future development, regardless of the distance a muscle must migrate from its site of origin. On this basis, all the special visceral musculature can be arranged in groups, together with the nerve supply, according to the branchial arch from which the muscles came.

From the first branchial arch arise the *muscles of mastication,* all innervated by the *trigeminal nerve* (V). In addition to these are the *mylohyoid, anterior belly of the digastric, tensor veli palatini,* and the *tensor tympani* muscles, also supplied by the fifth cranial nerve.

All the muscles of *facial expression,* including the *occipitalis, frontalis, muscles of the auricle,* and the *platysma,* develop from the second branchial arch and are innervated by the *facial nerve* (VII). The *posterior belly of the digastric muscle,* as well as the *stapedius muscle,* also comes from this arch and is similarly innervated.

The *stylopharyngeus* is the only muscle which has been proved to arise from the third arch. It is probable, however, that some of the *pharyngeal constrictors* also arise here. These muscles are innervated by the *glossopharyngeal nerve* (IX).

Most of the muscles of the *pharynx* and all the muscles of the *larynx,* innervated by the *vagus nerve* (X), arise from the fourth and fifth arches. The *glossopharyngeus, glossopalatine,* and *levator veli palatini* muscles are also believed to be derived from the fourth arch, since they are likewise supplied by the vagus nerve.

Like the somatic motor column of the head, this nuclear column is discontinuous along its rostrocaudal extent (Figs. 5-18, 16-1). The special visceral efferent nuclei assume an intermediate position between the somatic and general visceral columns in a transverse plane but lie ventral to both.[1]

[1] Actually, some of these nuclei may be drawn somewhat out of line because of the tendency for cell masses to migrate in the direction from which most of their stimuli arrive. This is the theory of *neurobiotaxis.*

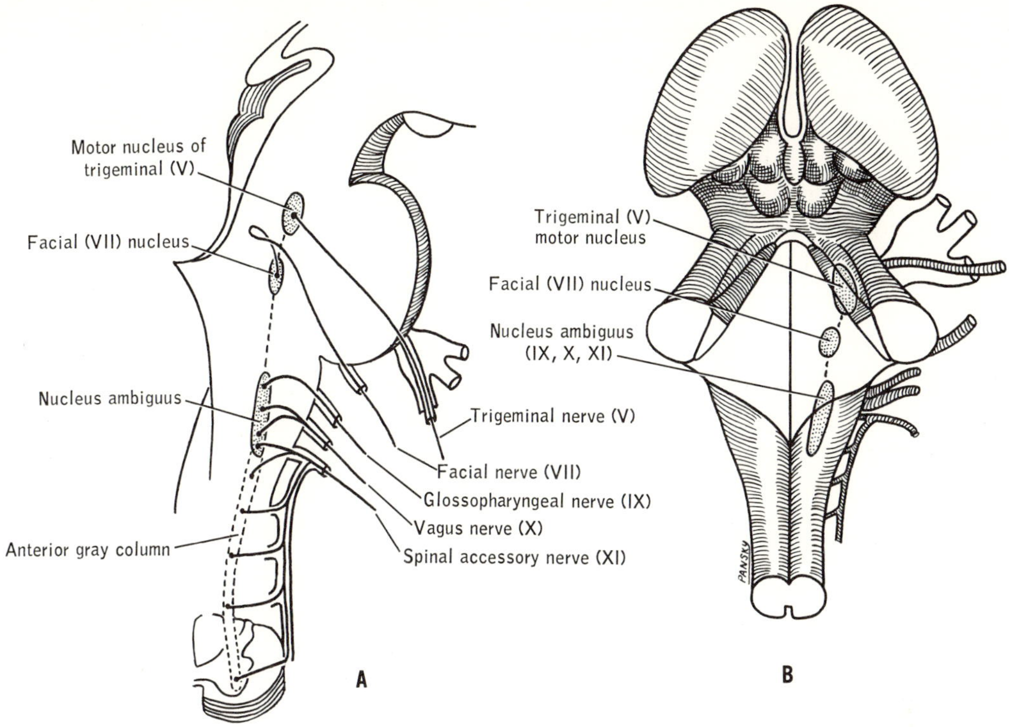

Fig. 16-1. Diagram of the special visceral efferent (SVE) nuclear column of the brain stem. *A.* Lateral view. *B.* Dorsal view.

PATHWAYS

Since this system is made up of fibers running in several cranial nerves, it is advantageous to describe each nerve individually.

Trigeminal Nerve (V)

Cell Body (Figs. 2-46, 16-2, 25-9.)

These are of the multipolar type, perhaps a little smaller than those in the somatic system. They are aggregated in the motor nucleus of the trigeminal nerve, located in the upper pons.

Axon (Figs. 2-46, 25-9.)

The single axons from each cell pass to the lateral aspect of the nucleus, where they encounter afferent fibers belonging to the trigeminal nerve. The motor fibers accompany the afferent fibers ventrolaterally across the pons to become superficial on its ventrolateral surface (Figs. 2-7, 2-8). Here, the motor fibers are collected in a bundle which is attached to the pons slightly rostral and medial to the larger mass of afferent fibers. The latter are spoken of as the *sensory root* or, since there are so many of them, the *portio major*. The efferents are collectively known as the *motor root* or *portio minor*.

After leaving the brain stem, the motor root lies along the medial side of the sensory root but not fused with it. It crosses the medial aspect of the posterior portion of the semilunar ganglion and continues downward along the mandibular division, to exit from the middle cranial fossa through the foramen ovale (Fig. 2-52). Just below the skull, the motor fibers actually become part of the mandibular root.

In response to the excitation of these fibers, a variety of activities ensues. The masseter and the pterygoid internus muscles close the jaw; the temporalis muscle closes the jaw and in part retracts the mandible; the pterygoid externus muscle is important in the grinding action, protruding the mandible and moving it from side to side. The anterior belly of the digastric muscle—and to a lesser degree the mylohyoid (when the hyoid bone is fixed)—depresses the mandible. The tensor tympani muscle increases tension on the tympanic membrane, while the tensor veli palatini muscle has a similar effect on the soft palate (Figs. 16-2, 17-18).

Facial Nerve (VII)

Cell Body (Figs. 2-47, 16-3, 25-8.)

These multipolar cells are grouped into a nucleus located in the ventrolateral portion of the pontine reticular formation not far from the caudal limit of the pons.

Axon (Figs. 2-47, 16-3, 25-7, 25-8.)

The axons from these cells pass dorsomedially from the nucleus in widely scattered bundles, the first part of the root of the facial nerve. These bundles approach the midline just beneath the floor of the fourth ventricle. Here they come together in a solid fascicle, the fibers now being directed rostrally along the medial side of the abducens nucleus, just dorsal to the medial longitudinal fasciculus. This portion is sometimes called the ascending part of the facial nerve. Near the rostral end of nucleus VI, the facial

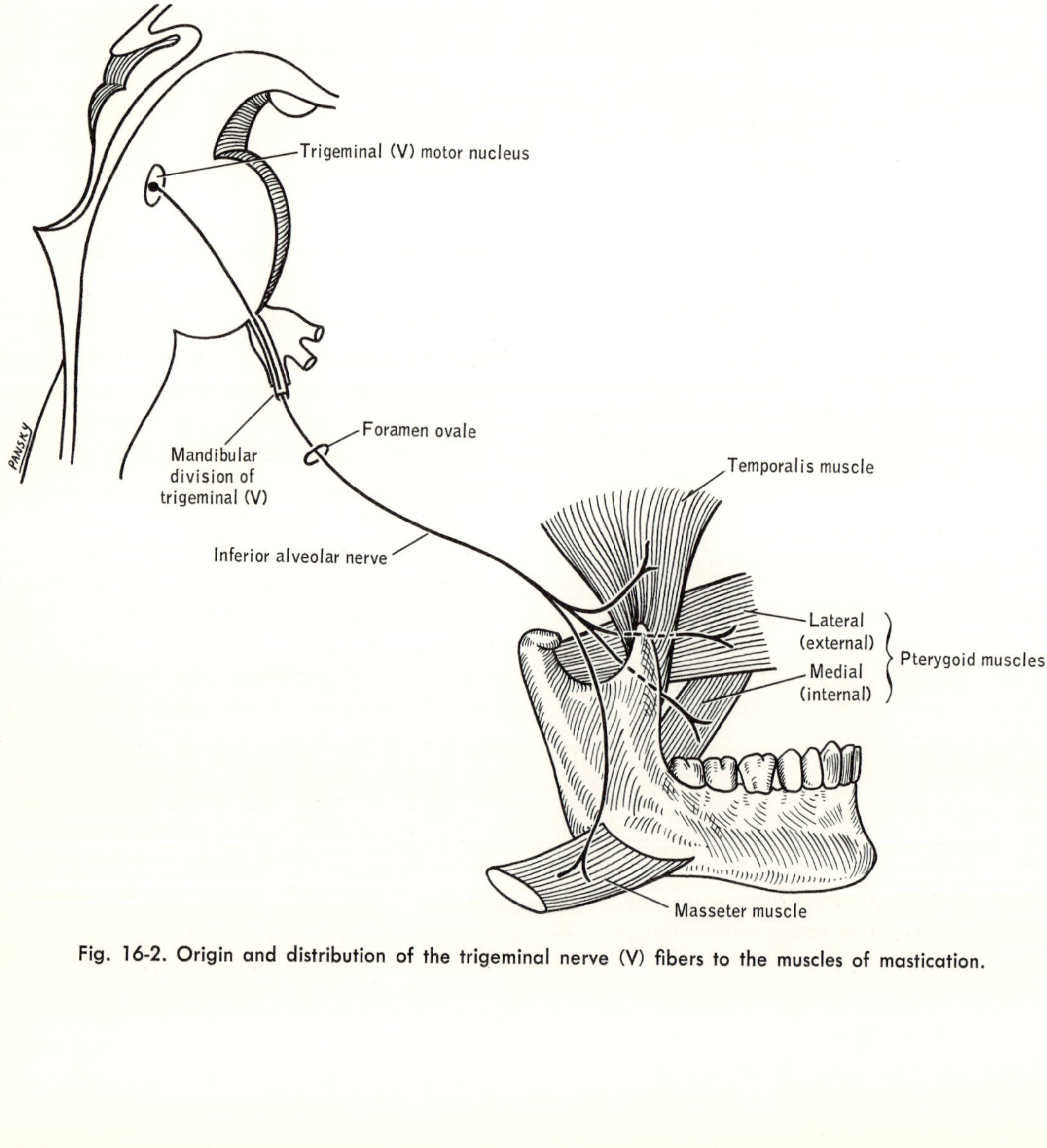

Fig. 16-2. Origin and distribution of the trigeminal nerve (V) fibers to the muscles of mastication.

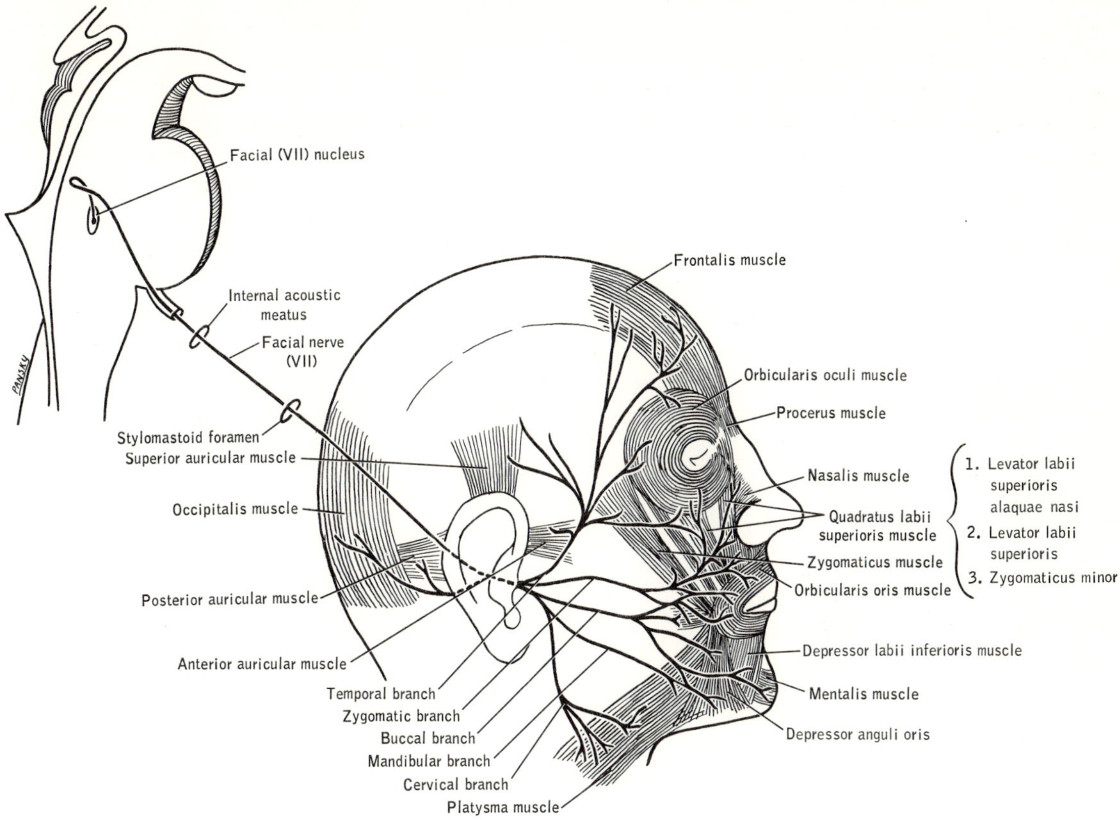

Fig. 16-3. Origin and distribution of the facial nerve (VII) to the muscles of facial expression.

fibers turn abruptly over the dorsal side of the abducens nucleus. This portion is known as the internal genu.[2] After crossing the abducens nucleus, the facial fibers are directed ventrolaterally with considerable caudal drift so that this group, called the second part of the root of the facial nerve, passes near the lateral side of the facial nucleus to exit from the lateral aspect of the caudal pons medial to the superficial attachment of the acoustic nerve (Figs. 2-7, 2-8). After leaving the brain stem, facial fibers run in close proximity to the acoustic nerve, the nervus intermedius lying between them. They continue laterally and enter the internal acoustic meatus (Figs. 2-52, 17-22).

[2] This is at least partially responsible for the elevation in the floor of the fourth ventricle called the *facial colliculus.* (Figs. 2-35, 2-36.)

The ability of the face to change expression, in response to impulses carried through the facial nerve, is well-known. The arrangement of the muscle fibers around the eyes and mouth has useful and important functions, especially in closing the eyelids (for protection), in moving the lips, in speaking, and in retaining food in the mouth while it is being masticated. The stapedius muscle puts tension on the stapes and, through it, on the membrane which supports it. This is an adjunct to hearing. The posterior belly of the digastric muscle helps to elevate and retract the hyoid, as in swallowing (Fig. 17-22).

Glossopharyngeal Nerve (IX)

Cell Body (Figs. 16-4, 25-5.)

The multipolar cells for this system are located in the nucleus ambiguus. This cell group is poorly circumscribed but has a considerable longitudinal extent (Fig. 16-1), located in the reticular formation throughout the length of the medulla oblongata. The cells of this nucleus are usually found scattered among the network of fibers in the lateral reticular formation between the inferior olive and the spinal trigeminal tract.

Axon (Figs. 16-4, 17-25, 25-5.)

These are from cells at the rostral end of the nucleus ambiguus. At first, they are directed dorsally. After a short distance they curve laterally and then pass ventrolaterally with some rostral drift to accompany afferents and general visceral efferents of nerve IX. On reaching the lateral aspect of the medulla, in company with the vagus nerve, they emerge along the posterolateral sulcus, dorsal to the olive (Figs. 2-7, 2-8). In company with the vagus and accessory nerves, the glossopharyngeal nerve courses caudally to leave the posterior cranial fossa through the jugular foramen (Fig. 2-52).

The action of the stylopharyngeus muscle in helping to elevate the pharynx and to increase the transverse diameter of the latter to receive the bolus of food from the mouth in the first part of deglutition, is of great importance (Fig. 16-4). Since it is not certain whether the glosso-

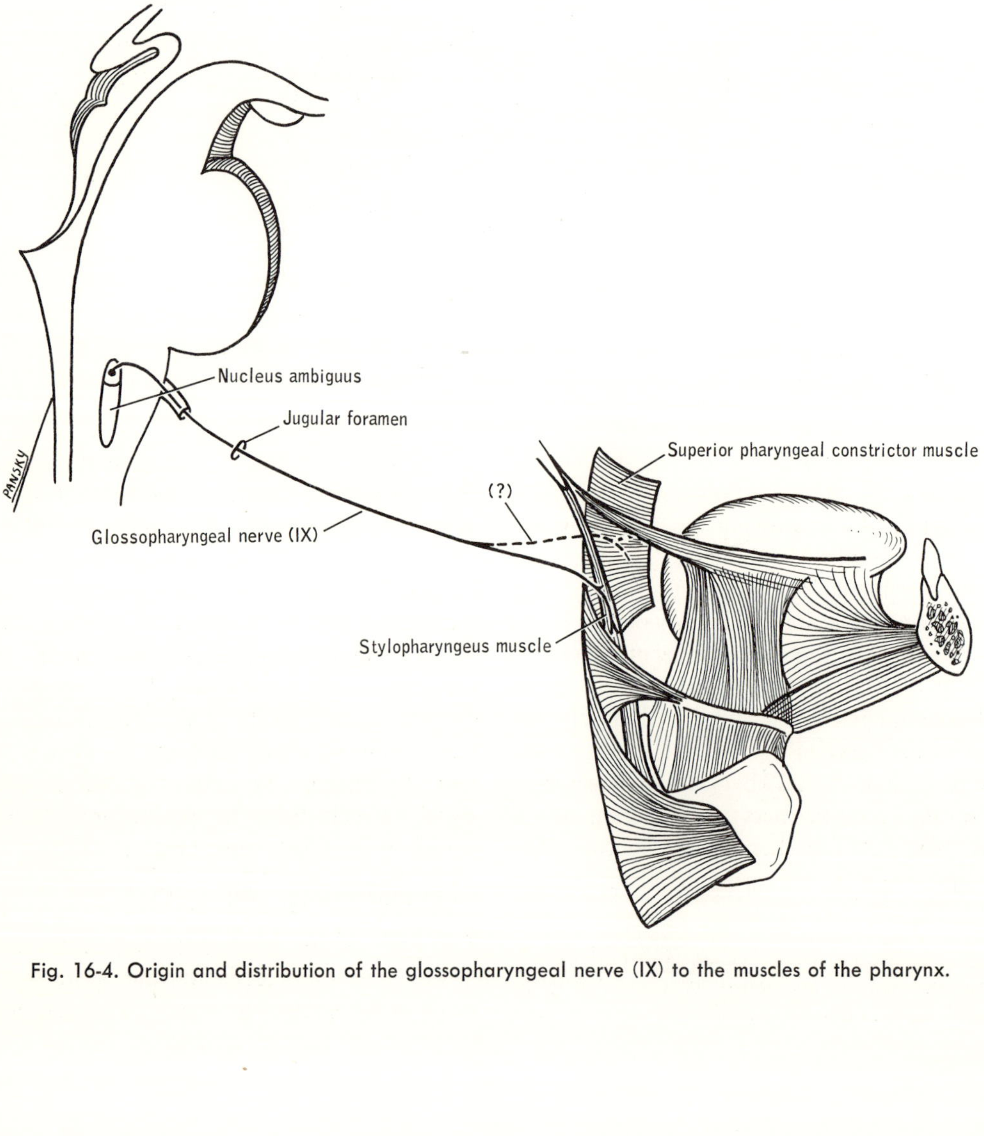

Fig. 16-4. Origin and distribution of the glossopharyngeal nerve (IX) to the muscles of the pharynx.

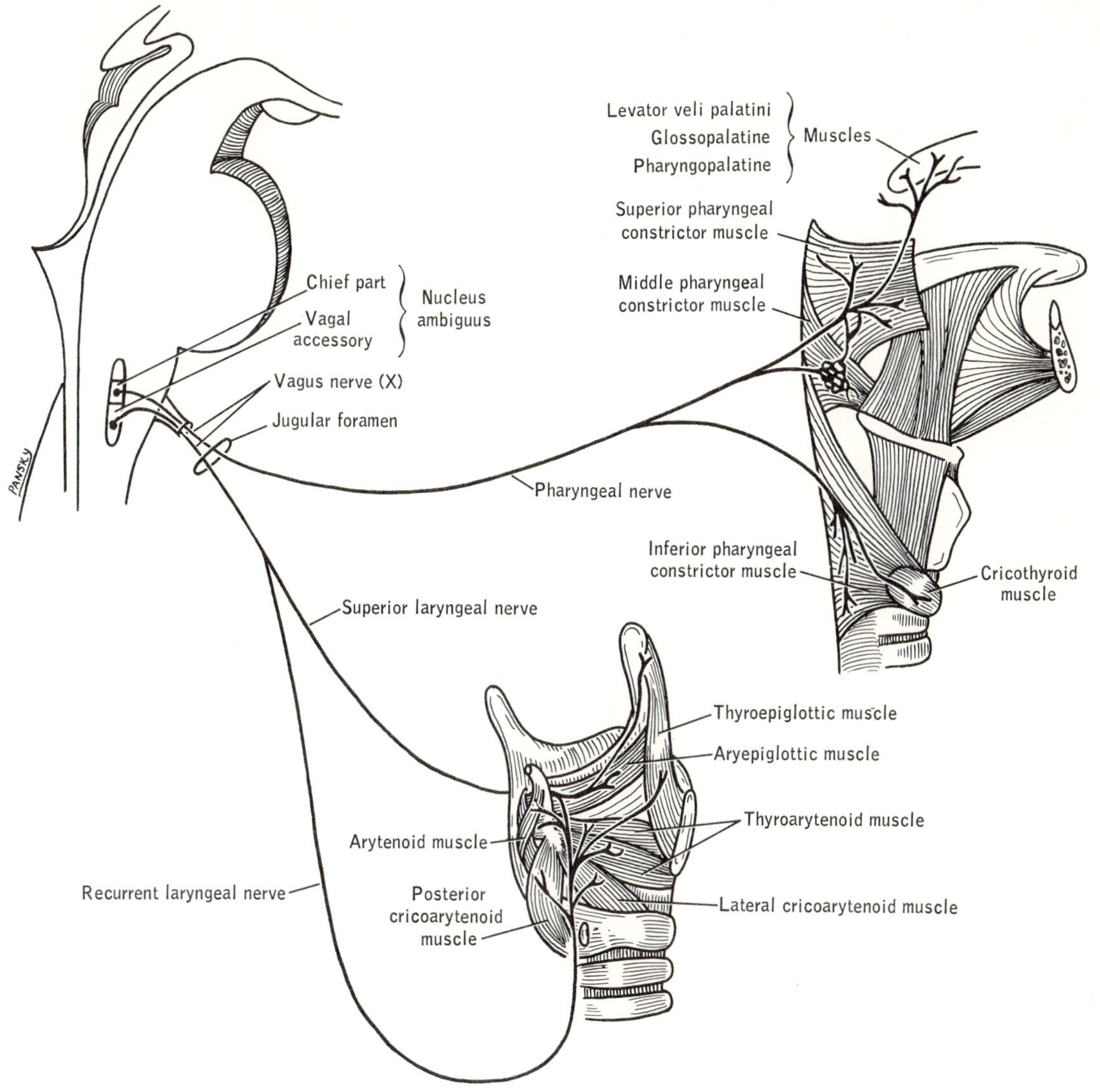

Fig. 16-5. Nucleus of origin and distribution of the SVE fibers of the vagus nerve (X) to the muscles of the palate, pharynx, and larynx.

pharyngeal nerve contributes to the innervation of the pharyngeal constrictors, their action will be discussed with the vagus nerve.

Vagus Nerve (X)

For the sake of convenience, the vagus nerve is considered as having two parts, a chief or rostral segment and a vagal accessory portion, not to be confused with cranial nerve XI.

Chief or Rostral Portions of the Vagus Nerve

Cell Body. (Figs. 2-48, 16-1, 16-5, 25-4.) The cells of this part of the vagus nerve lie in the lower rostral and intermediate portions of the nucleus ambiguus, its more rostral limit nearly overlapping the cells for the glossopharyngeal nerve.

Axon. (Figs. 2-7, 2-8, 2-52, 16-5, 25-4.)

The direction, course, and relations of these fibers, both within and outside the medulla, are similar to those already described for the glossopharyngeal nerve and need not be repeated.

The fibers of this part of the vagus nerve terminate in the pharyngeal constrictors, the levator veli palatini, the glossopalatine, and the pharyngopalatine muscles, which are essential for swallowing (Fig. 16-5). As the food mass moves from the tongue to glide over the epiglottis, the glossopalatine muscles, which act as constrictors of the fauces, contract behind the bolus, helping it move down and also preventing its return. At the same time, the levators of the palate raise the velum of the palate, both to accommodate the bolus and to prevent its passage into the nasopharynx. At the same time, the pharyngopalatine muscles are contracting to raise the pharynx over the bolus (Fig. 17-27).

Accessory Portion of the Vagus Nerve

Cell Body (Fig. 16-5.)

The cells of this portion also lie in the nucleus ambiguus, but in its caudal portion, only. No further comment need be made concerning this nucleus.

Axon (Figs. 2-7, 2-8, 2-52, 16-5.)

Their course within the brain stem is so similar to that described for the glossopharyngeal nerve and chief vagus nerve segment that no repetition is necessary. The extramedullary course is also similar to that of the nerves mentioned above, although a short distance below the exit from the brain stem, they are joined by the ascending spinal accessory nerve fibers, with which they exit from the skull through the jugular foramen. Just below the skull, the vagal accessory joins the rostral or chief segment to form a common trunk.

All the vagal accessory fibers terminate around the muscles of the larynx and either change the tension on the vocal cords or regulate the size of the aperture between them. Thus, the posterior cricoarytenoid, the lateral cricoarytenoid, and the lateral and oblique arytenoid muscles open or close the glottis, while the cricothyroid and the thyroarytenoid muscles regulate the tension (Fig. 16-5).

Accessory (Spinal Accessory) Nerve (XI)

This nerve, if it is to be considered an entity in itself and thus classified as one of the 12 cranial nerves, holds an equivocal position. There is no positive agreement as to whether the muscles it supplies come from the branchial arch mesoderm or from cervical somites. From the position of its nucleus, the point of emergence from the CNS, and its intimate relationship with a branchial motor nerve (X), it is likely that the upper part of both the trapezius and sternocleidomastoid muscles is dervied from branchial arches below five, arches which have disappeared long since in the process of evolution.

Cell Body (Figs. 2-50, 16-1, 16-6, 25-1.)

Most of the cells lie in the lateral part of the anterior gray column in the upper five segments of the cervical cord and persist in the lower medulla as far as the rostral limit of the pyramidal decussation.

Axon (Figs. 2-50, 16-1, 16-6.)

These are at first directed dorsolaterally, then laterally with rostral inclination, to emerge on the surface of the cord between the attachments of the dorsal and ventral roots of the upper cervical nerves. A short distance lateral to the edge of the cord these axons unite into a fascicle which runs rostrally beside the spinal cord (Figs. 2-7, 2-8, 16-1, 16-6) and enters the posterior cranial fossa through the foramen magnum (Fig. 17-29) to join the caudal fibers of the vagal accessory. Here the spinal accessory fibers swing laterally and then caudally to leave the skull with the vagal accessory through the jugular foramen (Fig. 2-52).

When the nerve is active, the upper part of

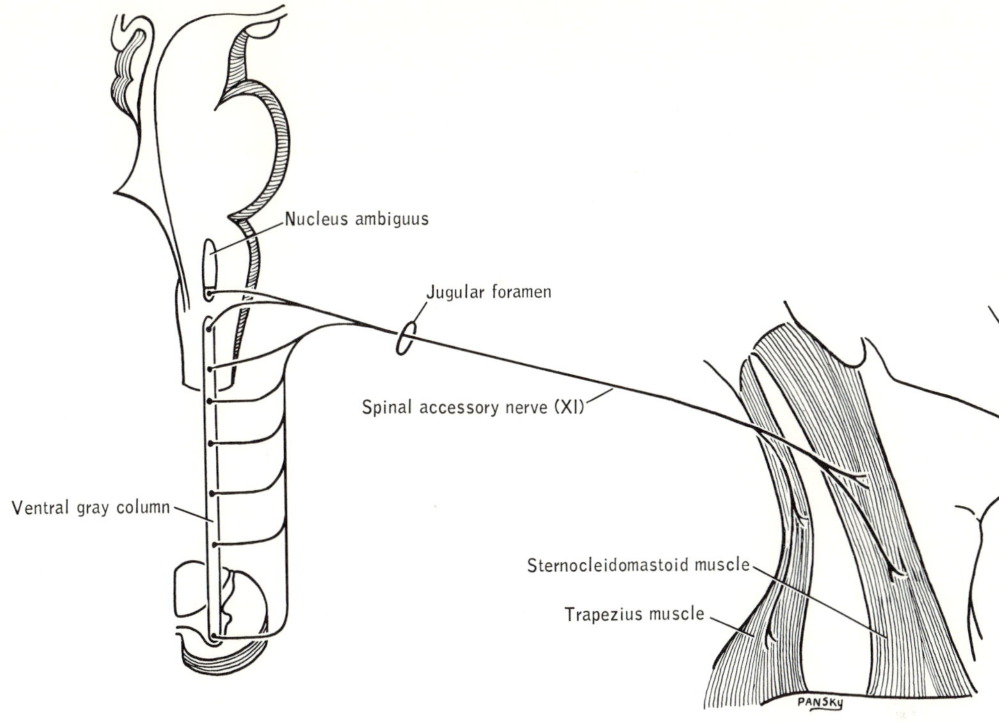

Fig. 16-6. Origin and distribution of the spinal accessory nerve (XI) to the muscles of the neck.

the trapezius muscle draws the head to the same side and turns the face to the opposite side. It also draws the scapula upward and braces the shoulders. The two sides acting together bend the head back. The sternocleidomastoid muscle, acting on one side alone, bends the cervical vertebral column to that side, so that the head approaches the shoulder. At the same time, the head is rotated, pointing the chin upward and to the opposite side.

CLINICAL CONSIDERATIONS

Testing

There are few actual tests to determine the integrity of the various parts of this system. Several observations can be made, however.

The examiner notes whether there is any deviation of the mandible. If the motor root of nerve V is damaged, the jaw may tend to deviate toward the side of the lesion.

The ability to move the mandible is tested by asking the patient to chew.

Since these muscles are also subject to atrophy when motor fibers are interrupted, the examiner looks for wasting in the masseteric area. Long-standing lesions in the trigeminal motor pathway would result in obvious shrinking in this region.

The examiner notes whether there is asymmetry of the face. In facial-nerve paralysis, the affected side will sag because the weight of the facial tissue will drag against the atonic and atrophying facial muscles. A smoothing out of the nasolabial fold may also be noted.

In this same connection, it should be noted whether the corner of the mouth droops.

Since the facial muscles are important in keeping substances in the mouth, one should look for evidence of, or inquire about, dribbling of saliva from the corners of the mouth. This would occur on the paralyzed side.

It should be determined whether the eye can

be blinked. Since the orbicularis oculi is the muscle performing eye closure, the eye cannot be closed on the affected side in cases of interruption or destruction of the facial nerve.

It is important to observe whether facial paralysis, when present, is total, i.e., whether the muscles above the eye (corrugator and frontalis), as well as those below, are affected. Total paralysis is indicative of disease either of the facial nucleus or along the course of its fibers. If the supraorbital muscles still contract, the lesion usually lies in the pathway of the upper motor neuron (Chap. 20).

One should notice whether there is difficulty in swallowing. Since nerves IX and X are responsible for the innervation of the palate and pharyngeal musculature, involvement of these nuclei would be extremely serious in this connection. Naturally, because of their much greater distribution, interruption of the vagal pathways is clinically more significant.

The physician should examine the pharynx and note whether there is deviation of the uvula. When the muscles on one side of the palate are paralyzed, the unopposed action of the normal muscles on the other side draws the uvula off center, away from the affected side. The palate droops on the paralyzed side, and gag reflexes on that side are diminished or absent. The examiner should also inquire about any tendency toward regurgitation from the mouth or pharynx into the nasal cavities.

One should listen to the voice. Since the vagus nerve supplies muscles of the larynx, lesions in this system lead to abnormalities in phonation. A laryngeal mirror or laryngoscope will show the vocal fold on the normal side to have a greater dorsolateral divergence from the midline.

General Pathology

The same conditions which adversely affect the somatic efferent system—tumors, either intra- or extramedullary; vascular accidents; or trauma—can also destroy or damage portions of the SVE mechanism. It is very rare, however, for such lesions to select isolated parts of this system without involving neighboring portions of other systems, some of which would present even more striking defects than are noticed in examinations just for SVE nerves. This is especially true when the pathologic condition lies within the CNS. Therefore, no attempt will be made to list all possible lesions or their locations in which the SVE fibers are included as a part of a much more generalized involvement. However, lesions including the facial and vagus nerves produce striking symptoms, the former because of the obvious differences between the two sides of the face; the latter because of the difficulties in swallowing and speaking.

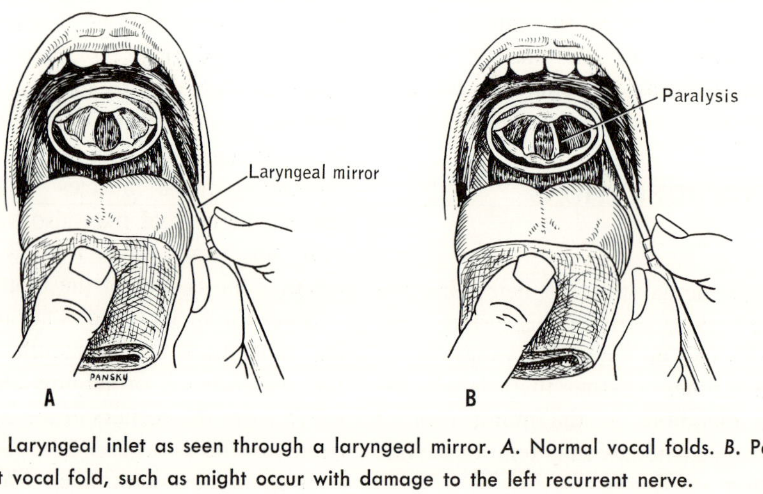

Fig. 16-7. Laryngeal inlet as seen through a laryngeal mirror. *A.* Normal vocal folds. *B.* Paralysis of the left vocal fold, such as might occur with damage to the left recurrent nerve.

Specific Pathology

Bell's Palsy

This is a general term applied to a facial paralysis, usually due to injury or disease in the peripheral part of nerve VII. Sometimes this results from an irritation, in which case, the paralysis may be only temporary. In disease and in surgery around the parotid gland, this nerve may be permanently damaged. Occasionally, in extensive disease of the middle ear followed by radical surgery on the middle ear, the facial nerve may be involved. This palsy is characterized by a lack of expression on the diseased side; the nasolabial groove is indistinct on that side; the palpebral fissure is larger on the diseased side; in chewing, food particles accumulate on the paralyzed side and the saliva may drip from the corner of the mouth. Depending on the location of the disease, certain autonomic reflexes, such as lacrimation and salivation, may be absent.

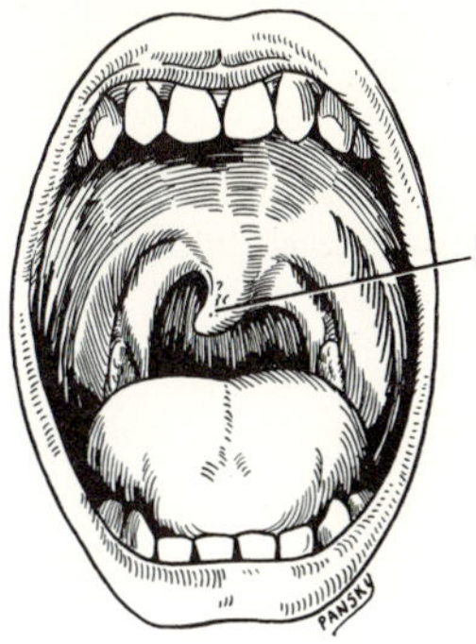

Fig. 16-8. Sagging of the left palate and pharyngeal wall, together with deviation of the uvula to the right, such as may occur with a lesion of the left vagus nerve. If the lesion occurs in the vagus nerve proximal to the origin of the recurrent nerve, this sign will be seen in conjunction with that shown in Fig. 16-7B. The muscles involved in this paralysis include levator veli palatini, glossopalatine, pharyngopalatine.

Trauma

In *surgery on the sensory root of the trigeminal (V) nerve* for the relief of trigeminal neuralgia (tic douloureux), the motor root, which adjoins the sensory root, on its medial side, may be inadvertently cut. This leads to paralysis of muscles of mastication with deviation of the jaw toward the paralyzed side and wasting away of the masseteric area on the side that has been operated upon.

In *surgery on the thyroid gland* for goiter, occasionally the recurrent laryngeal branch of the vagus nerve is destroyed. This leads to the paralysis of all the laryngeal muscles except the cricothyroid (Fig. 16-7). Abnormalities in the voice result. Should this occur bilaterally, normal phonation is impossible. There may also be difficulties in respiration because the rima glottidis cannot be altered.

Destruction of the nucleus ambiguus or emerging fibers of the vagus (X) nerve due to vascular thrombosis will lead to paralysis of the palatine and pharyngeal muscles on the side of the lesion. This results in difficulty in swallowing. On examination of the pharynx, the pharyngeal wall will be seen to sag on the side of the lesion and the uvula to deviate to the contralateral side (Fig. 16-8).

SUMMARY
Special Visceral Efferent

1. In the special visceral efferent column of the brain stem Motor nucleus of the trigeminal (V) in the upper pons Facial nucleus (VII) in the lower pons Nucleus ambiguus (nucleus for nerves IX and X): Rostral end Intermediate part Caudal end Accessory nucleus (XI) in lateral part of ventral gray column of the upper five cervical segments, and lower medulla, extending rostrally from this (as high as pyramidal decussation)	Cell body
2. From motor V, leaving brain stem through the portio minor into the mandibular division of the trigeminal (V) for distribution to masseter, temporalis, pterygoids, mylohyoid, anterior belly of the digastric, tensor veli palatini, and tensor tympani muscles From motor VII through the facial nerve (VII) to all muscles of facial expression, including the occipitalis and auricular group, plus the platysma, posterior belly of digastric, and the stapedius muscles From nucleus ambiguus: Rostral end, by way of the glossopharyngeal nerve (IX), to the stylopharyngeus (and superior pharyngeal constrictor?) Intermediate part, through the chief part of the vagus nerve (X), to the pharyngeal constrictors, the levator veli palatini, the glossopalatine, and pharyngopalatine muscles Caudal end, through the vagal accessory fibers (part of vagus nerve), to the muscles of the larynx From accessory nucleus through spinal accessory nerve (XI) to sternocleidomastoid and trapezius muscles	Efferent fiber
3. All in motor end plates in the skeletal muscle derived from mesoderm of branchial arch origin	Termination

17 SUMMARY OF FUNCTIONAL COMPONENTS OF PERIPHERAL NERVES

SPINAL NERVES

Although each spinal nerve may differ as to the number of fibers belonging to each of the functional components, they all contain at least some representatives of the GSA, GVA, GP, GSE, and GVE systems. Some of the information is so general that it will be given only once, under General Considerations, and will not be repeated for individual spinal nerves. The distribution of the receptors of the GSA system will be shown on the figures illustrating dermatomes (Figs. 17-1 to 17-3). The receptors for the GP system are distributed with the terminals of the GSE fibers and will, therefore, not be considered separately. In many cases, the fibers of the GVA system are sparse, their distribution is not definite, and their terminations are not clear. Therefore, it is not considered necessary (or even always possible) to list all components of each nerve. *Their presence is implied.* Only occasional mention will be made of some of these components when a point is to be emphasized.

FUNCTIONAL COMPONENTS OF SPINAL NERVES

General Considerations

I. Afferent components
- *A.* GSA (Chap. 8)
  - 1. Receptors
    - *a.* Types
      - (1). Free endings—for pain
      - (2). Bulbs of Krause and Ruffini—possibly for temperature
      - (3). Corpuscles of Meissner and Merkel—for touch
      - (4). Peritricheal arborizations—for touch
    - *b.* Location
      - (1). Epidermis
      - (2). Dermis
      - (3). Around hair follicles
    - *c.* Distribution—see dermatomes (Figs. 17-1 to 17-3)
  - 2. Cell bodies—in dorsal root ganglion of each nerve
  - 3. Terminations
    - *a.* Substantia gelatinosa—for pain and temperature
    - *b.* Body of dorsal column—for touch
  - 4. Symptoms of disease—anesthesia in area of distribution
- *B.* GP (Chap. 12)
  - 1. Receptors
    - *a.* Types
      - (1). Muscle spindles
      - (2). Tendon spindles
      - (3). Pacinian corpuscles
    - *b.* Location
      - (1). Among muscle fibers
      - (2). In fascia
      - (3). Along tendons
      - (4). In joint capsules

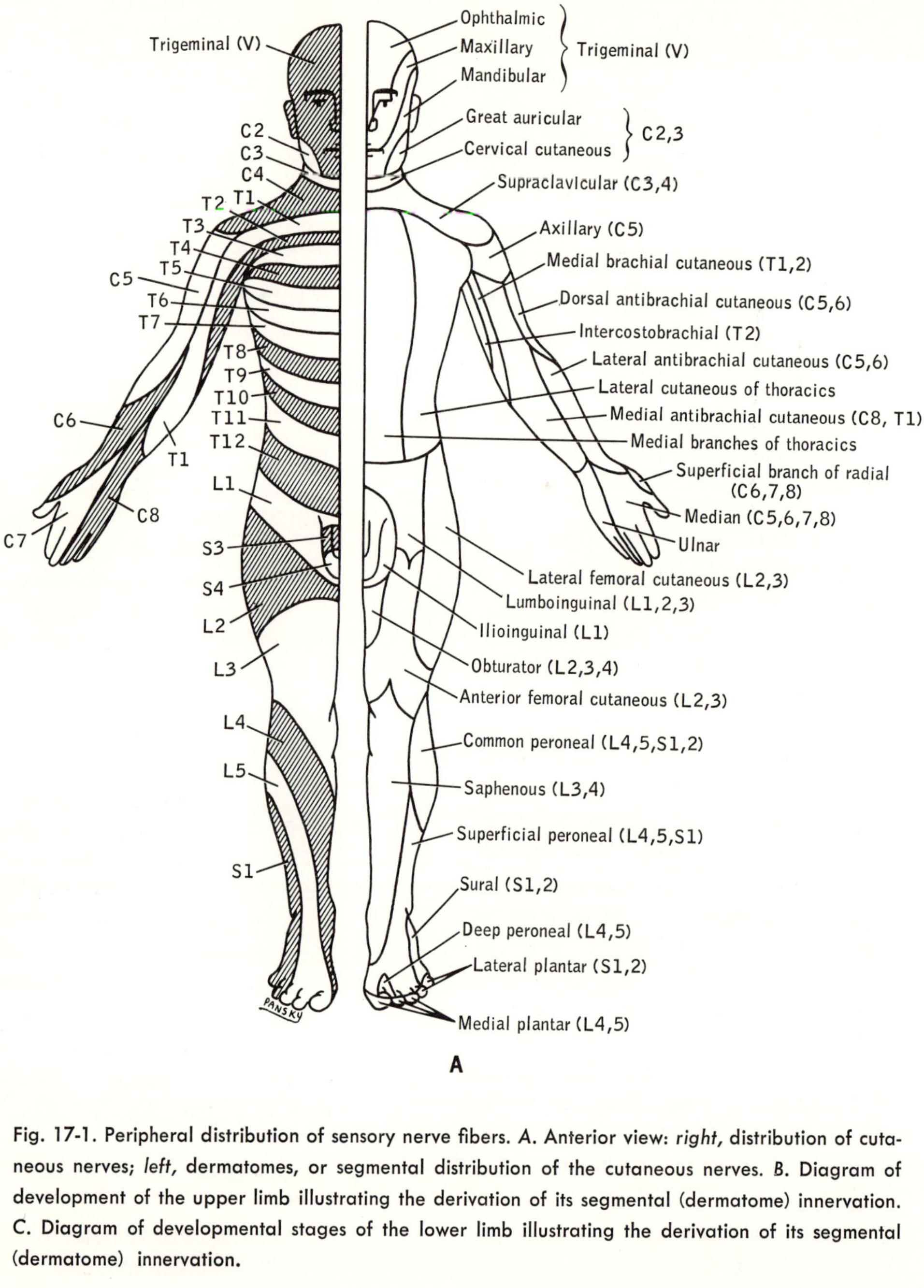

A

Fig. 17-1. Peripheral distribution of sensory nerve fibers. A. Anterior view: *right,* distribution of cutaneous nerves; *left,* dermatomes, or segmental distribution of the cutaneous nerves. *B.* Diagram of development of the upper limb illustrating the derivation of its segmental (dermatome) innervation. C. Diagram of developmental stages of the lower limb illustrating the derivation of its segmental (dermatome) innervation.

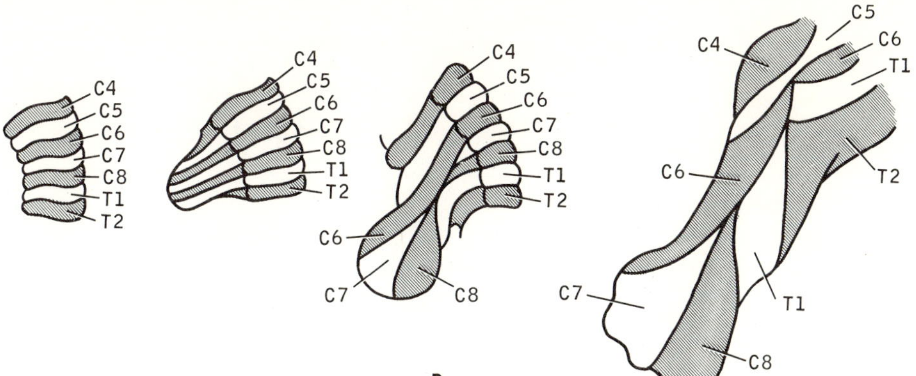

B

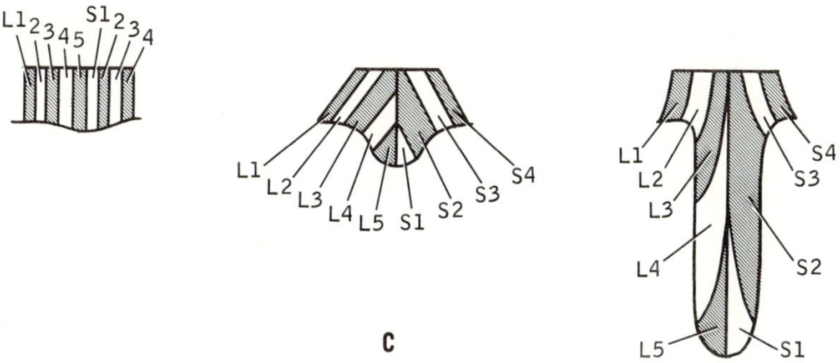

C

c. Distribution

(1). In same muscles supplied by GSE fibers of the nerve

(2). In articulations crossed by the nerve

2. Cell bodies—in dorsal root ganglion of each nerve
3. Terminations

a. Body of dorsal column

b. Clarke's column, T1 through L2

c. Lateral cuneate nucleus, for upper neck

d. Nucleus cuneatus, for upper half of body

e. Nucleus gracilis, for lower half of body

4. Symptoms of disease

a. Loss of tendon reflexes

b. Ataxia in muscles supplied

C. GVA (Chap. 10)

1. Receptors

a. Types

(1). Free

(2). Nets or tangles

(3). Pacinian corpuscles (?)

b. Location

(1). On mucous surfaces

(2). On serous surfaces

(3). Among muscle fibers

c. Distribution

(1). In walls of all viscera

(2). In supporting tissue, like mesenteries

(3). In body wall

2. Cell bodies—in dorsal root ganglia of each nerve
3. Termination—dorsal gray column of cord
4. Symptoms of disease—not clear-cut but perhaps some loss of proper reflex adjustments of the viscera

II. Efferent components.

A. GSE (Chap. 14)

1. Origin—from the ventral gray columns of the cord
2. Terminations—in the motor end-

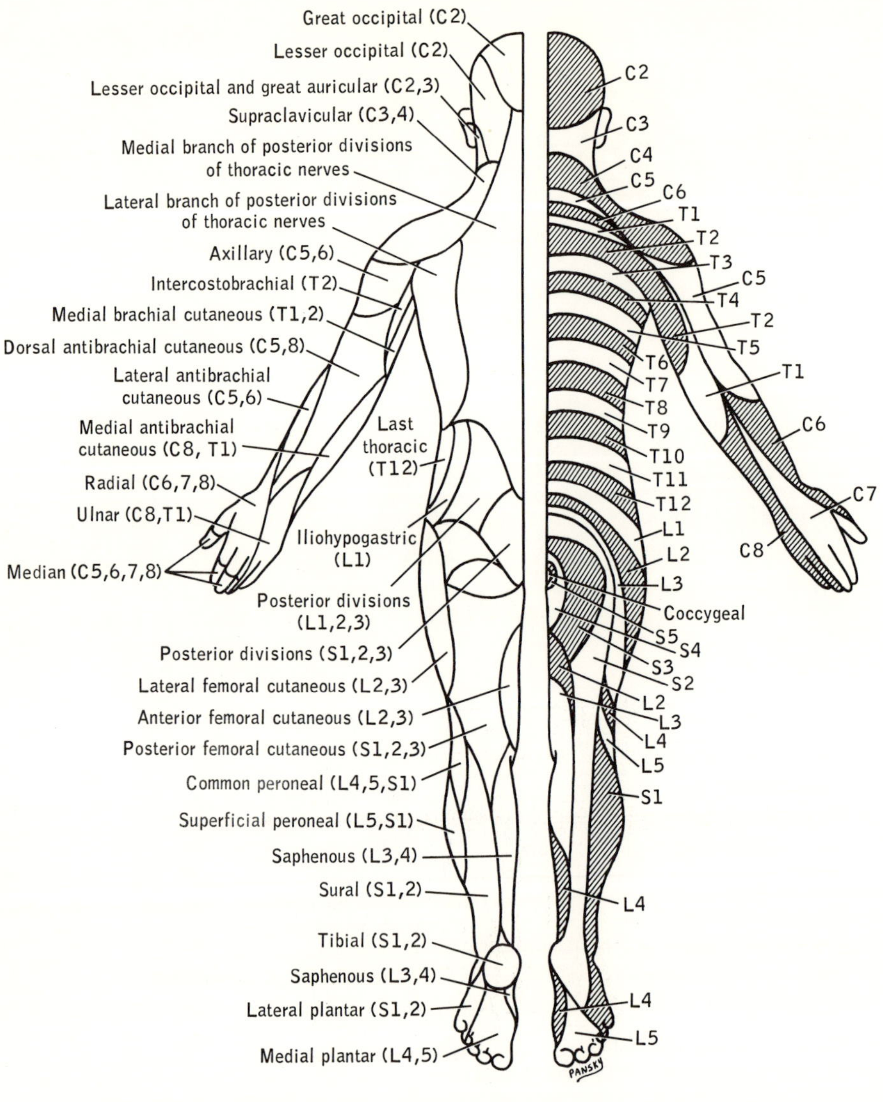

Fig. 17-2. Peripheral distribution of sensory nerve fibers showing the same features as in Fig. 17-1A, but from the dorsal side: dermatomes on the right, cutaneous nerves on the left.

plates of all skeletal muscle derived from somites

3. Distribution—in general, given with each nerve under Specific Considerations
4. Symptoms of disease
    a. Flaccid paralysis in muscles supplied
    b. Atrophy of muscles supplied

B. GVE—Sympathetic (Chap. 15)

1. Preganglionic
    a. Origin—intermediolateral gray column, T1 through L2
    b. Terminations
        (1). Ganglia of cervical sympathetic

(2). Chain ganglia
(3). Celiac ganglia
(4). Adrenal medula

2. Postganglionic
   a. Origin—any of ganglia listed under *B, b,* above
   b. Terminations
      (1). Smooth muscles and glands of head and trunk
      (2). Heart
      (3). Smooth muscle and glands of abdominal and thoracic viscera
3. Symptoms of disease: signs of hyperactivity or of hypoactivity, depending upon the specific characteristics of the organ innervated and upon the nature of the pathologic condition

C. GVE—Parasympathetic (Chap. 15)

1. Preganglionic
   a. Origin—intermediolateral cell column, S2 through S4
   b. Terminations
      (1). Ganglia in or on walls of pelvic viscera
      (2). Ganglia in walls of lower half of colon
2. Postganglionic
   a. Origin—in any of ganglia listed under *C, b,* above
   b. Terminations
      (1). Smooth muscle of pelvic viscera
      (2). Glands of pelvis
      (3). Muscle and glands of lower colon
3. Symptoms of disease—similar to those under *B,* 3, above but mainly referable to the pelvic viscera or genital apparatus

Specific Considerations

I. Cervical 1

A. GSE (Figs. 17-1, 17-2; Chap. 14)

1. Distribution
   a. Muscles of occipital triangle

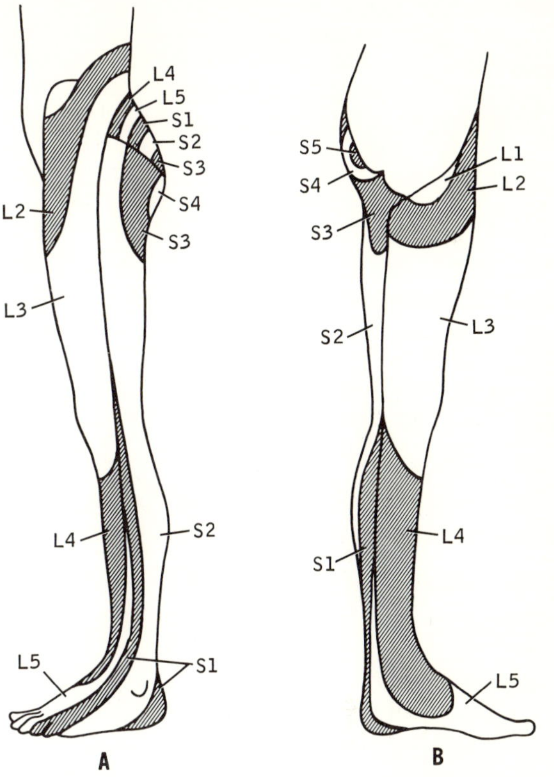

Fig. 17-3. Lower extremity showing the distribution of the dermatomes. *A.* Lateral view. *B.* Medial view.

   b. Through *descendens hypoglossi* to genio- and thyrohyoid muscles

II. Cervicals 2 through 4. *Cervical plexus* (Fig. 17-4)

A. GSE (Chap. 14)

1. Distribution
   a. From C2 and C3 through the *ansa hypoglossi* to infrahyoid muscles
   b. To longus and recti capitis
   c. From C3 and C4 to trapezius and sternocleidomastoid muscles
   d. From C4 through *phrenic nerve* to diaphragm

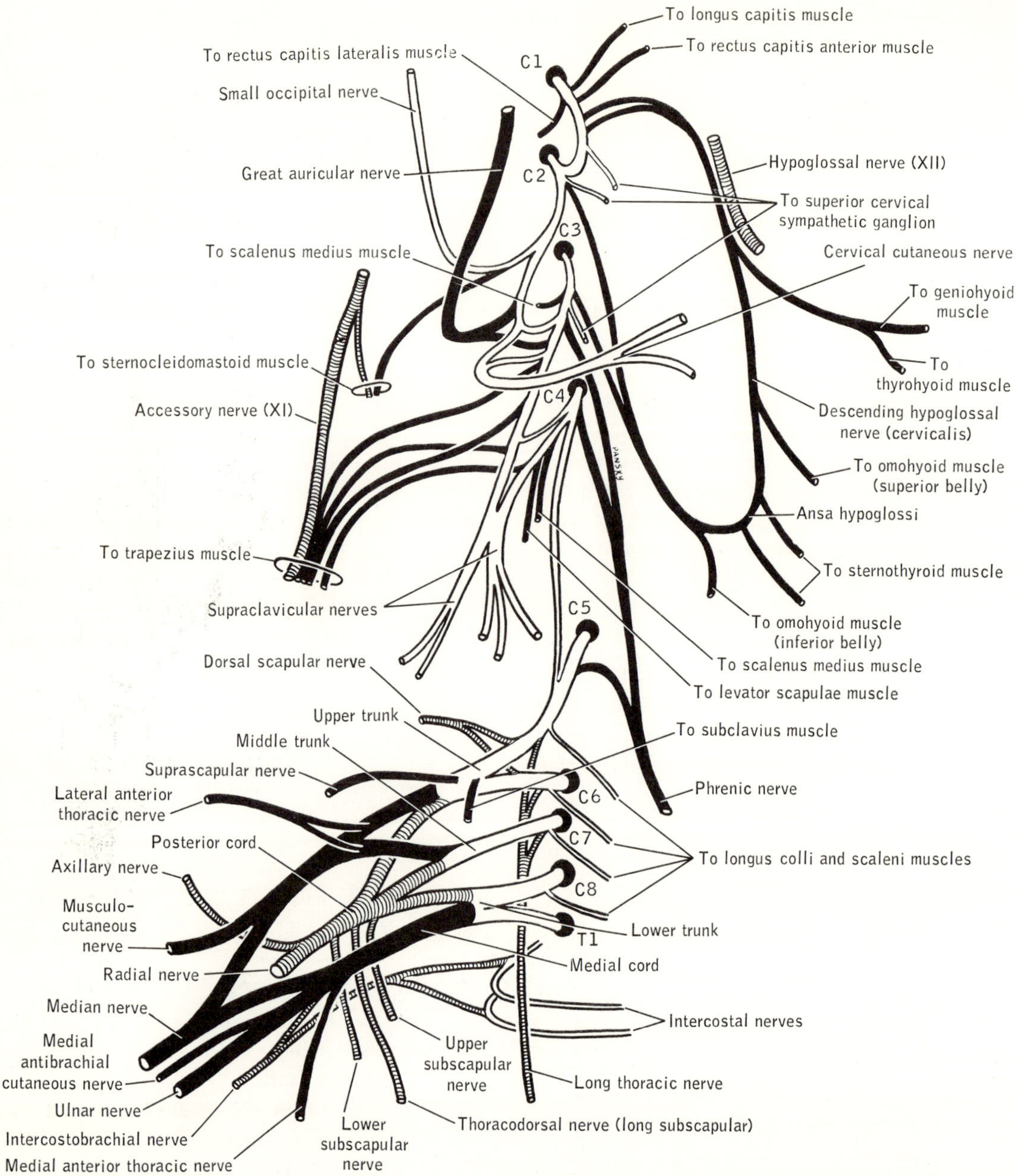

Fig. 17-4. Diagram of the formation and distribution of the cervical and brachial plexuses. In the brachial plexus, black denotes the anterior branches, striped fibers represent the posterior branches.

III. Cervicals 5 through 8 and T1. *Brachial plexus* (Fig. 17-4)
   A. GVA (Chap. 10)
      1. Distribution
         a. Blood vessels of upper extremity and neck
         b. Heart
   B. GSE (Figs. 17-4 to 17-9; Chap. 14)
      1. Distribution
         a. From C5 through *dorsal scapular nerve* to rhomboid muscles
         b. From C5 and C6 through *suprascapular nerve* to supra- and infraspinatus muscles
         c. From C5 and C6 through *subscapular nerves* to subscapularis and teres major muscles
         d. From C5, C6, and C7 through the *long thoracic nerve* to serratus anterior
         e. From C5, C6, and C7 through the *lateral anterior thoracic nerve* to the pectoralis major muscle
         f. From C8 and T1 through the *medial anterior thoracic nerve* to the pectoralis major and minor
         g. From C5, C6, and C7 through the *thoracodorsal nerve* to the latissimus dorsi
         h. From C5, C6, and C7 through the *musculocutaneous nerve* to biceps brachii, coracobrachialis, and brachialis muscles
         i. From C6, C7, C8, and T1 through the *median nerve* to most of flexors of wrist and fingers (see ulnar nerve); to the flexors, the short abductor, and opponens of the thumb; to the first and second lumbrical muscles
         j. From C8 and T1 through the *ulnar nerve* to flexor carpi ulnaris; ulnar half of flexor digitorum profundus; muscles of fifth finger; adductor and part of short flexor of thumb; all the interossei; and the third and fourth lumbrical muscles
         k. From C5 and C6 through the

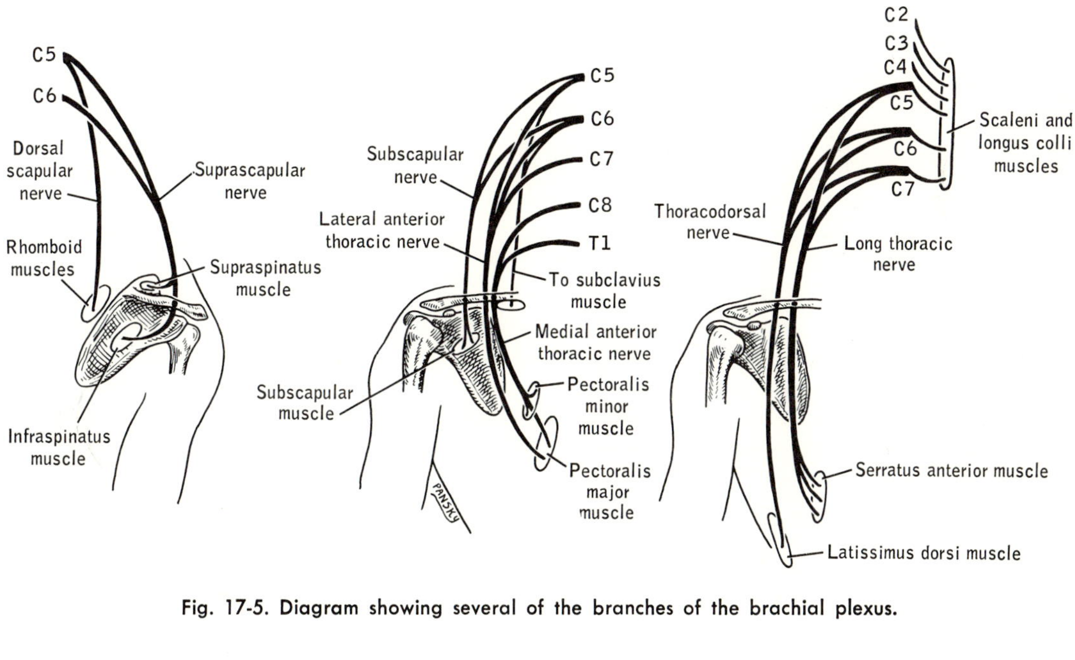

Fig. 17-5. Diagram showing several of the branches of the brachial plexus.

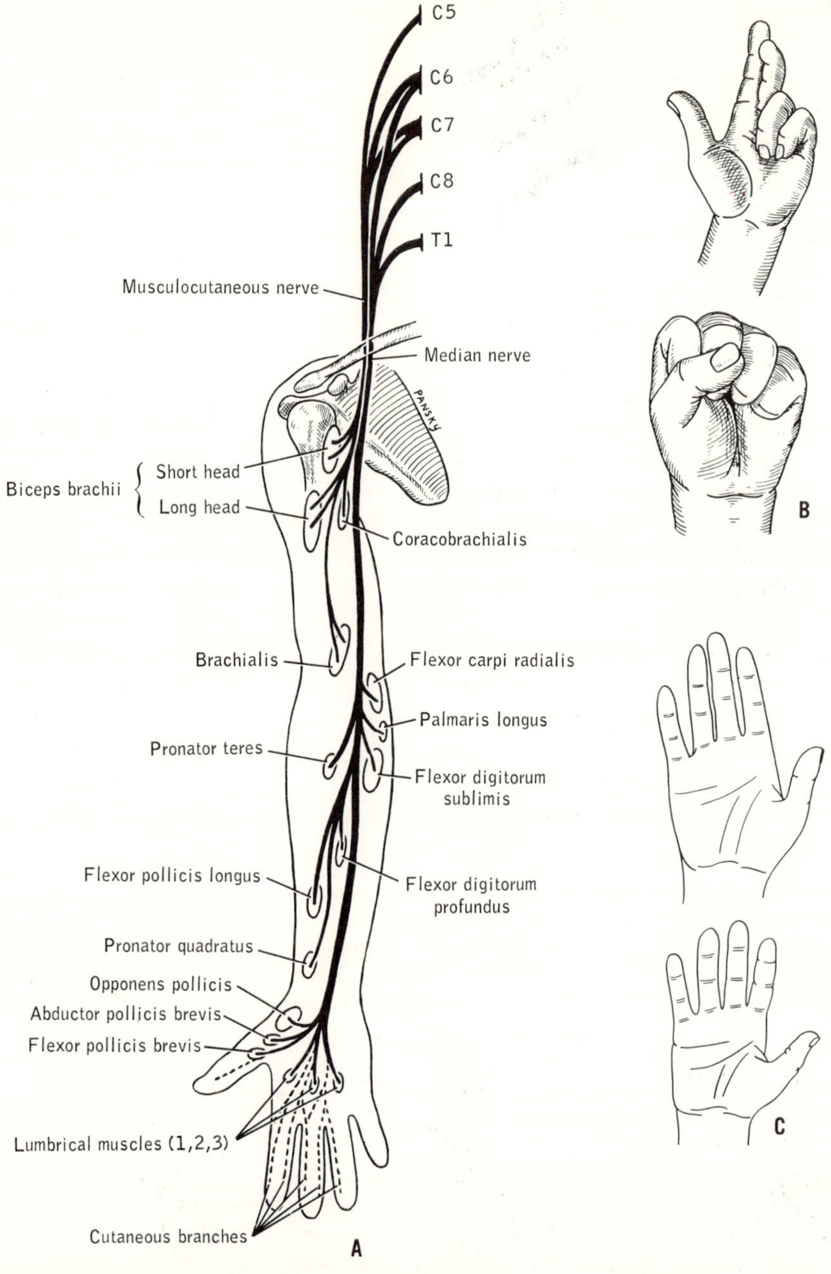

Fig. 17-6. Specific muscular distribution of two of the terminal branches of the brachial plexus. *A.* Motor distribution of the median and musculocutaneous nerves. *B.* Paralysis resulting from median nerve damage. *Top.* Hand of papal benediction. *Lower.* Normal fist. C. Paralysis resulting from median nerve damage. *Top.* Loss of opposition of the thumb—"ape hand." *Lower.* Normal.

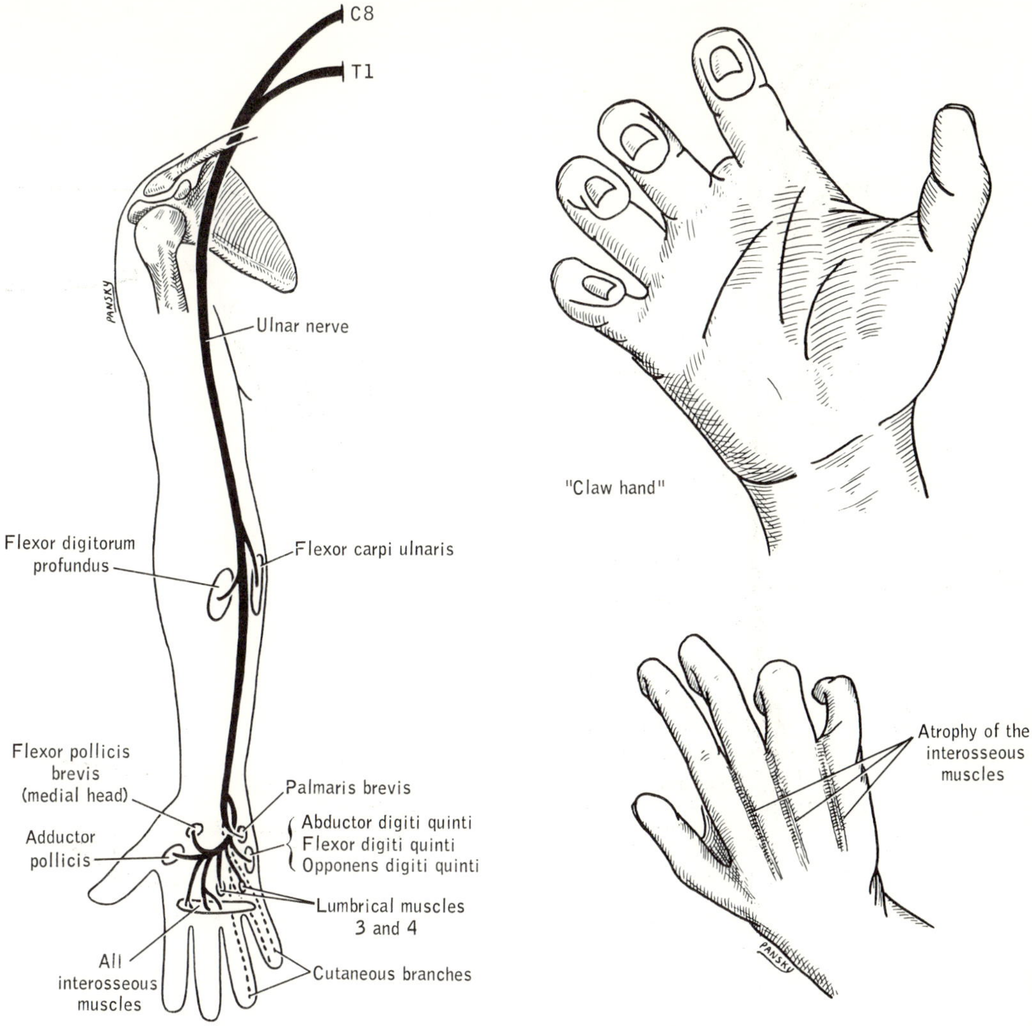

Fig. 17-7. Specific muscular distribution of one of the terminal branches of the brachial plexus showing distribution of the ulnar nerve and position of the hand in cases of ulnar nerve lesion.

axillary nerve to the deltoid and teres minor muscles

l. From C5, C6, C7, C8, and T1 through the *radial nerve* to the brachioradialis; triceps brachii; extensor carpi radialis; and all the extensors of wrist and fingers on the dorsal side of the forearm

C. GVE (Chap. 15)

1. Preganglionic

a. Origin—intermediolateral cell column of level T1

b. Terminations

(1). First thoracic chain ganglion

(2). Cervical ganglia of cervical sympathetic

2. Postganglionic

a. Origin—any of ganglia under *C, b,* above

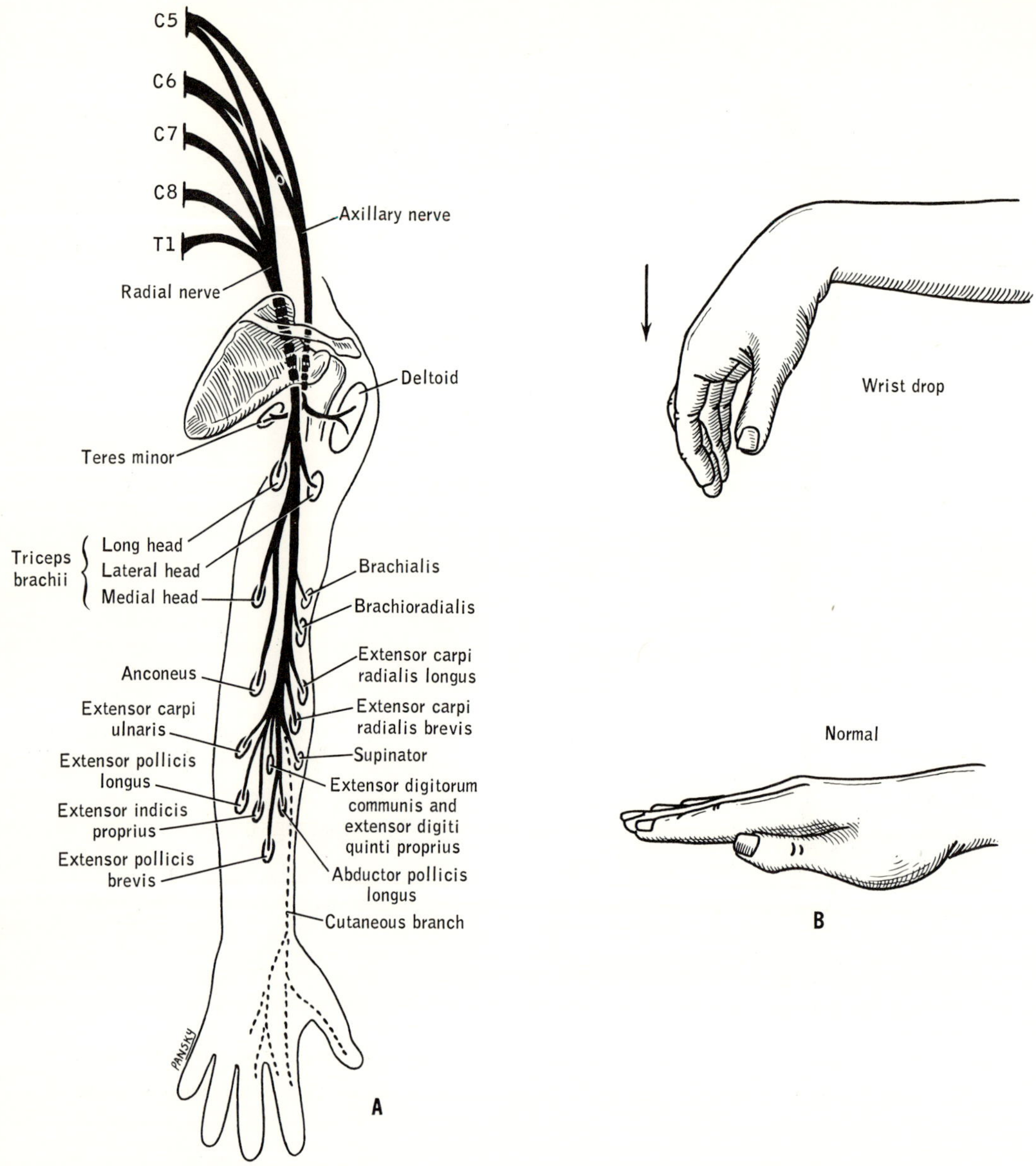

Fig. 17-8. Specific muscular distribution of the two terminal branches derived from the posterior cord of the brachial plexus. *A*. Muscular distribution of the axillary and radial nerves. *B*. Position of the hand in lesions of the radial nerve. In wrist drop the extensors are paralyzed and the flexors are unopposed.

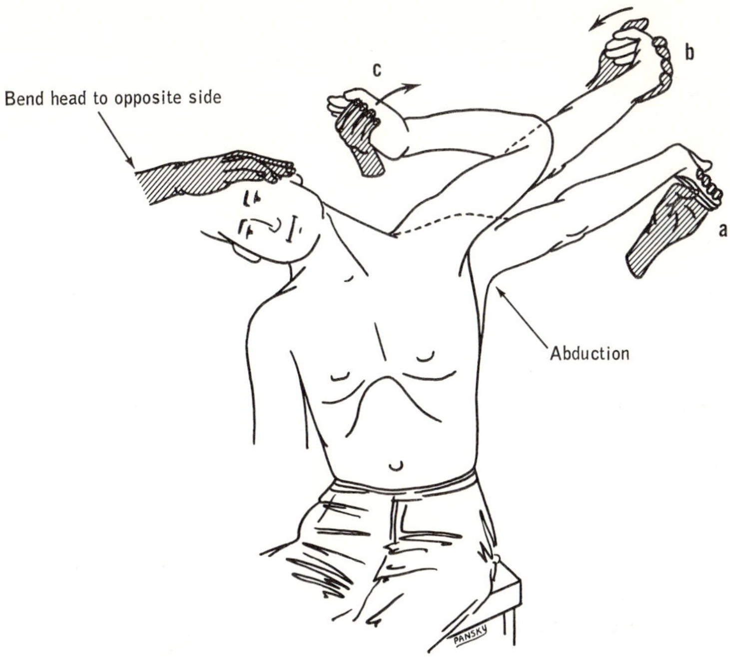

Fig. 17-9. Testing the median, radial, and ulnar nerves. *a.* Median: abduct shoulder, extend elbow, dorsiflex wrist. *b.* Radial: abduct shoulder, extend elbow, pronate wrist. c. Ulnar: abduct shoulder, flex elbow, dorsiflex wrist.

b. Terminations
(1). Vessels, glands, and smooth muscle of head and neck
(2). Vessels in upper extremity
(3). Heart

IV. Thoracics 2 through 6
A. GVA (Chap. 10)
1. Distribution—thoracic viscera, including the heart

B. GSE (Chap. 14; Figs. 17-1, 17-2)
1. Distribution
a. From each of these levels through *intercostal nerves* to intercostal muscles; serratus posterior superior; and upper external abdominal oblique

C. GVE (Chap. 15)
1. Preganglionic
a. Origin—intermediolateral cell column
b. Terminations
(1). Upper thoracic chain ganglia
(2). Cervical sympathetic ganglia

2. Postganglionic
a. Origin—any of ganglia under *C*, *b*, above
b. Terminations
(1). Dilator pupillae
(2). Glands of head and neck
(3). Walls of blood vessels of head, neck, upper extremity, and body walls (thorax)
(4). Heart
(5). Lungs

V. Thoracics 7 through 12
A. GVA (Chap. 10)
1. Distribution—abdominal viscera

B. GSE (Chap. 14; Figs. 17-1, 17-2)

1. Distribution—to all abdominal muscles

C. GVE (Chap. 15)

1. Preganglionic
   - *a*. Origin—intermediolateral cell column
   - *b*. Terminations
     - (1). Lower thoracic chain ganglia
     - (2). Through the *splanchnic nerves* to celiac ganglia
     - (3). Adrenal medulla
2. Postganglionic
   - *a*. Origin—under *b*, (1), (2), above
   - *b*. Terminations
     - (1). Blood vessels of abdominal wall
     - (2). All blood vessels of abdominal viscera
     - (3). Walls of all abdominal viscera

VI. Lumbar 1 through 4. *Lumbar plexus* (Fig. 17-10)

A. GVA (Chap. 10)

1. Distribution
   - *a*. Abdominal and pelvic viscera
   - *b*. Vessels of thigh

B. GSE (Figs. 17-10, 17-11; Chap. 14)

1. Distribution
   - *a*. From L1 through *ilioinguinal nerve* to the internal oblique
   - *b*. From L1 and L2 through the *genitofemoral nerve* to the cremaster muscle
   - *c*. From L2, L3, and L4 through the *obturator nerve* to the gracilis, obturator externus, and all adductor muscles of thigh
   - *d*. From L2, L3, and L4 through the *femoral nerve* to the iliacus, pectineus, sartorius, and all the quadriceps femoris (extensors of leg)
   - *e*. From L3 and L4 to iliacus and psoas
   - *f*. From L4 to form *lumbosacral trunk* with L5 (see VII, below)

C. GVE (Chap. 15)

1. Preganglionic
   - *a*. Origin—intermediolateral cell column, at levels L1 and L2 (possibly L3)
   - *b*. Terminations
     - (1). Ganglia of lumbar chain
     - (2). Celiac and inferior mesenteric ganglia
     - (3). Ganglia of pelvic plexus (?)
2. Postganglionic
   - *a*. Origin—any of ganglia under *C, b,* above
   - *b*. Terminations
     - (1). Blood vessels of thigh.
     - (2). Blood vessels of abdominal and pelvic viscera
     - (3). Walls of abdominal and pelvic viscera

VII. Lumbar V and sacrals 1 through 3. *Sacral plexus* (Fig. 17-10)

A. GVA (Chap. 10)

1. Distribution
   - *a*. Vessels of back of thigh; leg; foot
   - *b*. All pelvic viscera, mainly in S2 and S3 (also S4)

B. GSE (Figs. 17-10, 17-12 to 17-13; Chap. 14)

1. Distribution
   - *a*. From L4, L5, and S1 to quadratus femoris and gemellus inferior muscles
   - *b*. From L5, S1, and S2 to obturator internus and gemellus superior muscles
   - *c*. From S2 to piriformis muscle
   - *d*. From L4, L5, and S1 through the *superior gluteal* nerve to gluteus medius and minimus muscles
   - *e*. From L5, S1, and S2 through the *inferior gluteal* nerve to the gluteus maximus muscle
   - *f*. From L4, L5, S1, and S2 through the *common peroneal division* of the *sciatic nerve* to

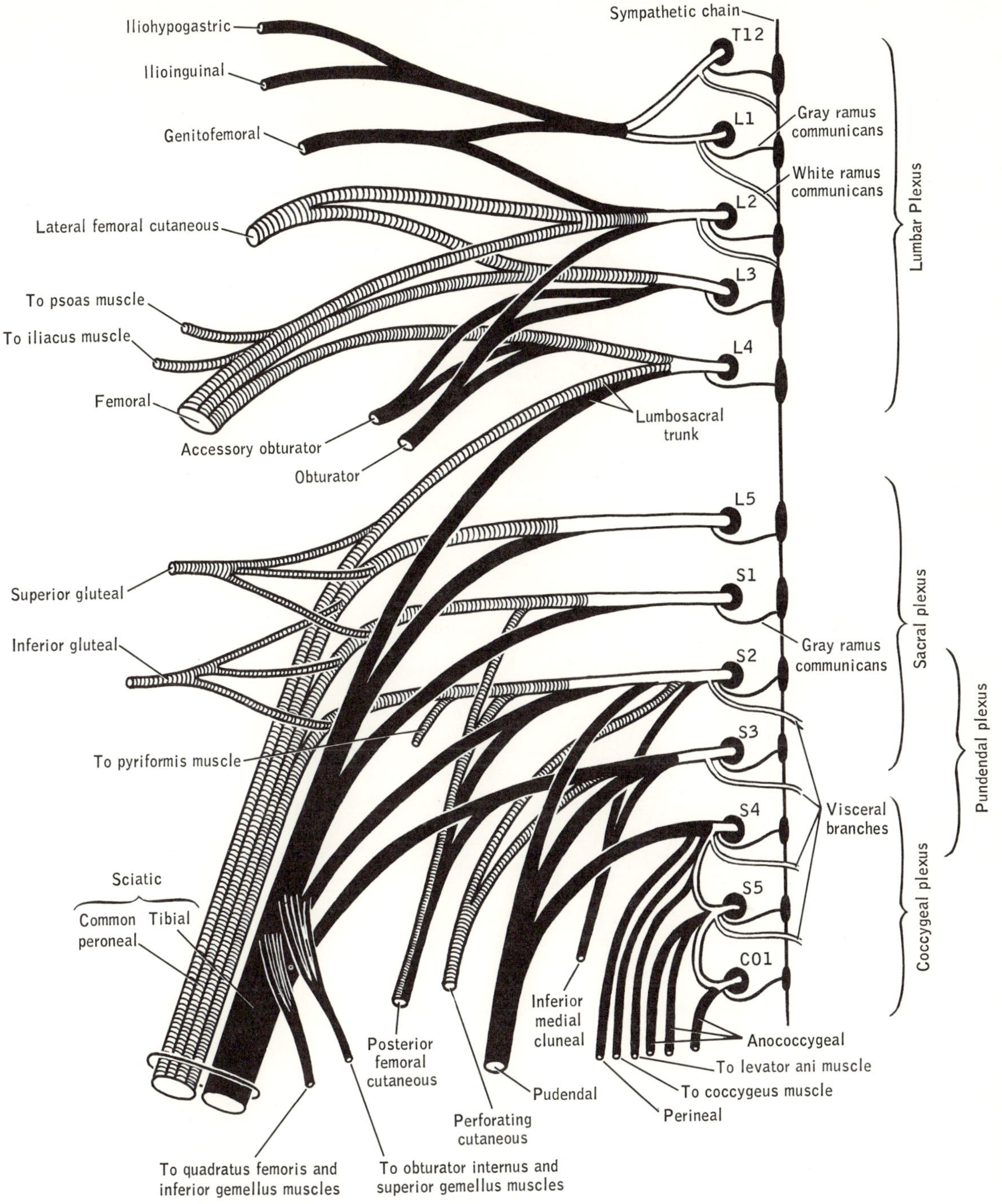

Fig. 17-10. Diagram of the formation of the lumbosacral, pudendal, and coccygeal plexuses. The anterior division is indicated in black, the posterior division is striped. (*Adapted from Schaeffer (ed.), Morris' Human Anatomy, 11th ed.,* McGraw-Hill Book Company, Inc., Blakiston Division, New York, 1953.)

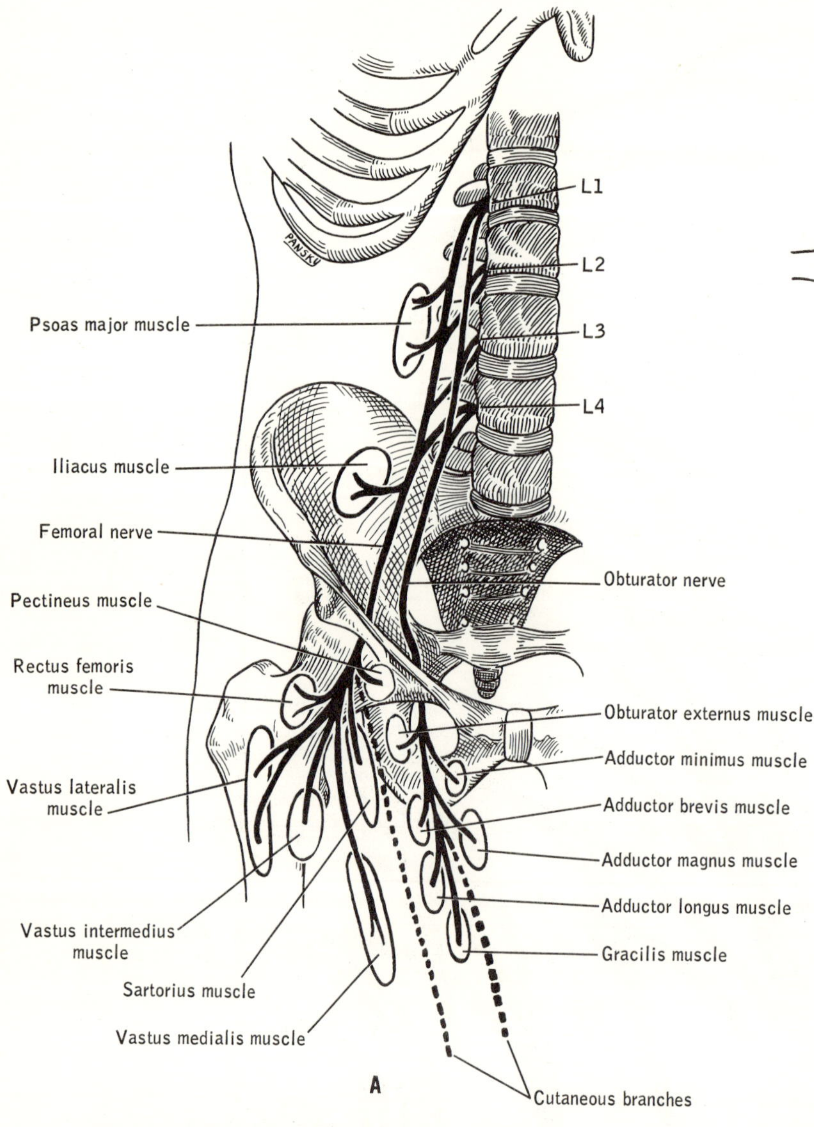

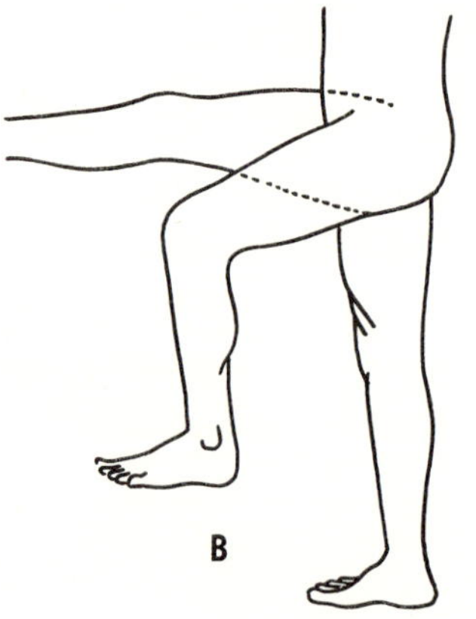

Fig. 17-11. Muscular distribution of two of the terminal branches of the lumbosacral plexus. *A.* Distribution of the motor fibers in the femoral and obturator nerves. *B.* Testing for femoral nerve paralysis—checking ability to extend leg at knee and to flex thigh at hip.

short head of biceps femoris; all peroneal muscles; extensors of the ankle; extensors of the toes; extensor of the large toe; and first two dorsal interosseous muscles

g. From L4, L5, S1, S2, and S3, through the *tribial division* of the *sciatic nerve* to all the hamstring muscles except short head of the biceps femoris (under *f*, above); all flexors of the ankle; all flexors of the toes, including the short muscles in the sole of the foot

C. GVE (Chap. 15)
1. Preganglionic
a. Origin—intermediolateral cell column at levels S2 and S3 (and usually S4)
b. Termination, through the pelvic splanchnic nerves, to
(1). Ganglia in or on walls of pelvic viscera
(2). Ganglia in wall of lower colon
2. Postganglionic
a. Origin—in any of ganglia under *C, b,* above
b. Terminations
(1). Pelvic viscera
(2). Colon, lower half
(3). Genitalia

VIII. Sacrals 4 and 5, with contributions from sacrals 2 and 3
A. GVA (Chap. 10)
1. Distribution
a. Genitalia
b. External sphincters
B. GSE (Chap. 14)
1. Distribution
a. From S4 (and also S3 and S5) to
(1). Muscles of pelvic diaphragm
(2). External anal sphincter
b. From S2, S3, and S4 through the *pudendal nerve* to all perineal muscles, including the external sphincters of anus and urethra
C. GVE (Chap. 15)
1. Preganglionic—none
2. Postganglionic
a. Origin
(1). For sympathetic outflow from inferior mesenteric and lumbar ganglia
(2). For parasympathetic outflow from ganglia of pelvic plexus
b. Termination—external genitalia

CRANIAL NERVES

Since the cranial nerves differ considerably in the representation of the various systems, and particularly because the special categories have been included, each nerve will be considered separately. However, in certain general respects they are similar to the spinal nerves and these items will not be repeated in each case. For example, the distribution of the GSA receptors will be shown on a figure; the GSA receptors for pain, temperature, and touch are the same type as those associated with the spinal nerves; the GP receptors are the same as those for the muscles of the limbs and trunk and have the same general distribution as the motor fibers supplying the cranial musculature; the symptoms of disease will be referable to the areas of distribution; and the receptors for the GVA are the same type except that with certain of the cranial nerves, chemoreceptors are utilized.

FUNCTIONAL COMPONENTS OF CRANIAL NERVES (Figs. 17-31, 17-32.)

Specific Considerations

I. Olfactory (Fig. 17-14)
A. SVA (Chap. 11)
1. Receptors
a. Type—hair cells
b. Location—nasal mucous membrane
c. Distribution upper third of nasal cavity
2. Cell bodies—in membrane
3. Termination—olfactory bulb
4. Symptoms of disease—anosmia

II. Optic [1] (Fig. 17-15)
A. SSA (Chap. 9)
1. Receptors
a. Types
(1). Rods
(2). Cones

[1] The so-called optic nerve, actually a part of the optic tract, arises in the ganglion cell layer of the retina and terminates in either the superior colliculus or the lateral geniculate nucleus (body) of the thalamus.

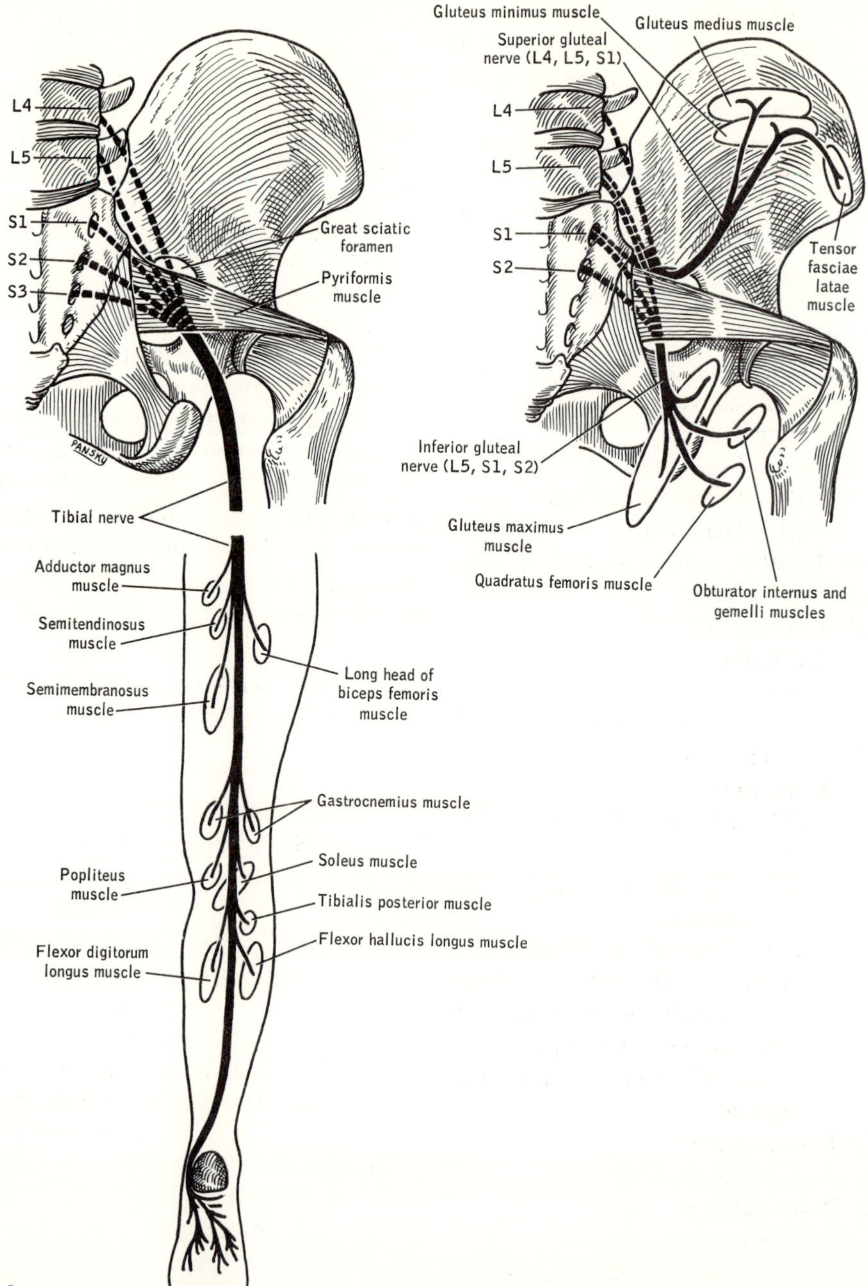

Fig. 17-12. Muscular distribution of one of the major divisions of the sciatic nerve. *A*. Muscular branches of tibial and gluteal nerves. *B*. Distribution of the tibial nerve to the muscles on the plantar side of the foot. C. Manifestations of tibial nerve lesions. *a* and *b*. Normal action with plantar flexion of foot and toes. *c*. In paralysis—lack of plantar flexion and excessively high arch.

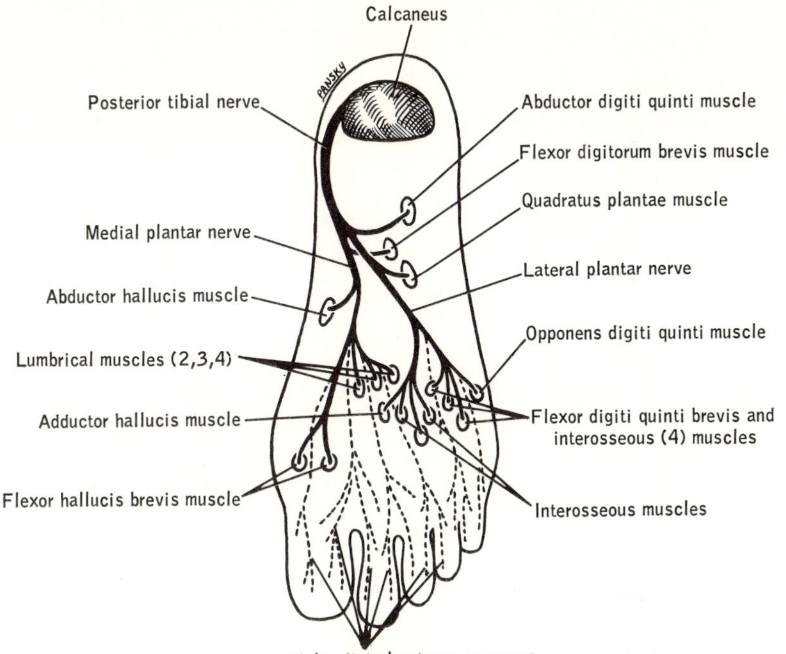

Fig. 17-12. B.

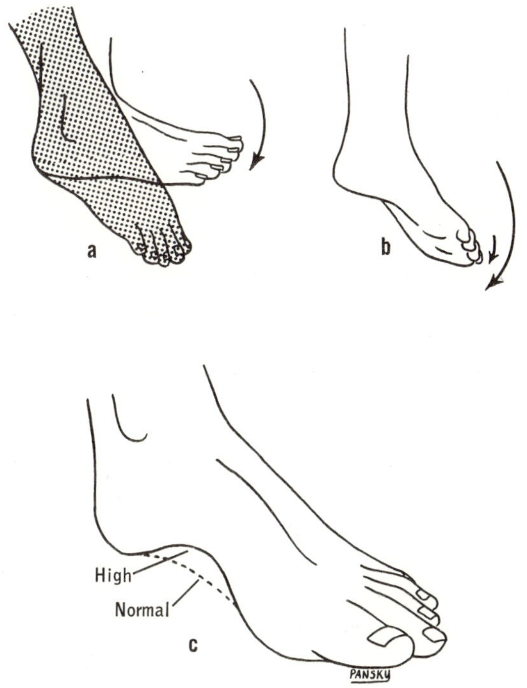

Fig. 17-12. C.

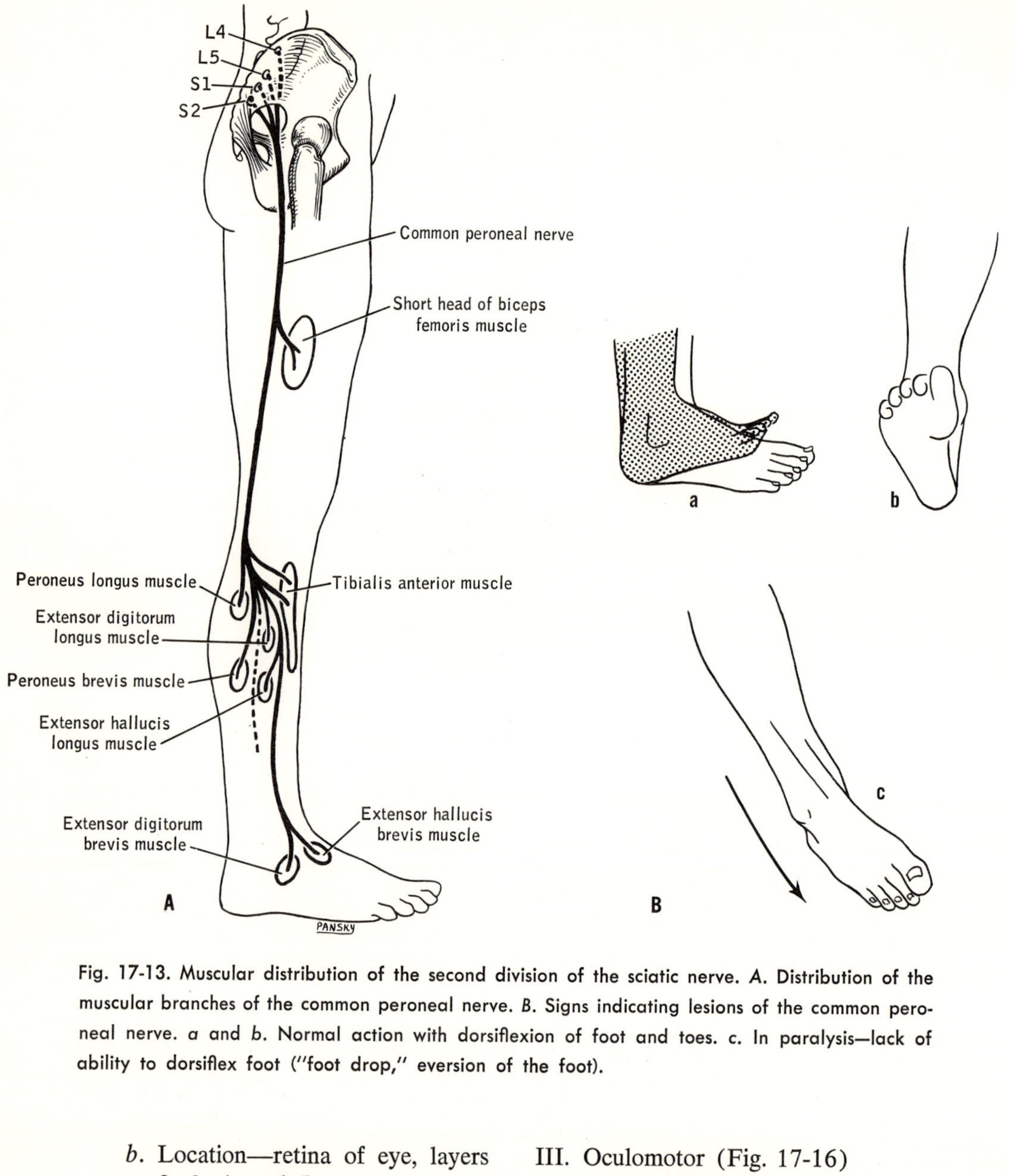

Fig. 17-13. Muscular distribution of the second division of the sciatic nerve. *A.* Distribution of the muscular branches of the common peroneal nerve. *B.* Signs indicating lesions of the common peroneal nerve. *a* and *b.* Normal action with dorsiflexion of foot and toes. c. In paralysis—lack of ability to dorsiflex foot ("foot drop," eversion of the foot).

b. Location—retina of eye, layers 2, 3, 4, and 5

c. Distribution—in sensory part of retina

2. Cell bodies—bipolar cells of retina
3. Termination—ganglion layer of retina
4. Symptoms of disease—anopsia

III. Oculomotor (Fig. 17-16)

A. GP (Chap. 12)

1. Receptors

a. Distribution—extrinsic eye muscles except lateral rectus and superior oblique

2. Cell bodies—mesencephalic nucleus of trigeminal

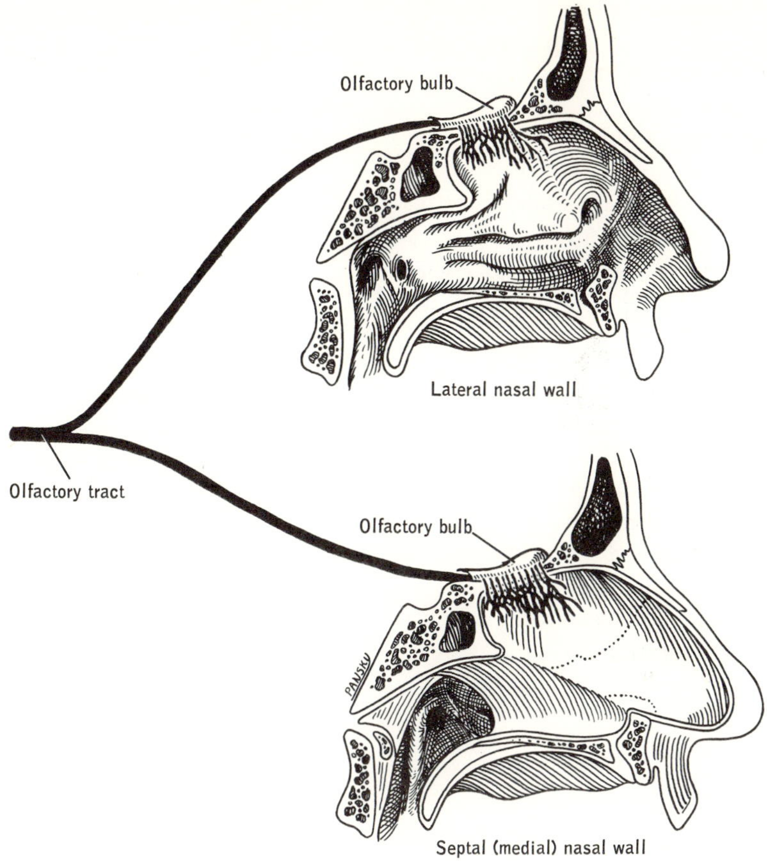

Fig. 17-14. The olfactory nerve (I) and the distribution of the olfactory receptors on the walls of the nasal chamber.

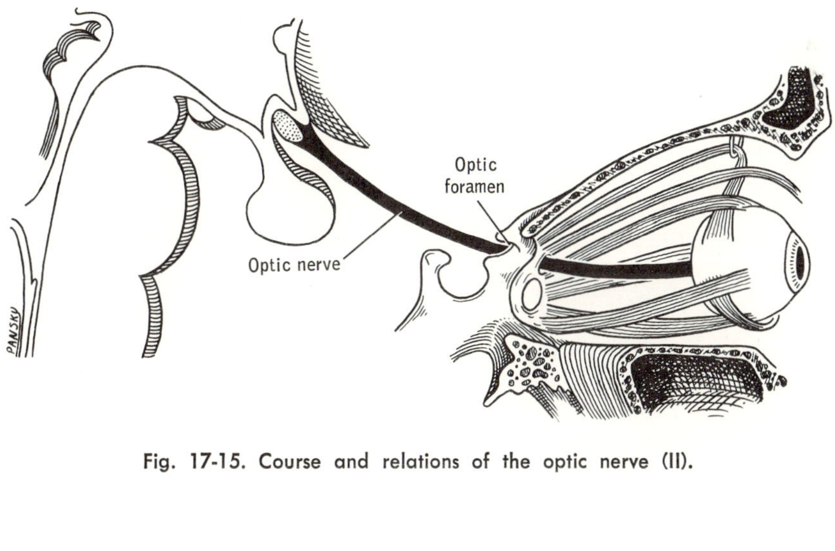

Fig. 17-15. Course and relations of the optic nerve (II).

3. Termination—through mesencephalic nucleus to reticular formation of brain stem

B. GSE (Chap. 14)

1. Origin—oculomotor nucleus
2. Termination—all extrinsic ocular muscles except the lateral rectus and superior oblique
3. Symptoms of disease—eye looks downward and outward with no convergence

C. GVE (Chap. 15)

1. Preganglionic
   a. Origin—Edinger-Westphal nucleus
   b. Termination—ciliary and episcleral ganglia
2. Postganglionic
   a. Origin—under *C, b,* above
   b. Termination—sphincter pupillae and ciliary muscle
3. Symptoms of disease—pupils do not constrict to light or for accommodation

IV. Trochlear (Fig. 17-17)

A. GP (Chap. 12)

1. Receptors
   a. Distribution—superior oblique
2. Cell bodies—mesencephalic nucleus of trigeminal
3. Termination—through mesencephalic nucleus to reticular formation of brain stem

B. GSE (Chap. 14)

1. Origin—trochlear nucleus
2. Termination—superior oblique muscle of eye
3. Symptoms of disease—eye tends to look slightly upward

V. Trigeminal (Figs. 17-18, 17-19)

A. GSA (Fig. 17-1*A*) (Chap. 8)

1. Receptors

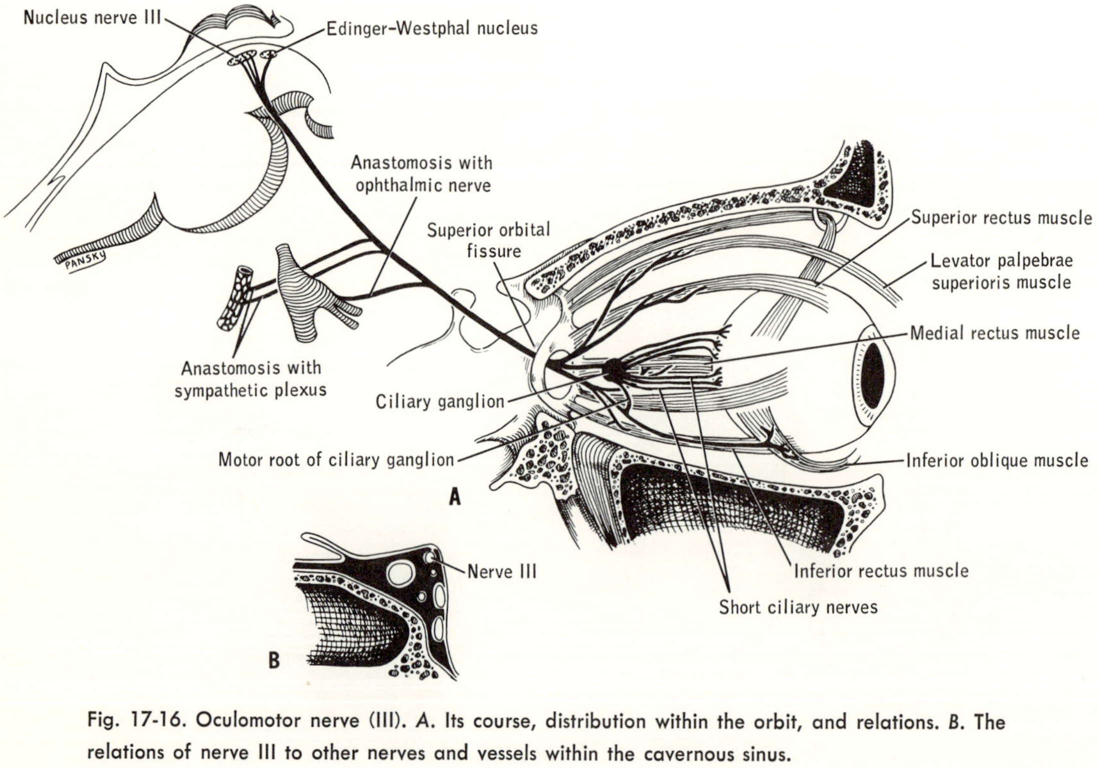

Fig. 17-16. Oculomotor nerve (III). *A*. Its course, distribution within the orbit, and relations. *B*. The relations of nerve III to other nerves and vessels within the cavernous sinus.

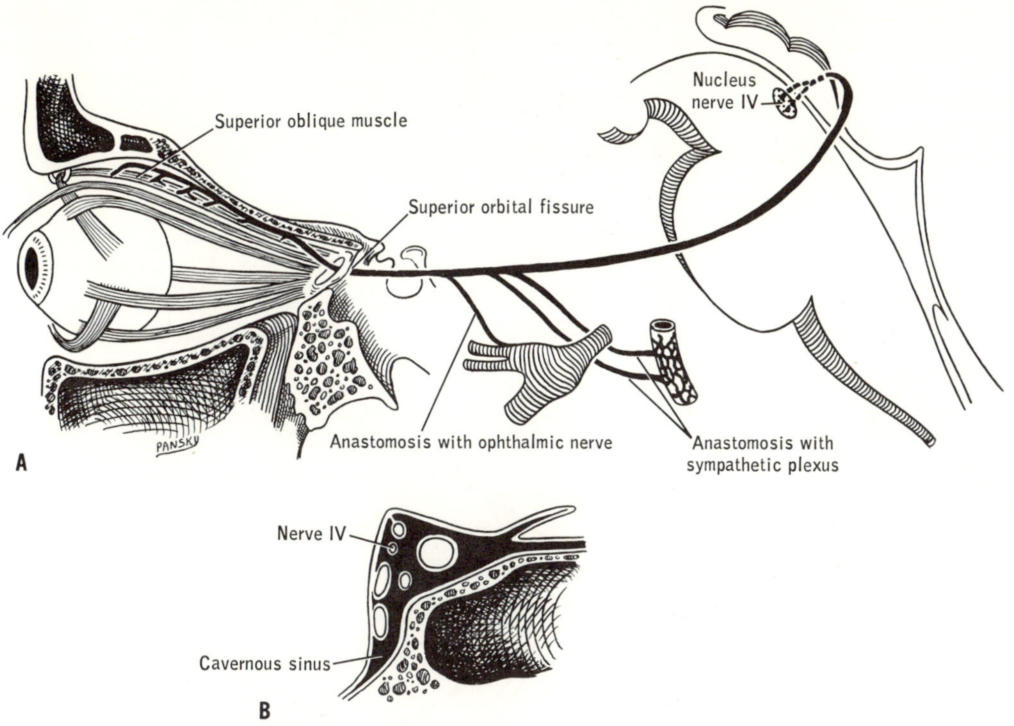

Fig. 17-17. Trochlear nerve (IV). *A*. Course, distribution, and relations. *B*. Its relations to other structures in the cavernous sinus.

a. Distribution—skin of face, conjunctiva and mucous membrane of nose and mouth

2. Cell bodies—semilunar (Gasserian) ganglion
3. Terminations
   a. Pain and temperature—spinal V nucleus
   b. Touch—chief sensory nucleus
4. Symptoms of disease—anesthesia in area of distribution

B. GP (Chap. 12)

1. Receptors
   a. Distribution
      (1). Muscles of mastication
      (2). Temporomandibular joint
      (3). Sockets of teeth
2. Cell bodies—mesencephalic nucleus
3. Termination—through mesencephalic nucleus to reticular formation of the brain stem

C. SVE (Chap. 16)

1. Origin—motor nucleus of trigeminal
2. Terminations
   a. Muscles of mastication
   b. Anterior belly digastric
   c. Tensor tympani
   d. Tensor veli palatini
   e. Mylohyoid
3. Symptoms of disease—paralysis of jaws

VI. Abducens (Figs. 17-20, 17-21)

A. GP (Chap. 12)

1. Receptors
   a. Distribution—lateral rectus muscle of eye
2. Cell bodies—mesencephalic nucleus of trigeminal

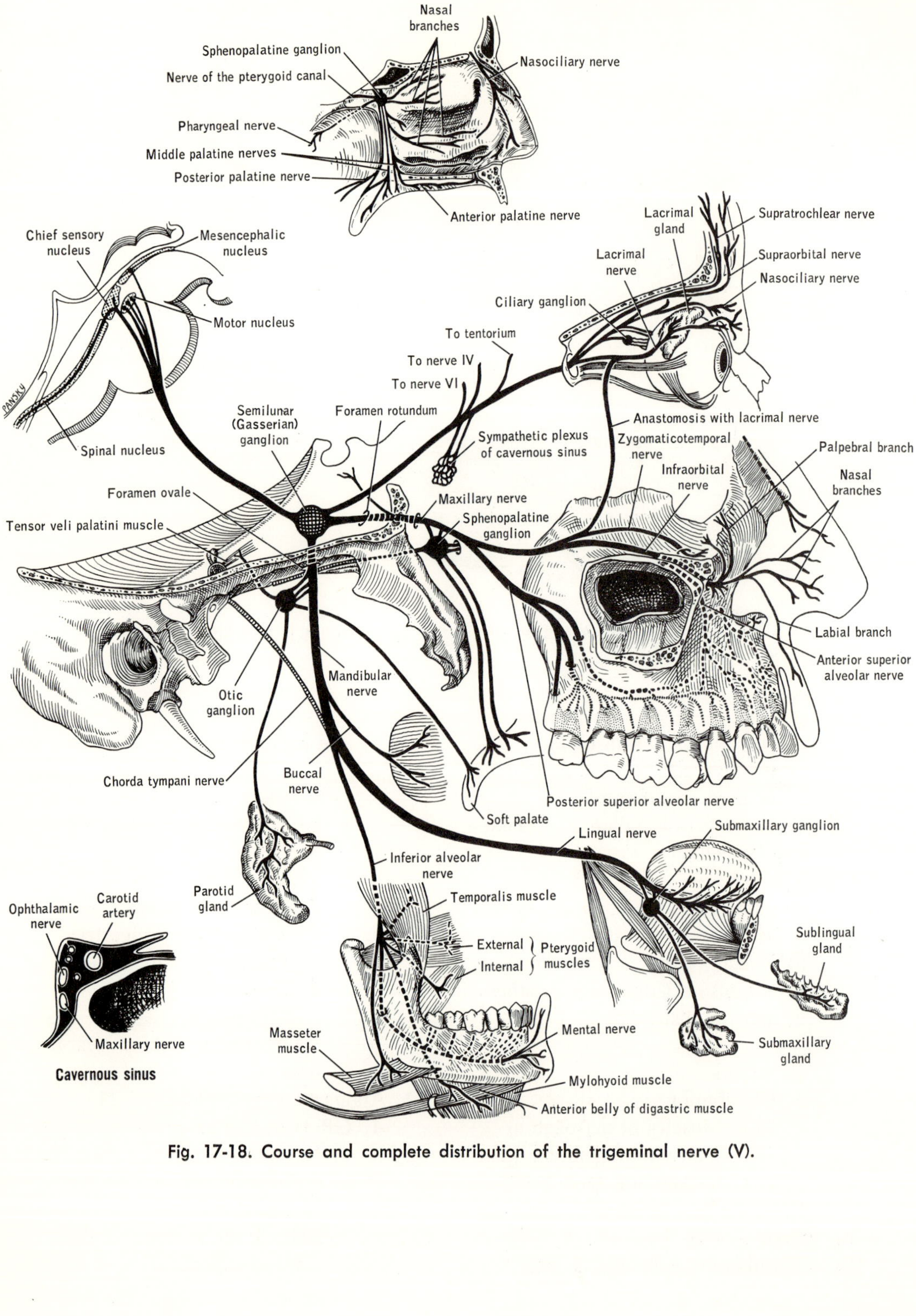

Fig. 17-18. Course and complete distribution of the trigeminal nerve (V).

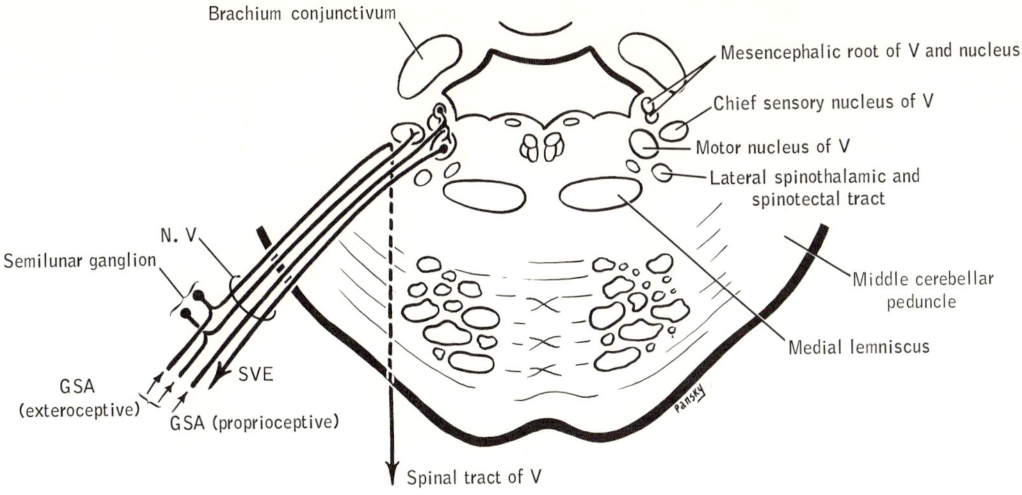

Fig. 17-19. Diagram of the functional components of the trigeminal (V) nerve.

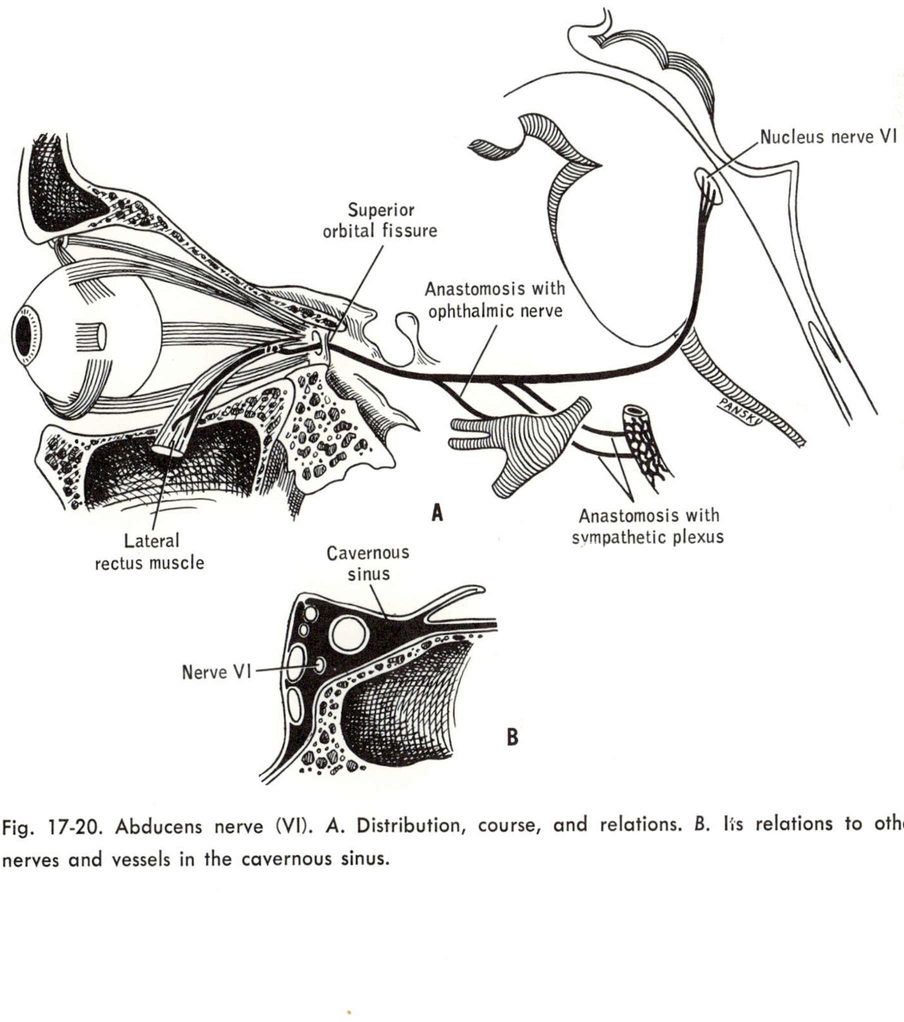

Fig. 17-20. Abducens nerve (VI). *A.* Distribution, course, and relations. *B.* Its relations to other nerves and vessels in the cavernous sinus.

3. Termination—through mesencephalic nucleus to reticular formation of brain stem

B. GSE (Chap. 14)

1. Origin—abducens nucleus
2. Termination—lateral rectus muscle of eye
3. Symptoms of disease—eye turns inward

VII. Facial (Figs. 17-21, 17-22)

A. GP (Chap. 12)

1. Receptors
   a. Muscles of facial expression
2. Cell bodies—mesencephalic nucleus of trigeminal
3. Termination—reticular formation of brain stem by way of the mesencephalic nucleus

B. GVA (Chap. 10)

1. Receptors
   a. Distribution—deep tissues of face
2. Cell bodies—geniculate ganglion
3. Termination—nucleus of tractus solitarius

C. SVA (Chap. 11)

1. Receptors
   a. Type—taste buds
   b. Location—in epithelium of tongue
   c. Distribution—anterior two-thirds of the tongue
2. Cell bodies—geniculate ganglion
3. Termination—nucleus of tractus solitarius (or gustatory nucleus)
4. Symptoms of disease—ageusia on anterior two-thirds of tongue

D. SVE (Chap. 16)

1. Origin—facial nucleus
2. Terminations
   a. Muscles of facial expression, including the platysma
   b. Posterior belly of digastric
   c. Stylohyoid
   d. Stapedius
3. Symptoms of disease—facial paralysis (Bell's palsy)

E. GVE (Chap. 15)

1. Preganglionic
   a. Origin

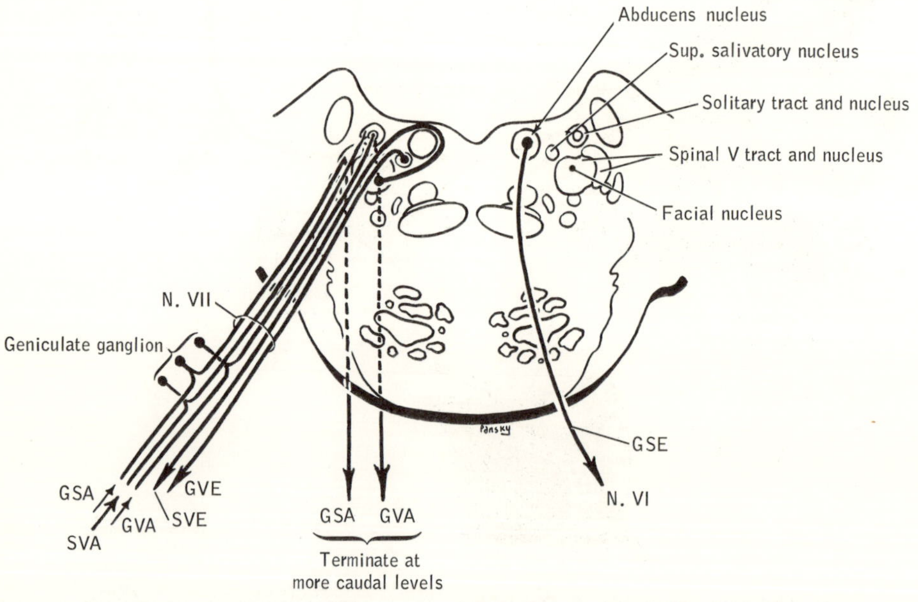

Fig. 17-21. Diagram of the functional components of the facial (VII) nerve.

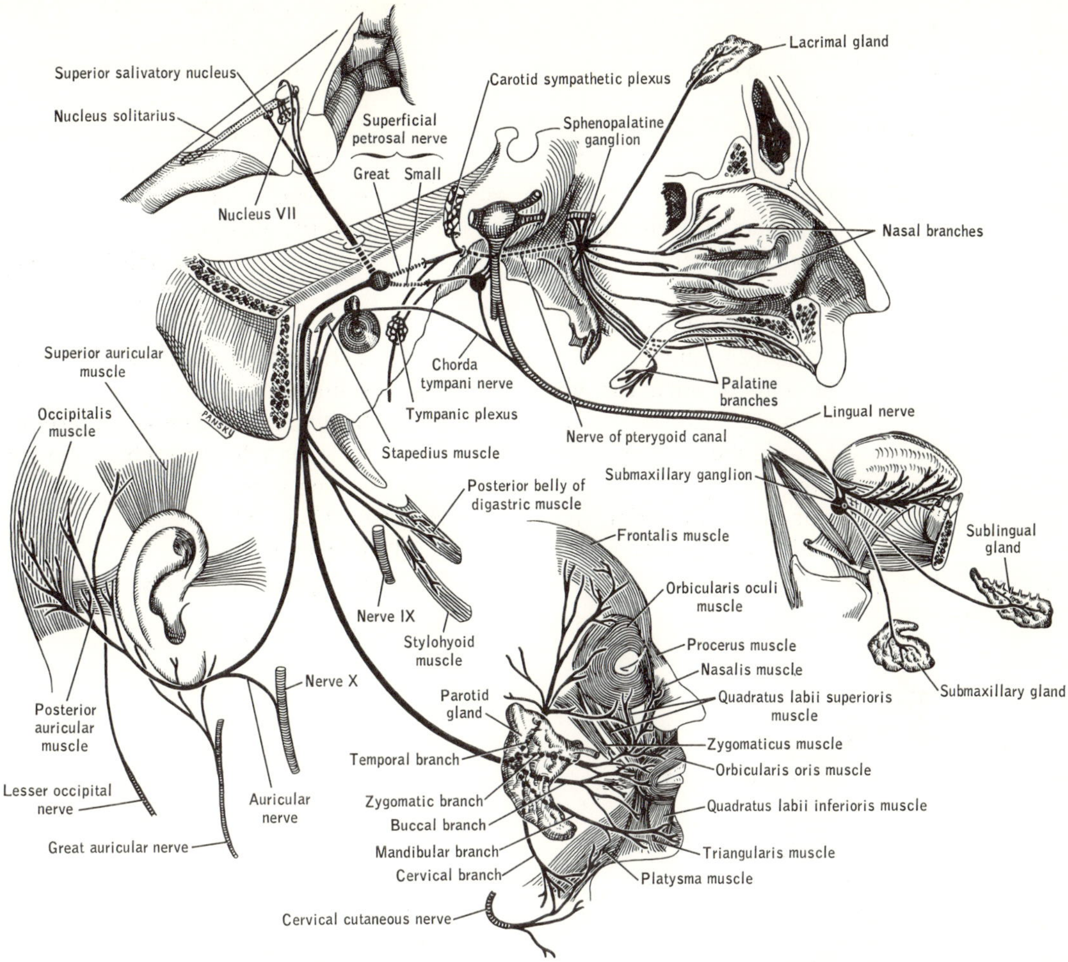

Fig. 17-22. Complete distribution, course, and relations of the facial nerve (VII).

(1). Superior salivatory nucleus
(2). Lacrimal nucleus

b. Terminations
(1). Submandibular ganglion
(2). Sphenopalatine ganglion

2. Postganglionic
   a. Origin, under *b*, (1) and (2), above
   b. Terminations
   (1). Submandibular and sublingual salivary glands—under *b*, (1), above
   (2). Lacrimal gland—under *b*, (2), above

3. Symptoms of disease—poor secretion from glands of termination

VIII. Acoustic (Figs. 17-23, 17-24)
A. SSA (Chap. 9)
1. Receptors
   a. Type—hair cells
   b. Location—organ of Corti
   c. Distribution—cochlear duct of inner ear
2. Cell bodies—spiral ganglion
3. Terminations
   a. Dorsal cochlear nucleus
   b. Ventral cochlear nucleus
4. Symptoms of disease—deafness

B. SP (Chap. 13)
  1. Receptors
    a. Type—hair cells
    b. Location
      (1). Cristae
      (2). Maculae
    c. Distribution
      (1). Ampullae of semicircular canals of inner ear, under *b,* (1), above
      (2). Utriculus of inner ear, under *b,* (2), above
      (3). Sacculus of inner ear, under *b,* (2), above
  2. Cell bodies—vestibular ganglion
  3. Terminations
    a. Vestibular nuclei (superior, medial, lateral, and spinal)
    b. Cerebellum

IX. Glossopharyngeal (Figs. 17-25, 17-26)
A. GVA (Chap. 10)
  1. Receptors
    a. Types
      (1). General
      (2). Chemoreceptors
    b. Distribution
      (1). Pharynx
      (2). Posterior third of tongue
      (3). Carotid sinus
  2. Cell bodies—petrosal ganglion
  3. Termination—nucleus of tractus solitarius
  4. Symptoms of disease—interference with the afferent limb of the swallowing reflex
B. SVA (Chap. 11)
  1. Receptors
    a. Type—taste buds

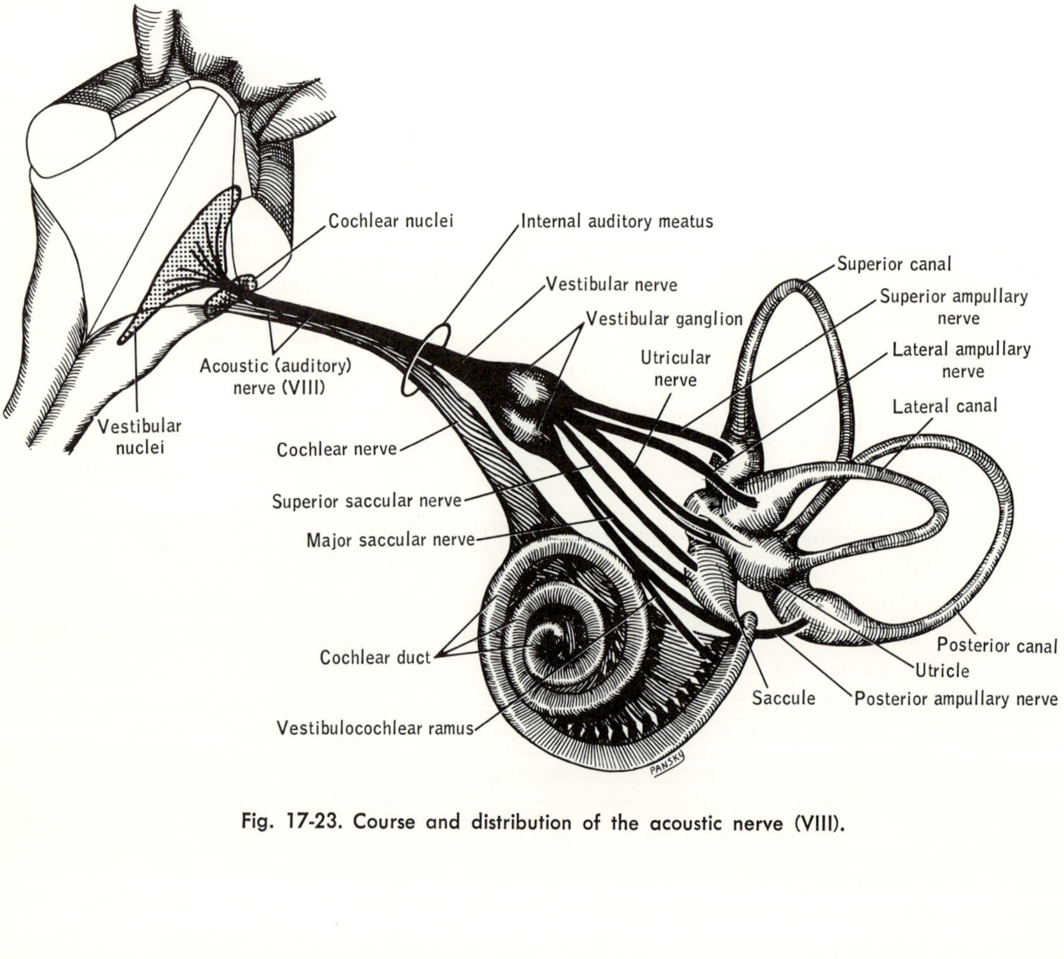

Fig. 17-23. Course and distribution of the acoustic nerve (VIII).

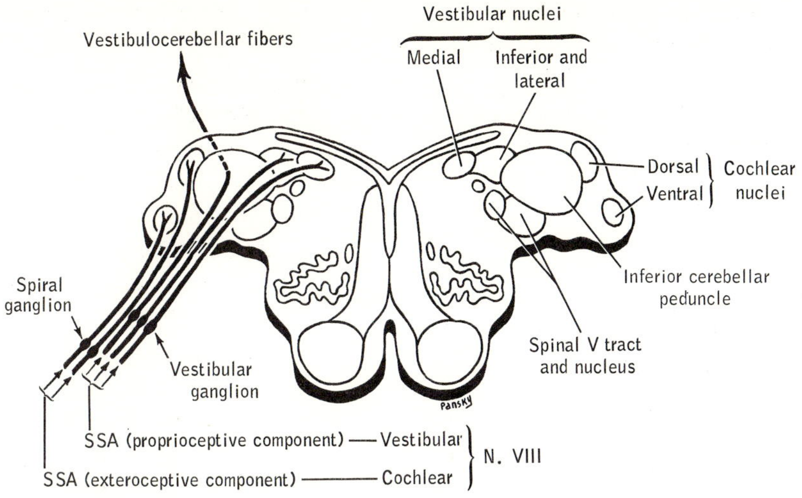

Fig. 17-24. Diagram of the functional components of the acoustic (VIII) nerve.

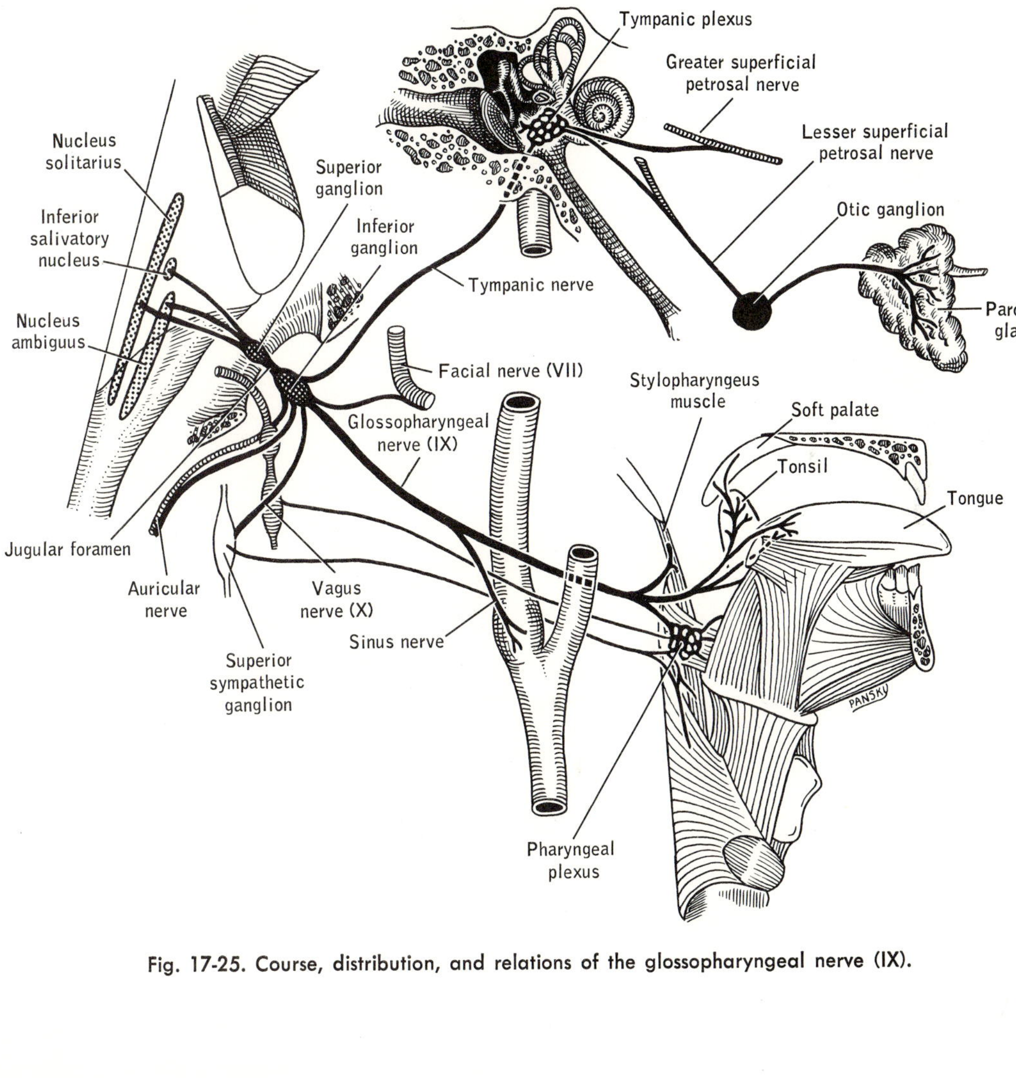

Fig. 17-25. Course, distribution, and relations of the glossopharyngeal nerve (IX).

b. Location—epithelium of tongue
c. Distribution—posterior third of tongue
2. Cell bodies—petrosal ganglion
3. Termination—nucleus of tractus solitarius (or the gustatory nucleus?)
4. Symptoms of disease—ageusia on posterior third of tongue

C. GVE (Chap. 15)
1. Preganglionic
a. Origin—inferior salivatory nucleus
b. Termination—otic ganglion
2. Postganglionic
a. Origin—under *C, b,* above
b. Termination—parotid salivary gland
3. Symptoms of disease—decreased secretion of the parotid

D. SVE (Chap. 16)
1. Origin—nucleus ambiguus
2. Terminations
a. Stylopharyngeus muscle
b. Superior pharyngeal constrictor (?)
3. Symptoms of disease—some difficulty in swallowing

X. Vagus (Figs. 17-27, 17-28)
A. GSA (Chap. 8)
1. Receptors
a. Distribution—external auditory meatus
2. Cell bodies—jugular ganglion
3. Termination—spinal V nucleus
4. Symptoms of disease—anesthesia in area of distribution

B. GVA (Chap. 10)
1. Receptors
a. Distribution
(1). Pharynx
(2). Respiratory system including larynx, trachea, bronchi
(3). Digestive system, esophagus through the middle of colon, inclusive
(4). Circulatory system including the heart, arch of the aorta, and carotid sinus
2. Cell bodies—nodose ganglion

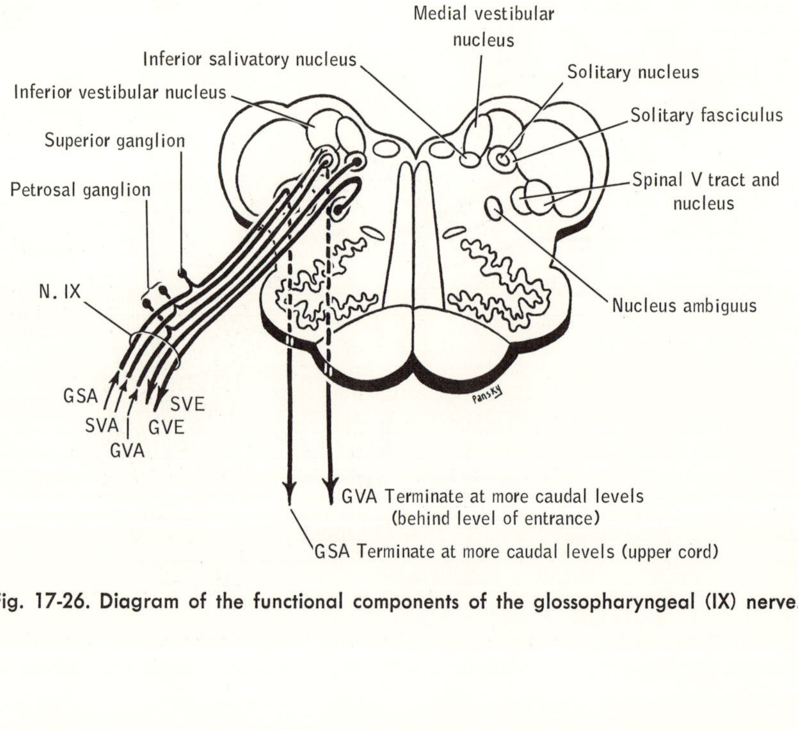

Fig. 17-26. Diagram of the functional components of the glossopharyngeal (IX) nerve.

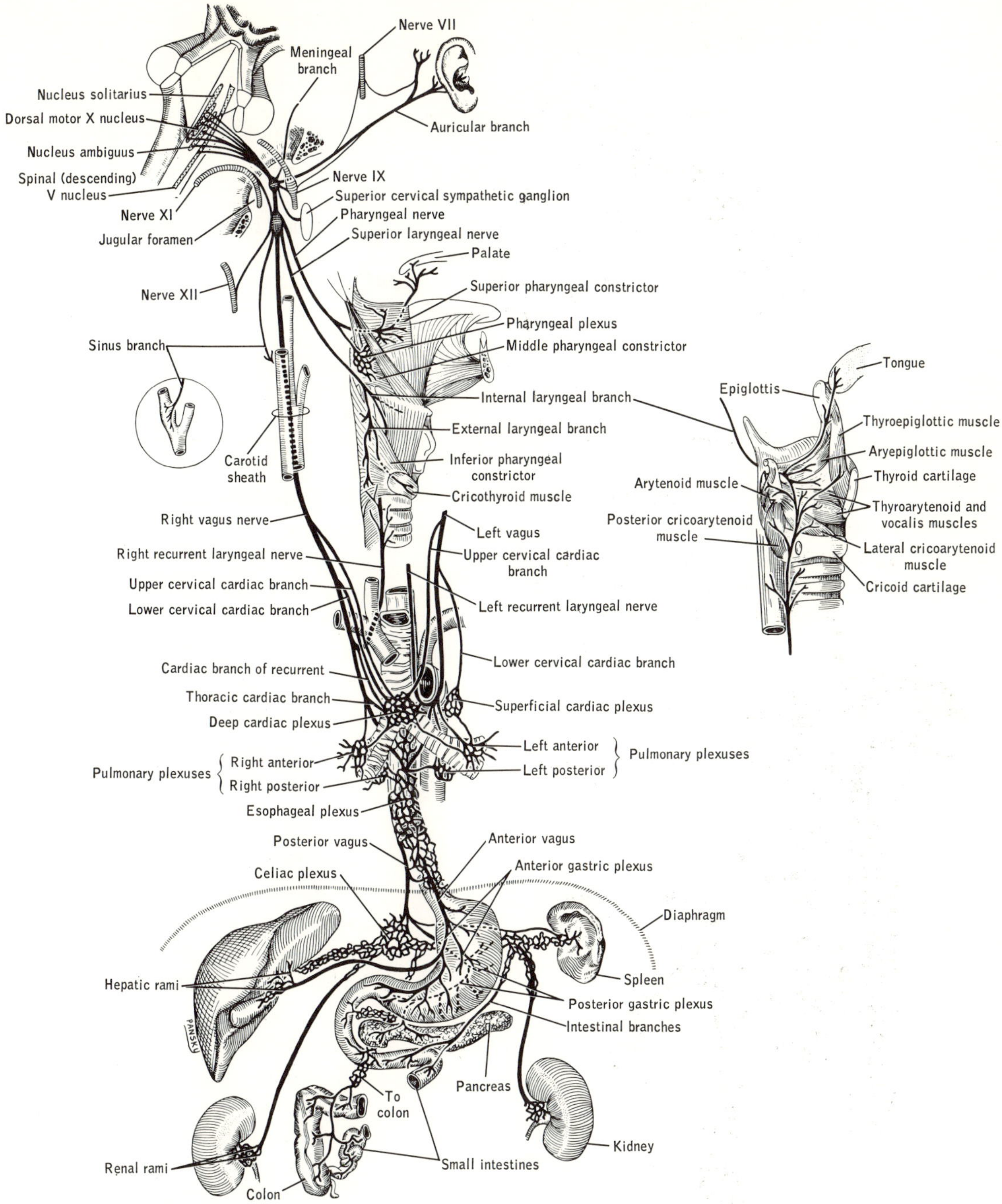

Fig. 17-27. Course, relations, and complete distribution of the vagus nerve (X).

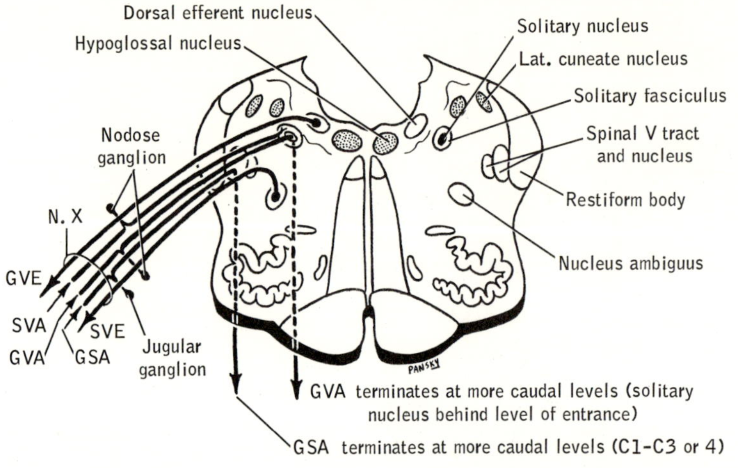

Fig. 17-28. Diagram of the functional components of the vagus (X) nerve.

3. Termination—nucleus of the tractus solitarius
4. Symptoms of disease
   a. Loss of reflex control of circulation (heart rate, etc.)

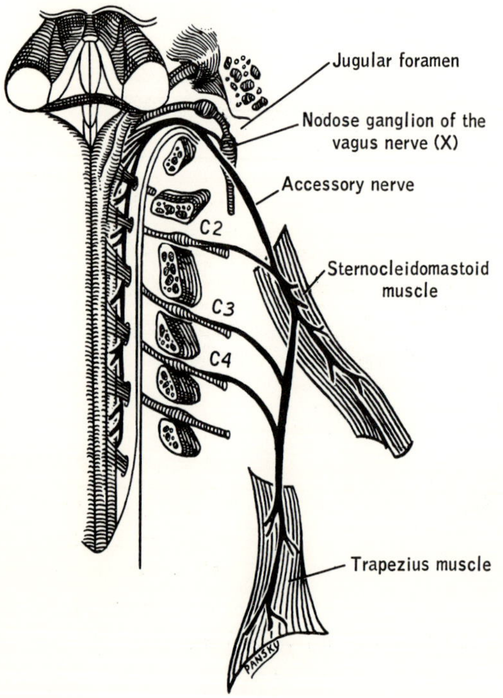

Fig. 17-29. Course, distribution, and relations of the spinal accessory nerve (XI).

   b. Disturbances in depth of respiration
   c. Poor digestion

C. SVA (Chap. 11)
1. Receptors
   a. Type—taste buds
   b. Location—in epithelium
   c. Distribution
      (1). Epiglottis
      (2). Tongue adjacent to epiglottis
      (3). Lower pharynx (?)
2. Cell bodies—nodose ganglion
3. Termination—nucleus of tractus solitarius (or gustatory nucleus?)
4. Symptoms of disease—anesthesia in area of distribution

D. GVE (Chap. 15)
1. Preganglionic
   a. Origin—dorsal motor nucleus of the vagus
   b. Termination—in terminal ganglia
      (1). Of cardiac plexuses
      (2). Of pulmonary plexuses
      (3). Of esophageal plexuses
      (4). In Auerbach's plexus in alimentary canal
      (5). In Meissner's plexus

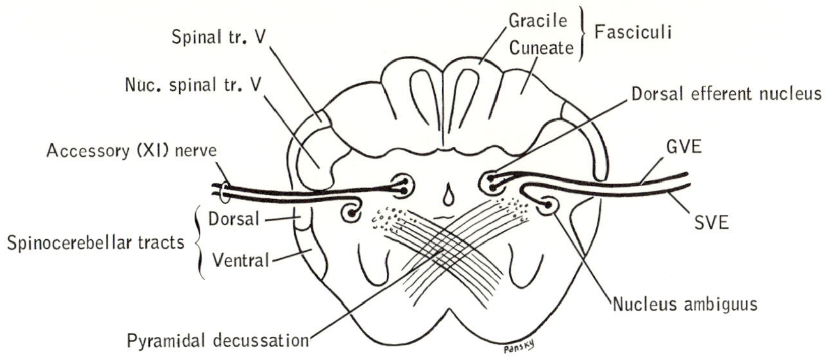

Fig. 17-30. Diagram of a section of the lower medulla at the level of the pyramidal decussation showing the components of the accessory (XI) nerve.

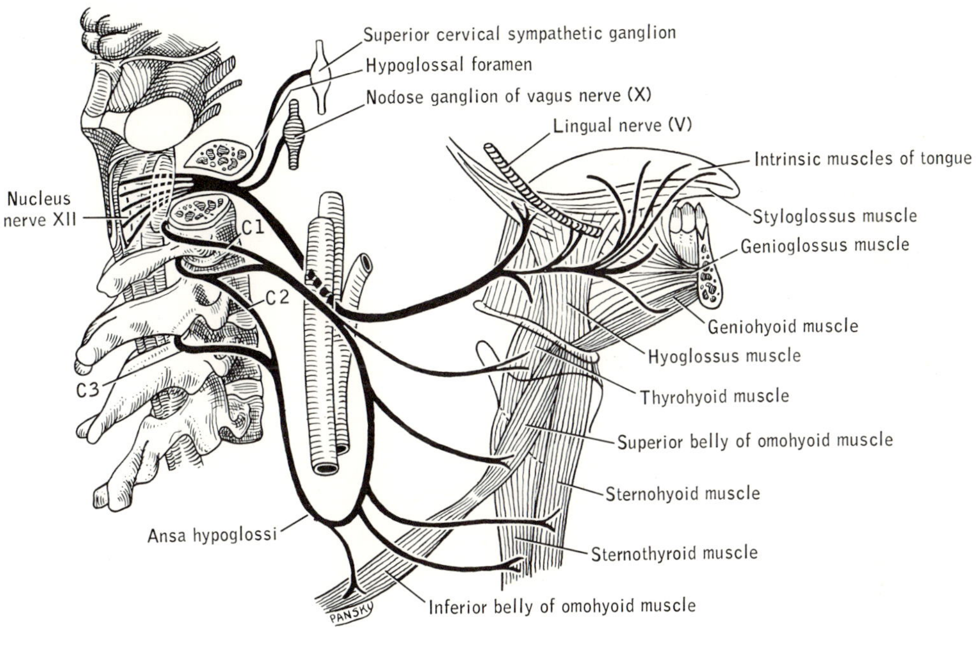

Fig. 17-31. Course, relations, and distribution of the hypoglossal nerve (XII).

2. Postganglionic
   a. Origin—in any of ganglia under *D,* 1, *b,* above
   b. Terminations
      (1). Heart
      (2). Smooth muscle and glands of trachea and bronchi
      (3). Muscle of esophagus
      (4). From Auerbach's plexus to smooth muscle of alimentary canal to midcolon
      (5). From Meissner's plexus to glands of walls of alimentary canal to midcolon
3. Symptoms of disease
   a. Loss of reflex control of circulatory system, as heart rate and blood pressure

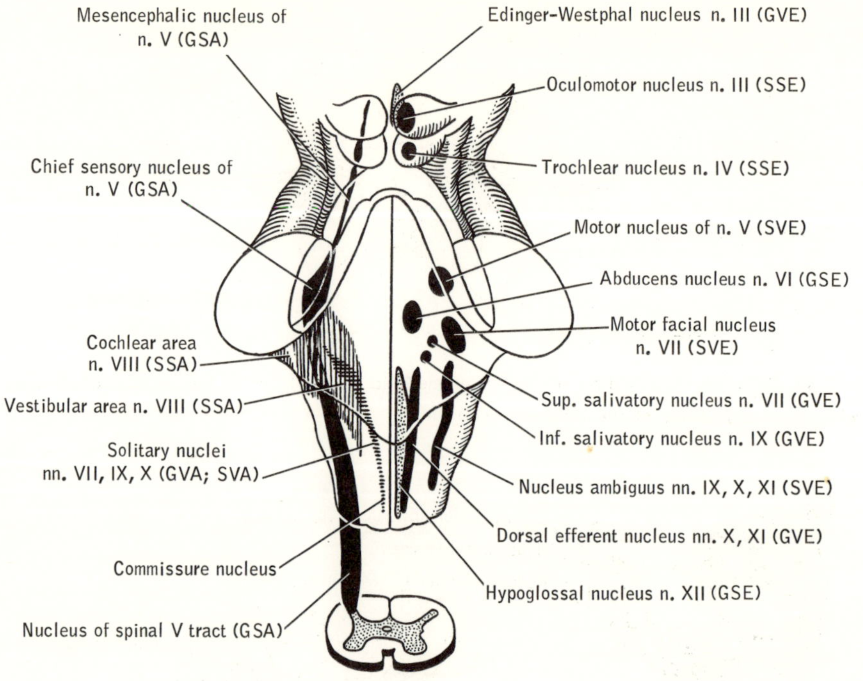

Fig. 17-32. Outline of the brain stem with a projection of the cranial nerve nuclei and their components. Afferents are shown on the left, efferents on the right.

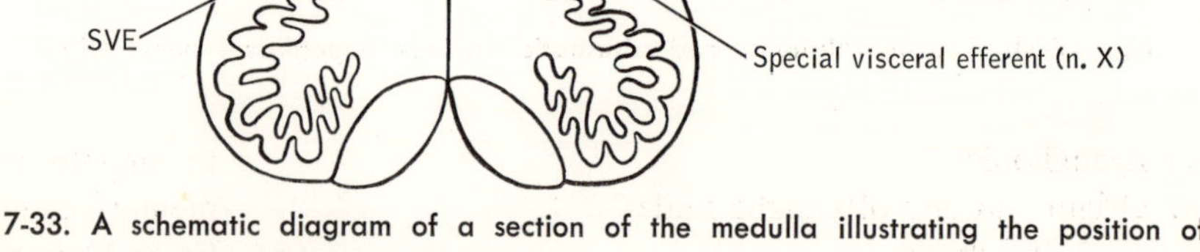

Fig. 17-33. A schematic diagram of a section of the medulla illustrating the position of the cranial nerve nuclei according to function.

   b. Poor digestion due to decreased secretion of digestive enzymes and slowing of peristalsis

E. SVE (Chap. 16)
1. Origin—nucleus ambiguus
2. Terminations
   a. Pharyngeal constrictors
   b. Muscles of larynx
   c. Muscles of palate
3. Symptoms of disease
   a. Difficulty in swallowing
   b. Difficulty in speaking

XI. Accessory (Figs. 17-29, 17-30)

A. GP (?) (Chap. 12)
1. Receptors
   a. Distribution—in muscles supplied by SVE

B. SVE (Chap. 16)
1. Origin
   a. Nucleus ambiguus
   b. Ventral horns of upper cervical cord
   c. Remnants of ventral horn in lower medulla
2. Terminations
   a. From *B*, 1, *a*, above, to larynx and pharynx with vagus
   b. From *B*, 1, *b* and *B*, 1, *c*, above, to the sternocleidomastoid and trapezius muscles
3. Symptoms of disease—difficulty in turning the head and possibly in swallowing

XII. Hypoglossal (Fig. 17-31)

A. GP (Chap. 12)
1. Receptors
   a. Distribution—muscles of tongue
2. Cell bodies—location uncertain
3. Termination—uncertain

B. GSE (Chap. 14)
1. Origin—hypoglossal nucleus
2. Termination—all muscles of tongue
3. Symptoms of disease—paralysis of tongue

C-5	C-6	C-7	C-8	T-1
BICEPS BRACHII . . . Musculocutaneous n. BRACHIALIS . . . Musculocutaneous and radial nn. BRACHIORADIALIS . . . Radial n. CORACOBRACHIALIS . . . Musculocutaneous n. DELTOID . . . Axillary n. INFRASPINATOUS . . . Suprascapular n. SUBSCAPULARIS . . . Upper and Lower Subscapular nn. SUPRASPINATUS . . . Suprascapular n. TERES MAJOR . . . Lower Subscapular n. TERES MINOR . . . Axillary n.				
	ABD. POLLICIS LONGUS . . . Deep Radial n. EXT. CARPI RADIALIS BREVIS . . . Deep Radial n. EXT. CARPI RADIALIS LONGUS . . . Radial n. EXT. POLLICIS BREVIS . . . Deep Radial n. FLEX. CARPI RADIALIS . . . Median n. PALMARIS LONGUS . . . Median n. PRONATOR TERES . . . Median n. SUPINATOR . . . Deep Radial n. EXT. CARPI ULNARIS . . . Deep Radial n. EXT. DIGITORUM . . . Deep Radial n. EXT. INDICIS . . . Deep Radial n. EXT. POLLICIS LONGUS . . . Deep Radial n. TRICEPS BRACHII . . . Radial n.			
		ANCONEUS . . .Radial n. EXT. DIGITI MINIMI . . . Deep Radial n. FLEX. DIGITORUM PROFUNDUS . . . Median and Ulnar nn. FLEX. DIGITORUM SUPERFICIALIS . . . Median n.		
			ABD. DIGITI MINIMI . . . Deep Ulnar n. ABD. POLLICIS BREVIS . . . Median n. ADD. POLLICIS . . . Deep Ulnar n. FLEX. CARPI ULNARIS . . . Ulnar n. FLEX. DIGITI MINIMI . . . Deep Ulnar n. FLEX. POLLICIS BREVIS . . . Median n. FLEX. POLLICIS LONGUS . . . Median n. INTEROSSEI . . . Deep Ulnar n. LUMBRICALES . . . Deep Ulnar and Median nn. OPPONENS DIGITI MINIMI . . . Deep Ulnar n. OPPONENS POLLICIS . . . Median n. PALMARIS BREVIS . . . Superficial Ulnar n. PRONATOR QUADRATUS . . . Median n.	

L-2 | L-3 | L-4 | L-5 | S-1 | S-2

ADD. BREVIS . . . Obturator n.
ADD. LONGUS . . . Obturator n.
GRACILIS . . . Obturator n.
SARTORIUS . . . Femoral n.

ILIACUS . . . Femoral n.
PSOAS MAJOR . . . Nn to Psoas

OBTURATOR EXTERNUS . . . Obturator n.
PECTINEUS . . . Femoral n.
QUADRICEPS FEMORIS . . . femoral n.

ADD. MAGNUS . . . Obturator and Sciatic nn.

TIBIALIS ANTERIOR . . . Deep Peroneal n.

GLUTEUS MEDIUS . . . Superior Gluteal n.
GLUTEUS MINIMUS . . . Superior Gluteal n.
INF. GEMELLUS . . . N. to Quadratus Femoris
LUMBRICALES . . . Medial and Lateral Plantar nn.
PLANTARIS . . . Tibial n.
POPLITEUS . . . Tibial n.
QUADRATUS FEMORIS . . . N. to Quadratus Femoris
TENSOR FASCIA LATAE . . . Superior Gluteal n.

SEMIMEMBRANOSUS . . . Sciatic n.
SEMITENDINOSUS . . . Sciatic n.

EXT. DIGITORUM LONGUS . . . Deep Peroneal n.
EXT. HALLUCIS LONGUS . . . Deep Peroneal n.
PERONEUS BREVIS . . . Superficial Peroneal n.
PERONEUS LONGUS . . . Peroneal n.
TIBIALIS POSTERIOR . . . Tibial n.

GLUTEUS MAXIMUS . . . Inferior Gluteal n.
OBTURATOR INTERNUS . . . N. to Obt. Internus
SOLEUS . . . Tibial n.
SUP. GEMELLUS . . . N. to Obt. Internus
BICEPS FEMORIS . . . Sciatic n.

ABD. DIGITI MINIMI . . . Lat. Plantar n.
ABD. HALLUCIS . . . Med. Plantar n.
ADD. HALLUCIS . . . Lat. Plantar n.
EXT. DIGIT. BREVIS . . . Deep Peroneal n.
EXT. HALLUCIS BREVIS . . . Deep Peroneal n.
FLEX. DIGITI MINIMI . . . Lat. Plantar n.
FLEX. DIGIT. BREVIS . . . Med. Plantar n.
FLEX. DIGIT. LONGUS . . . Tibial n.
FLEX. HALLUCIS BREVIS . . . Med. Plantar n.
FLEX. HALLUCIS LONGUS . . . Tibial n.
GASTROCNEMIUS . . . Tibial n.
INTEROSSEI . . . Lateral Plantar n.
PIRIFORMIS . . . N. to Piriformis
QUADRATUS PLANTAE . . . Lat. Plantar n.

18 CEREBELLAR MODIFICATION OF MUSCULAR ACTIVITY

The chief concern of the cerebellum is synergy, which is defined as "the faculty by which movements are properly grouped for the performance of acts requiring special adjustments." To appreciate fully what this means, it is necessary to analyze, in terms of muscular performance, the mechanics of movement. (1) The initiation of movement requires the contraction of a muscle or a group of muscles. Simultaneously, however, an opposing set of muscles must relax. (2) For the proper performance of a movement a definite amount of muscular contraction is required. This can be controlled only by an adjustment of the number of muscle fibers [1] involved in the reaction, which, in turn, is a function of the number of nerve fibers activated. (3) The proper duration of the nerve impulses for the completion of an act is important. (4) Especially when the action requires movement at several joints, it is essential for muscles to contract and relax in proper sequence.

In order to accomplish these things, certain basic connections must be present. First, the cerebellum must receive continuous information from the muscular system concerning tension states. Streams of impulses set up by movements must reach the cerebellum from the joints. Action currents from the vestibular receptors in the inner ear must reach the cerebellum. At the same time, the cerebellum must be in intimate relation to the streams of impulses leaving the voluntary motor centers of the cerebrum. Then, the cerebellum must contain an internal organization which will coordinate this information and must possess efferent pathways so that it can exert its influence upon the segmental apparatus and lower motor centers.

STRUCTURE OF THE CEREBELLUM

Gross (Figs. 18-1, 18-2)

The major structural features have already been given (Figs. 2-41 to 2-43). However, since reference is often made to divisions based upon evolutionary and developmental concepts, a description of the cerebellum would be incomplete without considering these aspects.

Early in phylogenesis, the cerebellum appears as lateral elevations of the ancient hindbrain which are almost a part of the primordial vestibular apparatus. Later, a median unpaired portion appears. This condition persists in animal forms without limbs. With the appearance of appendages, the median cerebellar body expands laterally. This expansion is the progenitor of the body of the cerebellum (hemispheres). At about the same stage of evolution, the two lateral parts of the original vestibular cerebellum join across

[1] According to the all-or-nothing law, a muscle fiber receiving a stimulus strong enough to cause a contraction at all will contract to its fullest. Therefore, the strength of the contraction of a muscle as a whole depends upon the number of contracting fibers, the latter being a function of the number of nerves carrying activating impulses.

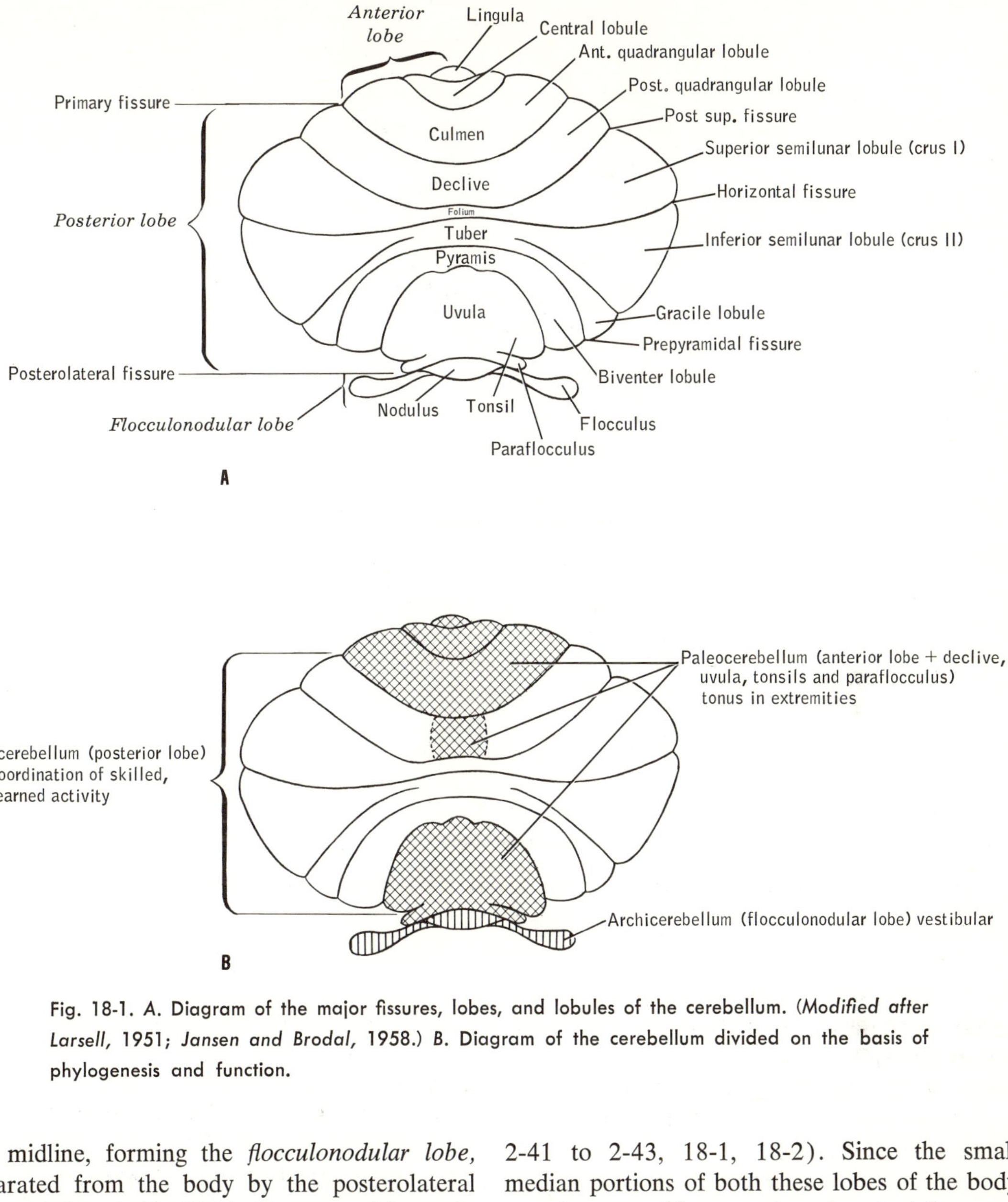

Fig. 18-1. A. Diagram of the major fissures, lobes, and lobules of the cerebellum. (*Modified after Larsell,* 1951; *Jansen and Brodal,* 1958.) B. Diagram of the cerebellum divided on the basis of phylogenesis and function.

the midline, forming the *flocculonodular lobe,* separated from the body by the posterolateral fissure (Figs. 2-43, 18-1). Because of its early phylogenetic appearance, the flocculonodular lobe is often referred to as the *archicerebellum.*[2]

Early in development, the body of the cerebellum lying rostral to the posterolateral fissure is divided into an anterior and posterior lobe by the appearance of the primary fissure (Figs. 5-7, 2-41 to 2-43, 18-1, 18-2). Since the small median portions of both these lobes of the body are also very old, appearing almost at the same time as the flocculonodular lobe, they are included as part of the archicerebellum. However, the lateral expansion of these parts, developing later, is referred to as the *paleocerebellum* [3] (Fig. 18-1).

[2] The prefix *archi-* denotes first or original.

[3] *Paleo-* means old but neither original nor as old as *archi-*.

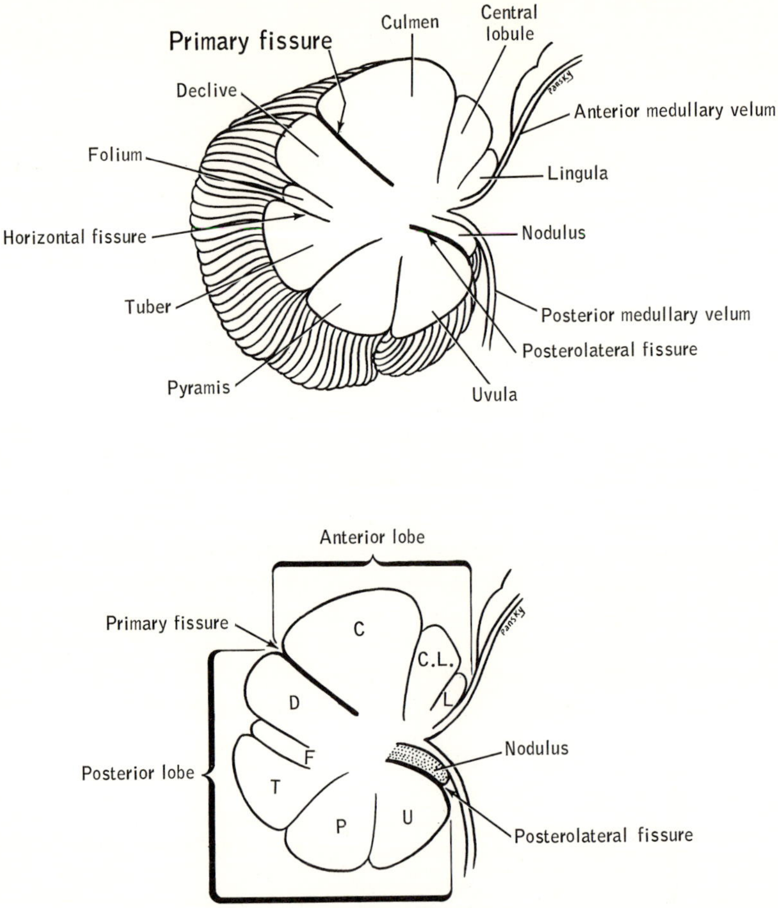

Fig. 18-2. Diagram of a sagittal section through the midline of the cerebellum showing the principal fissures and the divisions of the vermis.

Phylogenetically, the appearance of the cerebral hemispheres makes possible a tremendous range of voluntary actions. Therefore, there is an enlargement of the cerebellum, proportionate in extent to the size of the voluntary motor centers of the cerebrum. This is the *neocerebellum* [4] (Fig. 18-1), which accounts for the great size of the human cerebellum.

According to some authorities, the neocerebellum is the major and most rostral part of the posterior lobe of the cerebellum. According to others, the neocerebellum is represented by the middle lobe. Using the latter designation, that portion lying in front of the primary fissure, including the lingula, central lobule, culmen, and anterior quadrangular lobule, belongs to the anterior lobe (Figs. 2-41 to 2-43). The middle lobe, the rostral boundary of which is the primary fissure, includes (from front to back) the declive, with the posterior quadrangular lobule; the folium, with its lateral portion, the superior semilunar lobule; the tuber, and its extension, the inferior semilunar lobule. Just behind the tuber of the vermis, the prepyramidal fissure usually can be seen. This is the line dividing the middle from the posterior lobe. The latter is

[4] *Neo-* means new or recent.

made up, from front to back, of the pyramis and its biventer lobule; and the uvula, with its lateral extension, the tonsil.

Microscopic

Cortex

The superficial gray matter of the cerebellum is thrown into folds (folia), the long axes of which are arranged transversely from one hemisphere to the other. The center of each folium is composed of medullary substance through which all fibers enter or leave the cortex.

The arrangement of the cells and fibers within the cortex is an adaptation to functional requirements. First, the cerebellum must be able to disseminate its influence over the entire body musculature. To accomplish this, it must be possible for a single impulse to spread over, and thus activate, large areas of the cortex. Second, the influence of the cerebellum, in many instances, is reinforcing, enhancing, and perpetuating. For this to be possible, action currents leaving the cortex must be able to reactivate the same areas in the cortex from which they originally arose.

The cortex is composed of three layers (Fig. 18-3): the inner, or granular, layer; the middle, or Purkinje cell, layer; and the outer, or molecular, layer.

Granular (Inner) Layer. Two types of cells are found here. The predominant type is a small neuron called the *granule cell.* Its three to five dendrites spray out through this layer and terminate in small clawlike arrangements for the reception of afferent fibers entering the cerebellar cortex. The single axon passes outward through the Purkinje layer to enter the molecular layer, where it terminates in a T-shaped bifurcation. These branches are so arranged as to extend in the long axis of the folium. Thus, in their course, synaptic relations with dendrites of many Purkinje cells are facilitated. In addition to the granule cells, some larger cells (stellate) are found, particularly in that portion of the granule layer nearest the Purkinje cells. These cells have dendrites extending into the molecular layer. The axons are short and branch repeatedly into a plexiform arrangement within the granular layer itself.

Purkinje (Middle) Layer. This layer is one cell in thickness and contains one cell type, the Purkinje cell. The body of the cell is flask-shaped, the neck of the flask being directed superficially toward the surface of the cortex. From the neck arise one or two thick dendrites which enter the outer molecular layer. Within the molecular layer, the dendrites branch repeatedly, the branching taking place at right angles to the long axis of the folium. From the large end of the cell body, opposite the neck, a single axon extends across the inner granular layer, enters the white core of the folium, and terminates in one of the central nuclei. Within the granular layer, the axon gives rise to collaterals which pass backward through the layer to end in synaptic relations with adjoining Purkinje's cells. This facilitates spreading of the stimulation over wider cortical areas and adds strength and persistence to the total effect.

Molecular (Outer) Layer. It contains the dendrites of Purkinje cells, the axons of granule cells, and the fine dendrites of some of the larger cells of the granular layer. In addition there are also two cell types. One is a small neuron of the *Golgi type II class,* the processes of which apparently ramify in the more superficial part of the layer. The other is the *basket cell.* This has several branching dendrites, which extend into the outer portion of this layer, and a single axon which runs at right angles to the long axis of the folium. Each axon gives off several collaterals which bend inward toward the Purkinje cells, around which they form a network.

Fibers

These are classified according to the direction of their impulses.

Afferent. These fibers carry impulses into the cerebellum. Morphologically, they are of two types, *mossy* and *climbing* (Fig. 18-3). The *mossy fibers* are found in all parts of the cerebellum. They course and give rise to many branches within the granular layer. These branches terminate by forming mossy tufts, which

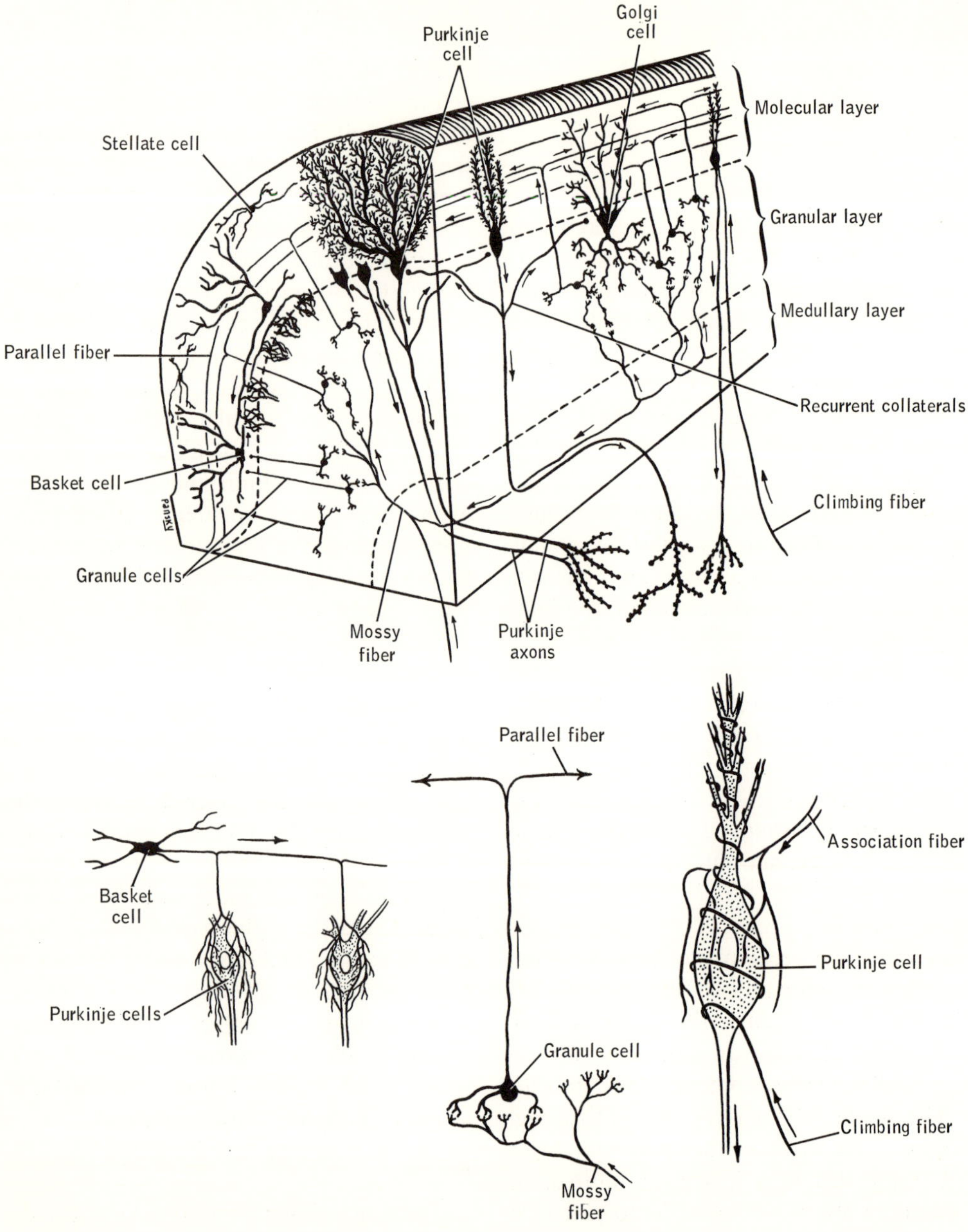

Fig. 18-3. A diagrammatic representation of a folium of the cerebellar cortex showing the arrangement of cells and fibers as seen both in longitudinal and transverse sections. The relationship between fiber types and cells is also illustrated.

are held in the clawlike dendrites of the granule cells. Impulses pass through the dendrites of the granule cells to come into synaptic relations with the dendrites of the Purkinje cells, many of which can be activated by an action current traveling in but one afferent fiber. It is now believed that mossy fibers represent the terminations of all fibers which enter the cerebellum from other portions of the CNS.

The *climbing fibers* are long and slender. They ascend through the granular and Purkinje layers to enter the molecular zone. Here, they climb, like a vine on a trellis, among the dendritic ramifications of Purkinje cells. These fibers may arise from certain cells in the central nuclei or from collaterals of axons leaving these nuclei, or they may be long, recurrent collaterals of the Purkinje cells themselves.

Efferent. There is only one set of fibers leaving the cerebellar cortex. These are all the axons of the Purkinje cells (Fig. 18-2) which pass through the molecular layer of the cortex to reach the white, medullary core of the folium. Continuing in the white substance, most of these axons end in one of the central nuclei. Few leave the cerebellum directly.

Medulla

Beneath the cortex, extending internally from the center of all the folia, is the medullary sub-

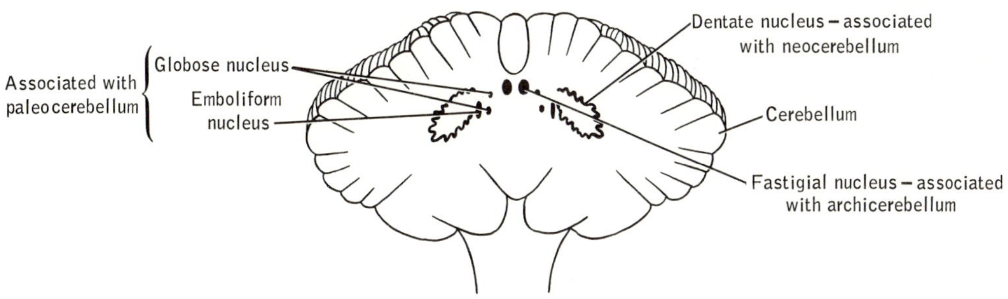

A

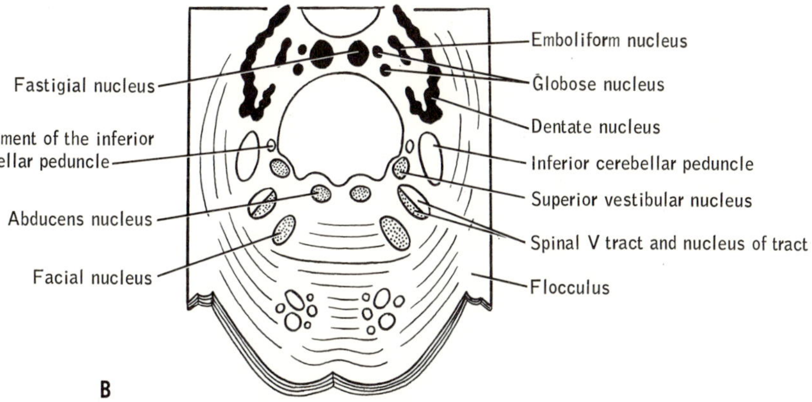

B

Fig. 18-4. A. Transverse section of the adult cerebellum illustrating the cerebellar nuclei. *B.* Vertical section through the adult cerebellum and brain stem at the level of the nuclei of the abducens (VI) and facial (VII) nerves. The fourth ventricle, inferior cerebellar peduncle, and cerebellar nuclei are also shown.

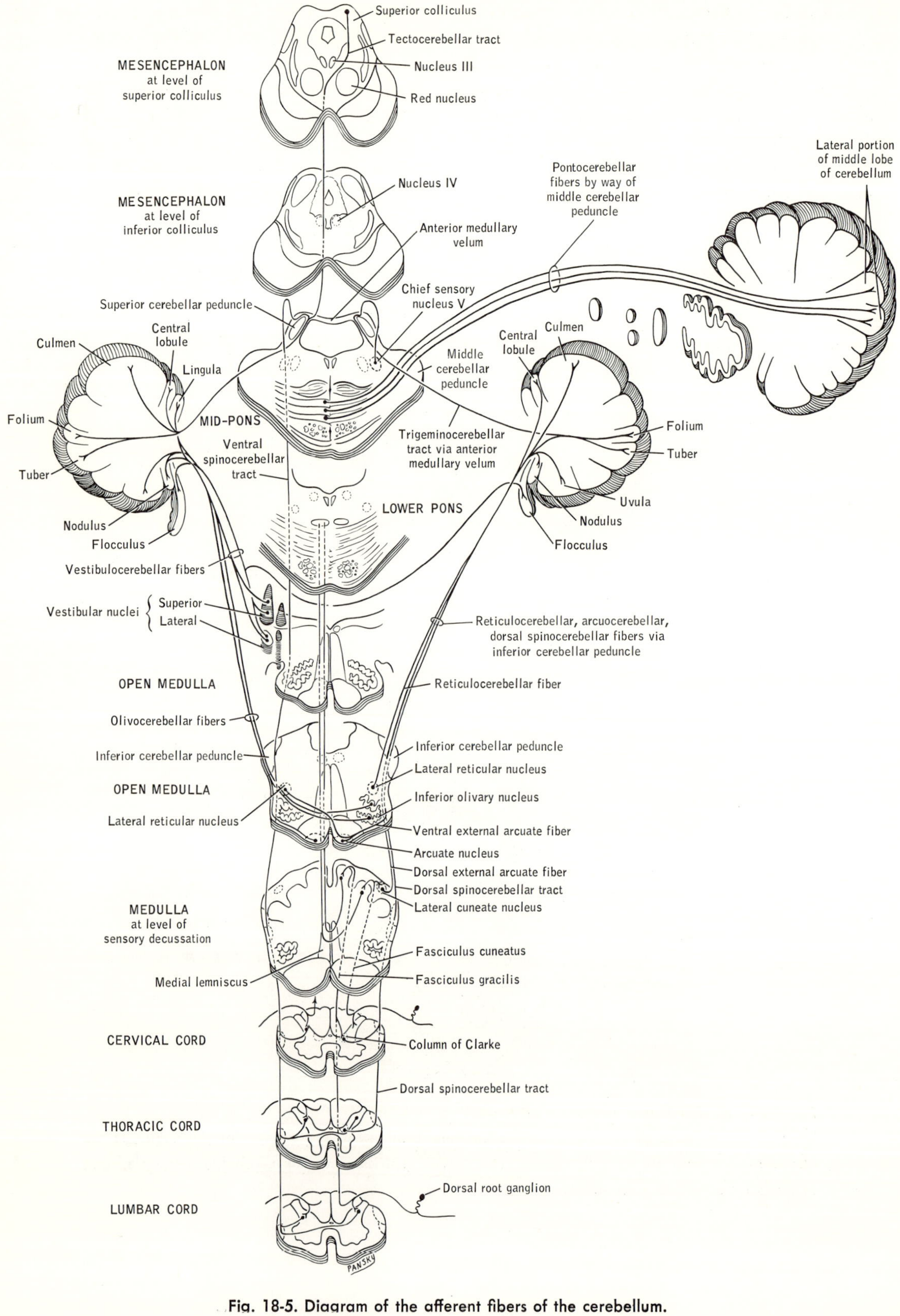

Fig. 18-5. Diagram of the afferent fibers of the cerebellum.

stance, composed of fibers carrying impulses to or from the cortex. The white matter of the cerebellum is somewhat treelike in its arrangement (Fig. 18-3). Four areas of cellular concentrations are embedded in the medullary substance. These areas are referred to as the central nuclei and from without inward are named dentate, emboliform, globose, and fastigial (Figs. 2-44, 18-4).

SPECIFIC CEREBELLAR CONNECTIONS

Afferent Tracts (Figs. 18-5 to 18-9.)

Spinocerebellar (Figs. 18-5, 18-6.)

These fibers are important in bringing into the cerebellum information concerning the tension states of muscles and the orientation of articulations. They travel in several different pathways from various points of origin. The *dorsospinocerebellar tract* arises from Clarke's column (Figs. 3-5, 12-2, 25-1) and terminates in the central lobule, culmen, and anterior quadrangular lobule of the anterior lobe and in the declive, uvula, and tonsil of the posterior lobe. This circuit may be concerned with activity initiated by the afferent limb of the stretch reflex. The *ventral spinocerebellar tract* arises from the cells near the base of the posterior column at all levels, most of the fibers crossing to the opposite side of the cord (Figs. 3-4, 3-5, 25-1 to 25-9). The majority of these fibers end in the central lobule and culmen of the anterior lobe. Some may enter the declive of the posterior lobe. This pathway may carry impulses initiated by tactile as well as proprioceptive receptors.

Dorsal External Arcuate Fibers (Fig. 18-8.)

The impulses carried by these fibers originate in the proprioceptors in the muscles and joints of the cervical region. These impulses are carried in the fasciculus cuneatus to the accessory (lateral) cuneate nucleus. From cells in this nucleus axons pass by way of the dorsal external arcuate fibers through the inferior cerebellar peduncle to be distributed to the same cortical areas as the fibers of the dorsal spinocerebellar tract (Fig. 25-3).

Vestibulocerebellar (Fig. 18-5.)

Fibers coming from the vestibular apparatus are of two sorts: (1) *direct,* representing a few of the ascending branches of the vestibular nerve

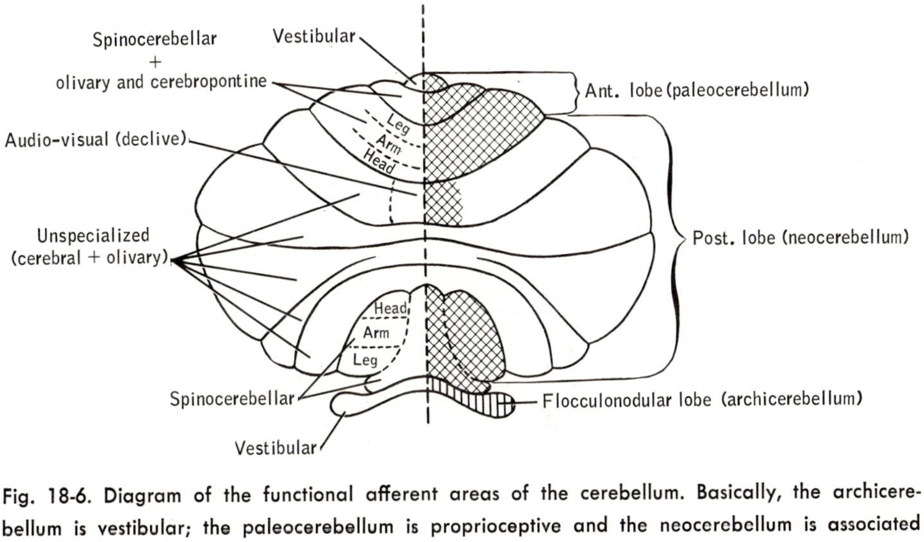

Fig. 18-6. Diagram of the functional afferent areas of the cerebellum. Basically, the archicerebellum is vestibular; the paleocerebellum is proprioceptive and the neocerebellum is associated with skilled movements. However, the boundaries are not sharp and there is some overlap. (*Modified after Elliott,* 1963.)

which course upward along the medial side of the inferior cerebellar peduncle proper to enter the homolateral flocculus, nodulus, and lingula; (2) secondary fibers arising in the medial, superior and inferior (spinal) vestibular nuclei. These fibers enter the cerebellum through the medial segment of the inferior cerebellar peduncle and end, in the flocculonodular lobe—especially on the contralateral side—in the uvula and in the fastigial nuclei of both sides.

Trigeminocerebellar (Fig. 18-5.)

Secondary proprioceptive fibers arising in the mesencephalic nucleus and terminating in the dentate and emboliform nuclei have been reported. Other sensory modalities, especially touch, have secondary fibers arising in the chief sensory nucleus of the trigeminal and ending in the anterior quadrangular lobule and tonsil. It is also possible that both crossed and uncrossed fibers may arise in the spinal nucleus of the trigeminal and ascend to these same areas of the cerebellum.

Reticulocerebellar (Figs. 18-5, 18-8.)

These fibers arise predominantly in the lateral reticular nucleus of the medulla but other nuclei (paramedian reticular, parahypoglossal and nucleus of the raphe) probably also contribute. From here, most of the fibers pass dorsolaterally to join the inferior cerebellar peduncle through which they are distributed chiefly to the vermis of the anterior lobe and perhaps to the flocculonodular lobe. Those fibers arising in the parahypoglossal and paramedian nuclei may also project to the pyramis and uvula. A few may pass ventrally through the median fissure as a part of the ventral external arcuate fibers and eventually join the dorsal spinocerebellar tract in the inferior peduncle. From the position of its cells of origin, this fiber system is in a position to receive impulses from several systems, among them being ascending fibers belonging to the sensory systems of the spinal cord, especially those running upward in the lateral funiculus. Furthermore, the reticulocerebellar system is believed to be interconnected with fibers descending from higher motor centers of the extrapyramidal system (Chap. 19).

Olivocerebellar (Figs. 2-50, 18-5, 18-7, 25-4.)

The inferior olivary complex is composed of a principal (chief) olivary nucleus, a dorsal accessory, and a medial accessory nucleus. The

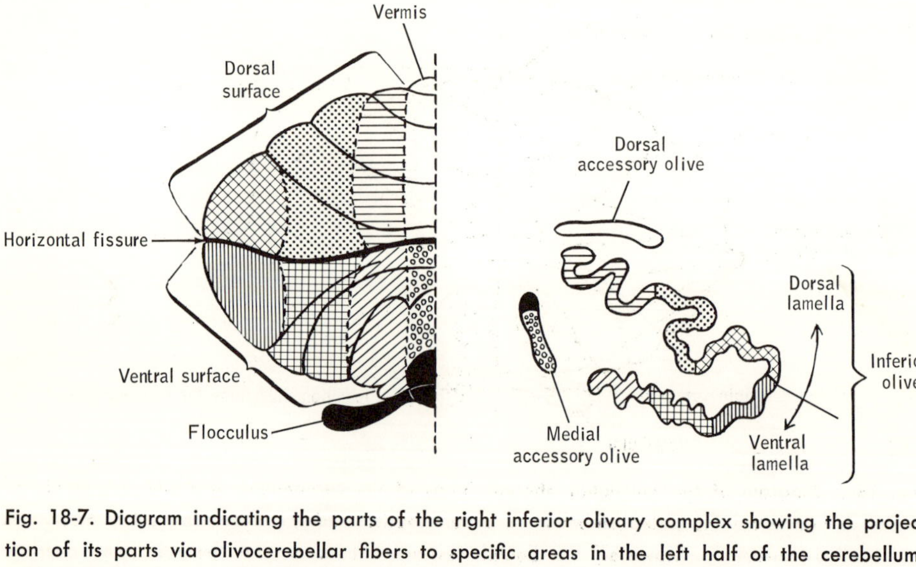

Fig. 18-7. Diagram indicating the parts of the right inferior olivary complex showing the projection of its parts via olivocerebellar fibers to specific areas in the left half of the cerebellum. (*Modified after Huber, 1899; Hamby and Gardner, 1935; Szentagothai, 1942.*)

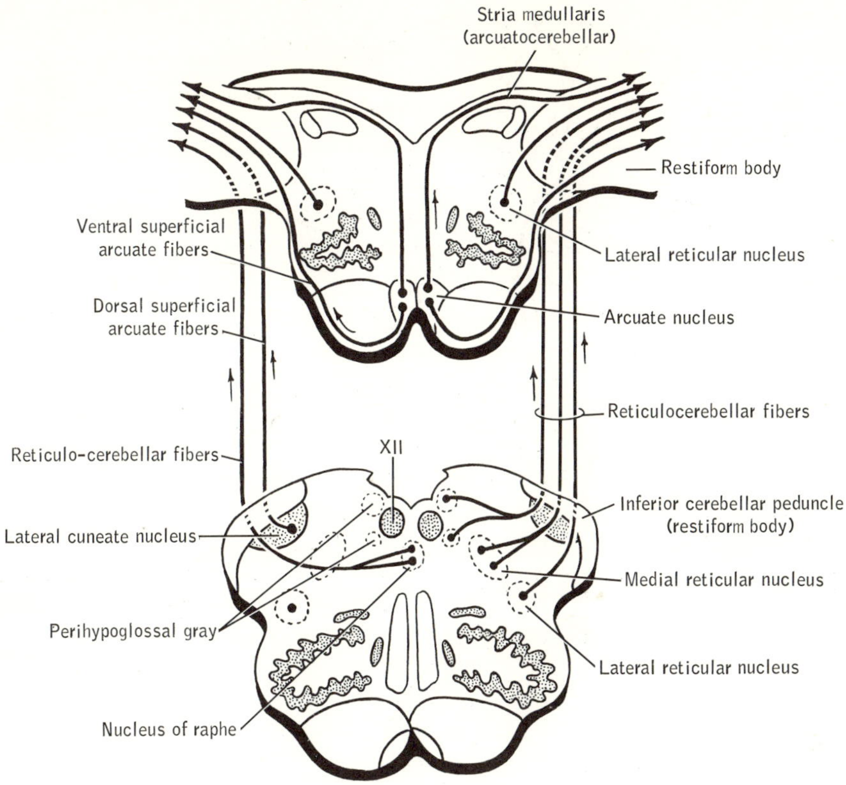

Fig. 18-8. Diagram to demonstrate some of the reticulocerebellar and arcuatocerebellar fibers of the brain stem. (*Modified after Crosby, Humphrey, and Lauer, 1962.*)

principal nucleus consists of a dorsal and ventral lamella, with a laterally placed interlamellar band connecting the two. Because of the descending fibers from the red nucleus and globus pallidus which end here, the olivocerebellar circuit may be closely allied to the subcortical portion of the extrapyramidal system (Chap. 19). The inferior olive is related to most of the spinal afferent systems by fibers ascending in the spino-olivary tract. The latter arises from cells in the dorsal column of the spinal cord on the side opposite to the tract. Olivocerebellar fibers arise from the entire complex, cross the midline, usually passing through the olive of the other side, and ascend into the cerebellum by way of the inferior cerebellar peduncle. Those which have their origin in the chief nucleus have a wide distribution to the hemispheres of both the anterior and posterior lobes. From the medial accessory olive, fibers terminate in the flocculonodular lobe, the pyramis, uvula, declive and the fastigial nucleus. The dorsal accessory olive sends most of its fibers to the vermian portions of the anterior lobe and to the declive and folium of the posterior lobe.

Pontocerebellar (Figs. 18-5, 18-9, 25-6 to 25-9.)

The mass of pontocerebellar fibers is concerned with the coordination of movements initiated in the motor cortex of the cerebrum. Descending fibers from the frontal, parietal tempero-occipital, and temporal association areas as well as collaterals of the pyramidal fibers arising in the precentral gyrus terminate among the pontine nuclei. The latter are scattered among the fascicles of the basal pons. Attempts

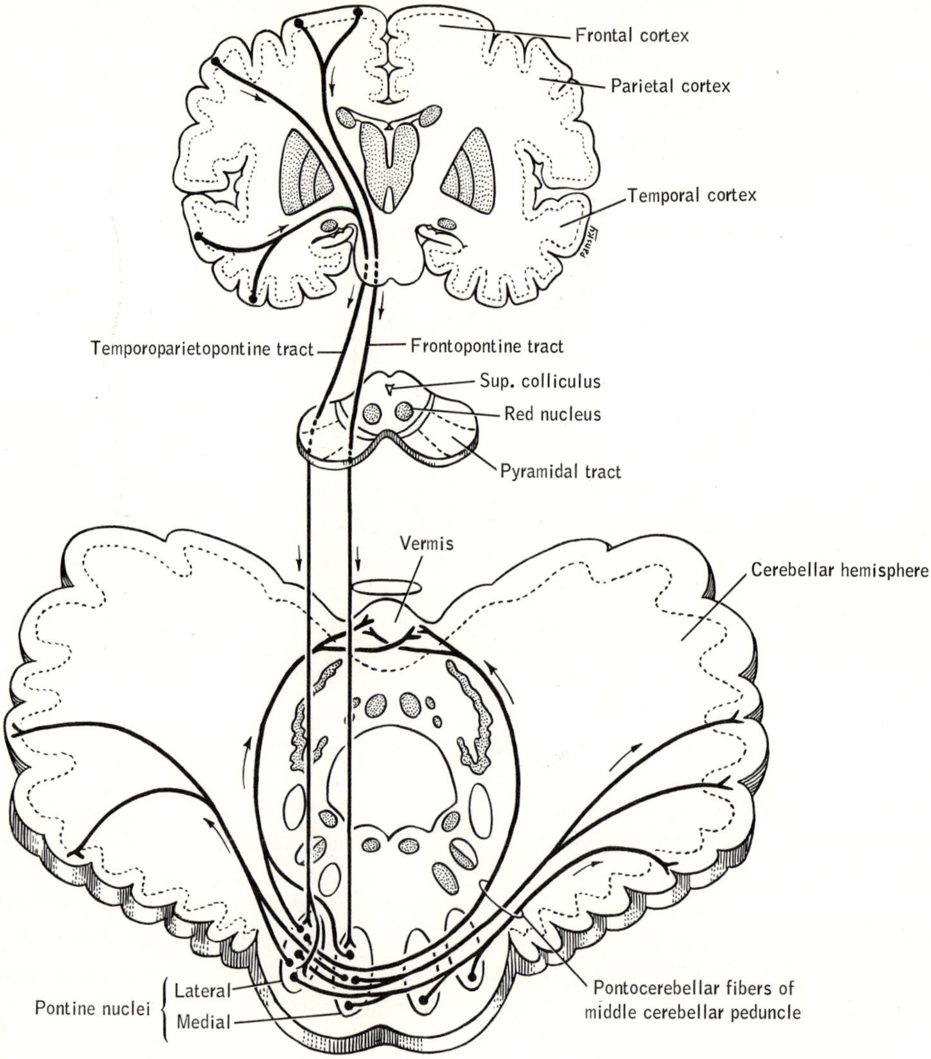

Fig. 18-9. Diagram of the cerebro-ponto-cerebellar circuit showing the origin of the fibers in the cerebrum, their position in the cerebral peduncle, the pontile nuclei, and the distribution of fibers to the cerebellar vermis and hemispheres.

have been made to subdivide the pontine gray into nuclear groups, i.e., dorsolateral, lateral, medial, and ventral, but they are so poorly circumscribed that only a general division will be made here—lateral and medial. From cells in these groups, fibers arise, most of which cross, to ascend into the cerebellum by way of the middle cerebellar peduncle. The vast majority of these terminate in the neocerebellar cortex, both of the hemispheres and the vermis. This includes most of the posterior lobe. There is also an overlap into the paleocerebellum of the anterior lobe, especially in the anterior quadrangular lobule and the culmen.

Arcuatocerebellar (Figs. 18-5, 18-8, 25-5.)

The arcuate nuclei from which these fibers arise are found on the ventral and medial surfaces of the pyramids of the medulla. Since it is believed that these nuclei have the same origin as those of the pontine gray and actually represent displaced pontine nuclei, this circuit acts as a supplement to the corticopontocerebellar pathway. Collaterals from the descending corticospinal tracts terminate among cells of the arcuate nuclei. Fibers arising in these nuclei leave in two streams: (1) the ventral external arcuates; (2) the arcuatocerebellar fibers. The former pass along the external ventral and lateral surfaces of the medulla, join the inferior cerebellar peduncle and enter the cerebellum. The latter run dorsally near the midline, to the floor of the fourth ventricle, whence they stream laterally as the striae medullares to enter the cerebellum by way of the inferior cerebellar peduncle. In general, it has been said that these fibers end in the flocculus. However, it seems likely that they may overlap the fibers in the pontocerebellar system.

Tectocerebellar (Fig. 18-5.)

These fibers probably arise both in the superior and inferior colliculi (tectum). From the caudal limits of the latter the fibers enter the anterior medullary velum where they are believed to undergo a partial decussation. In the cerebellum they terminate: in the anterior lobe, especially in the caudal part of the anterior quadrangular lobule; and in the posterior lobe, including the folium, tuber and pyramis; and in the most medial portion of the hemispheres adjoining these vermian regions. The tectum of the mesencephalon has been shown to be centers for visual and auditory reflexes, thus this pathway has to do with the coordination of the motor portion of these reflexes. It has been suggested that the tectocerebellar route is the most important pathway linking auditory impulses to the cerebellum. Visual impulses may have other routes such as a tectopontine-pontocerebellar or an occipitopontine-pontocerebellar pathways.

Efferent Tracts (Figs. 18-10 to 18-13.)

The efferent fibers are arranged in two major groups: (1) these arise in the cortex and, since they carry impulses away from the cortex, are called *corticifugal;* (2) this group of fibers arises in the *central nuclei* of the cerebellum and leaves the cerebellum proper.

Corticifugal

These are of two varieties: (1) the *direct* pass from the cortex into the brain stem; (2) the *corticonuclear* run from the cortex of the central nuclei.

Direct. (Fig. 18-10.) These fibers are relatively few. They arise in the flocculus and pass to the superior and lateral vestibular nuclei as the flocculovestibular tract or they ascend in the superior cerebellar peduncle as the flocculo-occulomotor tract. In addition to these, fibers arising in the nodulus and uvula of the posterior lobe and in the lingula, central lobule and culmen of the anterior lobe have also been traced to the vestibular nuclei. Direct fibers from the nodulus to the reticular formation of the medulla have also been described.

Corticonuclear. One group of these fibers has the *same cortical origin* as described for the direct fibers but terminates in the fastigial nuclei (Figs. 2-46, 18-10, 25-7). Another group arises in the biventer lobule, tonsil, medial part of the ansiform lobule, and the lateral part of the anterior lobe to terminate in the *emboliform* and *globose* nuclei [5] (Figs. 18-10, 25-7, 25-8). The lateral part of the ansiform lobule and perhaps the paraflocculus send their fibers to the dentate nucleus. According to a general rule, it may be said that: the vermis sends its fibers to the fastigial and globose nuclei; the cortex of the hemispheres adjacent to the vermis sends its fibers to the globose and emboliform nuclei; the lateral portion of the hemispheres send their fibers to the dentate nucleus.

Efferents from the Central Cerebellar Nuclei

Fastigiobulbar Tract (Fig. 18-1.)

This group of fibers is also known as the cerebellovestibular tract. They arise in the

[5] For practical purposes these two nuclei are frequently grouped together as the nucleus interpositus.

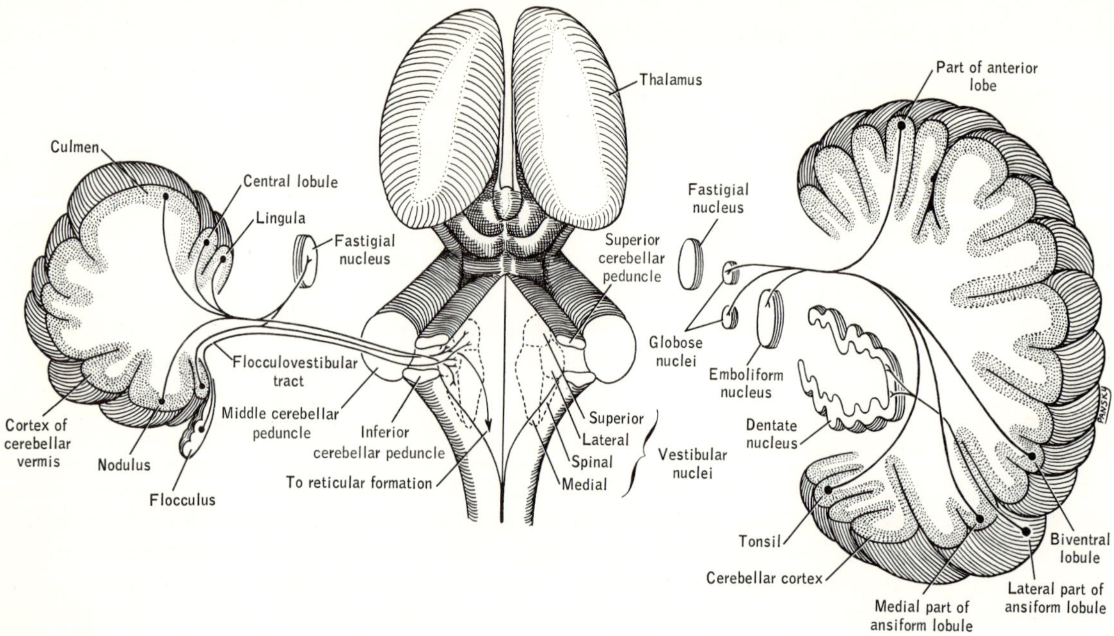

Fig. 18-10. Corticonuclear fibers of the cerebellum.

fastigial nucleus, some crossing while others remain on the same side. In either case, they descend to the brain stem in the medial segment of the inferior cerebellar peduncle and terminate in the lateral and superior vestibular nuclei. It is believed that perhaps other vestibular nuclei and the medullary reticular formation also receive fibers from this pathway.

Uncinate Bundle (*of Russell*) (Fig. 18-11.)

This fasciculus, also described as the cerebellospinal tract, arises from cells in the fastigial nucleus. The majority of fibers cross in the so-called inferior cerebellar commissure and ascend for a very short distance with the fibers of the superior cerebellar peduncle. They then curve around over the peduncle (hook over it, thus the name "uncinate") and descend from the cerebellum in the medial segment of the inferior cerebellar peduncle. On reaching the medulla, this bundle extends caudally past the vestibular nuclei and down into the spinal cord where it enters the anterior funiculus to become a part of the sulcomarginal fasciculus. Most of the fibers terminate on the cells in the anterior column of the cervical cord. As the tract lies in the brain stem, some fibers (or their collaterals) leave the tract to end upon the cells of the motor nuclei. Some of the fibers do not arch over the superior cerebellar peduncle but continue rostrally as a component of that peduncle to enter the central (periventricular) gray in the lower mesencephalon.

Dentatothalamic and Dentatorubrothalamic (Figs. 18-11 to 18-13.)

Although the names imply that these fibers arise exclusively in the dentate nucleus, both the emboliform and globose nuclei contribute to these groups. These fibers make up the bulk of the superior cerebellar peduncle which is the major efferent pathway of the cerebellum. It has been suggested that those fibers lying in the dorsal two-thirds of the peduncle come from the dorsal part of the dentate nucleus, the emboliform and globose nuclei while those in the

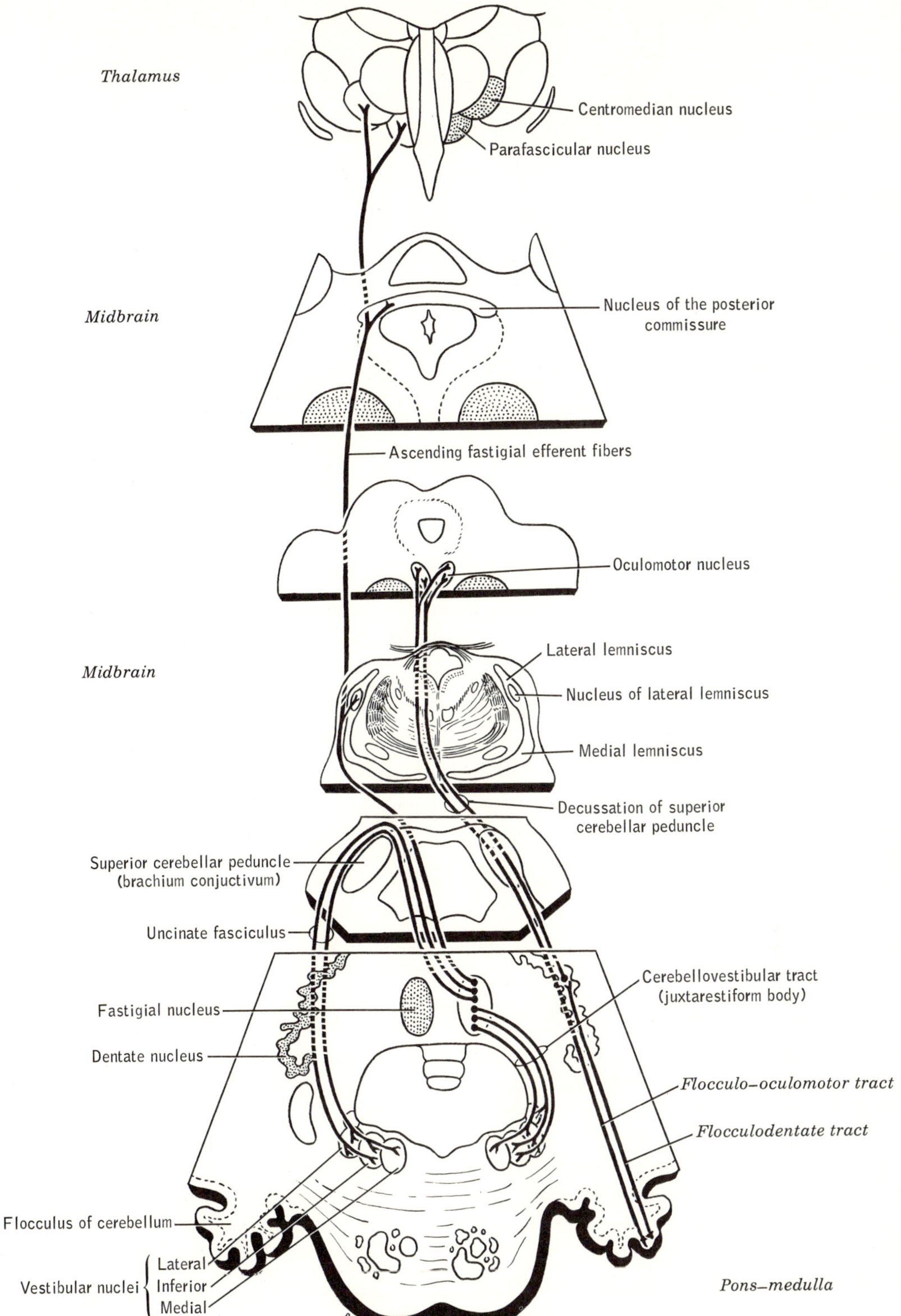

Fig. 18-11. Diagram of the efferent fibers of the fastigial nucleus illustrating both ascending and descending pathways. (*Based on Walberg, et al.,* 1962.) Also shown are the discharge pathways from the flocculus to the occulomotor nucleus. (*Modified after Wallenberg-Klimoff and Gerebtzoff,* 1941.)

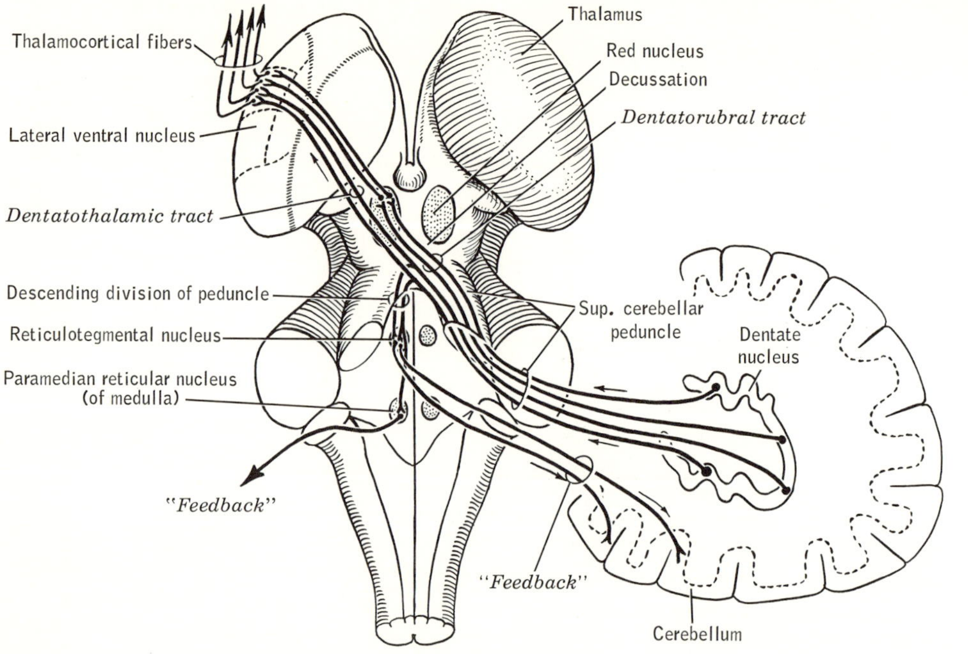

Fig. 18-12. Diagram of the dentatothalamic and dentatorubrothalamic pathways via the superior cerebellar peduncle. The "feedback" circuit via the reticular nuclei and reticulocerebellar fibers is also shown.

ventral third arise from the ventral and lateral part of the dentate. The peduncles pass rostrally out of the cerebellum and form the lateral walls of the superior portion of the fourth ventricle (Figs. 2-18, 2-38). In their forward course, the peduncles gradually sink into the pontine tegmentum and pass into the tegmental area of the midbrain. In the caudal part of the mesencephalon most of the fibers in the peduncles decussate. A few of the uncrossed fibers may end in the tegmental gray of the pons or in reticular nuclei lying farther caudad. After decussating, the peduncle breaks up into fascicles, the majority of which ascend. The descending fibers run for at least part of their course either in or closely adjacent to the central tegmental tract. Most of them terminate in the inferior olivary complex but collaterals have been traced into the tegmental reticular nuclei (cerebelloreticular tract). The latter may, at least in part, serve as synaptic centers in a "feedback" mechanism with reticulocerebellar fibers carrying a return flow to the cerebellar cortex (Fig. 18-12). There is some evidence that a few fibers continue caudalward into the spinal cord.

There are two major groups of ascending fibers: the cerebellorubral which arise chiefly in the dentate nucleus with contributions from both the globose and emboliform nuclei; and the dentatothalamic fibers which arise in the dentate nucleus. Rostral to the decussation, the former terminate in both the large and small-celled portions of the red nucleus, terminations among the large cells being more numerous. The dentatothalamic fascicles bypass the red nucleus and continue into the diencephalon where they end in the lateral ventral nucleus of the thalamus. Fibers arising in the red nucleus relay cerebellar impulses via rubrothalamic fascicles to the lateral ventral nucleus. From the latter, fibers ascend through the internal capsule to the motor and premotor cortex of the cerebrum. Fibers arising

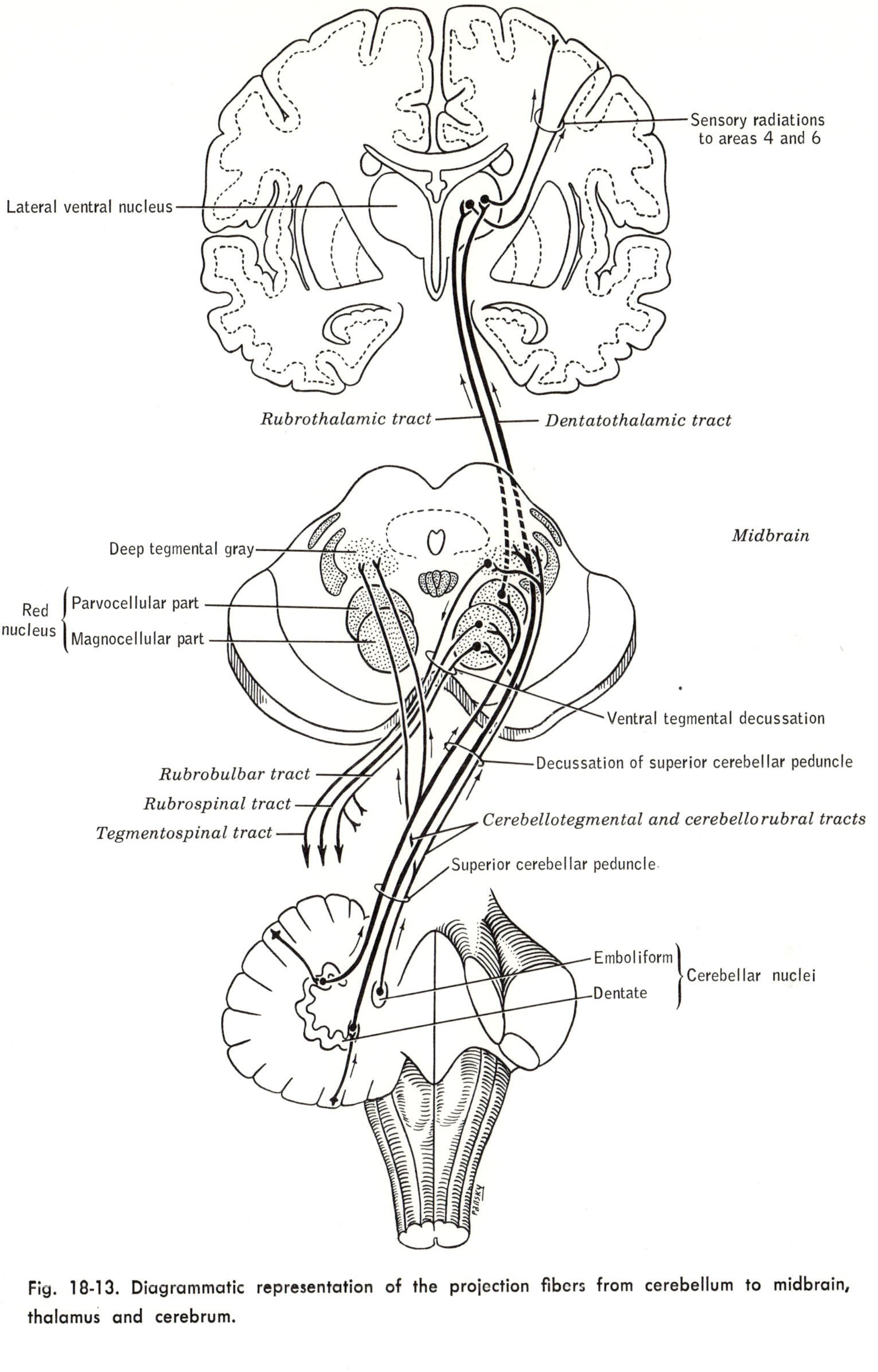

Fig. 18-13. Diagrammatic representation of the projection fibers from cerebellum to midbrain, thalamus and cerebrum.

in the red nucleus and descending to the dentate nucleus of this cerebellum have also been described.

CIRCUITS TO MOTOR CENTERS

It has just been shown that efferent cerebellar fibers carry streams of impulses to the vestibular nuclei, the reticular nuclei, the red nucleus, and the lateral ventral nucleus of the thalamus but that none of these fibers reaches motor centers directly. It is therefore necessary to describe the pathways by which the cerebellum eventually influences the primary motor nuclei.

Vestibular Pathway

In an earlier chapter (Chap. 13) it was demonstrated how the vestibular nuclei are related to the body musculature; the musculature of the trunk through the *vestibulospinal tract;* the motor centers of the neck musculature through the medial longitudinal fasciculus; and the motor centers of the brain stem, including those for the ocular muscles, through ascending and descending fibers of the medial longitudinal fasciculus.

Reticular Pathway

From cells in the various nuclei of the bulbar reticular formation, fibers may reach the motor nuclei of the brain stem and, through the *reticulospinal tract,* make contact with the cells in the ventral columns of the spinal cord.

Rubral Circuits

There are three possible routes through which the red nucleus may disseminate cerebellar influence. The first two are *descending,* the last is *ascending.*

Rubrospinal (Chap. 19.)

In man, this tract is a small group of fibers arising in the red nucleus. They leave the nucleus, decussate in the ventral tegmental decussation, and descend through the brain stem and upper spinal cord, sending collaterals into the ventral gray columns.

Rubroreticular (Chap. 19.)

A large number of fibers arising in the red nucleus enters the reticular formation, many probably synapsing among cells of the reticular nuclei. These cells give rise to other fibers, some of which pass to motor nuclei of the brain stem as *reticulobulbar,* while others become a part of the *reticulospinal tract* to terminate in the anterior gray columns of the cord.

Rubrothalamic

Some fibers ascend from the red nucleus carrying cerebellar influences still higher. Some reach the thalamus, as an adjunct to those fibers passing directly from the dentate nucleus, while others pass to the corpus striatum and thus exert their influence by way of the other extrapyramidal circuits (Chap. 19).

Thalamic Circuits

There are probably several ways through which the thalamus acts as an intermediary for the distribution of cerebellar influence.

Thalamocortical

Through this pathway, fibers arising in the lateral ventral nuclei may be distributed to both the pyramidal and extrapyramidal areas of the cortex (Chaps. 19, 20, 22, 23).

Thalamostriate and Thalamo-olivary

These fibers may also carry cerebellar influence into some of the subcortical extrapyramidal centers (Chap. 22).

EVALUATION OF THE CEREBELLAR CIRCUITS

Before attempting to understand how the cerebellum or any other suprasegmental center is able to effect or modify activity, it is essential to review the basic motor pattern (Chap. 14) and to recall the numerous descending fiber tracts which terminate within the anterior column of the spinal cord and the cranial motor nuclei.

In addition, it is necessary to know that: (1) due to an inherent quality in the descending fibers themselves, some will cause stimulation while others will inhibit these same cells; (2) the same descending fiber can not act directly as an activator and suppressor at the same time but, through a synapse with an intercalated neuron suppressor effect may be produced on another cell. Thus, a descending fiber may terminate directly on a motor fiber causing it to contract while at the same time, this same fiber may synapse on an intercalated neuron. The axon of the intercalated neuron ends on a cell in another part of the cell group which supplies the antagonistic muscle. This leads to a relaxation of the antagonist.

At this point, it might be useful to demonstrate the action of the cerebellar circuit using conjugate deviation of the eyes (Chap. 14) in response to a vestibular stimulus as an example. Thus, a particular movement of the head, due to the inertia of the endolymph in the semicircular canal (Chap. 12) stimulates the cristae of the left vestibule. As a result, volleys of afferent impulses stream through the left vestibular nerve to terminate in several of the vestibular nuclei (medial, spinal, and lateral). From here, association neurons cross the midline and enter the MLF. As the latter bundle passes the right abducens nucleus, either collaterals or terminals enter that nucleus. Typical somatic motor axons leave this nucleus, pass by way of the abducens nerve (VI) to the right lateral rectus muscle causing its contraction. However, as a part of this total action, the left medial rectus must also contract so that the left eye moves in the same direction as the right. Thus, fibers from the left vestibular nuclei terminate in the paraabducens nucleus from which fibers reenter the MLF of the left side and run to the medial part of the oculomotor nucleus (LII). Thence, fibers pass by way of the oculomotor nerve to the left medial rectus. However, this is only part of the story for, at the same time, there must be a compensatory relaxation of the right medial rectus and the left lateral rectus muscles. Now, it should be recalled that the same impulses set up in the left vestibular nerve which produced the activity described above are also carried both to the cerebellar cortex and to the left fastigial nucleus. From the latter, impulses are carried back to the vestibular nuclei via the fastigiobulbar tract. These cerebellar impulses apparently enhance and reinforce the nerve flow from the latter to the right lateral rectus and left medial rectus. At the same time, fibers from the left fastigial nucleus pass to the right vestibular nuclei either through the crossed fibers in the fastigiobulbar tract or in the uncinate bundle. These fibers tend to suppress the activity of the right vestibular nuclei which, in turn, leads to a diminution of tone in the left lateral and right medial rectus muscles. Thus, conjugate movement is facilitated.

Although the circuit described above only demonstrates a part of the vestibulo-ocular mechanisms, similar connections involving the motor nerves controlling the musculature of the neck and trunk which are important in maintaining balance are also present. In this case, cerebellar influences reach the vestibular nuclei through the fastigiobulbar tract and the uncinate bundle whence impulses are relayed caudalward both in the MLF and the vestibulospinal tract.

Reflexes initiated through the activity of the SSA system (both auditory and visual) apparently require cerebellar integration. For this reason, the tectocerebellar fibers link the reflex association centers of the mesencephalon with the cortex of the cerebellum. The latter then acts upon the motor centers by the pathways described through either the fastigial nucleus or nucleus interpositus, through reticular formation or possibly the dentate and red nuclei, and finally through the rubroreticular or rubrospinal route.

It is not altogether certain how the extrapyramidal motor apparatus is integrated through the cerebellum. Although it is possible that the cerebellum is linked to some of the subcortical motor centers, such as the corpus striatum, through the reticulocerebellar fibers, it seems likely that the inferior olivary complex is of great importance in this connection. A large fiber bundle is known to descend through the brain stem to terminate in the inferior olive. This bundle is sometimes referred to as the thalamo-olivary tract, a term which implies thalamic origin. Although it seems that at least a portion of these fibers do arise in the thalamus, they represent an intermediate station in the pathway from the striatum. Another name given to this bundle is the central tegmental tract, which appears to include fibers from several sources, including the striatum; the tegmental nuclei of the upper brain stem; the red nucleus; and the substantia nigra.

Since all the skilled, voluntary movements initiated in the motor cortex of the cerebral hemispheres require the highest degree of synergy, massive fiber pathways link the cerebrum and cerebellum. Thus one could visualize muscular activity as being initiated by impulses descending from the cerebral cortex instead of being initiated as a part of a reflex arc. Except for the use of different pathways, the modifying influences of the cerebellum would be the same. Descending from cerebral motor centers are the corticopontine fibers. These pass downward through the internal capsule (Fig. 2-16; Chap. 23) and the basis pedunculi to terminate in the homolateral pontine nuclei. Axons from the latter cross the midline, curve dorsally in the contralateral brachium pontis, and end chiefly in the neocerebellar cortex. The cerebellum then influences voluntary muscular activity in several ways: (1) through the red nucleus and then directly to motor centers via the rubrospinal tract or from the red nucleus indirectly, through the reticular formation and reticulospinal tract; (2) through the thalamus to the corpus striatum and then through the red nucleus or other extrapyramidal pathways. In either case, the action on the motor cells could be either facilitating or suppressing. It is also evident that the cerebellum can exert its influence on voluntary cortical centers directly by way of the dentatothalamic, thalamocortical circuit.

Through the use of electric recording devices, it has been possible to localize certain functional projection areas on the cerebellar hemispheres (in addition to the areas known to be associated with the general and special proprioceptive areas).

CLINICAL CONSIDERATIONS

Since the cerebellum is so intimately related to action and movements of all sorts, it is necessary to use examinations which help localize the lesion as being distinctly in the cerebellum and not, for example, in the posterior funiculi of the cord; in the inner ear; in the vestibular nerve or its nuclei; or in the pyramidal system somewhere along its course.

Before the procedure for examination is described, it is necessary to understand the terms used in connection with lesions of the motor systems. *Hypotonia, areflexia, ataxia,* and *nystagmus* have already been defined (Chap. 14). Other important terms are *hyporeflexia,* a weakening of reflexes, usually associated with hypotonia; *asynergia,* a loss of the facility to coordinate more or less complex movements which have a special function;[6] *asthenia,* a lack or diminution of muscular strength; *atelokinesia,* a term sometimes used for the intention or action tremor seen near the termination of a voluntary movement; *adiadochokinesia,* the inability to perform rapid, alternating movements; *dysmetria,* the improper measuring of distance in muscular acts. The latter is a disturbance in the power to control the range of movement, as in past pointing.

Testing

In this system, an attempt is made to localize the lesion in a very general way. For this purpose, it is found most convenient to classify the defects or disturbances under four categories: defective postural fixation; disturbances of skilled or voluntary acts; disturbed equilibrium; disturbances in gait and postural reflexes.

[6] In some patients, the different components of an act may not follow in the proper sequence, come at the proper time, or be of the proper strength.

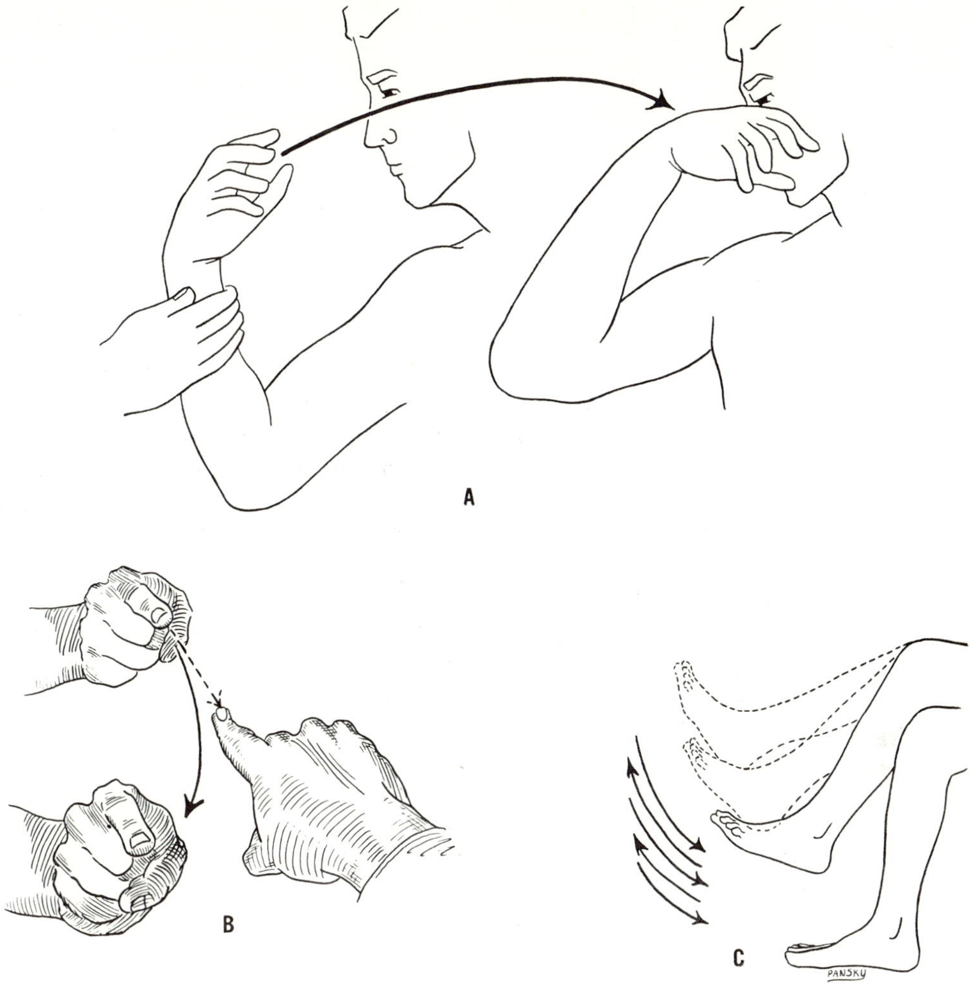

Fig. 18-14. Tests for cerebellar disease. *A.* Rebound phenomenon—in disease, there is no reciprocal antagonistic reaction to check the hand. *B.* Past pointing—deviation to the side of the lesion in unilateral cerebellar disease. *C.* Pendulum-like response. To-and-fro movement.

Postural Fixation

The muscles are palpated to see whether they are firm or flabby, flabbiness indicating hypotonia.

It is noted whether the extremity at rest appears to lie in an awkward position.

The examiner notes whether there is any loss in resistance to passive movement when he attempts to bend an extremity.

He notes whether the upper extremity flops about aimlessly when the shoulder is shaken.

When the patient is asked to close his eyes and extend both arms in front of him, the arm on the side of the lesion frequently is lower and less fully extended and tends to drift laterally. When the arms are extended to the side, the affected side tends to drift medially.

The patient is asked to sit on the edge of a table so that his legs hang down freely. If the examiner extends the patient's leg, then releases it, the leg on the diseased side will show an increase in the number of pendular swings (Fig. 18-14C).

The rebound phenomenon is checked by having the patient flex the arm against resistance which the examiner suddenly releases. In cerebellar disease, the arm often rebounds markedly before it is checked (Fig. 18-14A).

The patient is asked to sit on the bed with his legs extended and heels down on the bed. When he is instructed to lie down quickly, his feet fly into the air if cerebellar lesions are present.

Disturbances in Voluntary Skills

Such disturbances involve abnormalities in the rate, range, direction, or force of movement, frequently referred to as *dyssynergia.* These errors are sometimes accompanied by action or intention tremors. Thus, the examiner in the course of the tests given below will be watching to see whether a movement is slow in starting; whether the force and speed during movement are uneven; whether movement is slow in stopping and if it stops at the desired spot, without overreaching; whether there is slowness in starting successive components of more complex movements, i.e., whether the complex movement is decomposed into parts by a series of jerks; and whether there is any tremor present which becomes more marked near the end of a given movement.

The patient is asked to touch the tip of his nose with the index finger of either hand, starting with the extremity extended. This should be done simultaneously with both extremities.

The patient is instructed to touch the tip of his nose and the examiner's finger alternately, with the examiner changing the position of his finger from time to time. The patient later is asked to follow with his finger the moving finger of the examiner (Fig. 18-14B).

The patient is asked to place the heel of one foot to the knee of the other extremity.

The patient is asked to follow with his great toe the moving finger of the examiner, particularly in such a way that both thigh and leg will be flexed.

The patient is asked to perform certain tasks requiring alternation of movement, such as wiggling fingers, tapping the foot, or pronating and supinating the forearm. When certain cerebellar lesions are present, these acts are slow, the rhythm is poor, and the alternating action is clumsy, irregular, and variable in force.

Disturbed Equilibrium

In this category, no particular tests are necessary. Observation of the patient is usually sufficient. The examiner merely sees whether the patient can stand or sit, unsupported. Usually, if a cerebellar lesion is present, the patient tends to fall and his head wobbles and oscillates. If walking is possible at all, the gait is *reeling* and *drunken.* When equilibrium is disturbed the lesions are usually basal, involving either the archicerebellar cortex of the flocculonodular lobe or the median part of the posterior lobe.[7]

Disturbed Gait and Posture

Certain types of abnormality should be described. First, in a unilateral cerebellar lesion with the gait deviating toward the side of the lesion, the leg on the affected side shows incoordination of movement. The second type has been indicated under Disturbed Equilibrium as the reeling, drunken gait.

The third variety may sometimes be observed when there is a lesion of the anterior lobe, which is considered to control the synergies of walking.[8] The gait is wide-based, with bilateral deviation, and is often stiff-legged. These observations of gait should be made during the following tests.

The patient is asked to stand up, walk, stop quickly, turn quickly, and return.

The patient is asked to walk a line, heel to toe.

The patient is asked to lie recumbent in bed, and firm pressure is applied to the sole of his foot so that the examiner may feel for tonal increase in the muscles of the thigh.

[7] Disturbances in voluntary skills and often in postural fixation indicate a lesion in the lateral part of the hemispheres.

[8] As should be understood, in standing there has to be an excess tone in the extensor muscles. This is the positive supporting reaction. In walking, the legs must alternate in having and not having this extensor tone.

Nystagmus

Various clinical signs are often associated with cerebellar diseases but are not necessarily primary for lesions of the cerebellum. One of these is *nystagmus*. However, one of the three types of nystagmus is referable to the cerebellum alone. This is *deviation nystagmus,* characterized by four signs: (1) With the eyes in the midline position, there is a fine nystagmus with the quick component toward the side of the lesion. (2) When the eyes are fixed 10 to 30° to the side away from the lesion, there is no nystagmus. (3) When the eyes are shifted beyond 30° away from the lesion, nystagmus again occurs, with the quick component away from the lesion. (4) When the eyes are shifted well beyond the midline toward the side of the lesion, a very coarse nystagmus, with the quick portion toward the lesion side, occurs.

Specific Pathology

In addition to trauma, which may destroy parts of the cerebellum through externally applied force, certain other conditions may produce some or all of the above symptoms. These include certain congenital defects in which there is either agenesis or abnormal development; abscesses and tumors, either of the cerebellum or of surrounding parts which encroach upon the cerebellum; hemorrhage in one of its vessels or occlusions thereof; and cortical atrophy.

CORTEX OF CEREBELLUM

- I. Layers
  - *A*. Granular cells (inner)
    1. Granule—dendrites receive afferent cerebellar fibers; axons pass to molecular layer
    2. Stellate—dendrites spray out in molecular layer; axon branches in granular layer
  - *B*. Purkinje cells (middle)—dendrites spread out in molecular layer to synapse with axons of granule cells; axon leaves cortex, giving collaterals to adjoining Purkinje cells as it passes through the granular layer to reach the medullary core of cerebellum to end in the central nuclei
  - *C*. Molecular cells (outer)
    1. Basket—dendrites branch in outer part of layer; axon branches to synapse with rows of Purkinje cells
    2. Golgi type II—short dendrites and axon, extending horizontally in superficial part of the layer
- II. Fibers (morphologic types)
  - *A*. Mossy—afferent cerebellar fibers, ending with synapses among dendrites of granule cells in all parts of the cerebellum
  - *B*. Climbing—recurrent collaterals from axons of Purkinje cells; collaterals of axons of stellate cells; collaterals from axons of fibers leaving the central nuclei

SUMMARY OF CONNECTIONS

Cerebellar Afferents

- I. Through inferior peduncle (restiform body)
  - *A*. Dorsal spinocerebellar tract
    1. Origin: column of Clarke in dorsal gray of spinal cord
    2. Termination: central lobule, culmen, and posterior semilunar lobule
  - *B*. Dorsal external arcuate fibers
    1. Origin: accessory cuneate nucleus
    2. Termination: same as above
  - *C*. Reticulocerebellar fibers
    1. Origin: lateral reticular nucleus
    2. Termination: same as above
  - *D*. Olivocerebellar fibers
    1. Origin: inferior olivary nucleus
    2. Termination: all cerebellar cortex of the opposite side except the flocculus
  - *E*. Arcuocerebellar fibers
    1. Origin: arcuate nuclei via ventral external arcuate fibers
    2. Termination: opposite hemispheres of middle lobe

II. Through middle peduncle (brachium pontis)
   A. Pontocerebellar fibers
      1. Origin: pontine nuclei
      2. Termination: mainly in cortex of middle lobe on opposite side; to lesser extent, the vermis of middle lobe
III. Through juxtarestiform body
   A. Direct vestibulocerebellar fibers
      1. Origin: vestibular ganglion
      2. Termination: flocculus, nodulus, and lingula
   B. Indirect vestibulocerebellar fibers
      1. Origin: lateral and superior vestibular nuclei
      2. Termination: flocculus of both sides, nodulus, uvula, and lingula
IV. Through anterior medullary velum
   A. Ventral spinocerebellar tract
      1. Origin: body of dorsal gray column of the cord
      2. Termination: central lobule, culmen, and posterior semilunar lobule
   B. Trigeminocerebellar fibers
      1. Origin: chief sensory (and mesencephalic ?) nucleus of the trigeminal nerve (V)
      2. Termination: mainly in posterior semilunar lobule
   C. Tectocerebellar
      1. Origin: corpora quadrigemina
      2. Termination: tuber, folium, and posterior semilunar lobule

Cerebellar Efferents

I. Corticifugal
   A. Direct: cortex to brain stem nuclei
      1. Origin—flocculus
      2. Terminations: superior and lateral vestibular nuclei
      3. Origin: nodulus
      4. Terminations: vestibular nuclei and reticular formation
      5. Origin: uvula, lingula, central lobule, and culmen
      6. Termination: vestibular nuclei
   B. Corticonuclear (Indirect): cortex to central cerebellar nuclei
      1. Origin: from same cortical areas given above
      2. Termination: fastigial nucleus
      3. Origin: biventral lobule, tonsil, medial parts of superior and inferior semilunar lobules, and anterior semilunar lobule
      4. Terminations: emboliform and globose nuclei
      5. Origin: superior and inferior semilunar lobules
      6. Termination: dentate nucleus
II. Nuclear efferents
   A. Through juxtarestiform body
      1. Fastigiobulbar tract
         a. Origin: fastigial nucleus
         b. Terminations: crossed and uncrossed, in vestibular nuclei and reticular formation
   B. Through anterior medullary velum and peripeduncular route
      1. Uncinate bundle (of Russell)
         a. Origin: fastigial nucleus
         b. Terminations: crossed and uncrossed, in vestibular nuclei and reticular formation
   C. Through superior peduncle (brachium conjunctivum)
      1. Dentatorubral fibers
         a. Origin: dentate nucleus
         b. Termination: crossed, in opposite red nucleus
      2. Dentatothalamic fibers
         a. Origin: dentate nucleus
         b. Termination: crossed, in the opposite lateral ventral nucleus of thalamus
   D. Unnamed
      1. Origin: emboliform and globose nuclei
      2. Termination: same course and destination as the dentatorubral and dentatothalamic

SUMMARY

	VERMIS	HEMISPHERE
Anterior lobe	Lingula	
	Central lobule	Central lobule
	Culmen	Anterior semilunar lobule
	PRIMARY FISSURE	
Middle lobe	Declive	Posterior semilunar lobule
	Folium	Superior semilunar lobule
	Tuber	Inferior semilunar lobule
	PREPYRAMIDAL FISSURE	
Posterior lobe	Pyramis	Biventral lobule
	Uvula	Tonsil
	POSTEROLATERAL FISSURE	
Flocculonodular lobe	Nodulus	Flocculus

19 EXTRAPYRAMIDAL MODIFICATION OF MUSCULAR ACTIVITY

In its broadest sense, this mechanism includes all parts of the central nervous system concerned with motor activity except most of cortical area 4 and the fibers which descend from it.[1] According to another school of thought, it includes all the suprasegmental motor controls that pass by way of the reticular formation to the motor columns of the brain stem and spinal cord. The parts to be discussed here include the reticular system; rubral system; corpus striatum; globus pallidus; subthalamus; certain thalamic nuclei; and extrapyramidal portions of the cerebral cortex. It can be seen that this is a diverse, scattered group of loosely connected and functionally related structures rather than an anatomic unit.

In the first chapter it was stated that "with each step upward in the evolutionary series new parts are merely added to the old; sometimes they are modified and often almost obscured but nothing is thrown away." In a study of the parts and connections of the extrapyramidal system, one can trace the entire history of the motor mechanism. Perhaps this is one of the things that makes it so difficult to understand.

For a time, among the lower animal forms, the reticular formation and, later, the midbrain tegmental nuclei were sufficient for all motor activity. With the evolution of the fish, a nuclear mass—the paleostriatum—appears, corresponding to the globus pallidus of higher forms. Receiving mainly olfactory impulses, its efferents help to integrate movements important in feeding. Its connections to the hypothalamus indicate a measure of visceral control (and possibly defensive activity). In reptiles and birds, the neostriatum develops, corresponding to the caudate-putamen complex of man. It receives fibers from the thalamus which carry impulses from various sensory systems, for in birds and reptiles the cortical neopallium is rudimentary. It is evident that in animals without a cortex the corpus striatum is the chief integration center for all such normal but largely instinctive activities as locomotion, defense, feeding, and courting. Even in the higher animals, where the striatal complex becomes subservient to the neocortex, the corpus striatum is still utilized for the production of many automatic or semiautomatic movements concerned with postural adjustments, defense, feeding, etc. It has also been shown experimentally that most mammals can perform these functions after destruction of the pyramidal system.

Generally, the extrapyramidal system is thought to provide a background motor pattern. In other words, this system sets up approximate positions of the body parts through the adjustment of large muscle groups, while the more refined, precise, and specific activities of individual muscles (the nonpostural, modifiable movements which are the bases of acquired skills) are added by the pyramidal system. In other words, these two systems do not function independently but are in balance with each other. The smooth and

[1] Even fibers contained in the pyramids of the medulla, and perhaps even some in the corticospinal tracts of the cord, belong to this system.

effective performance of nonpostural, skilled, pyramidal activities demands a concomitant regulation by the purely postural circuits. Thus, within the province of the extrapyramidal system are the gross synergic movements of locomotion, expression, and postural adjustment, together with the semi-automatic movements associated with voluntary activities, such as swinging the arms when walking.

Because of the wide dispersion of its parts and the enormous complexity of its interconnections, these parts and connections will be considered only in a very general way in the text. For details, included for the sake of completeness, the reader is referred to the illustrations (Figs. 19-1 to 19-14) and to the summary at the end of the chapter.

PARTS AND CONNECTIONS

Extrapyramidal Cortex

The extrapyramidal system represents an ancient motor mechanism which has secondarily become dominated by cortical influences. Thus, certain regions of the cerebral cortex send downward large numbers of fibers, which ultimately exert their influence on motor activity. These areas are indicated on the cortical maps as 2, 4, 4s, 6, 8, 9, 19, and 24 (Fig. 23-14). At least area 4-s is a suppressor strip.

Corpus Striatum [2]

Structure (Figs. 2-14 to 2-17, 2-28, 25-18 to 25-20.)

The term *corpus striatum* is applied to the combined caudate nucleus and the outer part of the lenticular nucleus, called the *putamen*. Since these parts are more recently acquired, phylogenetically, than the medial part of the lenticular nucleus, they are also referred to as the *neostriatum*. Their anatomic proximity, as well as their structural and functional similarity, justifies considering them together. It is thought to be predominantly inhibitory in function.

Connections

Afferents. (Fig. 19-1.) Most of the fibers, arising in the extrapyramidal cortex, descend through the internal capsule [3] or subcallosal [4] bundle and end in the caudate nucleus. Some, however, end in the putamen. Fibers from certain thalamic nuclei [5] as well as collaterals from corticothalamic and corticospinal fibers also terminate in the striatum.

Efferents. (Fig. 19-2.) The majority leave the striatum and end in the globus pallidus; others terminate in the subthalamic nucleus or substantia nigra.

Globus Pallidus

Structure (Figs. 2-14 to 2-17, 2-27, 25-15 to 25-20.)

The term *globus pallidus* is applied to the medial portion of the lenticular nucleus. Since this is the older portion of that nucleus, it is referred to as the *paleostriatum*. The contracted term *pallidum* is frequently applied to it. It consists of an outer (larger) and inner (smaller) portion. This is said to function as an excitor.

Connections

Afferents. (Fig. 19-3.) Most of these fibers arise in the striatum,[6] but others, from the thalamus,[7] subthalamic nucleus, and cortical area 6,[8] also terminate here.

Efferents. (Fig. 19-4.) Such fibers may arise in either segment of the pallidum but chiefly

[2] The striate appearance is due to the intermingling of gray matter, interconnecting the ventral part of the head of the caudate and putamen with the fibers of the internal capsule.

[3] Passing through the internal capsule are thought to be corticocaudate fibers from areas 4s and 6. According to more recent evidence, areas 4s, 8, 19, 24, and 2 send their fibers to the caudate nucleus while areas 4 and 6 give fibers to the putamen.

[4] The subcallosal bundle lies on the ventricular surface of the angle between the corpus callosum and internal capsule. It contains corticocaudate fibers from frontal lobe areas 4, 6, 8, and 9.

[5] The medial nucleus and centrum medianum send fibers to the striatum through the inferior thalamic peduncle.

[6] Large numbers of striopallidal fibers enter the pallidum to terminate in both of its segments.

[7] Thalamopallidal fibers arise from the dorsomedial nucleus, centrum medianum, and possibly the anterior ventral nucleus, pass through the inferior thalamic peduncle, and end in both segments of the pallidum.

[8] Corticopallidal fibers descend through the internal capsule from area 6 and end in the inner segment of the pallidum.

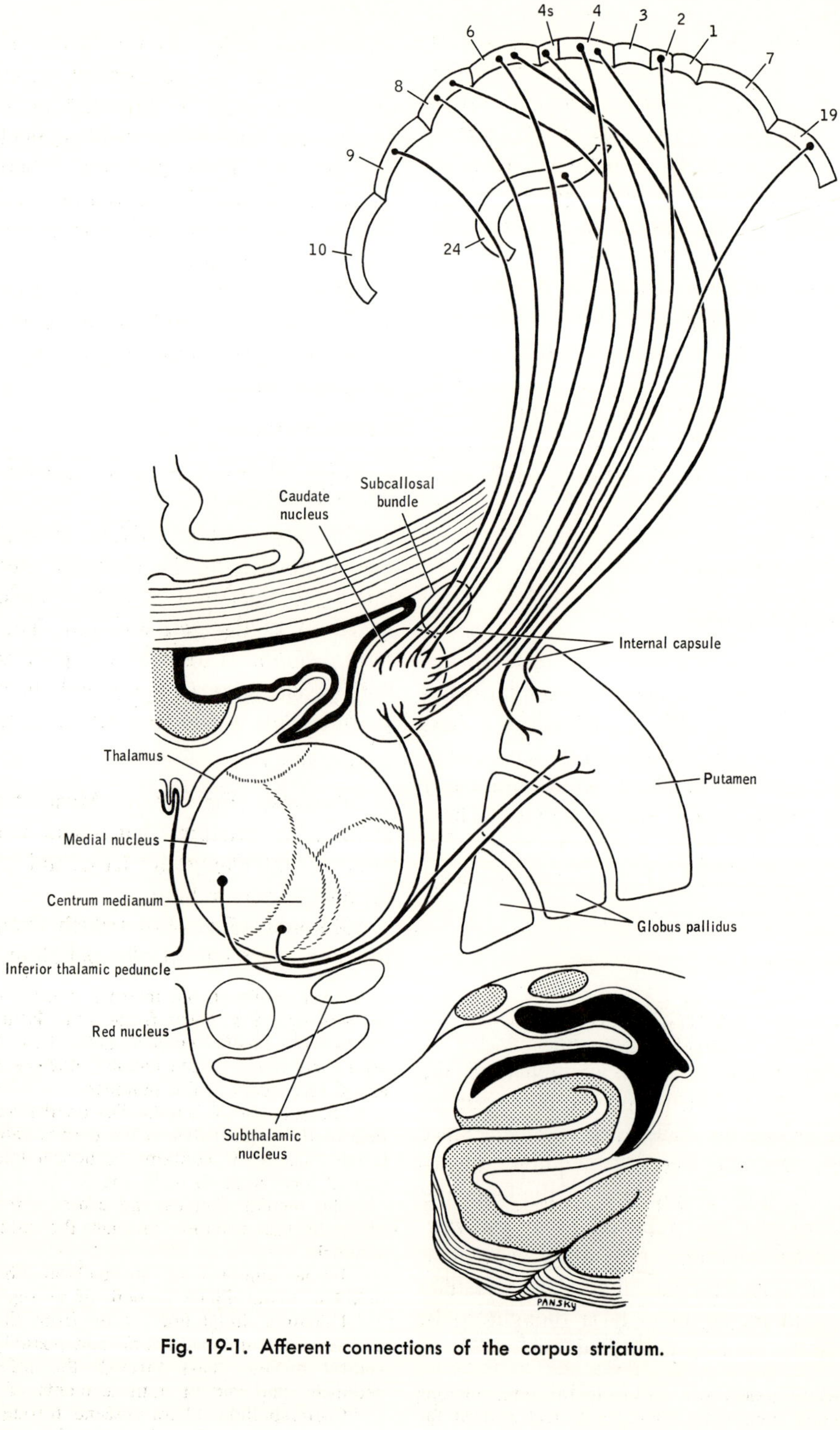

Fig. 19-1. Afferent connections of the corpus striatum.

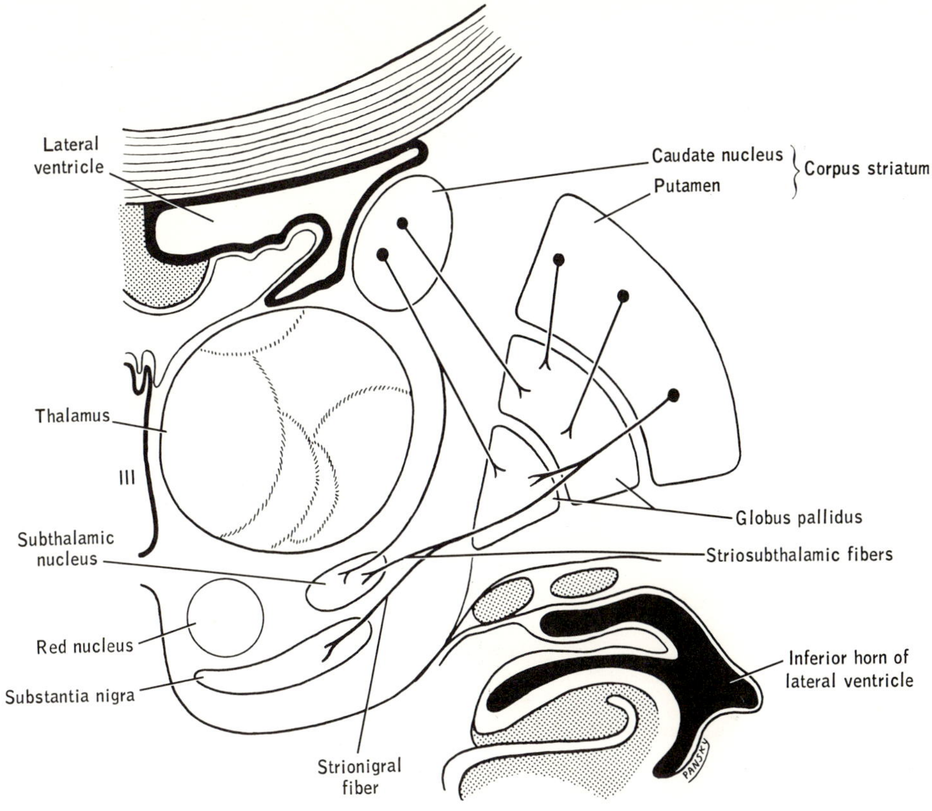

Fig. 19-2. Efferent fibers leaving the corpus striatum.

from the inner. In general, they are classified according to their destinations as *pallidothalamic, pallidosubthalamic, pallidohypothalamic, pallidoprerubral,* and *pallidorubral.*[9]

[9] These efferent fibers tend to leave the pallidum in three major streams. (1) *Ansa lenticularis* arises in the inner portion of the pallidum. Its fibers leave the ventral surface of this segment, turn medially, and then bend dorsally around the anterior border of the internal capsule to enter the subthalamic tegmentum (the latter region, together with its contained fiber bundles, is also referred to as Forel's tegmental fields H, H_1, and H_2). (2) *Fasciculus lenticularis* arises from both parts of the pallidum, but chiefly from the inner. The fibers emerge from the pallidum dorsally and take a dorsomedial course through the internal capsule to enter the subthalamus from the side. Here, they run between the zona incerta, dorsally, and the subthalamic nucleus, ventrally, to join the ansa. The large bundle formed by the union of ansa and fasciculus turns caudally into the prerubral field just rostral to the red nucleus. From the point where ansa and fasciculus join, a small bundle bends ventrally, passing over and around the column of the fornix to reach the hypothalamus (pallidohypothalamic). These fibers end in the paraventricular and dorsomedial hypothalamic nuclei but may go to others as well. As the combined ansa and fasciculus course caudally through the subthalamus, a large number of fibers diverge, coursing dorsally and laterally to form the *thalamic fasciculus.* These fibers end in the lateral ventral and anterior ventral nuclei of the thalamus. The remainder of the combined bundle actually terminates in the prerubral field, which contains large numbers of small cell bodies, which, according to some authorities, are considered to be a nucleus. The axons from the prerubral nucleus form the prerubral tract (prerubrorubral), which ends in the red nucleus. Some efferent pallidal fibers do not synapse in the prerubral field but go directly to the red nucleus. Also, some of the prerubral tract fibers bypass the red nucleus to end in the deep tegmental nucleus of the mesencephalon. (3) *Pallidosubthalamic fibers* arise, for the most part, in the outer portion of the pallidum but do not follow directly either the ansa or fasciculus lenticularis. Some perforate the internal capsule, while others pass ventrally and bend around the capsule (a few apparently travel with the fasciculus lenticularis). For the most part, all these fibers end in the subthalamic nucleus, although it is thought that some may continue caudally to the substantia nigra.

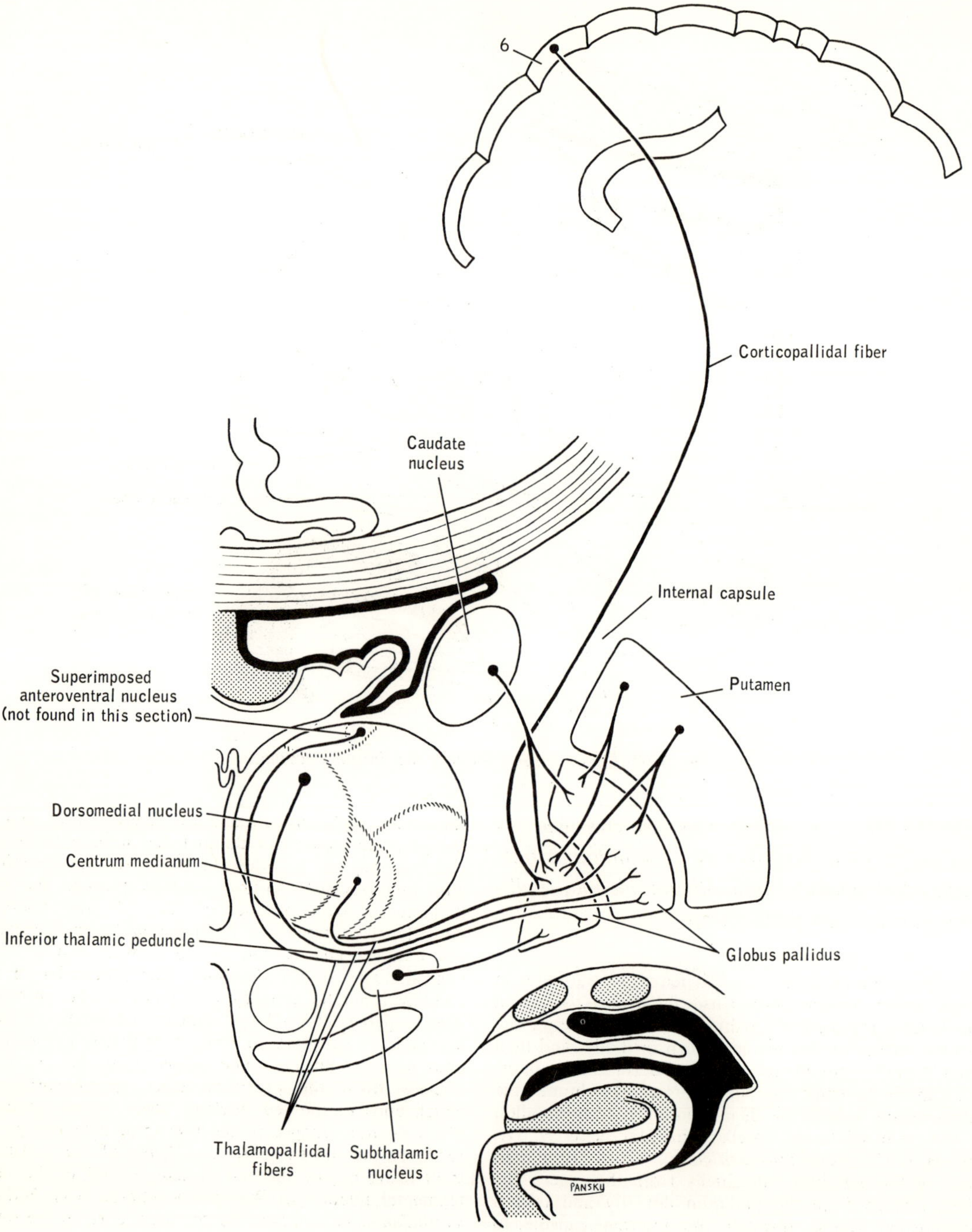

Fig. 19-3. Afferent fibers entering the globus pallidus.

Substantia Nigra

Structure

This nuclear mass forms a zone between the midbrain tegmentum and the basis pedunculi (Figs. 2-37 to 2-39, 25-11 to 25-16). At the level of the subthalamus it is almost continuous with the pallidum. It extends as far caudally as the pons. Its dorsal portion is *compact* and contains numerous neurons of moderate size which are pigmented with melanin. The more ventral, or reticular part, contains smaller cells and is somewhat intermingled with the peduncle. The evidence indicates that it has suppressor functions.

Connections

Afferents. (Fig. 19-5.) They are of several sorts. *Strionigral, pallidonigral,* and *subthalamonigral* fibers terminate at all levels of the substantia nigra. In addition, *corticonigral* fi-

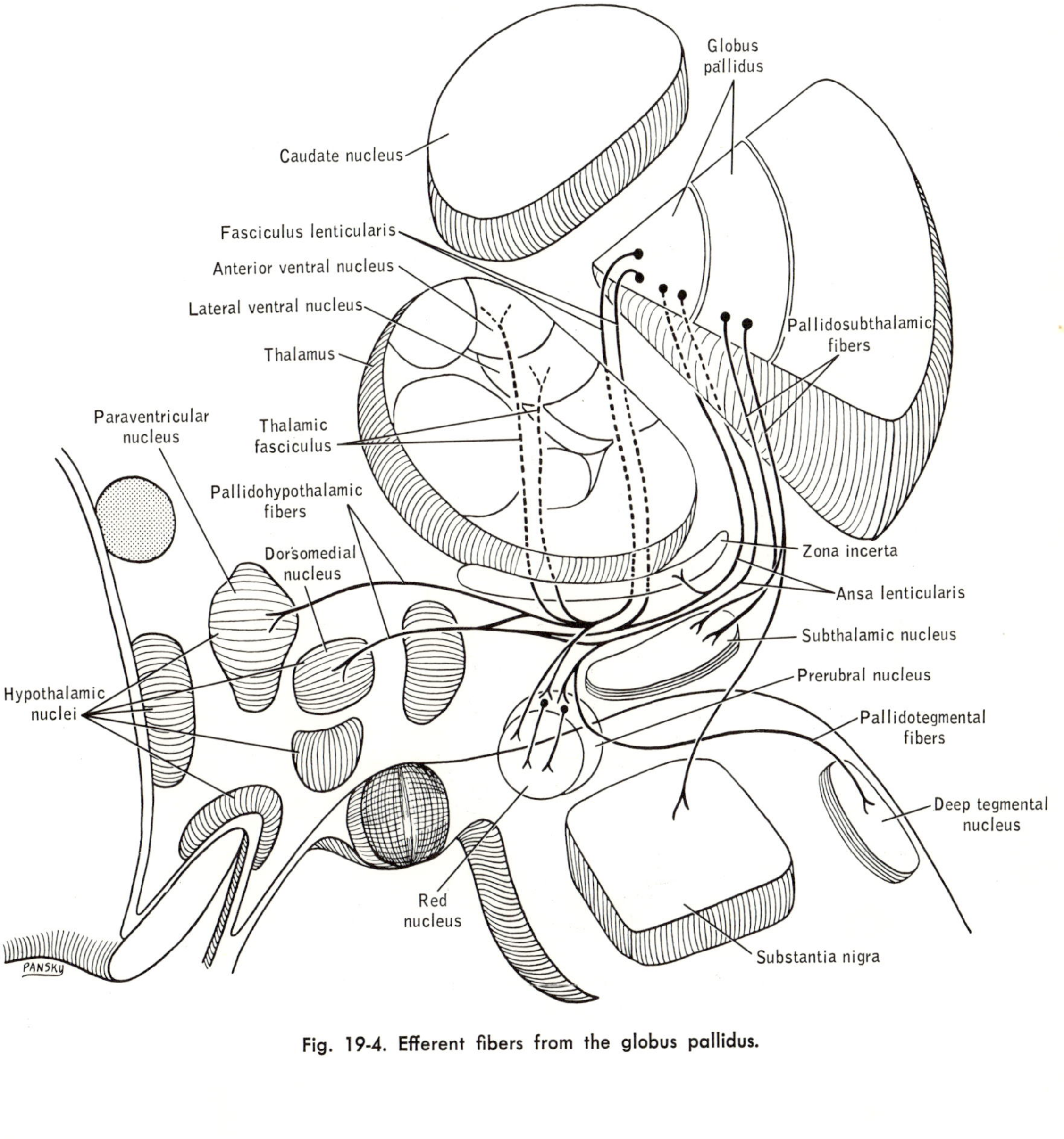

Fig. 19-4. Efferent fibers from the globus pallidus.

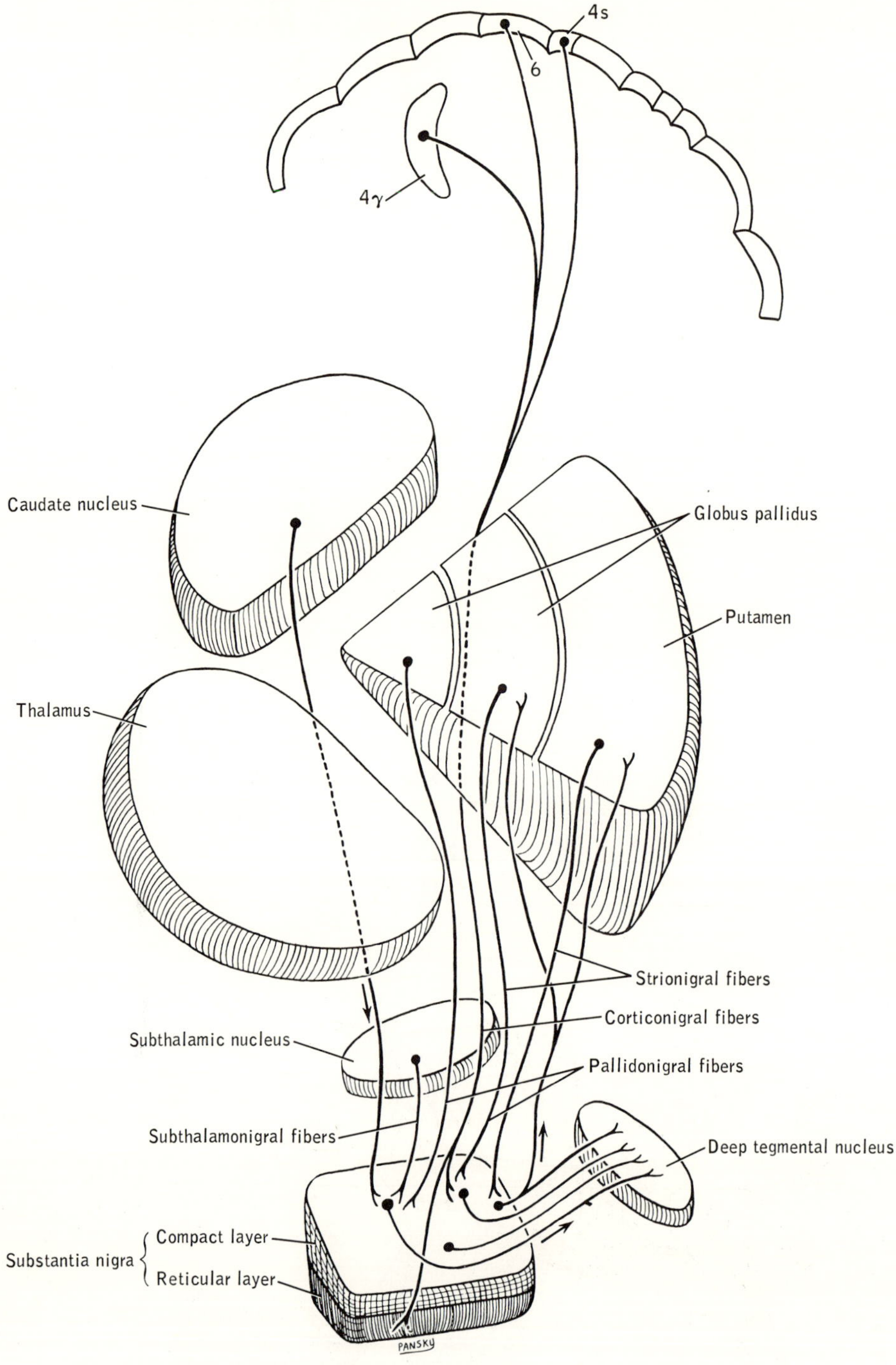

Fig. 19-5. Afferent and efferent connections of the substantia nigra.

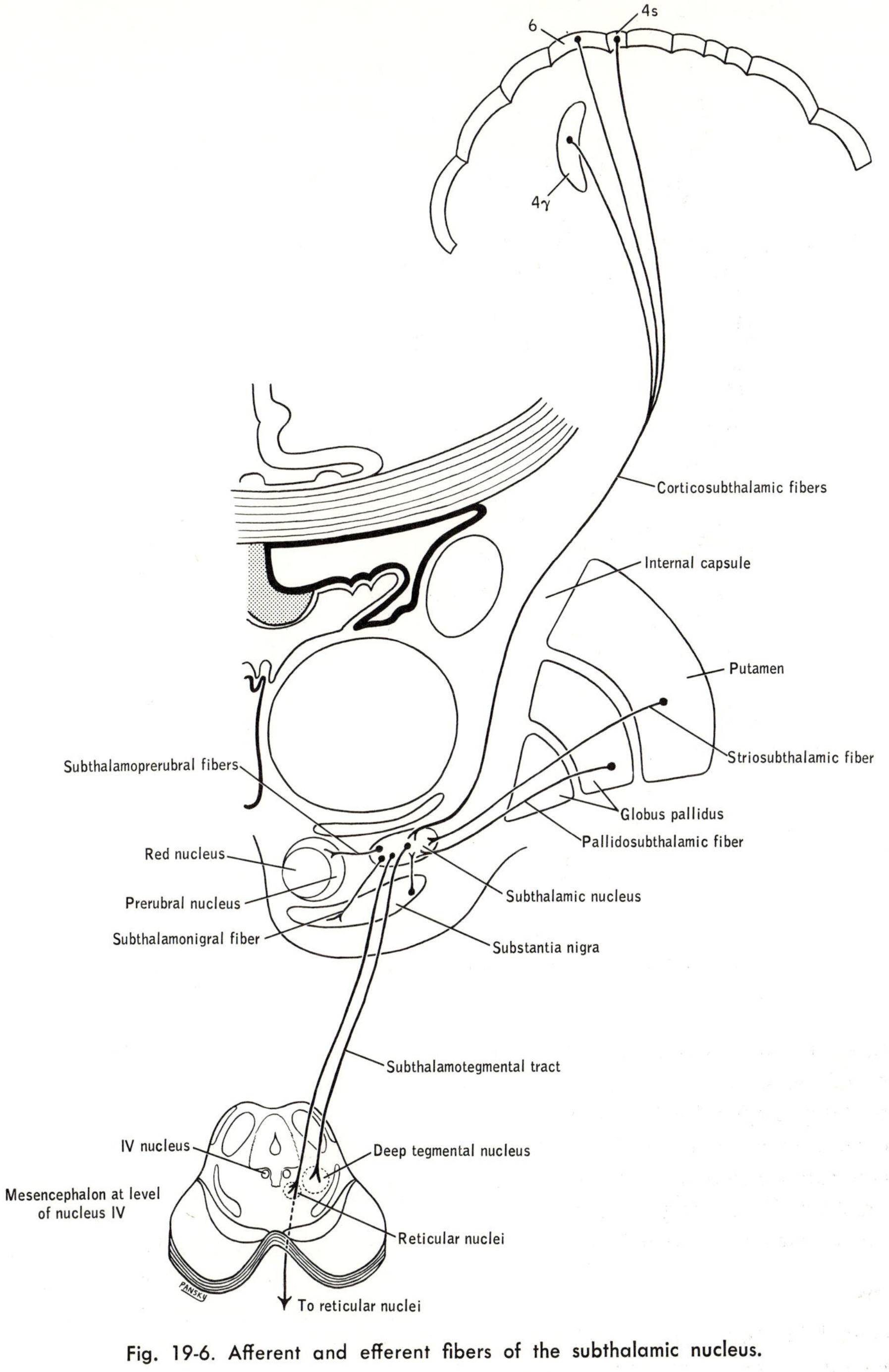

Fig. 19-6. Afferent and efferent fibers of the subthalamic nucleus.

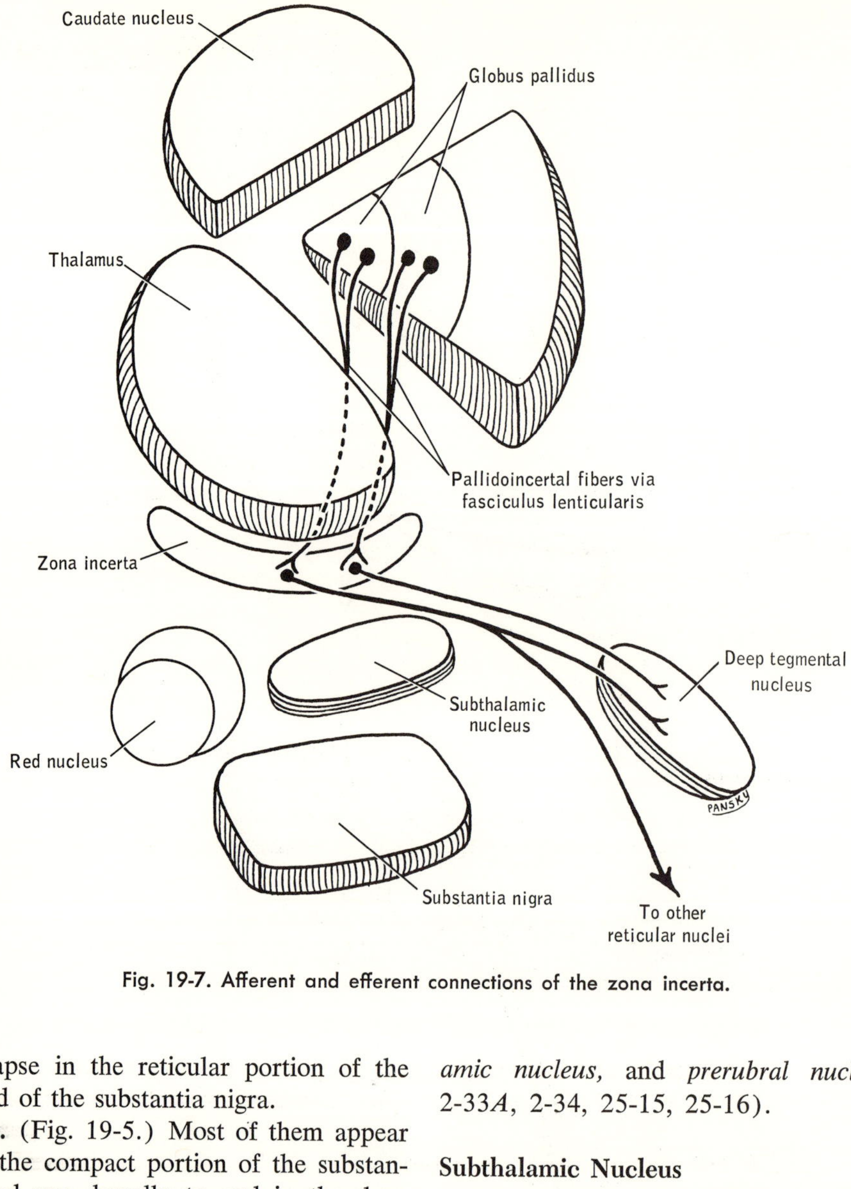

Fig. 19-7. Afferent and efferent connections of the zona incerta.

bers[10] synapse in the reticular portion of the cephalic end of the substantia nigra.

Efferents. (Fig. 19-5.) Most of them appear to arise in the compact portion of the substantia nigra and run dorsally to end in the deep tegmental nucleus. There may be ascending fibers back to the striatum and pallidum as well.

Subthalamus

This region, lying between the thalamus and the hypothalamus, extends from the red nucleus to the internal capsule. It contains several nuclear masses, among them the *zona incerta, subthalamic nucleus,* and *prerubral nucleus* (Figs. 2-33*A*, 2-34, 25-15, 25-16).

[10] These fibers arise mainly in areas 4γ, 4s, and 6.

Subthalamic Nucleus

Structure (Figs. 25-15, 25-16.)

It is a large, oval nucleus, its long axis being nearly horizontal. It is encapsulated by fibers, many of which terminate therein. Just dorsal to it is the fasciculus lenticularis. It appears to have suppressor functions and is an important part of the extrapyramidal system for stabilizing motor activity initiated in the cerebral cortex, perhaps because of the recurrent connections through the globus pallidus to the thalamus and thence to the motor cortex.

Connections

Afferents. (Fig. 19-6.) They arise in the corpus striatum, globus pallidus, and cerebral cortex.[11]

Efferents. (Fig. 19-6.) Many of them pass to the deep tegmental nucleus of the mesencephalon, while others descend still farther to reticular nuclei at lower levels. Some appear to terminate in the substantia nigra and the prerubral nucleus, the latter perhaps representing a relay in the pallidonigral pathway.

[11] These appear to come from areas 4γ, 4s, 6.

Zona Incerta

Structure (Fig. 25-15.)

It is a much smaller nuclear mass, separated from the subthalamic nucleus by the fasciculus lenticularis.

Connections

Afferents. (Fig. 19-7.) They are mainly from the globus pallidus.

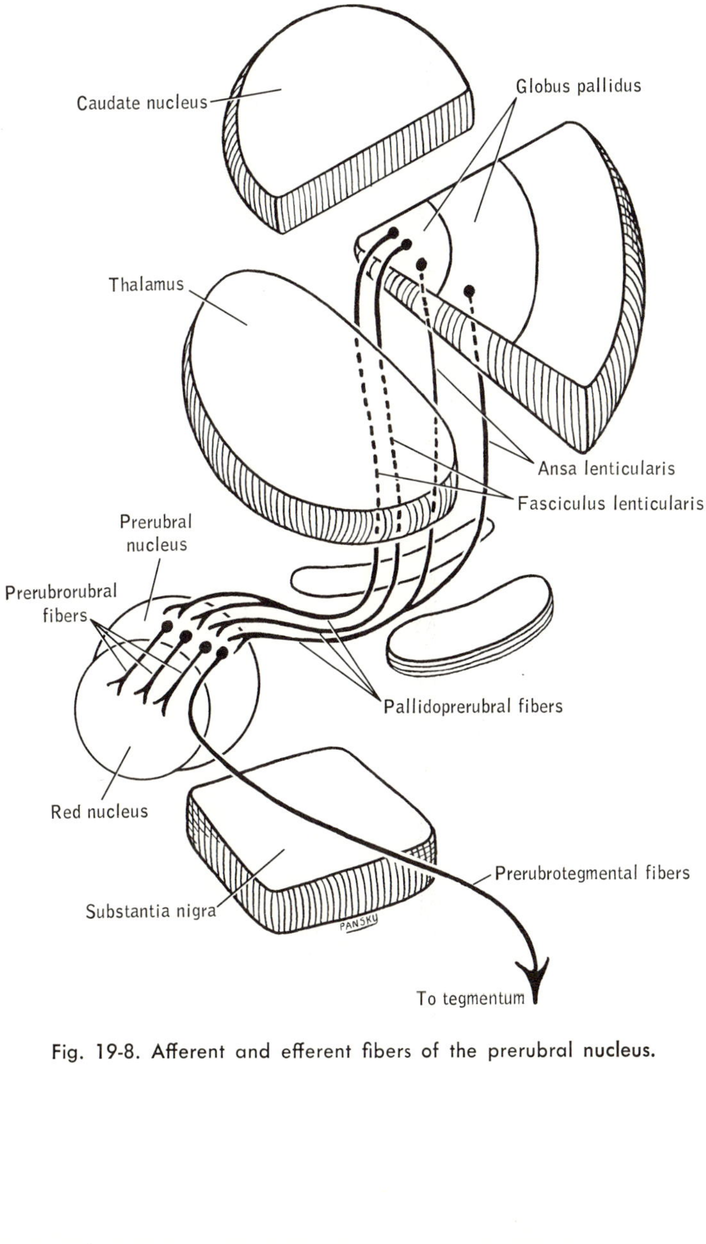

Fig. 19-8. Afferent and efferent fibers of the prerubral nucleus.

Efferents. (Fig. 19-7.) Most of them descend to the deep tegmental nucleus and other reticular cell groups. Thus, the zona incerta may be merely a relay station in the pallidotegmental pathway.

Prerubral Nucleus

Structure

It is located just rostral to the red nucleus and along its rostrolateral border.

Connections

Afferents. (Fig. 19-8.) They are mainly from the globus pallidus.

Efferents. (Fig. 19-8.) Most of them are short, acting as relays directly into the adjacent red nucleus. Some, however, appear to bypass the latter to terminate in the reticular nuclei of the tegmentum.

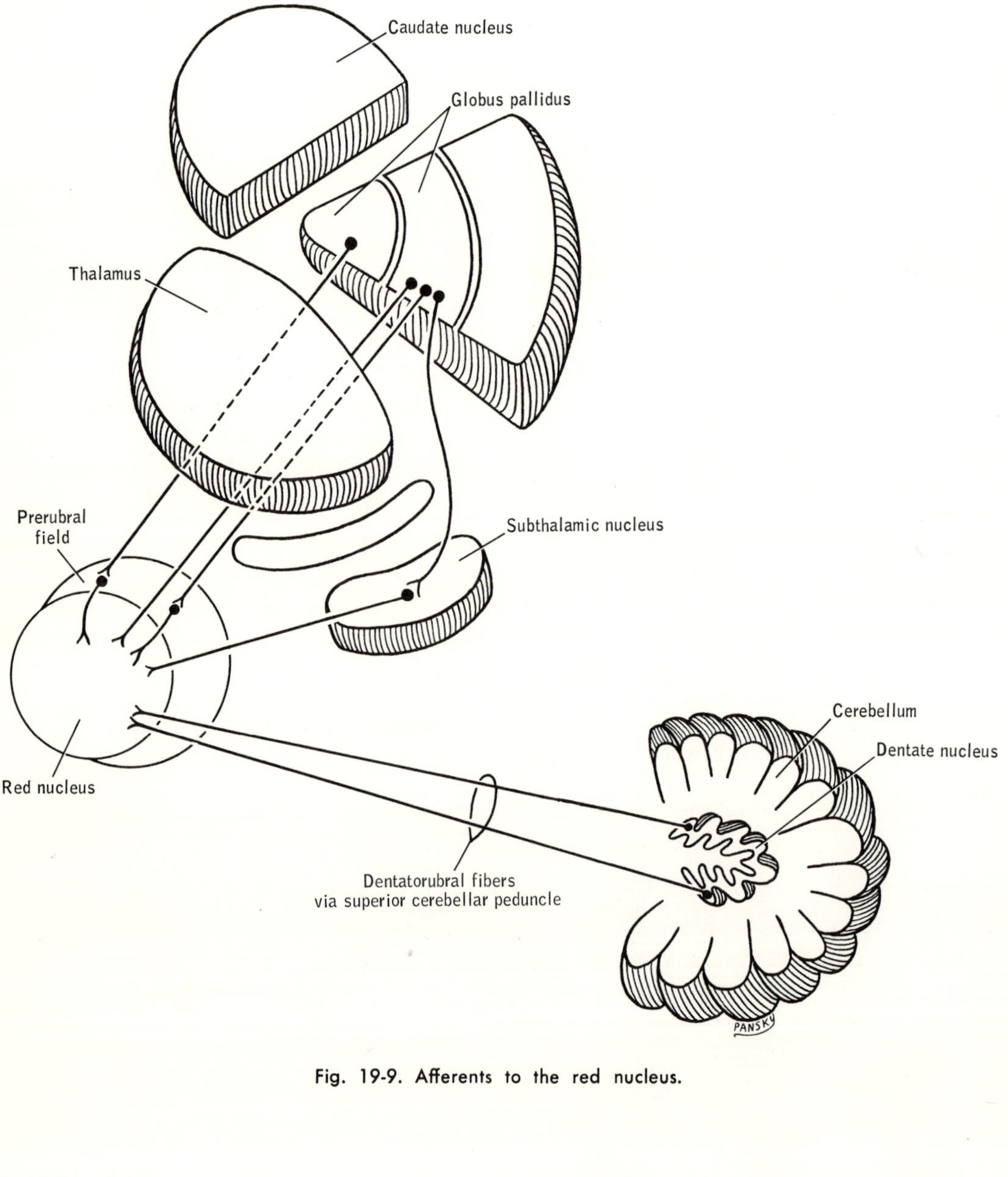

Fig. 19-9. Afferents to the red nucleus.

Red Nucleus

Structure (Figs. 2-33*A*, 2-34, 2-37, 2-38, 25-12, 25-14.)

It is a large, prominent cell mass, extending from the subthalamus through the tegmentum of the mesencephalon to the caudal level of the superior colliculus. It is frequently described as consisting of three parts: caudal, lateral, and medial. There are also two general cell types: (1) large, usually located in the more caudal part; (2) small to medium-sized, found further rostrally. The nucleus has a "capsule" made up of fibers entering and leaving its center.

Connections

Afferents. (Fig. 19-9.) Although there are some direct pallidorubral fibers, most of the afferent impulses are relayed from the prerubral field. Another large afferent contribution comes by way of the superior cerebellar peduncle from the dentate nucleus of the cerebellum.

Efferents. (Fig. 19-10.) Efferents from the red nucleus are widely distributed. Some enter the medial longitudinal fasciculus and are thus especially related to the nuclei of nerves III, IV, and VI. Some, but probably not many, at least in man, enter the *rubrospinal tract* (Figs. 3-7, 25-1 to 25-11) to be carried to the lower motor centers of the cord. Many, however, exert their influence over the segmental apparatus by first terminating in the reticular formation and then being relayed to lower levels through the *reticulobulbar* and *reticulospinal* tracts. There are also said to be connections through the reticular system with the inferior olive Ascending connections to the thalamus are also described.

Deep Tegmental Nucleus of Mesencephalon

Structure

This nucleus, deep in the midbrain tegmentum, extends from about the level of the posterior commissure to the caudal border of the inferior colliculus. It consists of neurons of all sizes, many diffusely scattered, while others are aggregated into relatively distinct groups.

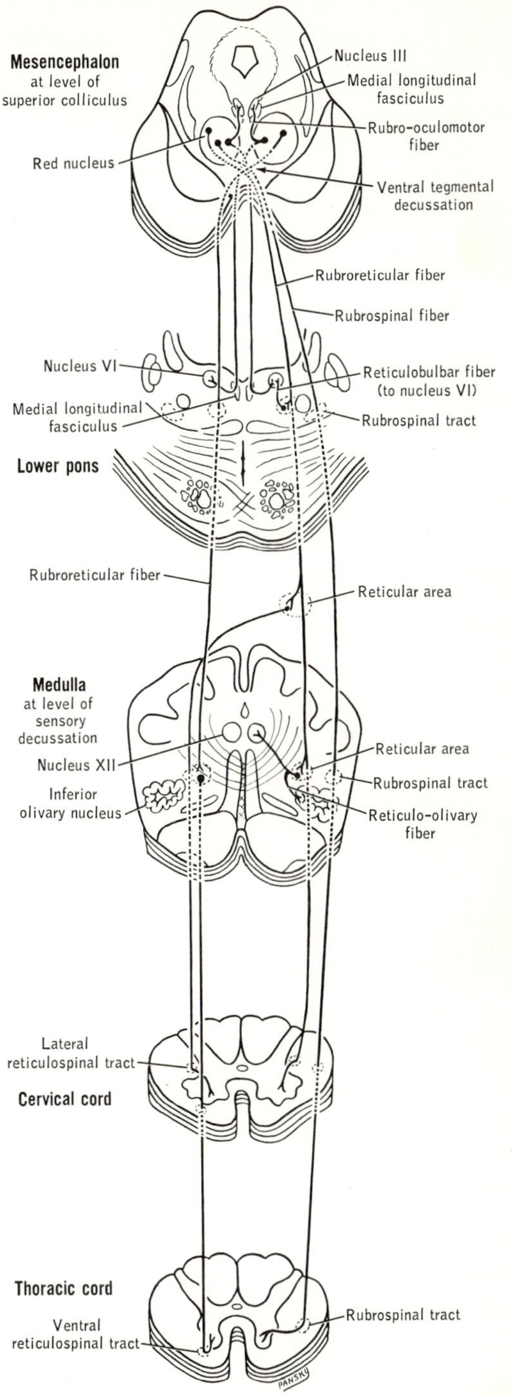

Fig. 19-10. Efferents from the red nucleus, particularly the rubrospinal and rubroreticular tracts.

Connections

Afferents. (Fig. 19-11.) This nucleus is an important relay center. It receives fibers from the pallidum, subthalamus, rubral fields, substantia nigra, and certain extrapyramidal cortical areas.[12]

Efferents. (Fig. 19-11.) The efferents from this nucleus go either into the reticular nuclei of medulla and pons or to the inferior olive.

Reticular or Tegmental Nuclei and Tracts of Medulla and Pons

Structure

The reticular formation is spread throughout the brain stem between the tracts and nuclei thereof, making up the bulk of tissue in the central portions of the tegmentum of the medulla, pons, and midbrain. Originally, it consisted mainly of the axons of association neurons interconnecting sensory and motor nuclei. Later in phylogenesis, as the spread of impulses over a wider area became necessary and a modicum of suprasegmental control over the purely segmental activity of the spinal motor mechanisms became essential, nuclear groups developed within the fibrous reticulum. Since this formation already was interconnected to the efferent system, suprasegmental motor control units became associated with these groups as well. The role of the reticular system in the mesencephalon, of which the red nucleus and the deep tegmental nucleus of the midbrain are a part, has already been discussed. Although many so-called reticular nuclei and their connections are present, only those concerned in the relays of the extrapyramidal system will be considered here.

Central Tegmental Reticular Nucleus of Pons

Structure

This is such an extremely diffuse mass that it is sometimes called the *dissipated reticular nucleus.* It is located in the lateral and central pontine tegmentum and extends from the lower midbrain to the caudal pons (Fig. 19-12).

[12] Areas 4, 4s, and 6 send fibers to this nucleus. It is also said that areas 2, 8, 19, and 24 have efferents terminating here.

Connections

Afferents. (Fig. 19-12.) Descending fibers from the more rostral portions of the extrapyramidal system, probably mainly from the deep tegmental nucleus of the mesencephalon, terminate here. (Some may come from the red nucleus directly or from the subthalamus.)

Efferents. This nucleus contributes fibers to both the *medial* and *lateral reticulospinal tracts,* as well as short relays to other reticular nuclei.

Central Reticular Nucleus of the Medulla

Structure (Fig. 19-13.)

It extends from a plane at the level of the eighth cranial nerve rostrally to the level of the motor nucleus of the trigeminal nerve. It lies along the raphe and in an area somewhat lateral to it.

Connections

Afferents. (Fig. 19-13.) Fibers reach this nucleus from the pallidum, cortex, red nucleus, or more rostral tegmental reticular nuclei.

Efferents. Most of these fibers enter the medial reticulospinal tract.

Inferior Medial Reticular Nucleus of the Medulla (Magnocellular Nucleus)

Structure (Fig. 19-14.)

It is the larger of the inferior medullary nuclei. It extends from below the inferior olive to a rostral point near the level of entrance of the vestibular part of the acoustic nerve. It occupies the area from just dorsal to the inferior olive to a point medial and slightly ventral to the spinal trigeminal tract.

Afferents. These fibers come mainly from the more rostral extrapyramidal nuclei.

Efferents. This nucleus may have a few relay fibers in the reticulospinal tract.

Inferior Lateral Reticular Nucleus of the Medulla

Structure (Fig. 19-14.)

This is a smaller and more circumscribed nucleus than the former. It occupies the region

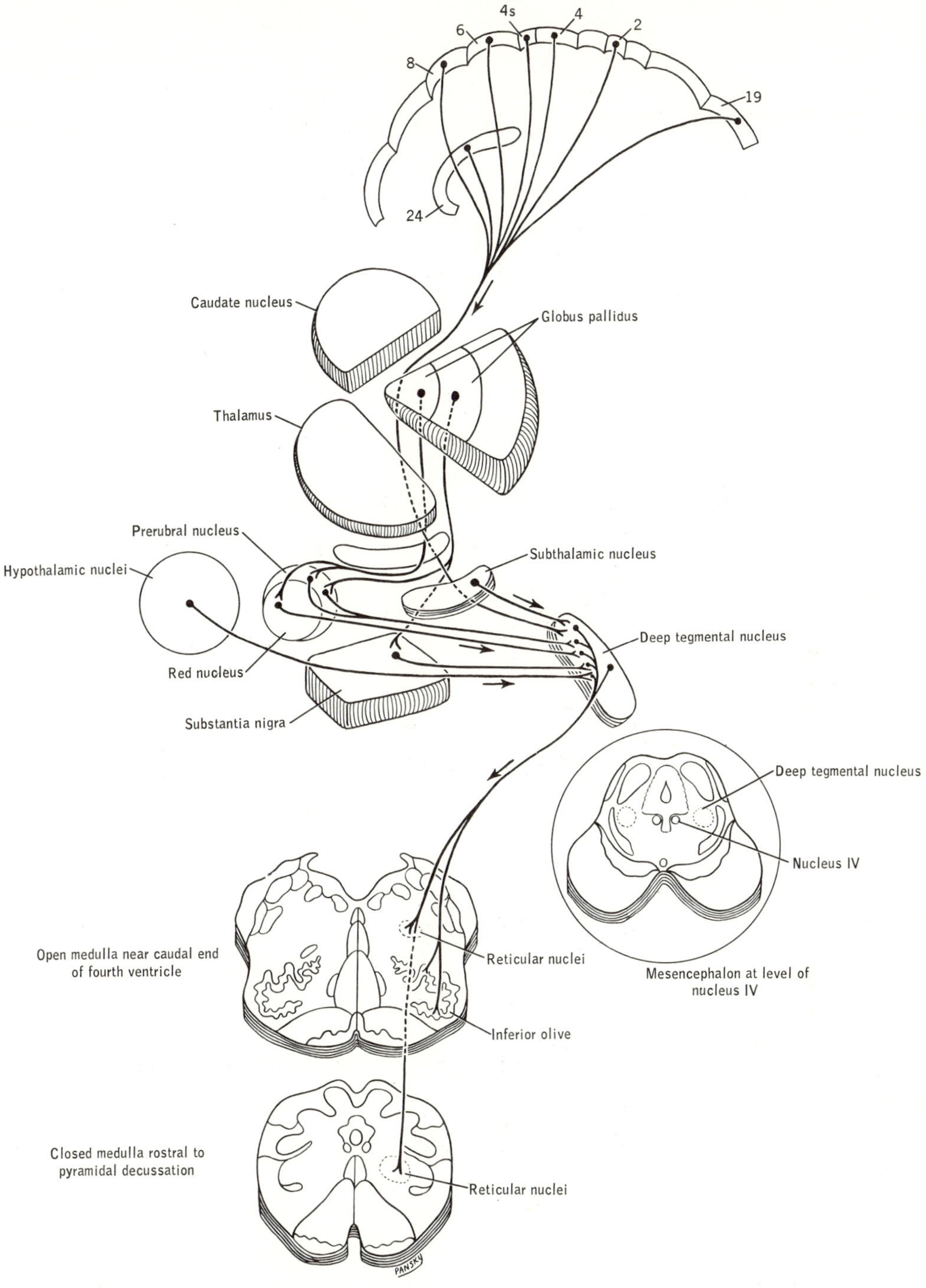

Fig. 19-11. Afferent and efferent connections of the deep tegmental nucleus of the mesencephalon.

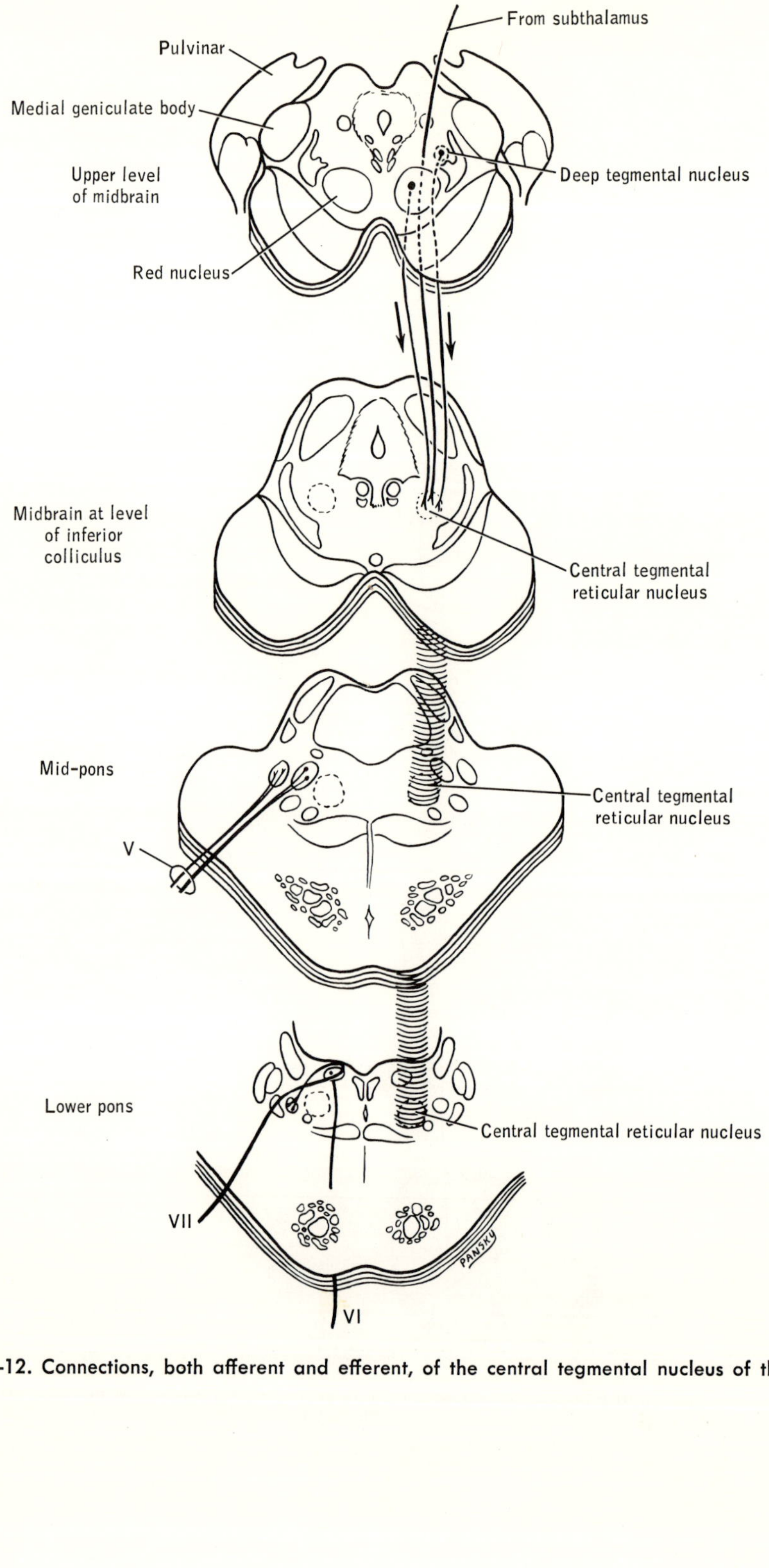

Fig. 19-12. Connections, both afferent and efferent, of the central tegmental nucleus of the pons.

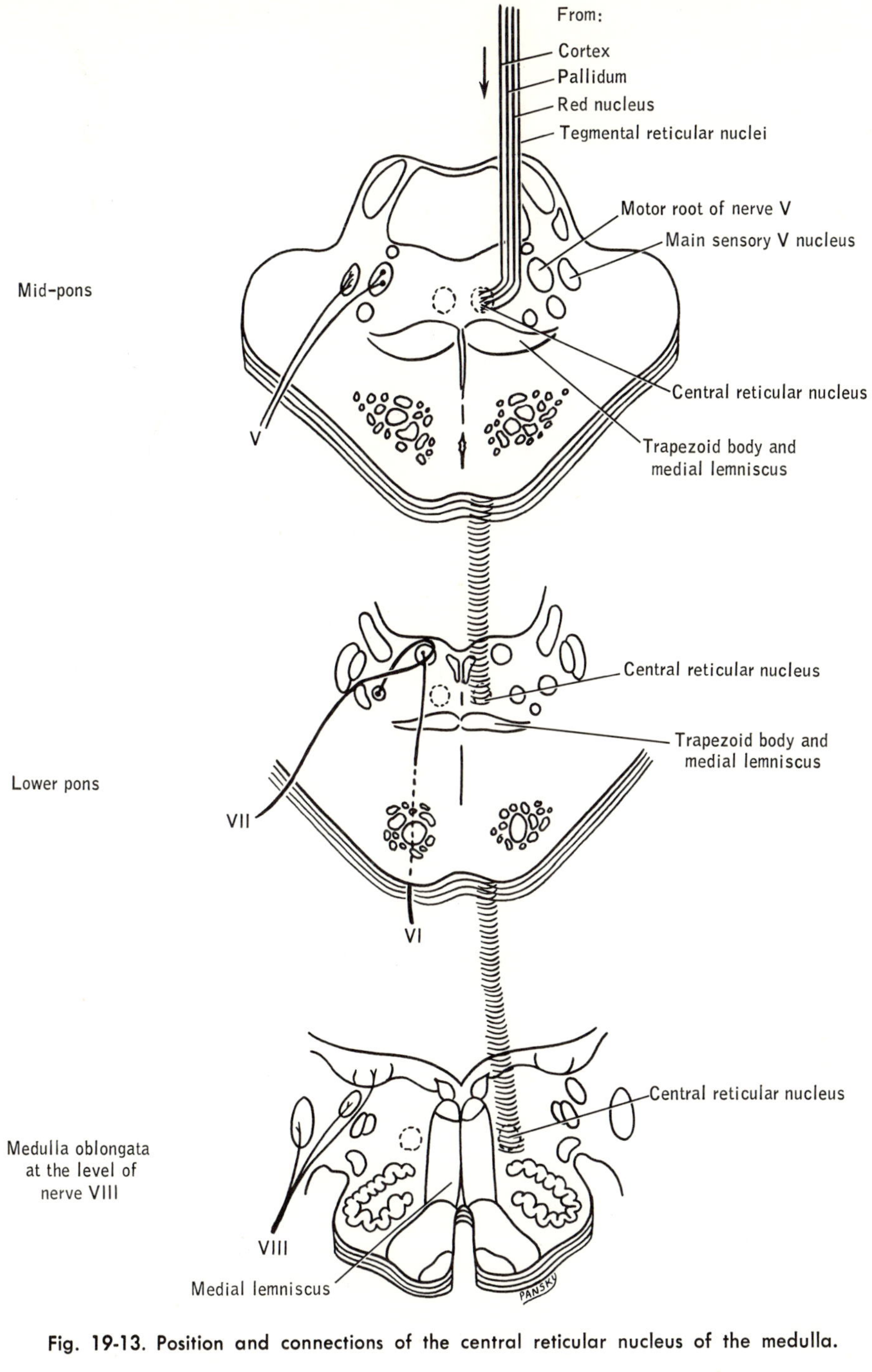

Fig. 19-13. Position and connections of the central reticular nucleus of the medulla.

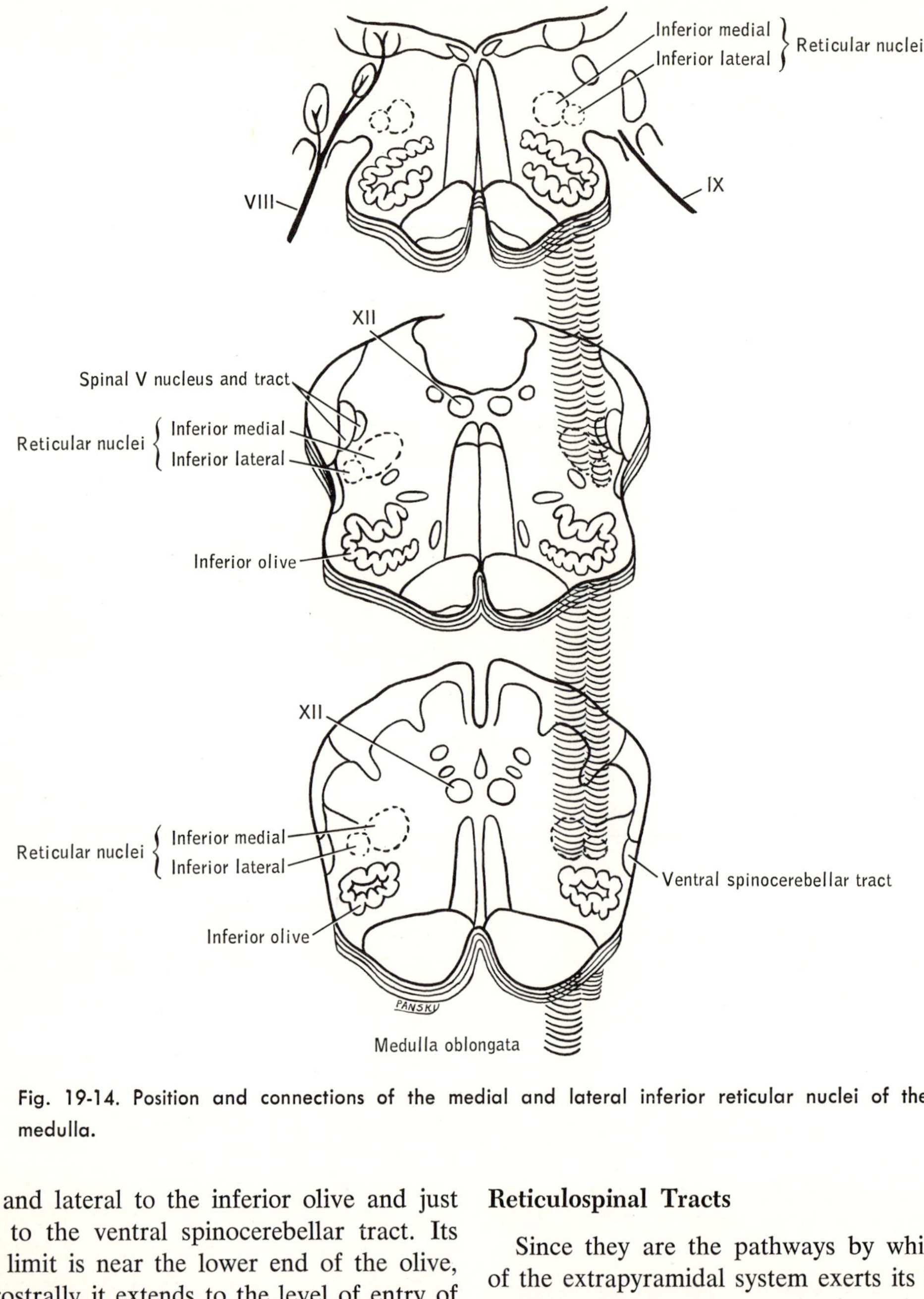

Fig. 19-14. Position and connections of the medial and lateral inferior reticular nuclei of the medulla.

dorsal and lateral to the inferior olive and just medial to the ventral spinocerebellar tract. Its caudal limit is near the lower end of the olive, while rostrally it extends to the level of entry of the ninth cranial nerve.

Afferents. Fibers come from the more rostral nuclei of the reticular system.

Efferents. They may lie in the medial reticulospinal tracts. Reticulocerebellar fibers also arise here.

Reticulospinal Tracts

Since they are the pathways by which much of the extrapyramidal system exerts its influence over the spinal motor mechanism, their origin and course must be understood.

Medial Reticulospinal Tract

Fibers of the tract arise from several sources, particularly the central tegmental nucleus of the pons, the central reticular nucleus of the medulla, the inferior medial reticular nucleus of the medulla, and possibly the inferior lateral reticular nucleus of the medulla. From these nuclei fibers collect slightly ventral and lateral to the medial longitudinal fasciculus and descend into the cord, coming to lie in the anterior funiculus near the medial side of the anterior gray column.

Lateral Reticulospinal Tract

This tract takes origin from the central tegmental nucleus of the pons and perhaps one of the inferior medullary reticular nuclei. These fibers pass caudally through the brain stem in a position ventromedial to the spinal trigeminal tract and nucleus. On entering the cord they descend in the lateral funiculus close to the border of the gray substance.

EVALUATION OF THE EXTRAPYRAMIDAL CIRCUIT (Fig. 19-15.)

No system in human neuroanatomy is so difficult to evaluate from a physiological point of view. There are many reasons for this, the first of which is already evident—the wide dispersion of its parts and the multiplicity of its connections. In the second place, the inaccessibility of many of its centers and the relations of both centers and their interconnections to other parts of the CNS makes it difficult to approach experimentally without the possibility of adversely affecting unrelated areas. Third, it is dangerous to extrapolate conclusions based upon animal experimentation since the enormous development of the human cortex exerts more extensive control over subcortical centers than is the case in lower forms. Fourth, stimulation experiments are hard to adjust and control. Fifth, even in human patients where it has been possible to relate the lesions to the symptoms, it is almost impossible to find a pathological process, whether CVA or tumors, which confines itself to a specific part of a specific pathway.

Since we know so little about the actual function of its component parts, we can make only a few general comments concerning the entire system. First, it consists of an interrupted descending pathway which passes through a complex series of relays. Two, there are basically two functional but physiologically opposing parts—one an excitor and the other an inhibitor with normal activity depending upon a balance of the two.

As has already been stated, the extrapyramidal system is mainly the regulator of large muscle masses of the trunk, girdle, and proximal parts of the limbs, while the pyramidal mechanism controls the muscles of the distal portions of the extremities. In order to produce activity, it is essential for one set of muscles to become active while the opposing set is inhibited. Thus, this system must provide for the passage of activating impulses from higher centers to motor neurons of the agonist muscle groups; the facilitation (enhancement) of such impulses; and the complete suppression of the activity of the antagonist muscle groups.

The pathways from the cortex and striatum, through which direct activation is accomplished, have already been described. The facilitation-suppression mechanism requires further discussion.

Facilitation

When certain portions of the cerebrum are stimulated in the absence of area 4 or its projections, mass muscular movements result. These are areas 1, 2, 3, 5, 6α, 6β, 7, 8, 19, and 22.

A center in the medulla which appears to facilitate spinal motor activity has also been found. It lies in the more lateral portion of the reticular formation in both the medulla and pons. Impulses from these levels also course in both reticulospinal tracts to the motor cells of the cord. Its activity is influenced through discharge of the subthalamus, pallidum, and cerebellum.

Stimulation, particularly of the medullary facilitory center, will increase motion initiated as part of a reflex. It has also been shown that stimulation of certain other regions (hypothalamus, subthalamus, and the central gray area of the mesencephalon), as well as the pontine and medullary reticular formation, facilitates cor-

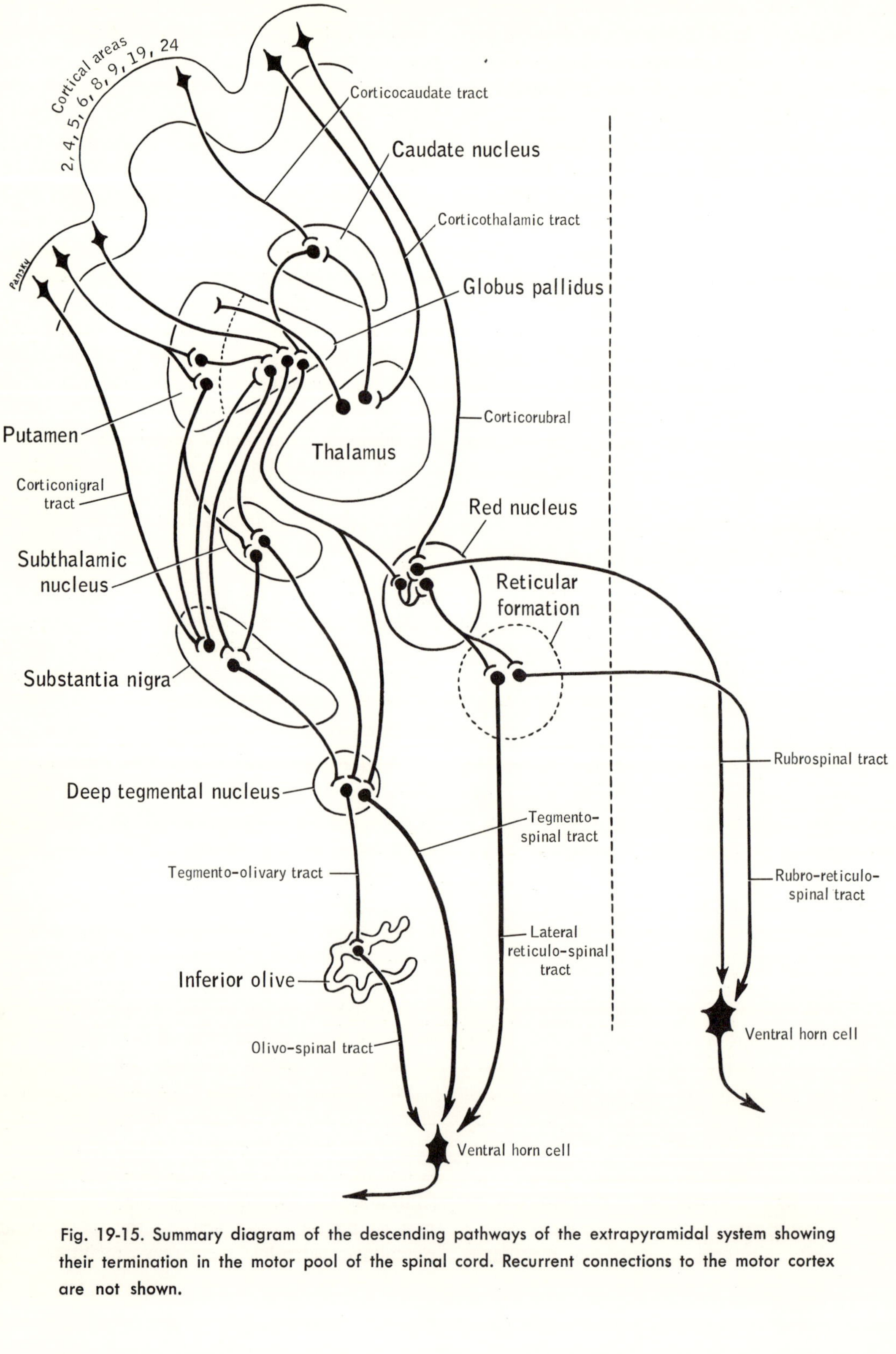

Fig. 19-15. Summary diagram of the descending pathways of the extrapyramidal system showing their termination in the motor pool of the spinal cord. Recurrent connections to the motor cortex are not shown.

tically induced movement. The evidence indicates that there may be a series of facilitating centers, each of which, up to a certain level of the brain stem,[13] may be destroyed without impairing function.

It also appears that the facilitatory mechanism also includes ascending fiber pathways. The presence of such fibers has been indicated. They may in some way affect the cortex. In this connection, it has been suggested that the fibers ascending in the reticular system to the thalamus and cortex send a continuous stream of impulses to the cortex, thus activating it. Since the reticular formation does receive, through collaterals and association fibers, impulses from all sensory systems, a steady supply of activating influences is always present.

Suppression

Apparently the neurons belonging to the medial reticular nuclei, particularly in the rostral portion of the medulla,[14] act as a powerful inhibiting influence on the spinal motor activity, whether the activity is induced through a purely reflex circuit or from cortical centers. Thus, this area is called the *bulbar inhibitor center*. It receives afferents from the cerebrum, basal ganglia, and cerebellum and exerts its influence by way of both medial and lateral reticulospinal tracts.

The stimulation of certain cortical areas either will produce no muscular activity or will suppress movement already started. The first area mapped out was 4s, the stimulation of which leads to the release of extensor tone. Other regions of the cortex were found also to be capable of suppressing motor responses elicited by a previous stimulation of the primary voluntary motor cortex (area 4). These areas are 2s, 19s, and 24s, the most powerful of which appears to be 24s.

There are at least two possible pathways by which the extrapyramidal suppressor areas depress motor activity. The first passes from the suppressor cortex through the corticostriate fibers to the caudate nucleus, thence to the pallidum. From here fibers are distributed to the lateral ventral and anterior ventral nuclei of the thalamus. The former, in particular, projects back to the cortex, primarily to areas 4 and 6, thus depressing activity of the motor cortex.

A second pathway, more direct, descends through various possible relays (see description above) to reach the bulbar inhibitor center and thence over the reticulospinal tracts to the motor columns of the cord.

[13] This level appears to be in the region of the pons-medulla junction, since massive destruction here results in less facilitation.

[14] Electrical stimulation of this area eliminates the exaggerated extensor tone seen in decerebrate animals.

CLINICAL CONSIDERATIONS

From the foregoing it seems obvious that normal muscular activity depends upon a balance between facilitation and suppression. If anything upsets this balance, the results are expressed in abnormalities of motor function. In practice, three general types of abnormality are seen: loss of certain movements; involuntary movements; aberrations in states of muscle tone, i.e., hypotonia, spasticity, or rigidity.

Abnormalities of Motor Function

Tone

Abnormalities in tone may take one of two directions: exaggererated, as in hypertonicity (rigidity); and decreased, as in hypotonia. The disorder of tone most frequently encountered is one of increase. Sometimes the degree of hypertonia is so great that volitional and emotional movements are almost completely suppressed. The patient may *appear* paralyzed but tests will prove that he *is not*. The face is masklike, the expression is changed infrequently and then only with difficulty, and the patient does not blink his eyes. He does not swing his arms in walking. Part of his difficulty is due to actual increased tone and part to the suppression of accompanying voluntary movements of the limb. In spasticity the increase in tone is observed for the most part in the antigravity muscles and may be the consequence of an interference with area 4s or its projection to the bulbar inhibitor center. When there is widespread pathologic change over much of the frontal lobe or to a large segment of subcortical extrapyramidal centers, increased tone is seen in practically all muscle groups. In contrast to the picture seen in spasticity, the tendon reflexes are usually not found to be increased. When the hypertonia is so general, the condition is usually called *rigidity*. Rigidity is classified as *plastic* or *cogwheel*.

Plastic Rigidity. In such cases, the hypertonia is constant and the examiner can feel a constant, continuous, and smooth resistance to passive stretching.

Cogwheel Rigidity. In this case an examiner will find that the resistance to passive stretch is not smooth but is discontinuous; there is an alternation of resistance and lack of resistance. This condition may actually be due to a milder form of the same pathological changes responsible for the plastic type of rigidity, but in this case not so much of the suppressor mechanism is interrupted.

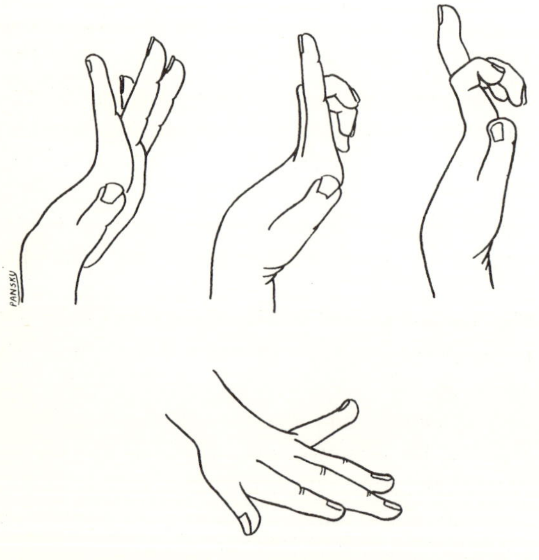

Fig. 19-16. Athetoid movements of the hand.

Involuntary Movements

Several of these movements are encountered. Among them are tremors, choreiform movements, athetosis, hemiballism, and dystonia. The underlying cause is unknown.

Tremors. Tremors are of various sorts, depending upon when they occur. When they appear while the body is at rest they are called *postural* (*static,* or *alternating*). This tremor consists of the alternating contraction of opposing muscle groups—flexors and extensors, abductors and adductors. In the hands this tremor is characterized by thumb opposing fingers in the "pill-rolling" maneuver. In most cases this type of tremor is suppressed during voluntary acts and may disappear in sleep. It is more severe in emotional states. *Action,* or *intention, tremors* always appear during voluntary acts, increasing in severity near the end of the action. They are not seen at rest.

Choreiform Movements. These movements are rapid, dancing, and jerky. They appear somewhat purposeful. There may be a rapid flexion of a finger, abduction of the arm, elevation of a shoulder, a grimace around the mouth, or a twitching of the facial muscles. They may occur at rest and may also accompany voluntary acts.

Athetosis. (Fig. 19-16.) This is a slow pattern of movement rather than an isolated act. It may occur either at rest or in the course of voluntary action. The movement begins slowly and is often seen in the distal part of the upper extremity, where there are alternating hyperextension and flexion of the fingers, usually with abduction. The wrist may slowly flex and pronate. The arm is often retracted. This is referred to as "serpentine movement." Grimaces of the face frequently occur simultaneously with the limb action. The muscles are hypertonic during the active phase of the movement but are hypotonic at rest. Most frequently the striatum and cortex are involved. However, lesions have been seen in the globus pallidus and thalamus. The site of the lesion is usually contralateral to that of the abnormal movement.

Dystonic Movements. These movements are slow, writhing, and involuntary, with bizarre, grotesque tortions and twistings of the shoulder and pelvic girdles as well as of the trunk. There are spasmodic alterations of muscle tone, first hypertonus, then hypotonus predominating. There may be rigidity, scoliosis, and lordosis.[15]

Ballism. This is characterized by involuntary movements of the entire limb, beginning in the proximal portions and passing in waves down the extremity. There may be wild swinging of the arms. Rolling, wavelike patterns seem to flow down the arm from time to time. When both limbs of the same side are involved, this is called hemiballism, when only one is involved, it is monoballism. Like chorea and atetosis, this is thought to be a release phenomenon. In other words, lesions in one center or pathway have removed the regulating influences which the diseased structure normally had upon related, normal portions of the system. Thus, with the regulatory influence gone or diminished, overactivity of the normal part results.

It seems probable that in the case of choreiform and choreoathetoid movements where degeneration in the caudate nucleus and putamen is observed, the lesion has interrupted interconnections between the suppressor strips of the hemisphere and the motor cortex in areas 4 and 6.

Testing

Few specific tests need to be made for this system. Much depends on merely observing the patient to see whether there is evidence of any of the abnormal movements of the type given above. Facial expression should be noted, to see if there are changes under different conditions. The patient should be watched while he is walking to see if the normal associative movements, such as swinging of the arms, occur in a normal way.

One specific type of test should be performed, however. It involves the manipulation of the extremities to get an impression of the muscle tone and of resistance to passive movement. At this time, the presence or absence of rigidity can be determined, and if it is present, its type—plastic or cogwheel—can be ascertained. The type may sometimes best be brought out by alternately pronating and supinating the forearm.

Specific Pathology

Although the various nuclear groups and their interconnections which make up the extrapyramidal system have been described in some detail, it is difficult to localize the particular portion of the system involved on the basis of symptoms seen among patients. It might be said that any successful skillful motor performance is the result of the integration of the entire motor mechanism. This represents not only a balance between facilitatory and inhibitory effects but a balance which can be subject to rapid alterations with the initiation of a specific action. Thus, if any portion of the system is destroyed or otherwise blocked, the resulting movement will represent the product of the parts still capable of function. For example, a pathologic process may involve the facilitatory mechanism. This, therefore, leads to a lack of influx of activating influences, together with an unchecked suppressor system. Conversely, disease in the inhibitory system removes the inhibitor impulses and leaves unchecked the facilitatory apparatus. However, since many of the nuclear masses and their interconnections are close together or even intermingled, it is obvious that lesions of the central nervous system will inevitably damage parts of both the facilitatory and inhibitory apparatuses simultaneously. Thus, the resulting motor performance will be the product of the undamaged parts of both systems. In the specific considerations listed below, an attempt has been made, where possible, to correlate the physical signs with the pathologic change of the CNS as determined after post-mortem examination.

Hemiballism

The movement pattern has already been discussed. It is the only one of the "diseases" of

[15] Scoliosis is an abnormal lateral curvature of the spinal column. Lordosis is a curvature of the spinal column with a forward convexity.

this system the onset of which may be sudden. It is frequently the result of destruction of the contralateral subthalamic nucleus from vascular or other disorders. Lesions involving the pallidosubthalamic fibers may also produce these symptoms.

Paralysis Agitans (*Parkinson's Disease*) (Fig. 19-17.)

In these cases, extensive degeneration of the globus pallidus and substantia nigra and cortex is seen. The putamen and caudate are involved to a lesser degree. By some, the substantia nigra is considered to be most important. The etiology is unknown. This disease is characterized by rigidity of both the plastic and cogwheel types. The trunk may be especially affected and this may lead to the assumption of a flexed posture. Postural tremor is present and is especially marked in the distal extremities, with a rate of about five tremors per second. These occur at rest and disappear with voluntary movement.

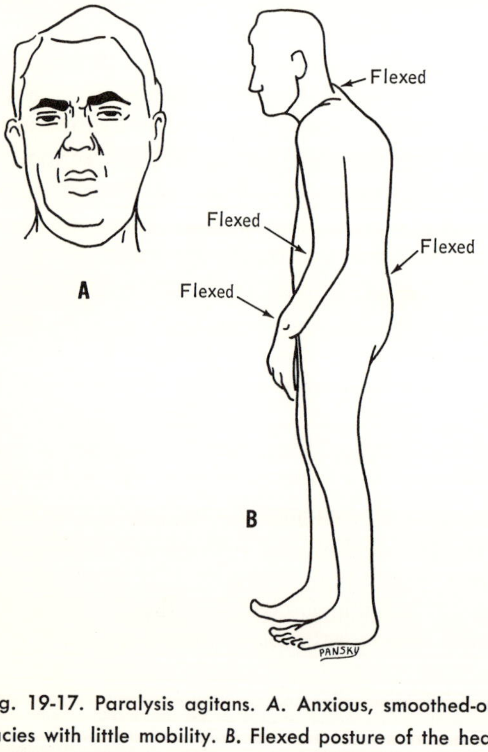

Fig. 19-17. Paralysis agitans. A. Anxious, smoothed-out facies with little mobility. B. Flexed posture of the head and trunk; flexion of the arms; pill-rolling position of the hand.

Encephalitis

While parkinsonism usually occurs later in life, encephalitis may lead to the appearance of these signs at any age. There may be trunk flexion, and the tremor in these cases occurs at the rate of about eight per second. It has been found that when rigidity is the most striking feature, the most severe damage is in the globus pallidus and the reticular portion of the substantia nigra. If tremor is the dominant sign, the compact zone of the substantia nigra shows more extensive pathologic change, while the pallidum exhibits less.

Hepatolenticular Disease (*Wilson's Disease*)

This is a rare, familial disease, usually fatal, occurring in young people. It is characterized clinically by an intention tremor, athetoid movements, rigidity, dysarthria, dysphagia, contractures, muscle weakness, progressive dementia, and emaciation.[16] In many cases, a peculiar golden-brown pigmented ring (Kayser-Fleischer ring) is seen at the outer margins of the cornea. The neuropathologic process is essentially limited to the corpus striatum. It consists of bilateral, symmetric, and visible cavitation, with degeneration of the putamen. Pathologic changes have also been found in other widely scattered areas of the brain, including the lateral ventral nucleus of the thalamus, the midbrain tegmentum and the substantia nigra. Like parkinsonism, the tremor disappears with sleep.

Sydenham's Chorea

This is a disease of children or adolescents, often associated with rheumatic fever. There are quick, irregular, involuntary, asymmetric, purposeless movements, increased by emotional or other stimuli. The pathologic changes have never been adequately studied, but petechial lesions in the striatum and cortex have been described.

[16] Dysarthria is imperfect articulation in speech. Dysphagia is difficulty in swallowing. Dementia is a mental deterioration.

Huntington's Chorea

This is an adult disease, onset of which occurs between the ages of 35 and 40 (sometimes earlier). Moderate to severe choreiform movements are coupled with progressive mental deterioration. There is degeneration in both the cortex and the basal ganglia (caudate and putamen). The disease is definitely hereditary.

Dystonia Musculorum Deformans (Torsion Spasm) (Fig. 19-18.)

Dystonic movements have been observed frequently as a sequel to epidemic encephalitis. In these cases, however, other signs and symptoms betray the acute, inflammatory origin of the disease. In the syndrome as described by one group of neurologists, these dystonic movements constitute practically the whole clinical picture. It is a chronic, progressive disease, usually beginning between the ages of 8 and 15. It appears to occur most commonly among Russian Jews. In typical cases, the diagnosis can be made at a glance. Slow, pattern-like movements, twisting of the pelvis, spasmodic torticollis, scoliosis, and contractures of the feet (striatal foot) point to the nature of the condition. The few cases which have come to autopsy have shown degenerative changes in practically every part of the brain, including basal midbrain, pons, cerebellum, and cerebral cortex.

As pointed out earlier, diseases of the extrapyramidal system destroy only portions of the system so that an imbalance exists between excitation and inhibition. Since it is patently impossible to restore the damaged part, most therapy attempts to destroy a portion of the normal or overactive region as a counterbalance. For example, it has been found that destruction of parts of the globus pallidus relieves contralateral rigidity, while destruction of parts of the thalamus helps to relieve contralateral tremor. Lesions placed in these same areas tend to ameliorate dystonic symptoms. It might also be noted that intension tremors encountered in certain cerebellar diseases may be relieved by placing lesions in the ventral lateral nucleus of the thalamus.

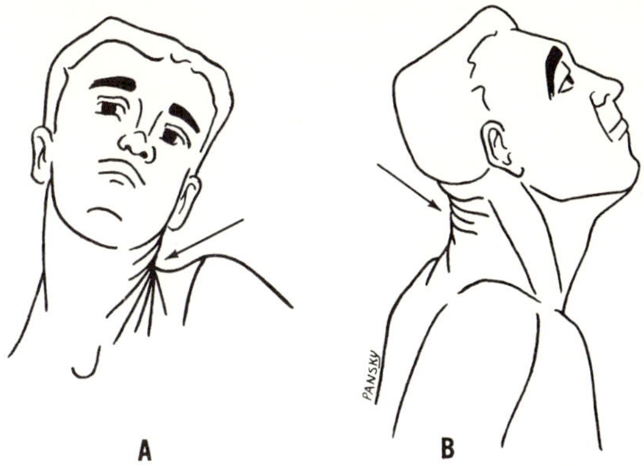

Fig. 19-18. Extrapyramidal disease. *A.* Spasmodic dystonia. *B.* Dystonia—postencephalitic.

SUMMARY

I. Parts
- *A.* Cortex: area 2, 4γ, 4s, 6, 8, 9, 19, and 24
- *B.* Basal nuclei
  1. Corpus striatum
     - *a.* Caudate nucleus
     - *b.* Putamen (outer segment of the lenticular nucleus)
  2. Globus pallidus (inner portion of the lenticular nucleus)
     - *a.* Outer segment
     - *b.* Inner segment
- *C.* Subthalamus
  1. Subthalamic nucleus
  2. Zona incerta
  3. Prerubral nucleus
- *D.* Mesencephalon
  1. Red nucleus
  2. Substantia nigra
  3. Deep tegmental nucleus
- *E.* Pons—central tegmental nucleus
- *F.* Medulla
  1. Central reticular nucleus
  2. Inferior medial reticular nucleus
  3. Inferior lateral reticular nucleus

II. Connections and descending pathways
- *A.* Extrapyramidal cortex
  1. From areas 2, 4s, 8, 19, and 24 to caudate nucleus of corpus striatum

2. From areas 4γ and 6 to putamen of corpus striatum
3. From area 6 to globus pallidus
4. From areas 4γ, 4s, and 6 to substantia nigra
5. From areas 4γ, 4s, and 6 to subthalamic nucleus
6. From areas 4γ, 4s, and 6 to deep tegmental nucleus of mesencephalon

B. Corpus striatum (caudate nucleus and putamen)
1. Receives afferents from
   a. Extrapyramidal cortex, areas 2, 4s, 8, 19, and 24 (caudate)
   b. Extrapyramidal cortex, areas 4γ and 6 (putamen)
   c. Medial nucleus and centrum medianum of the thalamus
2. Sends efferents to
   a. Outer segment of globus pallidus
   b. Inner segment of globus pallidus (few)
   c. Subthalamic nucleus
   d. Substantia nigra

C. Globus pallidus
1. Receives afferents from
   a. Extrapyramidal cortex (area 6)
   b. Striatum (chiefly to outer segment)
   c. Anterior ventral, dorsomedial, and centrum medianum of the thalamus (to both segments)
2. Sends efferents by three streams
   a. Ansa lenticularis, from inner segment, to join
   b. Fasciculus lenticularis, from both segments. The combined streams give
      (1). Thalamic fasciculus (pallidothalamic) fibers to the lateral ventral and anterior ventral nuclei of the thalamus
      (2). Pallidorubral fibers (few) red nucleus
      (3). Pallidoprerubral fibers to prerubral nucleus
      (4). Pallidohypothalamic fibers to dorsomedial and paraventricular nuclei of the hypothalamus
   c. Pallidosubthalamic fibers to
      (1). Subthalamic nucleus
      (2). Substantia nigra

D. Substantia nigra
1. Receives afferents from
   a. Extrapyramidal cortex (areas 4γ, 4s, and 6)
   b. Striatum
   c. Pallidum
2. Sends efferents to deep tegmental nucleus of mesencephalon

E. Subthalamic nucleus
1. Receives afferents from
   a. Extrapyramidal cortex (areas 4γ, 4s, and 6)
   b. Striatum
   c. Pallidum
2. Sends efferents to
   a. Deep tegmental nucleus of mesencephalon
   b. Reticular nuclei at lower levels

F. Zona incerta
1. Receives afferents from globus pallidus
2. Sends efferents to
   a. Red nucleus
   b. Reticular nuclei at lower levels

G. Prerubral nucleus
1. Receives afferents from globus pallidus
2. Sends efferents to
   a. Red nucleus
   b. Reticular nuclei

H. Red nucleus
1. Receives afferents from
   a. Globus pallidus, directly
   b. Prerubral nucleus
   c. Dentate nucleus of cerebellum
2. Sends efferents to
   a. Medial longitudinal fasciculus and thence to nuclei III, IV, VI, and XII

- *b.* Reticular formation and thence to all motor nuclei of brain stem
- *c.* Rubrospinal tract, directly to ventral gray column of spinal cord
- *d.* Reticular nuclei and thence to ventral gray column of the spinal cord over the reticulospinal tracts

I. Deep tegmental nucleus of the mesencephalon
- 1. Receives afferents from
  - *a.* Extrapyramidal cortex (areas 4γ, 4s, and 6)
  - *b.* Globus pallidus
  - *c.* Subthalamic nucleus
  - *d.* Red nucleus
  - *e.* Substantia nigra
- 2. Sends efferents to
  - *a.* Reticular nuclei of pons and medulla
  - *b.* Inferior olive

J. Central tegmental nucleus of pons
- 1. Receives afferents from
  - *a.* Deep tegmental nucleus of mesencephalon
  - *b.* Subthalamic nucleus
  - *c.* Red nucleus
- 2. Sends efferents to brain stem and spinal cord via medial and lateral reticulospinal tracts

K. Central reticular nucleus of medulla
- 1. Receives afferents from
  - *a.* Globus pallidus
  - *b.* Red nucleus
  - *c.* Deep tegmental nucleus of mesencephalon
  - *d.* Central tegmental nucleus of the pons
- 2. Sends efferents to brain stem and cord through medial reticulospinal tract

L. Inferior medial reticular nucleus of medulla
- 1. Receives afferents from any of more rostral reticular nuclei
- 2. Sends efferents to cord, probably through reticulospinal tracts

M. Inferior lateral reticular nucleus of medulla
- 1. Receives afferents from any of more rostral reticular nuclei
- 2. Sends efferents to lower brain stem and cord through medial reticulospinal tract

III. Reticulospinal tracts

A. Medial
- 1. Origin
  - *a.* Central tegmental nucleus of pons
  - *b.* Inferior medial reticular nucleus of medulla
- 2. Termination: ventral gray column of the cord, through the anterior funiculus

B. Lateral
- 1. Origin
  - *a.* Central tegmental nucleus of the pons
  - *b.* One of the inferior reticular nuclei of the medulla (?)
- 2. Termination: ventral gray column of the cord, through the lateral funiculus

20 PYRAMIDAL CONTROL OF MUSCULAR ACTIVITY

Muscular activity is controlled from two levels of the central nervous system: (1) by neurons arising from the brain stem and cord—lower motor neurons, or final common path (Chap. 14); (2) by upper motor neurons, arising from the motor cortex of the cerebrum and descending through long projection pathways to synapse with the lower motor neurons.

Functionally and anatomically, it is difficult to define a "true pyromidal system, since long projection fibers of both pyramidal and extrapyramidal system travel in close association with each other. It has been shown that the extrapyramidal system sets up approximate positions of gross adjustment, is the background of the motor system, is related to tonic control, and may be either activator or inhibitor. The pyramidal system, on the other hand, stimulates muscular activity and is responsible for the precise and specific movements necessary for all fine and skillful activities. Thus, extrapyramidal and pyramidal systems combine their influences upon the lower motor neurons so that volitional impulses are modified and amplified to result in an orderly muscular response.

PARTS AND CONNECTIONS

Pyramidal Cortex

The cells of origin, the giant pyramidal cells (of Betz) (Fig. 6-1) lie in the pyramidal, or motor cortex, which lies in the anterior lip of the central sulcus. It extends onto the lateral surface of the precentral gyrus superiorly, where it occupies more than half the precentral gyrus, and onto the medial side of the hemisphere, covering the rostral portion of the paracentral lobule. This area is roughly in the form of an attenuated triangle, with the base directed superiorly and the apex lying just above the lateral fissure, where much of the motor cortex lies deep in the central sulcus. On the cortical maps, this strip is designated as area 4 (Fig. 23-12).

Experimental evidence indicates that the entire body musculature has a specific orientation within the motor area (Fig. 23-7). Of interest, however, is the great disparity in size or extent of the various muscle areas within the motor cortex. By far the largest area is that representing the hand, and within this division, the thumb occupies the largest portion. Although not so large as that of the hand, the foot area is larger than that for the thigh, while areas for the mouth and face are proportionately larger than those for the arm, leg, or foot. Thus, it becomes apparent that cortical extent is not proportional to the total muscle mass but rather to the elaborateness and delicacy of movements of the parts.

Pathways

From the giant pyramidal cells of area 4, efferent fibers descend by way of the *corticospinal* and *corticobulbar* pathways to reach the ventral columns of the cord and the cranial motor nuclei, respectively. However, these tracts may contain fibers originating from smaller cells in area 4 as well as area 6 (and perhaps other regions).

Corticospinal Fibers (Fig. 20-1.)

These arise chiefly in the dorsal half to two-thirds of the precentral gyrus and the paracentral lobule. They pass through the corona radiata into the posterior limb of the internal capsule, where those fibers destined for the upper extremity lie in the rostral portion, nearest the genu, while those of the lower limb lie more caudally. At the rostral border of the mesencephalon they join other descending cortical fibers in the formation of the cerebral peduncles (basis pedunculi or pes pedunculi) and occupy the middle three-fifths of the peduncles (Figs. 2-38, 2-39, 25-12). The latter enter the rostral end of the pons, through which they descend in irregular bundles lying in the ventral portion of the pons (Figs. 2-45 to 2-47, 25-10). At the caudal end of the pons, these fiber bundles recombine to form the medullary pyramids, which extend throughout much of the length of the medulla (Figs. 2-48, 20-1, 25-4, 25-5). Just above the cord-medulla junction, 80 to 90 per cent of the fibers leave each pyramid and cross the ventral fissure. This is known as the motor decussation (pyramidal decussation) (Figs. 2-50, 20-1, 25-1). Thus both crossed and uncrossed fibers continue in the spinal cord.

Crossed Fibers. From the region of the decussation these fibers continue in the contralateral lateral funiculus of the cord in a circular bundle which lies between the fasciculus proprius and the dorsal spinocerebellar tract (Fig. 3-7). This is designated as the *lateral corticospinal tract.* Although this tract gradually becomes smaller as it descends, because of the continuous terminations of its fibers at higher levels, it may be traced to the caudal limits of the cord. In the lower lumbar and sacral regions it lies superficially along the lateral edge of the lateral funiculus, because of the absence of the dorsal spinocerebellar tract at these levels. Although terminations of this tract may be directly upon the motor cells of the ventral column, there is a feeling among investigators that the terminations actually lie in the dorsal column, the motor cells being activated by the internuncial neurons which run from the dorsal to ventral gray columns at the level of termination of the cortical fibers.

Uncrossed Fibers. Many of the uncrossed fibers continue downward into the cord in a direct line with the pyramids, entering the ventral funiculus and occupying a small area adjoining the ventral fissure of the cord (Fig. 3-7). This is the *ventral corticospinal tract.* Although many of its fibers are said to continue throughout the cord, it is difficult to trace it as a tract below thoracic levels. Before the fibers terminate, they cross through the anterior white commissure to end among the motor cells of the opposite ventral column.

In addition to these, a small group of uncrossed fibers apparently diverges somewhat laterally into that region of the cord neighboring on the ventral spinothalamic tract. This is the *ventrolateral corticospinal tract* (Barnes's tract). Its fibers apparently end directly upon ventral column cells without crossing.

Corticobulbar Fibers[1] (Fig. 20-2.)

The cells of origin lie predominantly in the lower quarter of the motor cortex. However, some of the fibers, particularly those which help to regulate speech, may actually arise in the caudal end of the inferior frontal gyrus, while those concerned with the eye movements come from the caudal part of the middle frontal gyrus. All converge as they pass through the corona radiata and come to lie in the genu of the internal capsule. Continuing downward, they enter the cerebral peduncle, where they lie just medial and dorsal to the corticospinal fibers.

Just caudal to the subthalamus, corticobulbar fibers separate into two main groups. One of these accompanies the corticospinal fibers through the pons and medullary pyramids, giving off fibers to motor nuclei at successively lower levels. Some may actually continue beyond the

[1] Although the term *bulb* usually refers only to the pons and medulla, these fibers also terminate in the mesencephalon.

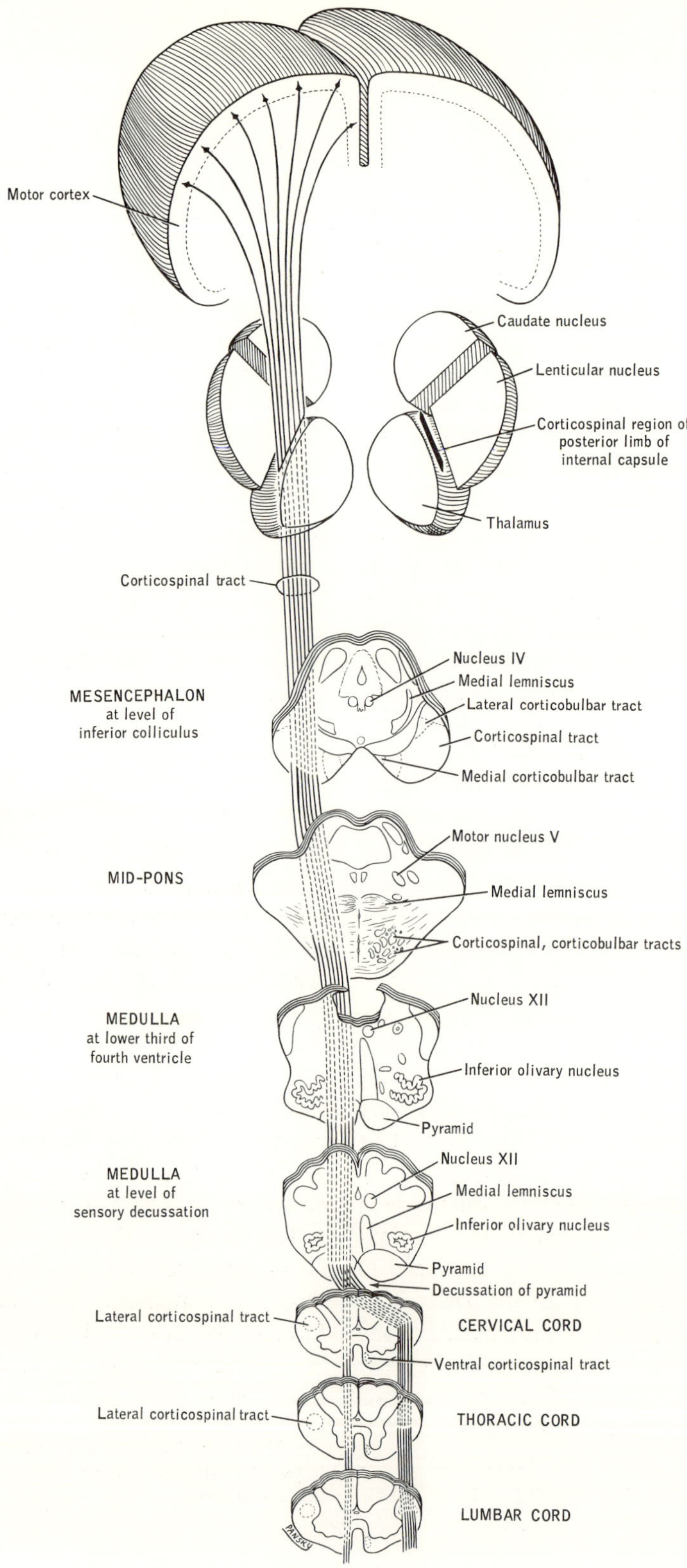

Fig. 20-1. Diagram of the corticospinal pathway.

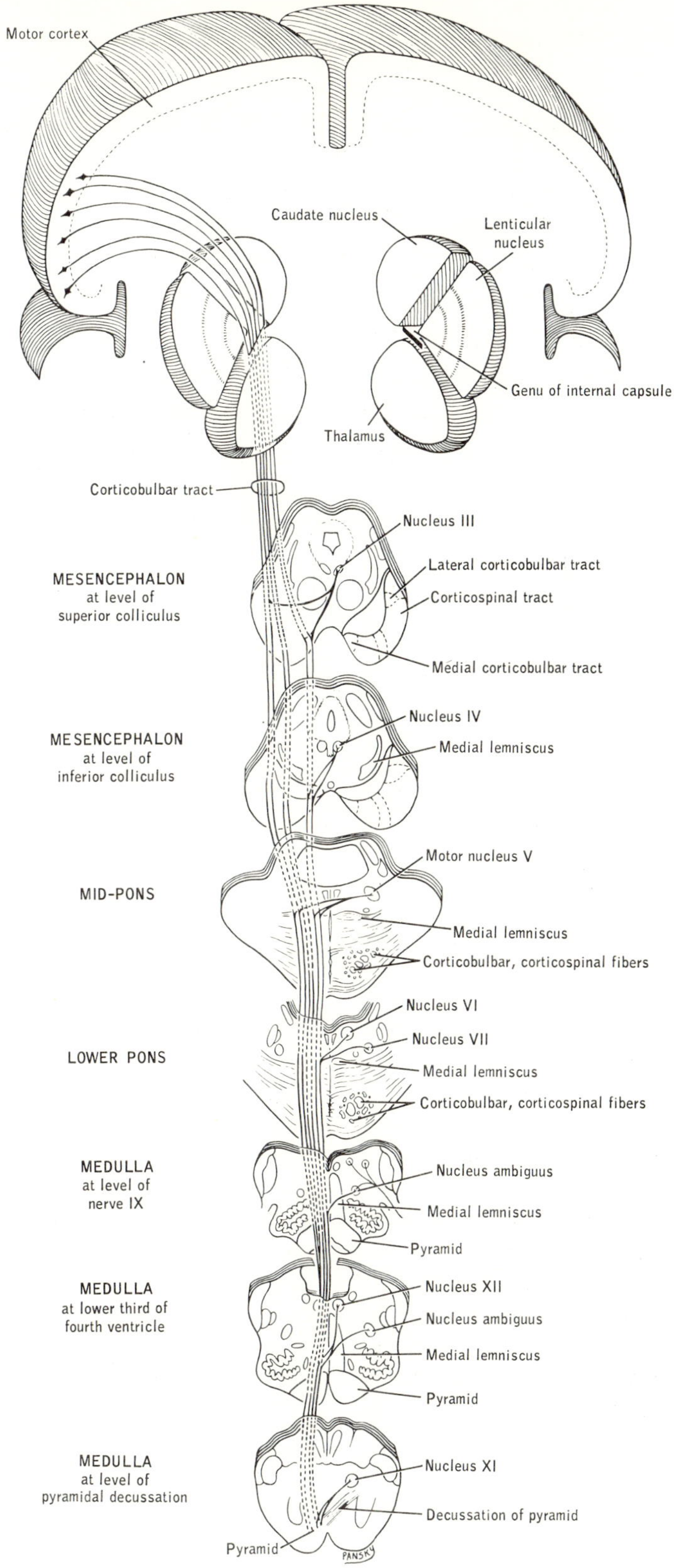

Fig. 20-2. Diagram of the corticobulbar pathway.

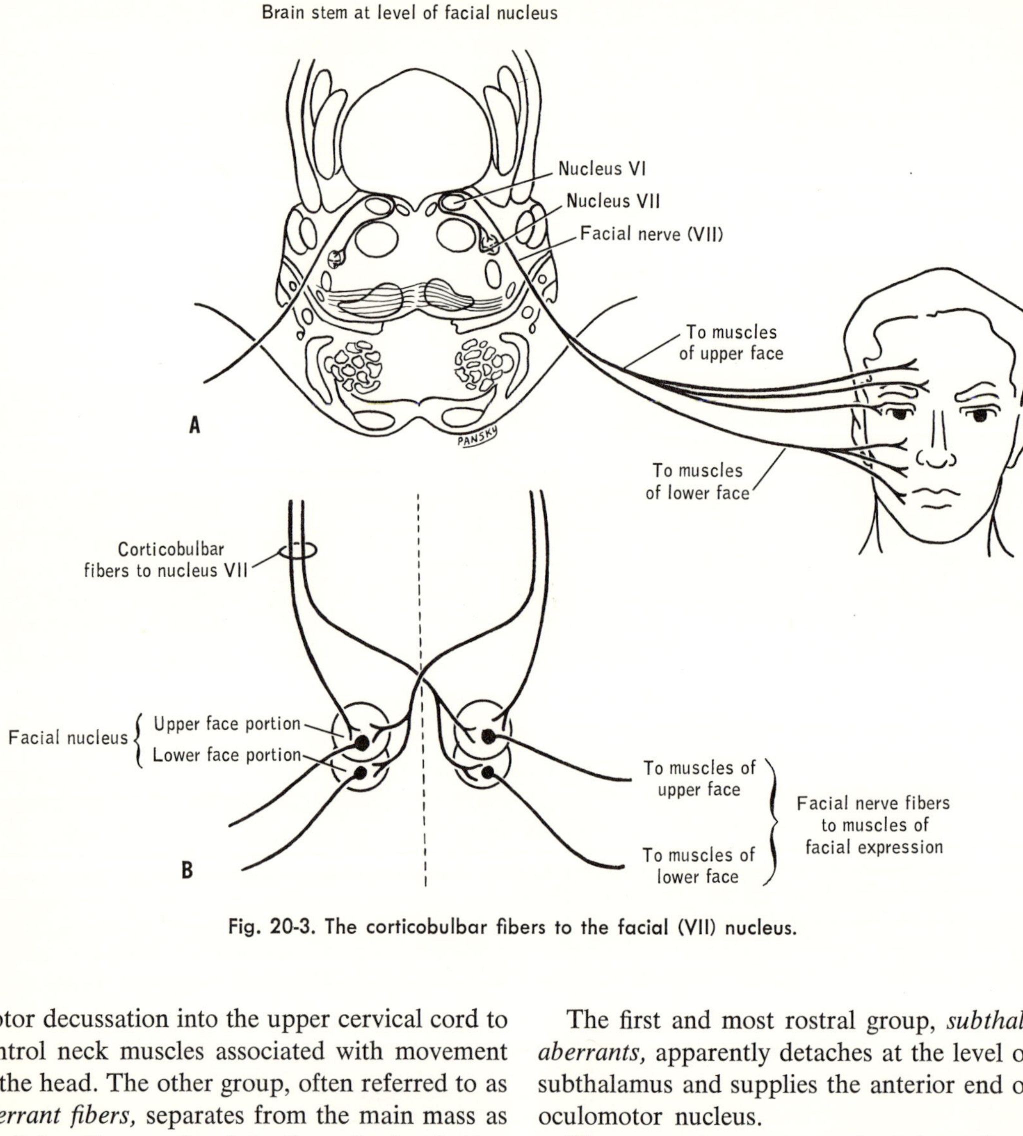

Fig. 20-3. The corticobulbar fibers to the facial (VII) nucleus.

motor decussation into the upper cervical cord to control neck muscles associated with movement of the head. The other group, often referred to as *aberrant fibers,* separates from the main mass as small bundles passing into the reticular formation. Of these, some course dorsomedially and cross the midline to reach motor nuclei of the opposite side, others go to nuclei of the same side. Some detach from the main pyramidal bundle quite a distance above the nucleus for which they are destined and descend in the region of the medial lemniscus. They usually do not cross until they reach the level of the nucleus to be supplied. Several groups of aberrant fibers are usually described.

The first and most rostral group, *subthalamic aberrants,* apparently detaches at the level of the subthalamus and supplies the anterior end of the oculomotor nucleus.

The second group, *peduncular aberrants,* diverges in the rostral mesencephalon, enters the medial lemniscus, sending off terminals to the oculomotor (III), trochlear (IV), abducens (VI),[2] and accessory (XI) cranial nerves and perhaps the upper cervical cord.

[2] It has been suggested that the cortical aberrant fibers that eventually terminate in nuclei III, IV, and VI may pass from the region of the medial lemniscus, enter the vestibular nuclei, progress to the medial longitudinal fasciculus, and are then distributed to these nuclei by way of this fasciculus.

The third group, the *aberrants of the pons,* comes off in the rostral portion of the pons. These fibers also join the medial lemniscus. Their endings lie in the contralateral nucleus of the trigeminal nerve (V) and the nucleus ambiguus.

The fourth group is formed at the pons-medulla junction. These fibers pass to the nucleus ambiguus and to the nuclei of the facial (VII) and hypoglossal (XII) nerves.

In general, most of the cranial motor nuclei receive both crossed and uncrossed cortical fibers. However, though the rostral part of the facial nucleus, which supplies the muscles of the face above the eye, receives both crossed and uncrossed fibers, the caudal part of the nucleus receives crossed fibers only (Fig. 20-3). The abducens nucleus is said to receive only crossed fibers.

CLINICAL CONSIDERATIONS

In cases of lesions involving the pyramidal system, certain findings are commonly encountered: (1) all the cortical types of conditioned reflex are eliminated, loss being most apparent in the hands and in the speech apparatus; (2) since the motor nerves (lower motor neurons) are intact, there is no degeneration of muscle, although some diminution of muscular size occurs owing to disuse.

One chief difficulty is the problem of whether flaccid (Chap. 14) or spastic paralysis is most commonly found when a lesion involves the pyramidal system. Spastic paralysis is characterized by hypertonia, increased resistance to passive movement, and exaggerated reflexes. It seems probable that since the pyramidal fibers are mainly excitatory, a lesion affecting only the *true pyramidal* cells or fibers would lead to the flaccid type of paralysis. This has been demonstrated under strictly experimental conditions. However, in clinical practice, the pyramidal and extrapyramidal systems are so closely associated that lesions involving one will invariably encompass both. Thus, it is usual to observe, at least in the early stages (whether the condition occurs from a vascular accident or trauma), a state of flaccidity, due both to loss of pyramidal excitation and to shock. Days and perhaps even weeks later, this early condition is superseded by a permanent spasticity, apparently owing to the loss of the inhibitor fibers normally part of the extrapyramidal system. With these inhibitors removed, the lower motor neurons are exposed directly to the innumerable impulses traveling to them via the many association neurons derived from afferent systems; thus hyperreflexia and hypertonia result.

Testing

The examiner checks for the ability to perform voluntary, skilled activities as directed.

The deep reflexes are examined as described in the chapter on proprioception (Chap. 12). In upper motor lesions, these reflexes are exaggerated.

Superficial reflexes, particularly on the abdomen, are checked by stroking the skin lightly. The abdominal and cremasteric reflexes are both eliminated in upper motor neuron lesions, since they travel in an arc through the cortex.

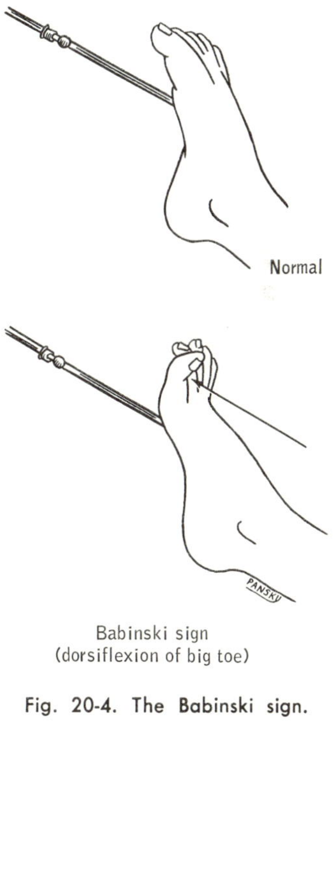

Fig. 20-4. The Babinski sign.

The plantar surface of the foot is stroked in the heel to toe direction. In upper motor neuron lesions, the toes are spread apart and the great toe is dorsiflexed (Babinski sign) (Fig. 20-4). It is possible that this reaction represents a reversion to the more primitive reaction which actually may be dorsiflexion, since it is seen in infants before cortical control is established.

Although the foregoing tests will suffice to indicate whether pathologic change involves the upper motor neurons of the pyramidal system, they are not adequate to localize the lesions within the CNS. Lesions of only one pyramidal tract produce the same symptoms irrespective of the level at which the damage occurs, whether in the cortex, internal capsule, midbrain, pons, or

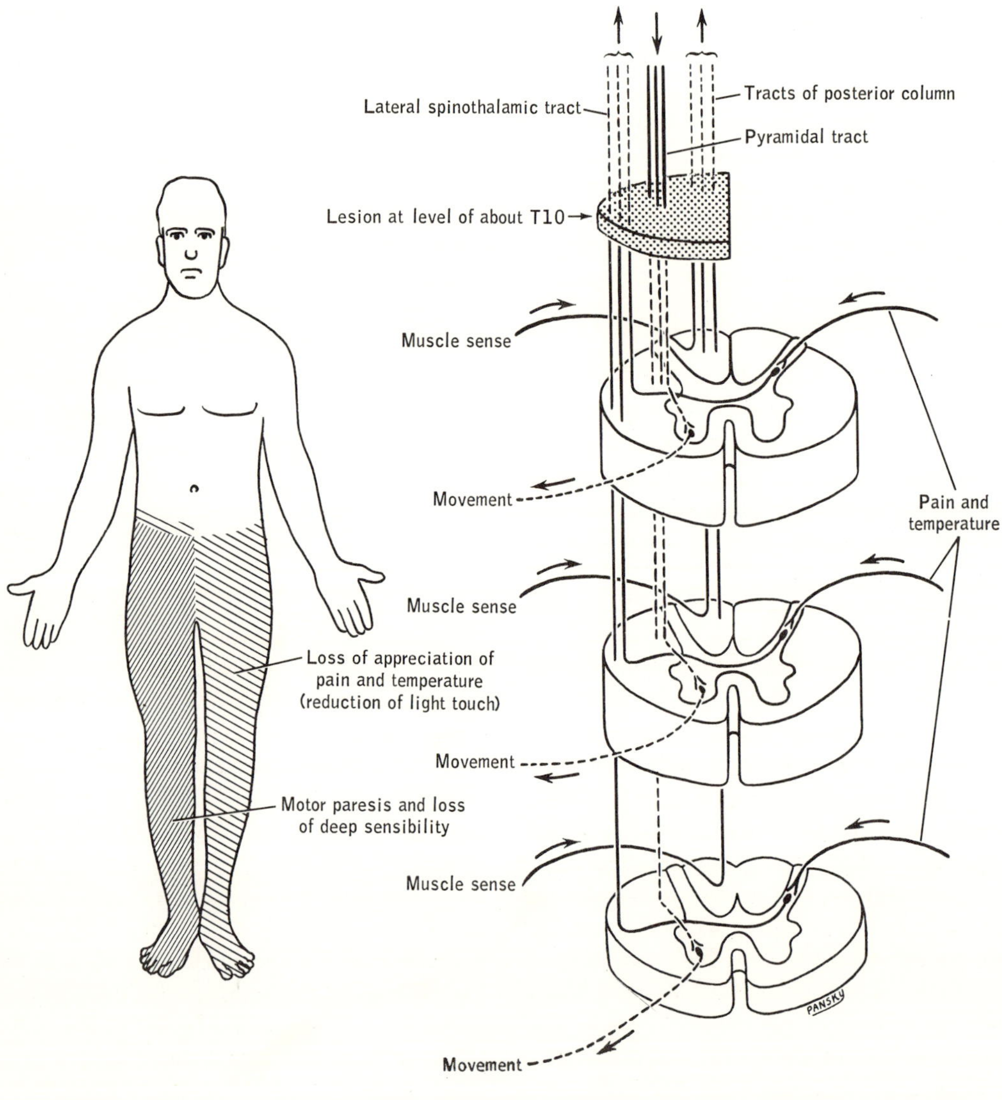

Fig. 20-5. The Brown-Séquard syndrome, resulting from a lesion on the right half of the spinal cord in the region of T10. Note: motor paralysis on the same side; deep anesthesia and cutaneous hyperesthesia on the same side; cutaneous anesthesia on the opposite side.

medulla. Criteria other than pyramidal tract signs are thus needed to determine the level of the lesion. In the brain stem such supplementary information can be gained by noting disturbances in the function of cranial nerves III through XII. Such disturbances may be upper motor neuron in nature and are significant in localizing the lesion because of the differences in level at which corticobulbar fibers diverge from the corticospinal tract. They may also be lower motor neuron in type, involving either the nucleus of origin or emerging fibers of the cranial nerves. This is particularly important since sites of cranial nerve nuclei have been well established. Furthermore, since it should be clear that within the brain stem and cord, focal lesions in the corticospinal pathways are virtually impossible, sensory tracts may also be involved, and examinations of these systems may also contribute to the localization of the lesion (Fig. 20-5).

Specific Pathology

Specific pathologic changes may be the result of direct trauma either from wounds about the head involving the motor cortex directly or from damage to the spinal cord (resulting from fracture of the spine, gunshot wounds, etc.) which interrupts the upper motor neuron pathway in its descent. Other changes are due to some form of vascular accident in which the blood supply is cut off, either from cell bodies or from their long processes.

Before discussing particular conditions, it is necessary to define certain terms. *Monoplegia* refers to paralysis of one part (upper or lower extremity). *Hemiplegia* is the paralysis of both the upper and lower extremities on the same side (Fig. 20-6). *Tetraplegia* is the paralysis of all four extremities. *Paraplegia* signifies the paralysis of both lower extremities.

Hemiplegia

Lesions which produce this condition may occur in several locations. When the lesion is in the motor cortex, sensory involvement may or may not appear, the size of the lesion determining the extent of the paralysis. When the lesion is in the internal capsule, general sensibilities are always involved and if the lesion is large enough, vision and hearing may be affected. Lesions of the central portion of the cerebral peduncles may give pure hemiplegia without interruption of the sensory system and may or may not involve the cranial nerves. Lesions in the basal portion of the pons may give very few symptoms unless the area of pathologic change is extremely large, since the corticospinal fibers are here split up into scattered bundles.

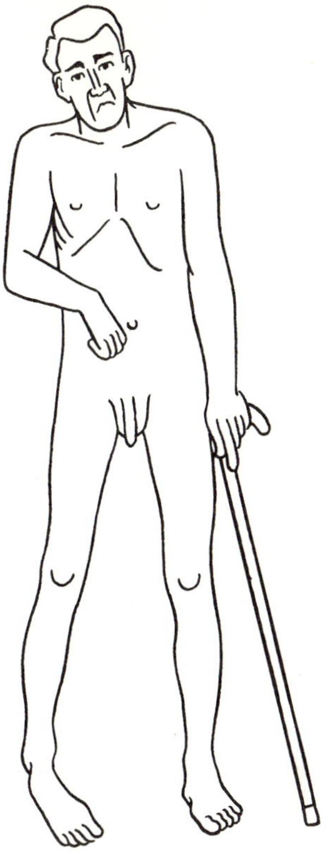

Fig. 20-6. Hemiplegia. Paralysis on the right side due to a lesion in the pyramidal pathway above the decussation.

Hemiplegia Cruciata. (Fig. 20-7.) This is due to a lesion involving the lateral aspect of the pyramidal decussation where crossed fibers to the lower extremities and uncrossed fibers to the upper extremities are passing. It results in paralysis of the homolateral arm and contralateral leg.

Hemiplegia Alternata (**Alternating Hemiplegia**). (Fig. 20-8.) This is a symptom com-

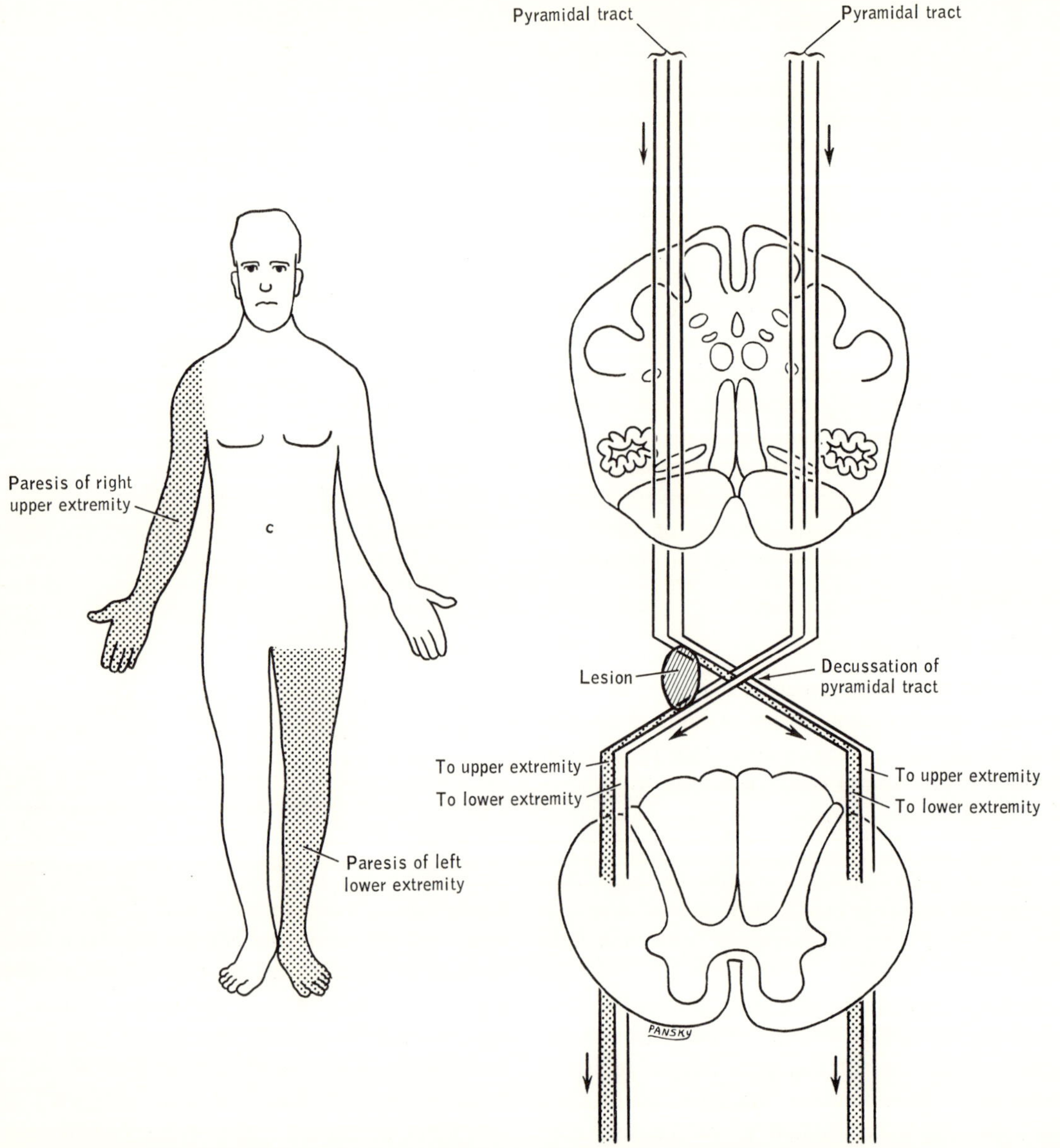

Fig. 20-7. Hemiplegia cruciata due to a lesion on the right side of the pyramidal decussation.

plex in which there is an altered function of cranial nerves of the same side and an altered function of one of the long pathways connected with the opposite side. There are several patterns of this type, depending on the location of the lesion.

When the lesion is in the *cerebral peduncle,* there is an oculomotor paralysis of the homolateral side, owing to an interruption of the emerging fibers of the third cranial nerve, and a contralateral paralysis of the lower face, tongue, and extremities, owing to interruption of the cortico-

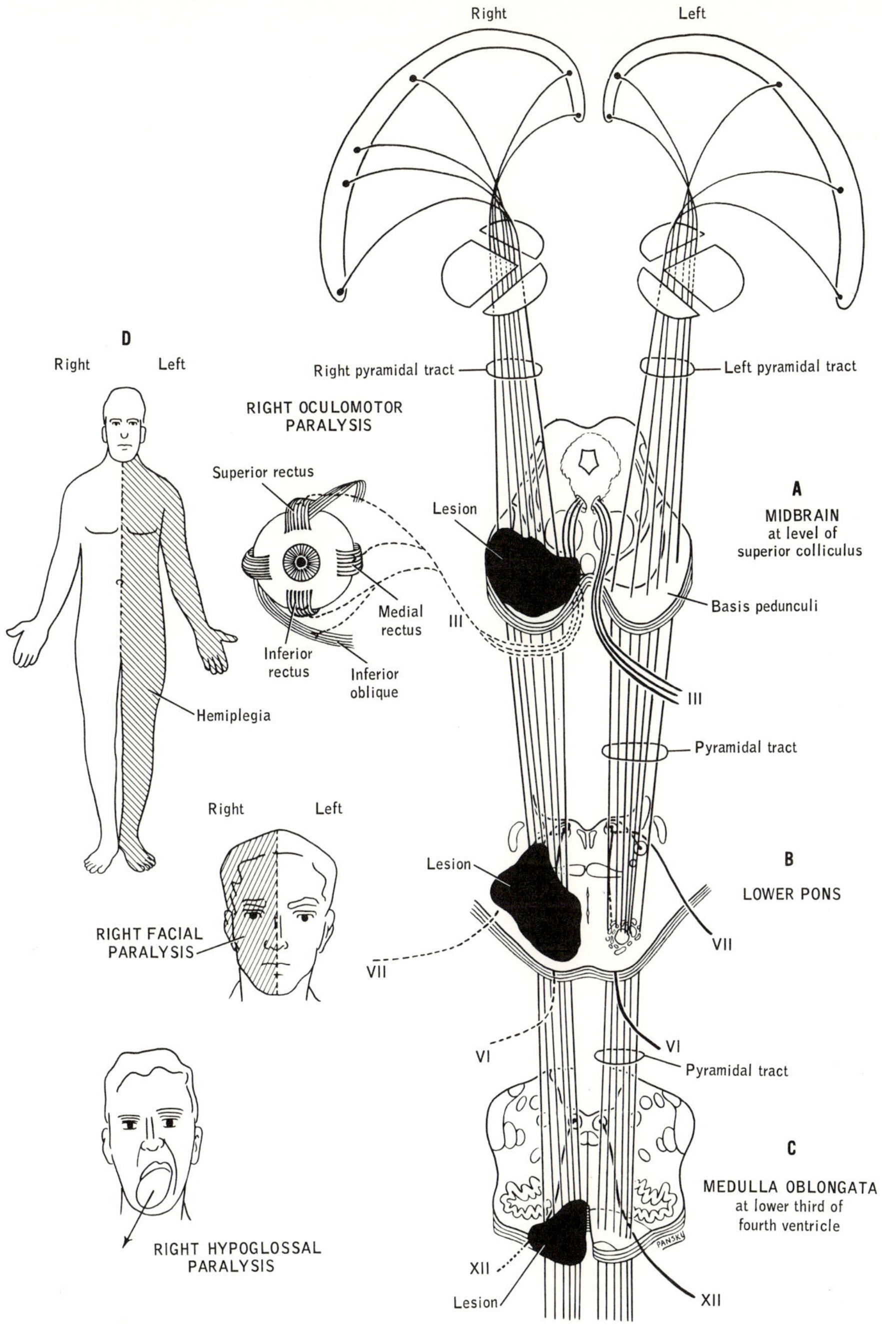

Fig. 20-8. Hemiplegia alternata, with lesions at various levels. *A*. At the level of the emerging fibers of nerve III, involving this nerve and a portion of the adjoining cerebral peduncle. *B*. At the level of nerve VII. C. At the level of nerve XII, involving emerging fibers of the hypoglossal nerve and the adjoining pyramid. *D*. Area of body paralysis with lesions at levels *A*, *B*, or *C*.

spinal and corticobulbar fibers. This condition is called *crossed oculomotor paralysis* or *Weber's syndrome.*

Lesions of the caudal portion of the pons may produce a *hemiplegia alternata facialis* or *crossed facial paralysis* (*Millard-Gubler syndrome*), which results in a homolateral facial paralysis plus contralateral paralysis of tongue and extremities.

Foville's syndrome appears when the lesion is so large as to include the abducens (VI) nucleus and the center for conjugate lateral ocular deviation, which lies near it. In this case, besides the symptoms associated with the Millard-Gubler syndrome, there are also paralysis of the lateral rectus muscle and absence of conjugate ocular deviation to the side of the lesion.

Lesions in the medulla may lead to paralysis of the homolateral half of the tongue and a paralysis of the contralateral extremities, *hemiplegia alternata hypoglossica,* or crossed hypoglossal paralysis.

Tetraplegia

The small caliber of the medulla oblongata accounts for the fact that small, unilateral foci, especially in the posterior portions, give rise to extensive disturbances in function which are often bilateral in distribution. Thus, the pyramids lie so close together in the medulla that a small lesion in this region may cause tetraplegia. However, death usually occurs rapidly owing to involvement of the respiratory or cardiac centers, the tetraplegia often going unnoticed.

Jacksonian Epilepsy

This condition appears as involuntary muscular reactions which may begin with the involvement of relatively few muscles or muscle groups but eventually may spread to include most of them on one side of the body. This condition arises as a result of an irritative lesion at some point on or near the motor cortex. A clue to its exact location is given by noticing which muscles react at the beginning of the attack.

SUMMARY
Pyramidal System

Trunk		Head
1. Giant pyramidal (of Betz)	Cell type	1. Same as for trunk
2. Paracentral lobule and upper two-thirds of precentral gyrus (area 4)	Location	2. Lower third of the precentral gyrus
3. In order: corona radiata; posterior limb of the internal capsule; middle three-fifths of cerebral peduncle; scattered fascicles in the pons; pyramids in upper medulla In the lower medulla, 80 to 90 per cent cross to the opposite side of the brain stem through the decussation of the pyramids to become the lateral corticospinal tracts which descend through the spinal cord in the lateral funiculus In the lower medulla, 10 to 20 per cent remain uncrossed, descending on the same side of the brain stem and passing through the spinal cord in the anterior funiculus as the ventral corticospinal tract	Course	3. In order: corona radiata; genu of the internal capsule; cerebral peduncles, dorsal and medial to the corticospinals. From here, fibers may either continue caudally with the corticospinal fibers or form aberrant bundles at various levels in the subthalamus, mesencephalon, pons, or medulla
4. From the lateral corticospinal tract fibers may terminate either directly around motor cells in the ventral gray columns of the cord, or around cells of intercalary neurons in the dorsal gray columns, which, in turn, send their axons to synapse with motor cells in the ventral gray columns From the ventral corticospinal tract, fibers pass medially and cross to the opposite side of the cord through the anterior white commissure, just before terminating around motor cells of the ventral gray column	Termination	4. Those running with corticospinals end in ventral gray columns of upper cervical cord Subthalamic aberrants go to the rostral end of nucleus III Peduncular aberrants pass to nuclei III, IV, V, and XI Pontine aberrants pass to contralateral V and nucleus ambiguus, for nerves IX and X Medullary aberrants pass to nuclei VII and XII

21 HYPOTHALAMIC CONTROL OF VISCERAL FUNCTION

The hypothalamus is the highest integration center for the autonomic nervous system. Its rostral part is concerned particularly with the craniosacral portion of the system, its caudal portion is important for the thoracolumbar part. The interaction of these parts is essential for three basic physiologic processes: heat regulation, water metabolism, and general metabolism.

STRUCTURE OF THE HYPOTHALAMUS

Gross

The gross structure and relations have been described elsewhere (Chap. 2).

Hypothalamic Nuclei (Figs. 21-1, 21-2.)

The hypothalamus is broken up into several nuclear groups. Among the most definite of these groups are the preoptic, supraoptic, paraventricular, ventromedial, dorsomedial, and mammillary. In addition there are three other regional divisions, designated merely as *anterior, lateral,* and *dorsal areas.*

CONNECTIONS

Afferent Pathways

Fornix (Figs. 2-19, 11-2, 11-4, 21-3, 25-13 to 25-19.)

The origin of these fibers from the hippocampus and dentate gyrus has been indicated in the special visceral afferent system, and their course has also been described (Chap. 11). These fibers terminate especially in the lateral portion of the mammillary bodies.

Medial Forebrain Bundle (Figs. 11-6, 21-3.)

At least a portion of its fibers arise in the olfactory brain, particularly the ventromedial part, in the vicinity of the olfactory stria and perhaps other parts of the adjoining frontal cortex. Some of them terminate in the preoptic nuclei.[1] Then the bundle passes on through the lateral hypothalamic area, some fibers apparently ending there, others descending to end in the lateral portion of the mammillary body. What is left of the bundle continues caudally into the tegmentum of the mesencephalon.

Thalamohypothalamic Fibers (Fig. 21-4.)

These fibers arise in the dorsomedial nucleus of the thalamus and perhaps in other midline and reticular nuclei of the thalamus. They course chiefly ventrally to end in the anterior area of the hypothalamus.

Strio- and Pallidohypothalamic Fibers (Fig. 19-4.)

Some of these fibers arise in the putamen, but probably the majority begin in the globus pallidus to terminate particularly in the ventro-

[1] These nuclei may also contribute fibers which continue caudally in the medial forebrain bundle.

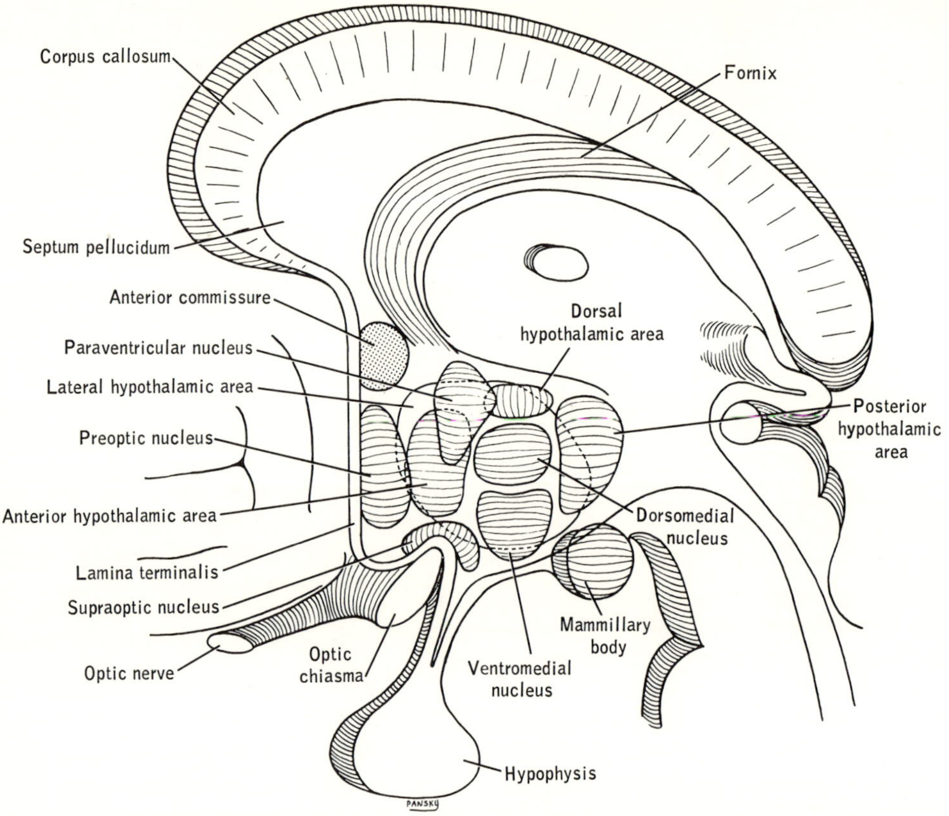

Fig. 21-1. Hypothalamic nuclei. Three-dimensional reconstruction of the hypothalamus.

medial, dorsomedial, paraventricular, and possibly the mammillary hypothalamic nuclei. Some of the strio- and pallidohypothalamic fibers also cross through the anterior hypothalamic commissure (Ganser's) to the hypothalamic nuclei on the opposite side.

Stria Terminalis (Figs. 11-2, 11-6, 21-3.)

The position and course of these fibers have already been described (Chap. 11). They begin in the amygdaloid complex and terminate in the preoptic nucleus and the anterior hypothalamic area.

Mammillary Peduncle (Fig. 21-5.)

This tract arises in the midbrain tegmentum, the latter probably acting as a relay center for impulses arising in various lower brain stem centers. It is believed that ascending fibers from the spinal cord play into this bundle by way of the medial lemniscus. Collaterals from other secondary sensory systems may also makes their way through the tegmental reticular substance to be carried in this peduncle. Special visceral afferent fibers for taste, arising in the gustatory nucleus, and general visceral afferent fibers from the nucleus of the tractus solitarius, both traveling in the tegmentum, are carried to the hypothalamus by way of this peduncle. It terminates chiefly in the lateral part of the mammillary body.

Corticohypothalamic Fibers (Fig. 21-6.)

Fibers from cortical area 6, relayed probably through the rostral septal area and the medial forebrain bundle, are reported in the literature. They apparently end in mammillary nuclei, the lateral hypothalamic area, and the posterior nucleus. The posterior orbital cortex of the frontal lobe has been shown to connect with the paraventricular and ventromedial nuclei. Still other cortical fibers seem to end in the supraoptic nucleus. The prefrontal cortex also may influence the hypothalamus indirectly by relaying through the dorsomedial nucleus of the thalamus and the paraventricular fibers. The gyrus cinguli (area 23) also has descending connections with the anterior thalamic nucleus, which, in turn, sends some fibers downward along the mammillothalamic tract to the medial mammillary nucleus.

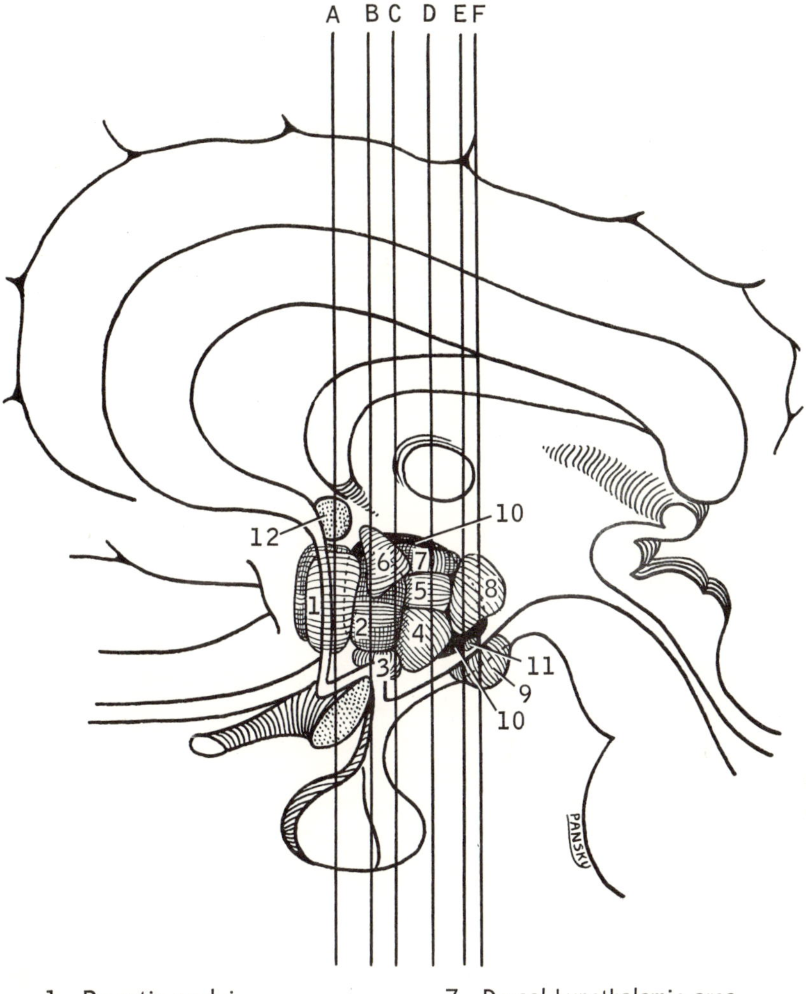

1. Preoptic nuclei
2. Anterior hypothalamic area
3. Supraoptic nucleus
4. Ventromedial nucleus
5. Dorsomedial nucleus
6. Paraventricular nucleus
7. Dorsal hypothalamic area
8. Posterior hypothalamic area
9. Mammillary body
10. Lateral hypothalamic area
11. Intercalated nucleus
12. Anterior commissure

Fig. 21-2. General topography of the hypothalamus, the first part indicating the planes for the vertical sections shown in parts *A, B, C, D, E, F.* (*After Netter Ciba Clinical Symposia.*)

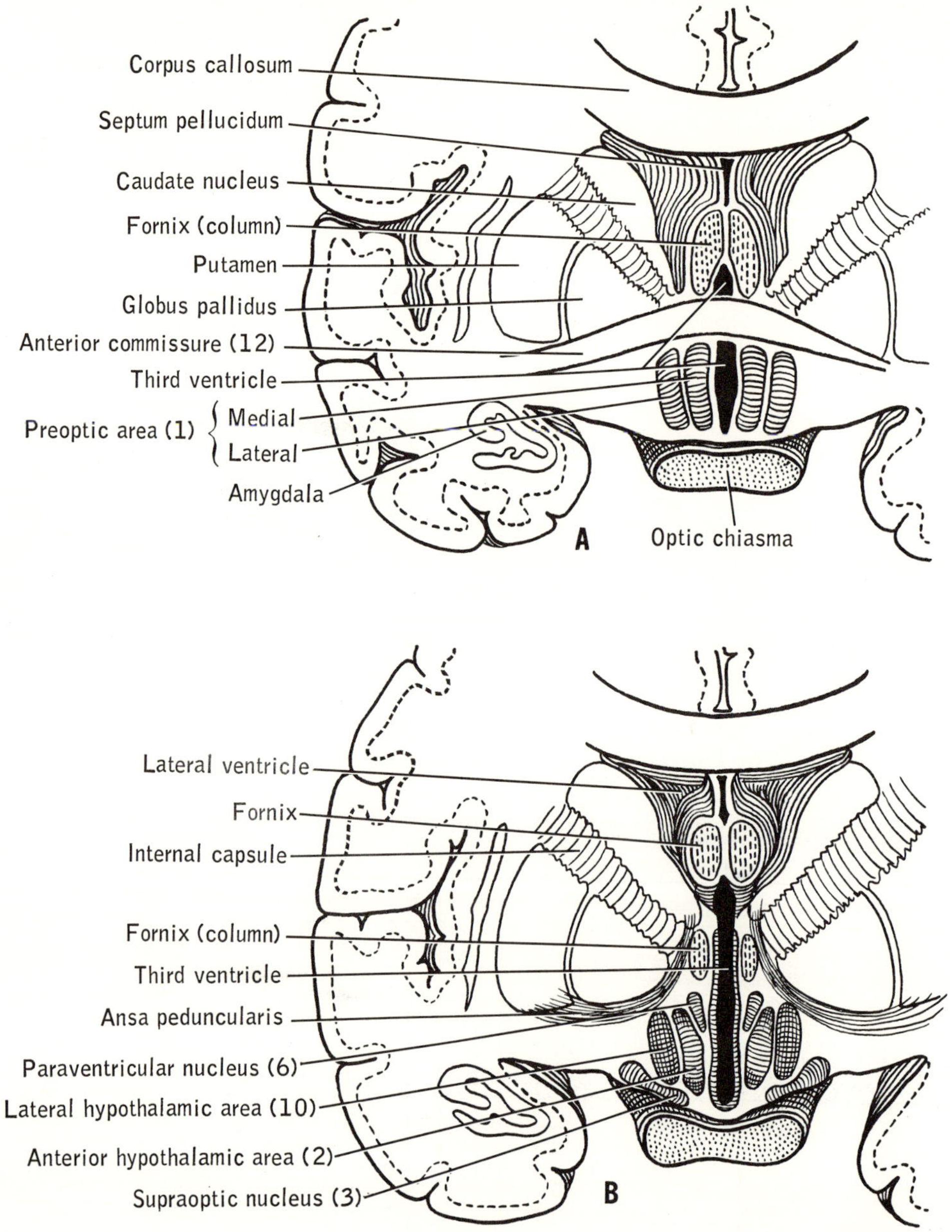
Corpus callosum
Septum pellucidum
Caudate nucleus
Fornix (column)
Putamen
Globus pallidus
Anterior commissure (12)
Third ventricle
Preoptic area (1)
Medial
Lateral
Amygdala
A
Optic chiasma
Lateral ventricle
Fornix
Internal capsule
Fornix (column)
Third ventricle
Ansa peduncularis
Paraventricular nucleus (6)
Lateral hypothalamic area (10)
Anterior hypothalamic area (2)
Supraoptic nucleus (3)
B

Fig. 21-2. A, B.

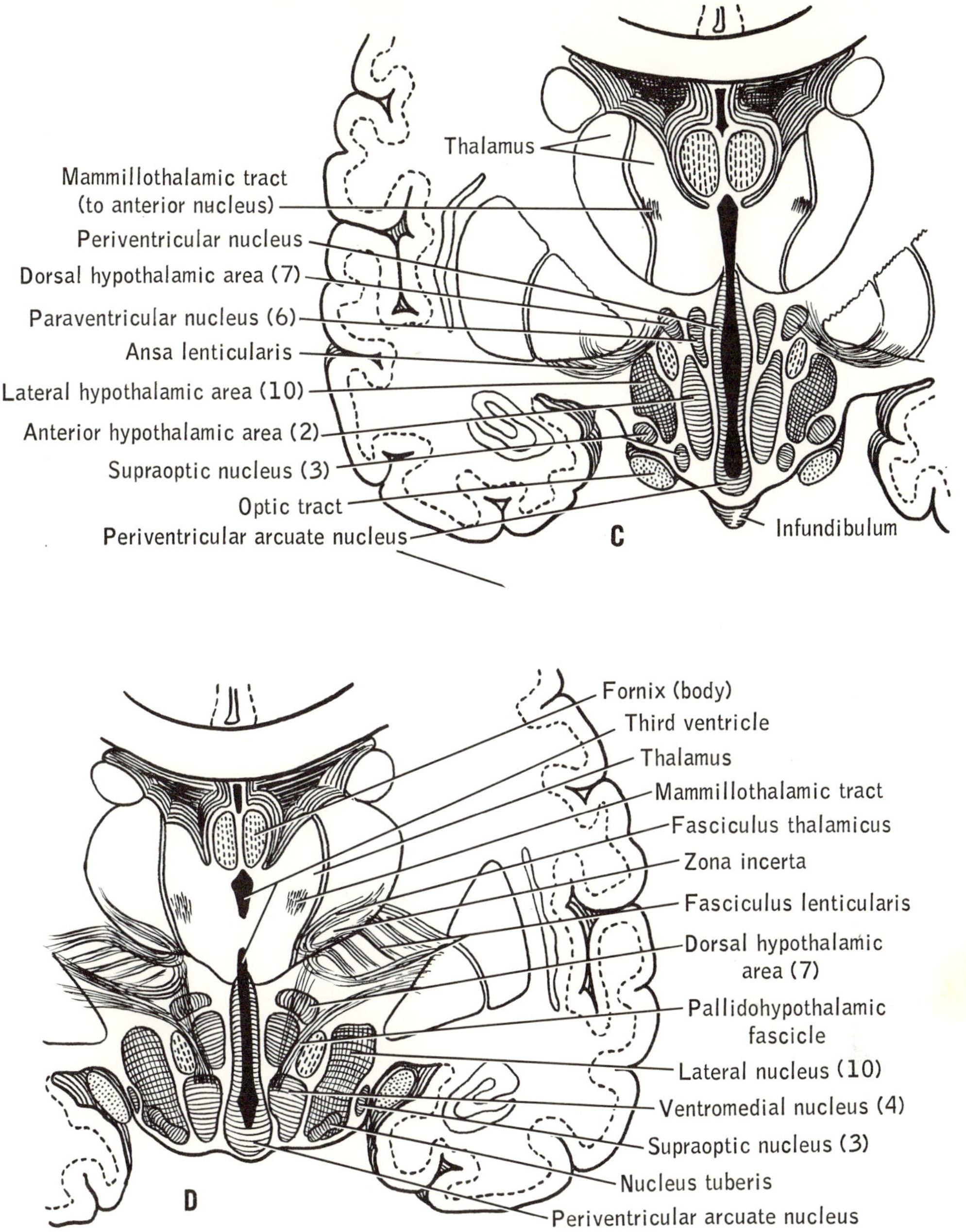
Thalamus
Mammillothalamic tract
(to anterior nucleus)
Periventricular nucleus
Dorsal hypothalamic area (7)
Paraventricular nucleus (6)
Ansa lenticularis
Lateral hypothalamic area (10)
Anterior hypothalamic area (2)
Supraoptic nucleus (3)
Optic tract
Periventricular arcuate nucleus
C
Infundibulum
Fornix (body)
Third ventricle
Thalamus
Mammillothalamic tract
Fasciculus thalamicus
Zona incerta
Fasciculus lenticularis
Dorsal hypothalamic
area (7)
Pallidohypothalamic
fascicle
Lateral nucleus (10)
Ventromedial nucleus (4)
Supraoptic nucleus (3)
Nucleus tuberis
Periventricular arcuate nucleus
D

Fig. 21-2. C, D.

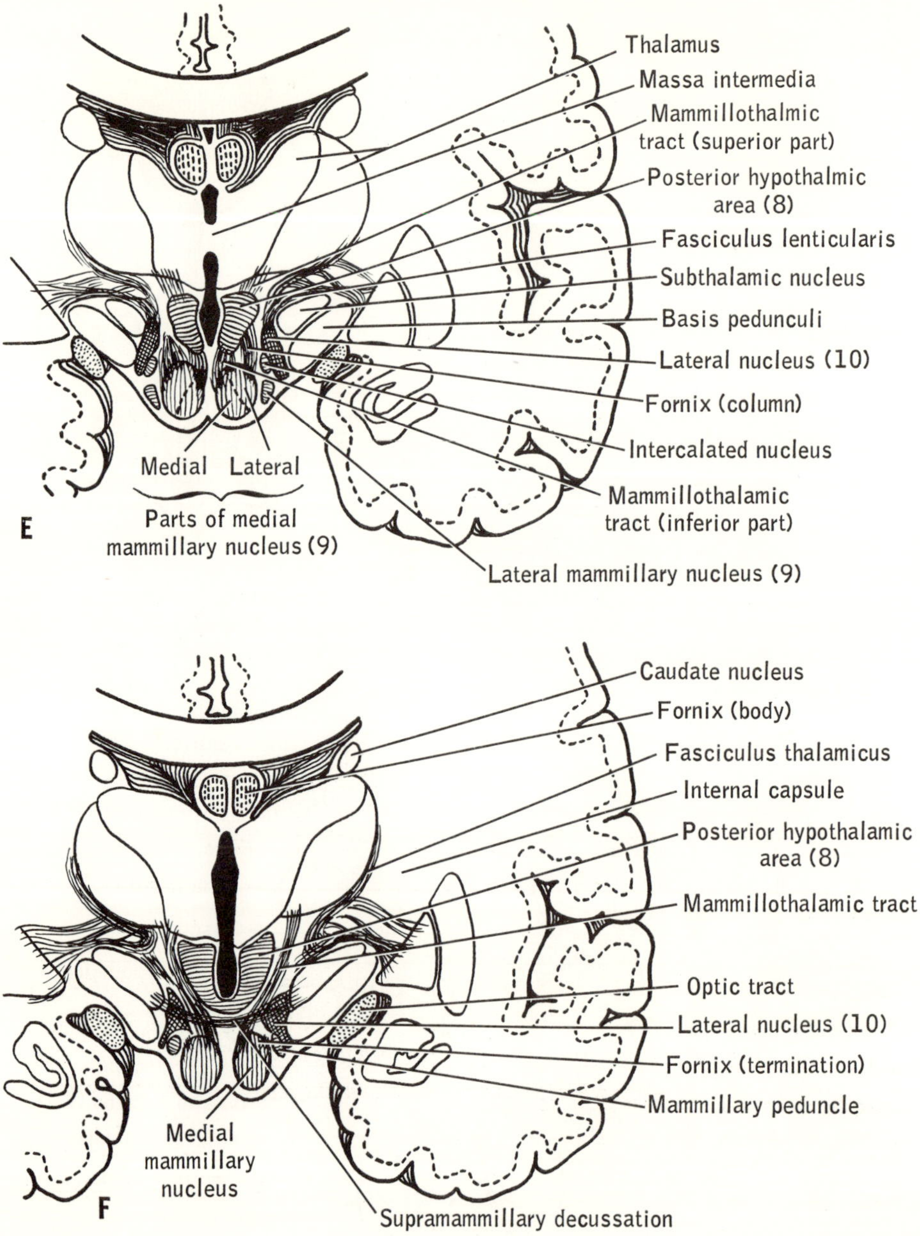
Thalamus
Massa intermedia
Mammillothalmic tract (superior part)
Posterior hypothalmic area (8)
Fasciculus lenticularis
Subthalamic nucleus
Basis pedunculi
Lateral nucleus (10)
Fornix (column)
Intercalated nucleus
Mammillothalamic tract (inferior part)
Lateral mammillary nucleus (9)
Medial Lateral
Parts of medial mammillary nucleus (9)
E
Caudate nucleus
Fornix (body)
Fasciculus thalamicus
Internal capsule
Posterior hypothalamic area (8)
Mammillothalamic tract
Optic tract
Lateral nucleus (10)
Fornix (termination)
Mammillary peduncle
Medial mammillary nucleus
Supramammillary decussation
F

Fig. 21-2. E, F.

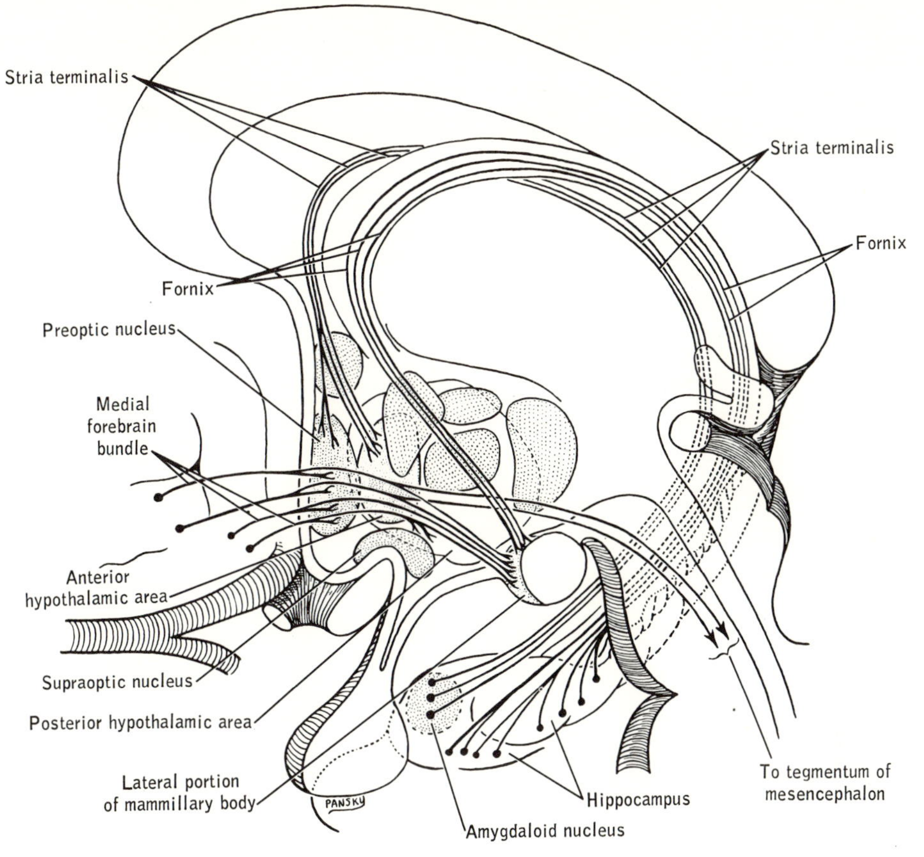

Fig. 21-3. Some of the afferent pathways to the hypothalamus, showing in particular the fornix, medial forebrain bundle, and the stria terminalis.

Mammillothalamic Tract (*Bundle of Vicq d'Azyr*) (Figs. 21-7, 25-16, 25-17.)

Most of these fibers take origin in the medial portion of the mammillary body. The aggregate forms a prominent bundle which courses cephalically, with rostral inclination, to reach the anterior nucleus of the thalamus. This, in turn, gives rise to ascending thalamocortical fibers to the gyrus cinguli. Thus, it can be seen that a circular circuit—hypothalamus, thalamus, cortex, thalamus, hypothalamus—is established.

Mammillotegmental Tract (Fig. 21-7.)

The fibers of this tract also take origin in the medial portion of the mammillary bodies. Coursing caudally through the mesencephalon, some crossing to the opposite side, they terminate in the lateral and central reticular nuclei of the tegmentum (Figs. 19-11, 19-13). From here, by way of relays in the reticular formation, the cranial autonomic nuclei are activated. This influence is continued to the intermediolateral column of the spinal cord through the reticulospinal tract.

Periventricular Fibers (Fig. 21-8.)

These are said to arise in the posterior hypothalamic nucleus, the tuberal nuclei, and the supraoptic nucleus. From here, they pass dorsally into the gray substance adjoining the third ventricle. Some of them end in the dorsomedial and midline nuclei of the thalamus. The majority of periventricular fibers are descend-

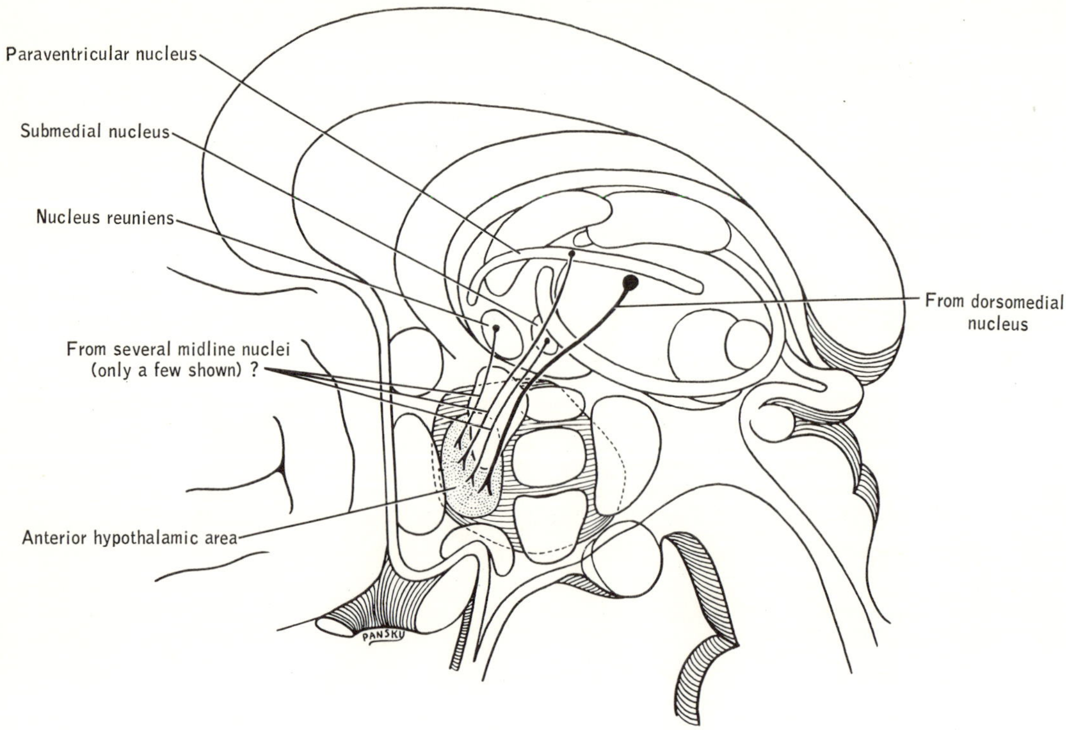

Fig. 21-4. The thalamohypothalamic connections.

ing, however. Some end in the tegmental reticular nuclei of the mesencephalon. Others continue caudally, either scattered diffusely in the lateral portions of the tegmentum or aggregated in the *dorsal longitudinal fasciculus* (*of Schütz*), which descends through the midbrain, pons, and medulla just ventral to the aqueduct and the fourth ventricle. These fibers terminate throughout the brain stem in parasympathetic nuclei and in the vital centers (cardiac, respiratory) in the medullary reticular formation. Many, either directly or through reticular system relays, enter the cord through the reticulospinal tracts in both the ventral and lateral funiculi and terminate about the cells of the intermediolateral cell column.

Hypothalamicohypophyseal Fibers (Fig. 21-9.)

Most of the fibers of this system terminate in the neurohypophysis.[2] Many fibers arise in the supraoptic and paraventricular nucleus, traverse the infundibular stem, and terminate in the neural lobe. It appears that many of those fibers arising in the paraventricular nuclei terminate in the supraoptic nucleus and the tuber cinereum, only a few going all the way to the neural lobe. There are also some fibers running in the lateral and posterior portions of the infundibular stalk which arise from tuberal nuclei—*the tuberohypophyseal fibers*. It is improbable that any of the fibers from the hypothalamus pass into the anterior lobe of the pituitary.

EVALUATION OF HYPOTHALAMIC CIRCUITS

Fibers ascending from the cord and brain stem, especially those belonging to the GVA

[2] This includes the neural lobe of the pituitary and the infundibulum, which consists of an infundibular stem running cephalically from the neural lobe and the median eminence of the tuber cinereum to which the stem attaches.

system, and the gustatory fibers, belonging to the SVA system, enter the hypothalamus through the mammillary peduncle. In this way, information about the presence and nature of substances in the alimentary canal and pressure states within the circulatory system is brought to the hypothalamus. After integration through the intrahypothalamic connections, the appropriate adjustments of visceral activity are attained through the fibers descending from the hypothalamus by way of *periventricular fibers* (especially those in the *dorsal longitudinal fasciculus*) and the *mammillotegmental tract*.

Impulses arising in the olfactory apparatus of the SVA system are also carried into the hypothalamus by way of the *median forebrain bundle,* or the *fornix*. It is probable that here in the hypothalamus the intimate blending of smell and taste occurs. There is little doubt that the visceral reflex responses, such as salivary secretion initiated by smell, are facilitated by some descending hypothalamic fibers.

The interconnections between the hypothalamus and certain of the basal nuclei belonging to the extrapyramidal system establish a closer cooperation between visceral and somatic motor

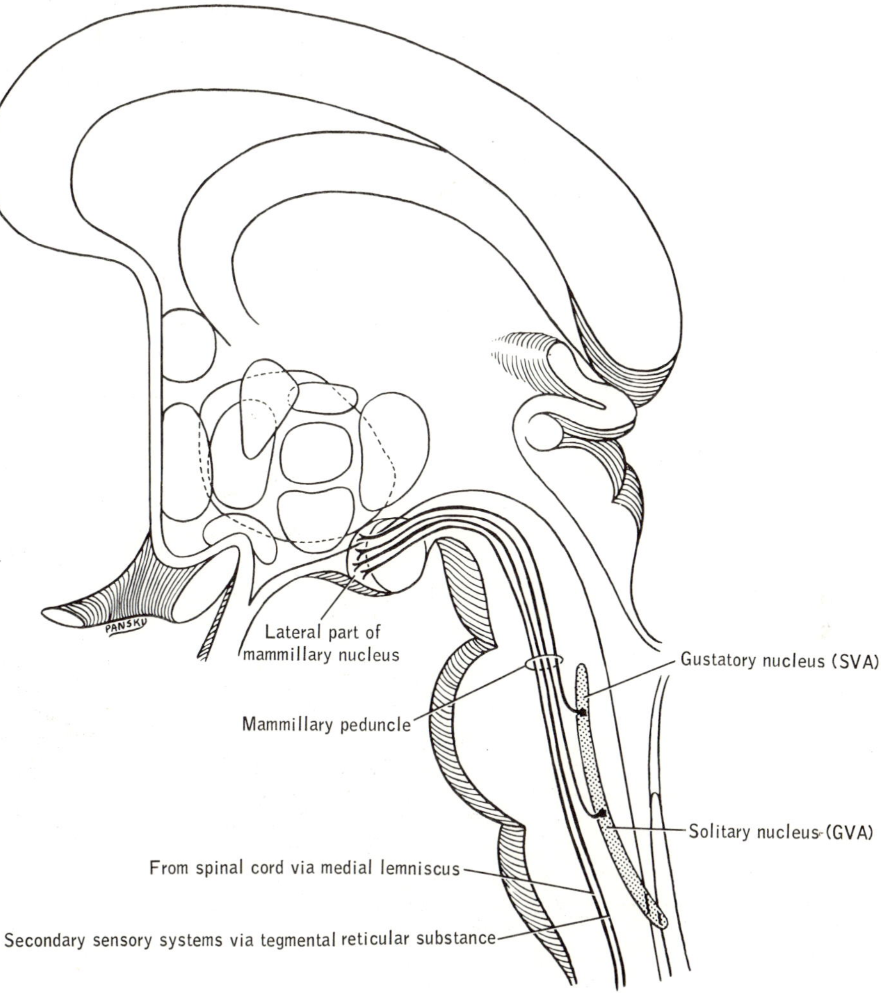

Fig. 21-5. Diagrammatic representation of the mammillary peduncle.

activity. Although not so significant in man as in lower forms, reflexes of the somatic musculature initiated by visceral afferents and associated with feeding and defense are relayed through the hypothalamus.

The fibers descending from the hypothalamus to the neural hypophysis strongly indicate the importance of the hypothalamus in the activation of the posterior lobe of the pituitary. Evidence also indicates that the hypothalamus can influence (if not control) the secretion of the adenohypophysis. However, since there are few, if any, descending fibers from the hypothalamus to the anterior lobe and since the fibers brought to the anterior lobe through the autonomic nervous system do not appear significant enough to control secretion, some other mechanism must be found to account for these influences. The most recent evidence supports the contention that the functional interrelation between the adenohypophysis and the hypothalamus is a neurovascular linkage. The acceptance of this tenet, however, is dependent upon the acceptance of the theory of neural secretion. Certainly there is much to support this concept. Further, it has been established that the hormones attributed to the posterior pituitary are the products of the nervous tissue which make up the neural hypophysis, with the possibility that such secretions may even be produced in the hypothalamus itself. The actual manner by which hypothalamic secretions are brought to bear on the cells of the anterior lobe is best indicated diagrammatically (Fig. 21-10).

With the advent of the neopallium, descend-

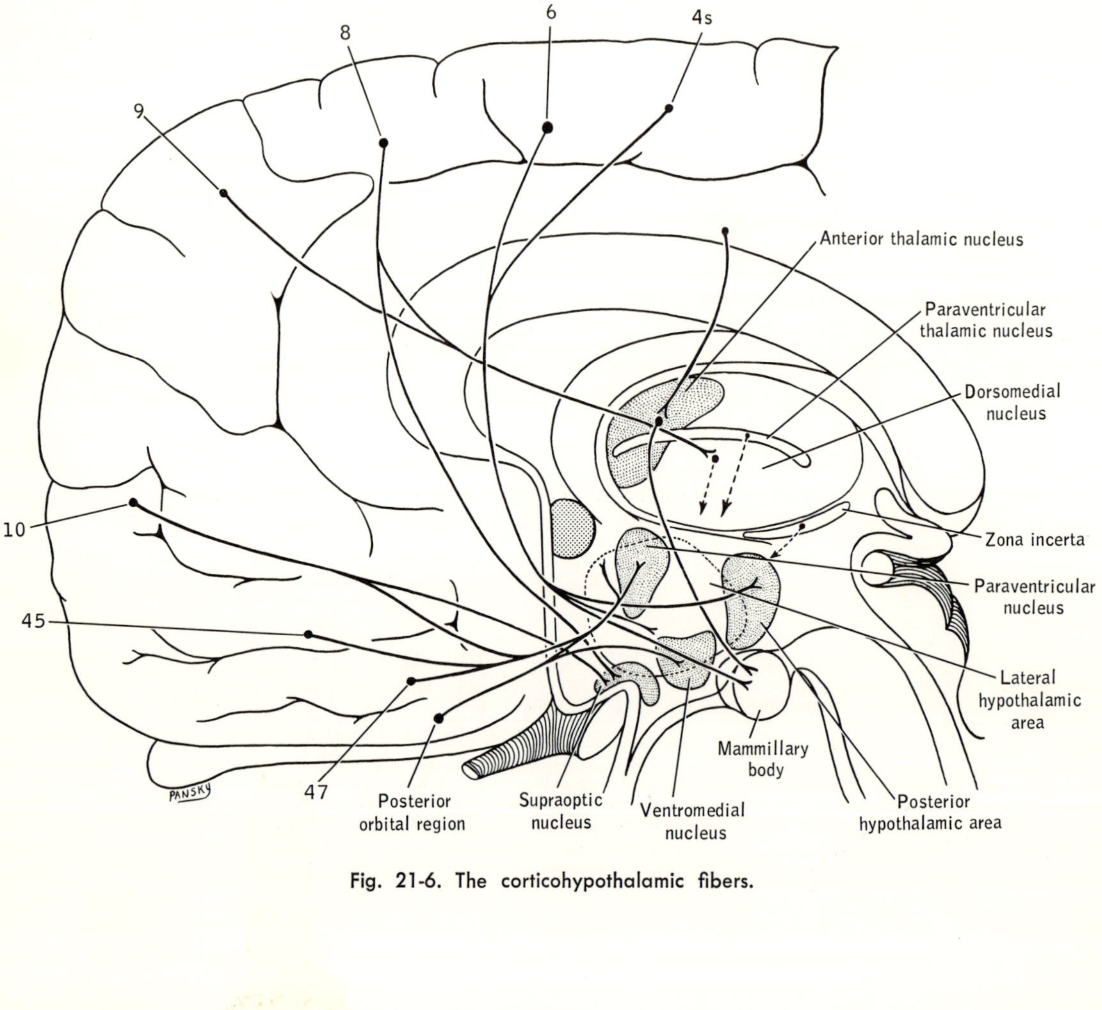

Fig. 21-6. The corticohypothalamic fibers.

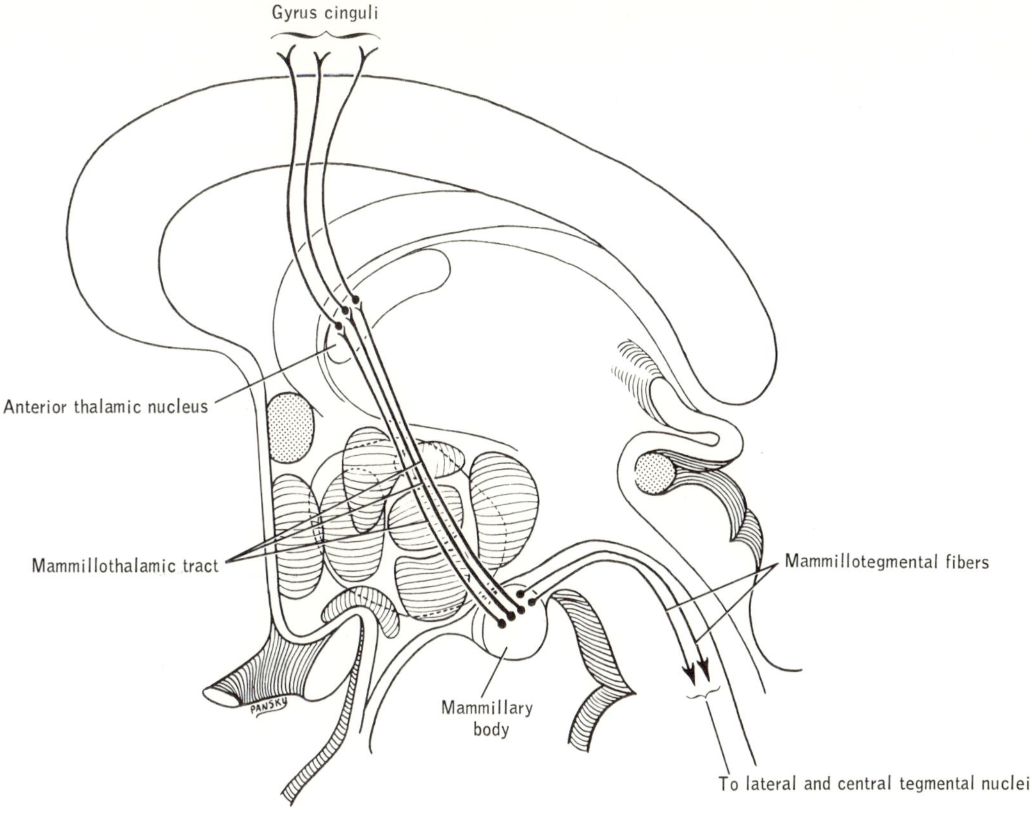

Fig. 21-7. The mammillothalamic tract and the mammillotegmental connections.

ing fibers, arising in the neocortex, pass to the more ancient hypothalamus, and, conversely, ascending fibers run from the hypothalamus back to the cortex. The former circuit (corticohypothalamic) in no way implies that the hypothalamus is under cortical control, but it does explain how the hypothalamus is influenced by higher centers. On the one hand, one cannot command the heart to speed up or slow down; the blood pressure to rise or fall; the body temperature to increase or decrease; or the food to digest through the voluntary control of glandular secretions. On the other hand, it is equally obvious that certain thoughts may lead to the erection of the penis; worry inevitably leads to indigestion; and fear may cause fluctuations in temperature. The hypothalamus, then, exerts its control over visceral function through its efferent fibers (mammillotegmentals, including the dorsal longitudinal fasciculus and relays in the reticular formation).

The ascending fibers in the mammillothalamic tract are part of the reciprocal circuit through which the hypothalamus influences the cerebral cortex. This pathway serves several purposes, one of which is the usual reinforcement and enhancement typical of reverberating circuits found in many parts of the CNS. A second might be considered to be in the nature of a cortical activation mechanism important in the wakeful state.

FUNCTIONS OF THE HYPOTHALAMUS

Emotion

Although it is in no way implied that the hypothalamus is the emotional center, it can be

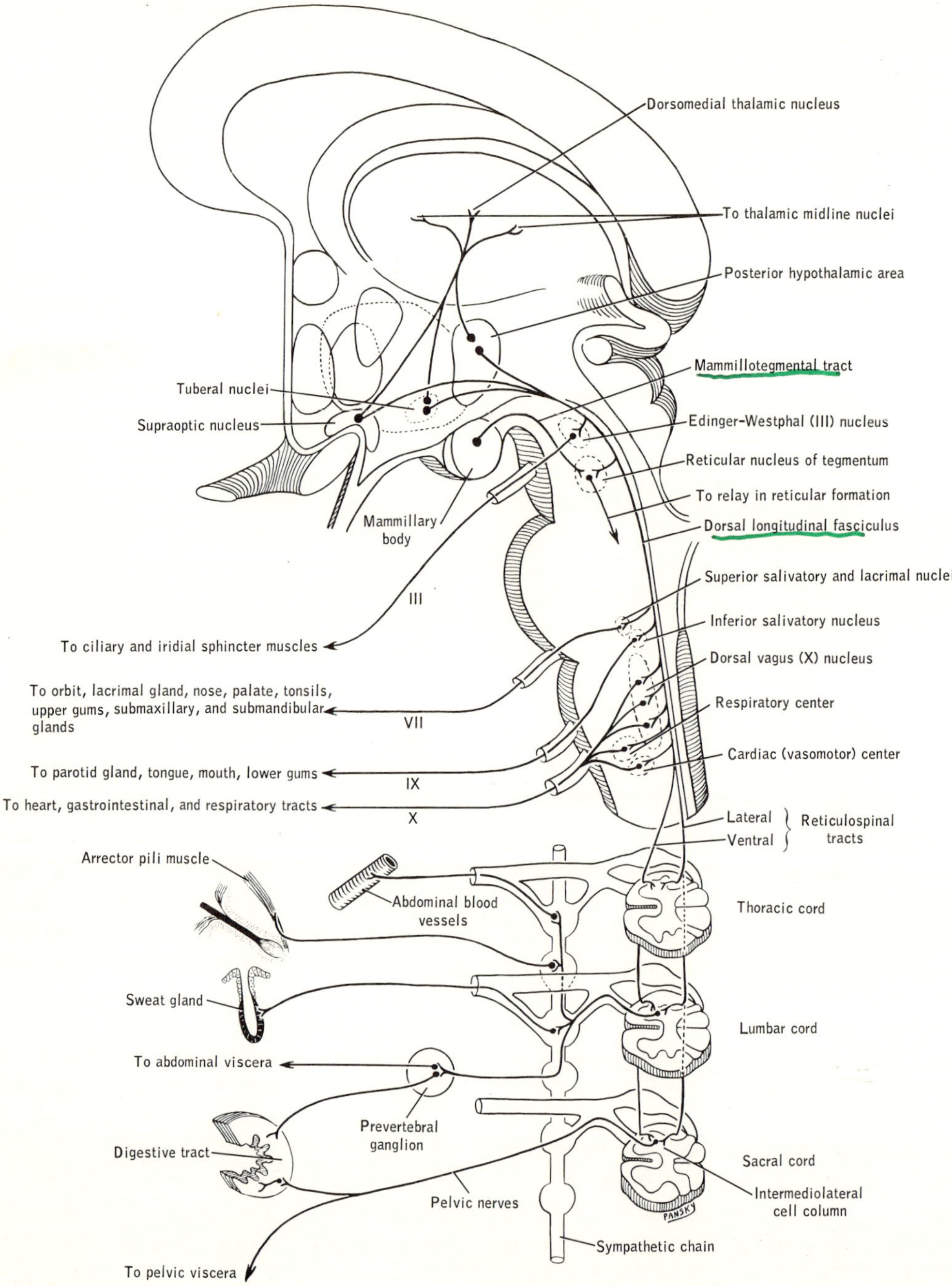

Fig. 21-8. The periventricular fibers of the hypothalamus.

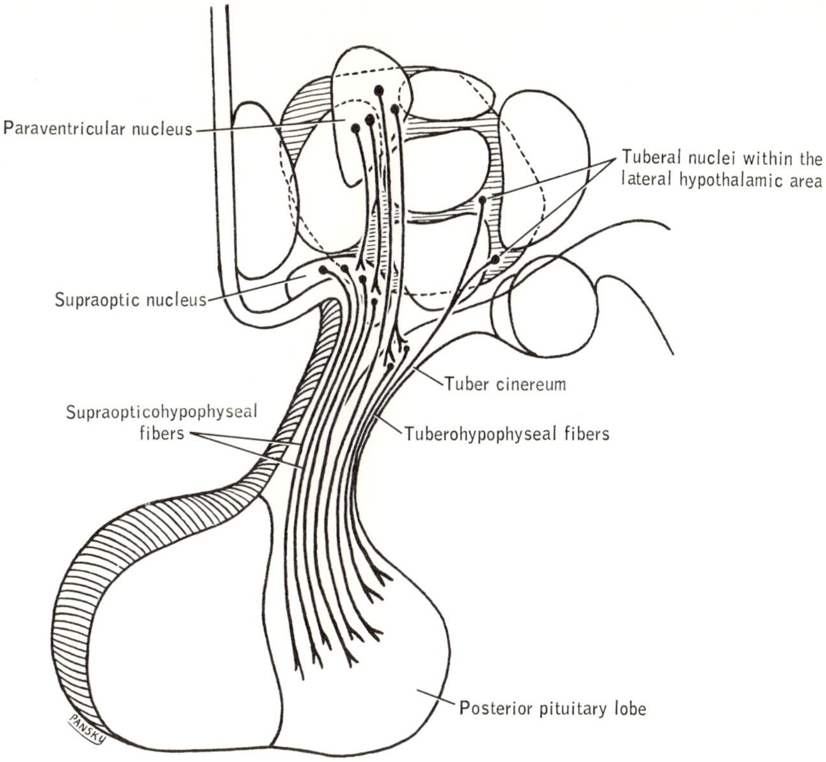

Fig. 21-9. Hypothalamicohypophyseal paths.

said that it does take part in the activities of the autonomic system which accompany emotion. There is good evidence that certain areas of the cerebral cortex act as an inhibitor for these activities. Through cortical destruction (bilateral frontal lobe lesions just above the optic chiasma or lesions in the bilateral olfactory tubercles), cats can easily be induced to demonstrate behavior usually seen in rage, provided the posterior hypothalamus is intact. The behavior includes dilation of the pupil; erection of the hair; increase in the cardiac rate and blood pressure; increase in salivation. Since this is simulated rage, produced in the absence of the normal cortical inhibiting influence, it is usually classified as "sham rage." More recently, however, other experiments have indicated that sham rage does not depend upon the removal of the neocortex alone. In these experiments it was shown that the removal of parts of the neocortex leads to placid states, provided parts of the gyrus cinguli are intact. Conversely, in a placid animal, a rage state can be induced through the ablation of the amygdaloid complex and the pyriform lobe, the former being considered the center through which all inhibitory influences can be expressed. However, it should be pointed out that most normal human beings under the proper set of circumstances will experience typical rage reactions (Figs. 21-11, 21-12).

Renal Outflow (Water Excretion) (Fig. 21-13.)

Some years ago it was shown that among the substances secreted by the posterior pituitary is the *antidiuretic hormone*. The absence of this secretion leads to a clinical condition known as *diabetes insipidus,* characterized by the excretion of excessive amounts of low specific gravity urine. The antidiuretic hormone, which apparently keeps water excretion within physiologic

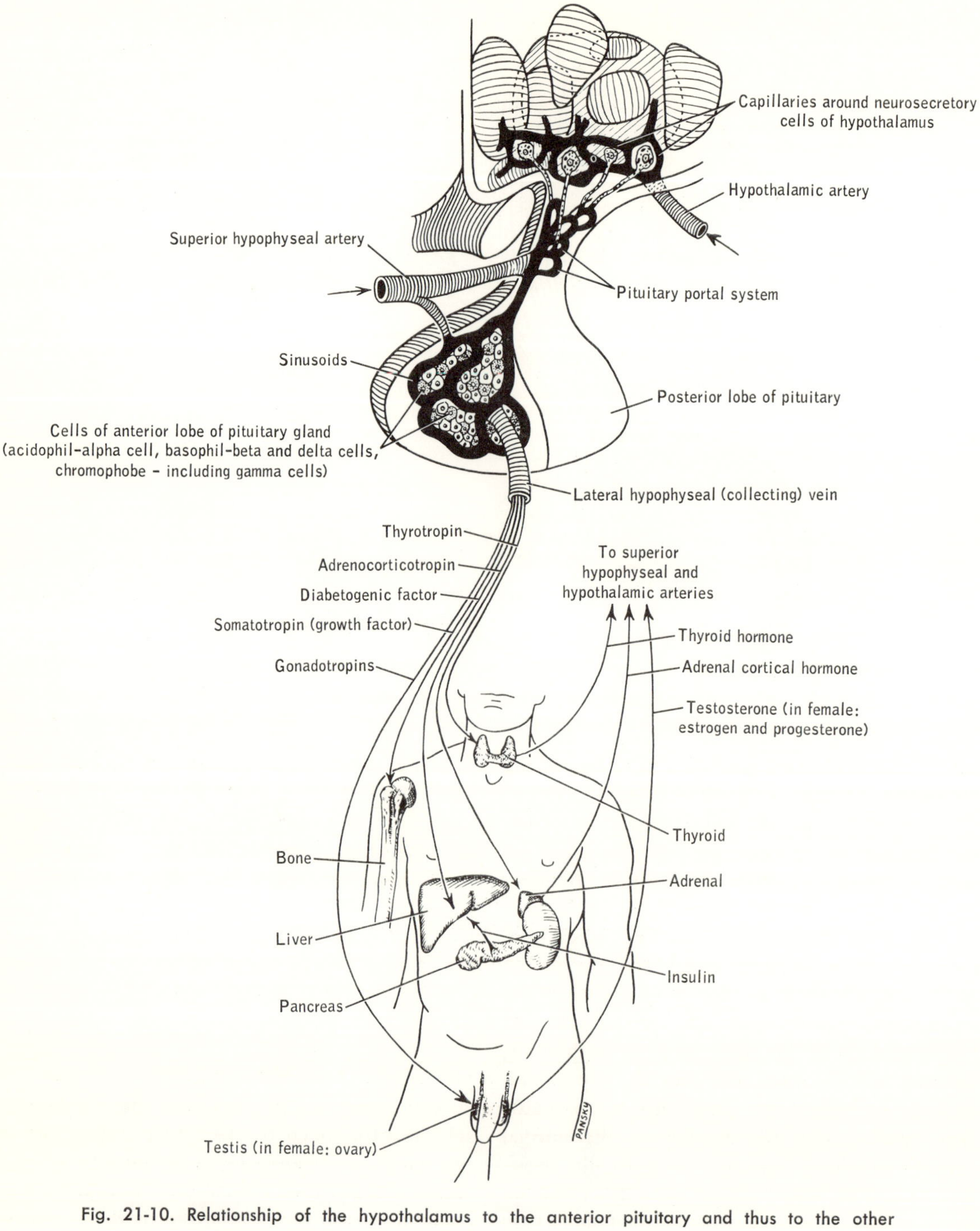

Fig. 21-10. Relationship of the hypothalamus to the anterior pituitary and thus to the other endocrines, the liver, and the bone marrow. (*After Netter Ciba Clinical Symposia.*)

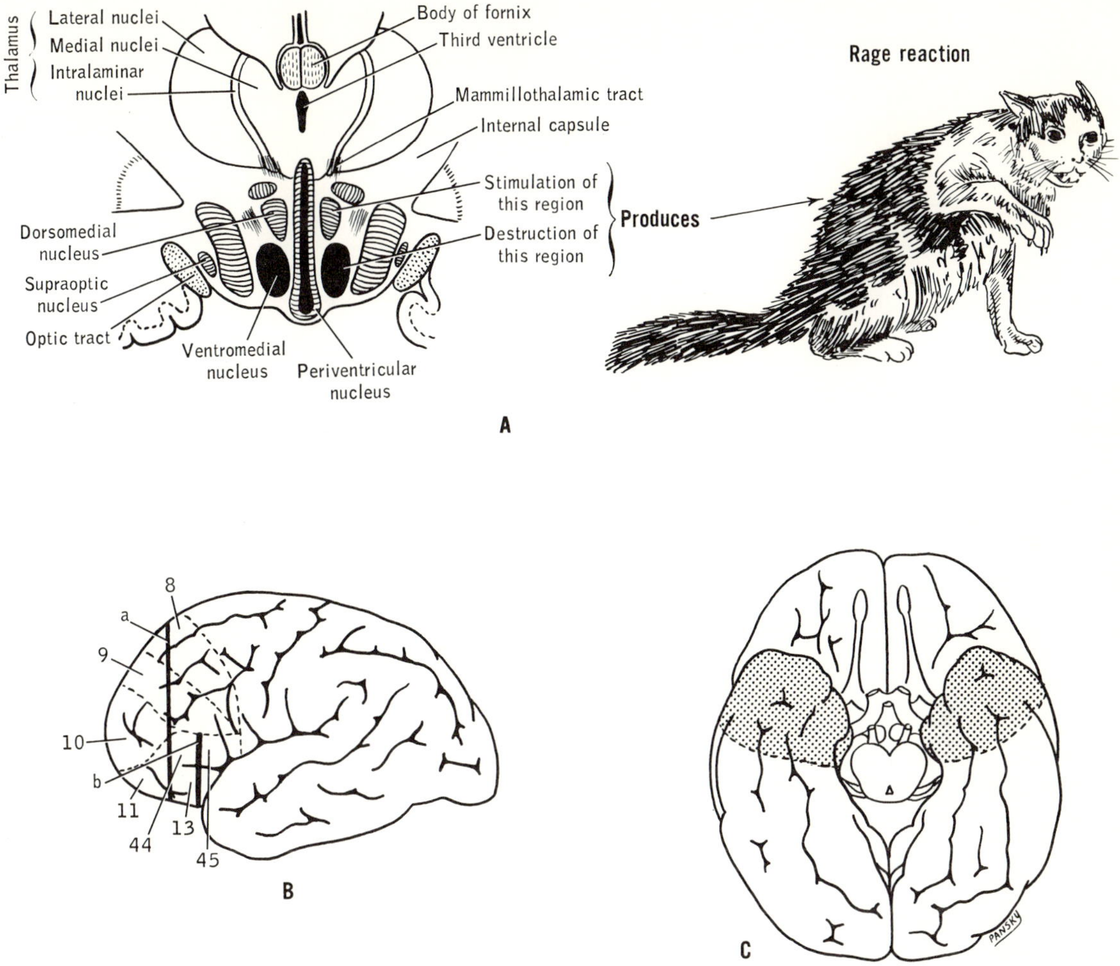

Fig. 21-11. *A.* Hypothalamic mechanism in emotional behavior. *B.* Lobotomy. *a.* Incision may relieve severe schizophrenia possibly interfering with intellect. *b.* Incision (through posterior orbital gyri) may relieve less severe states not interfering with intellect. (Some frontal cortical areas are indicated by numbers.) C. Lesions in amygdaloid nuclei and adjacent rhinencephalon (dotted area) may produce in some species (rat, cat, monkey) gentle, tame, fearless animals with the males in sexually hyperactive state. (*After Netter Ciba Clinical Symposia.*)

limits, passes into the capillaries of the infundibular stalk. Most recent evidence indicates that this hormone is a neurosecretion, produced by the cells of the supraoptic nucleus of the hypothalamus.[3] The secretion migrates along the axons of this tract, to be discharged into the capillaries of the posterior lobe. The amount of secretion may be regulated in two ways: (1) nervous influences are carried to the nucleus by way of afferent hypothalamic fiber systems, which may account for variations in urine output in different emotional states; (2) the cells of the supraoptic nucleus respond to changes in blood and tissue fluids surrounding them. In other words, if tissue

[3] It was once believed that this substance was secreted by the glioid pituicytes of the posterior lobe of the pituitary activated by the fibers descending from the supraoptic nucleus as the supraopticohypophyseal tract.

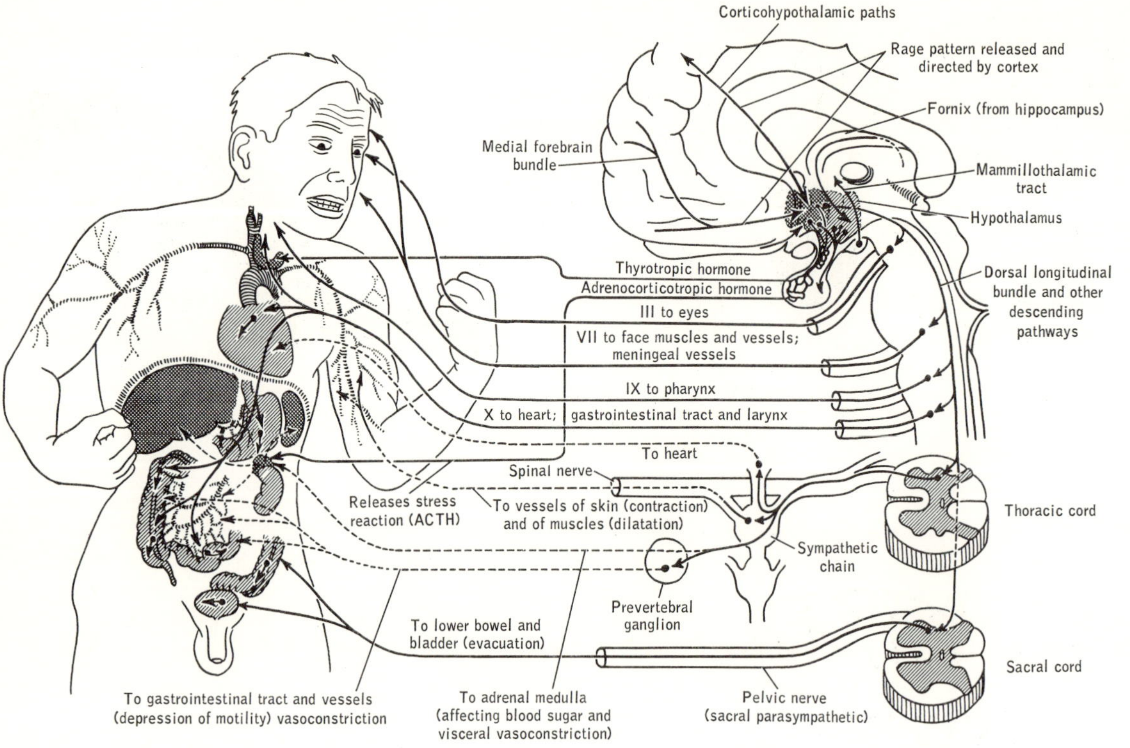

Fig. 21-12. Neurogenic and hormonal pathways in the rage reaction. (*After Netter Ciba Clinical Symposia.*)

fluid is in excess in the hypothalamus (which would be a reflection of the condition over the entire body), less antidiuretic hormone would be indicated so that the overabundance of intercellular fluid could be drained off through the kidneys. In this connection it has been shown that there are receptors, probably within the supraoptic nucleus, capable of detecting changes in osmotic pressure (osmoreceptors), since the injection of hypertonic saline solution into the internal carotid artery leads to antidiuresis.

It is believed that the target of the antidiuretic hormone is the distal convoluted tubule of the kidney. The target is reached through regulation of the amount of water resorbed into the blood stream from the glomerular filtrate. For example, when hypertonic saline solution is injected into the internal carotid artery, the blood in the hypothalamic arterial branches becomes hyperosmotic, simulating a condition of dehydration seen in patients after hemorrhage or hyperemesis. This causes an increase of production and release of the antidiuretic factor into the capillaries of the infundibular stalk. The factor is then carried through the systemic circulation to the kidneys, the distal convoluted tubules of which respond by resorbing more water in order to help reestablish isotonicity in the blood.

Temperature Regulation (Fig. 21-14.)

The maintenance of a constant body temperature (the homothermic state) depends upon a balance between heat loss and heat production and/or conservation. This balance is apparently brought about through the activity of two different neuron groups. One of these groups is affected by a rise in temperature of the blood, the other by a decline in temperature. Since the neurons having similar sensitivities to temperature change are grouped together in specific areas,

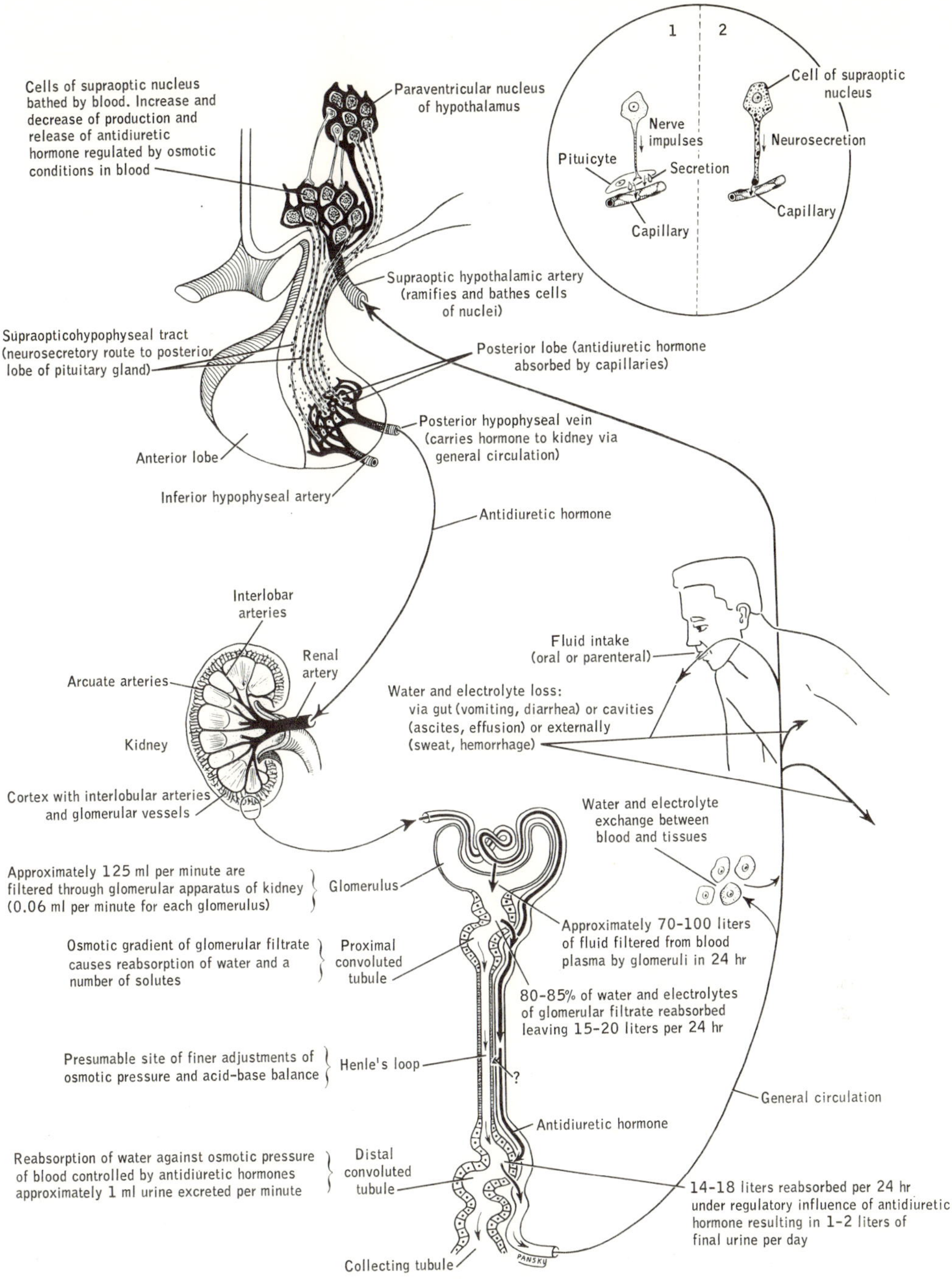

Fig. 21-13. Control of water excretion and water balance. Theories of origin of antidiuretic hormone. (1) Pituicytes release hormone under nervous influence. (2) Hormone produced as neurosecretion by cells in supraoptic nucleus and conducted by nerve fibers to posterior lobe for storage or absorption. (*After Netter Ciba Clinical Symposia.*)

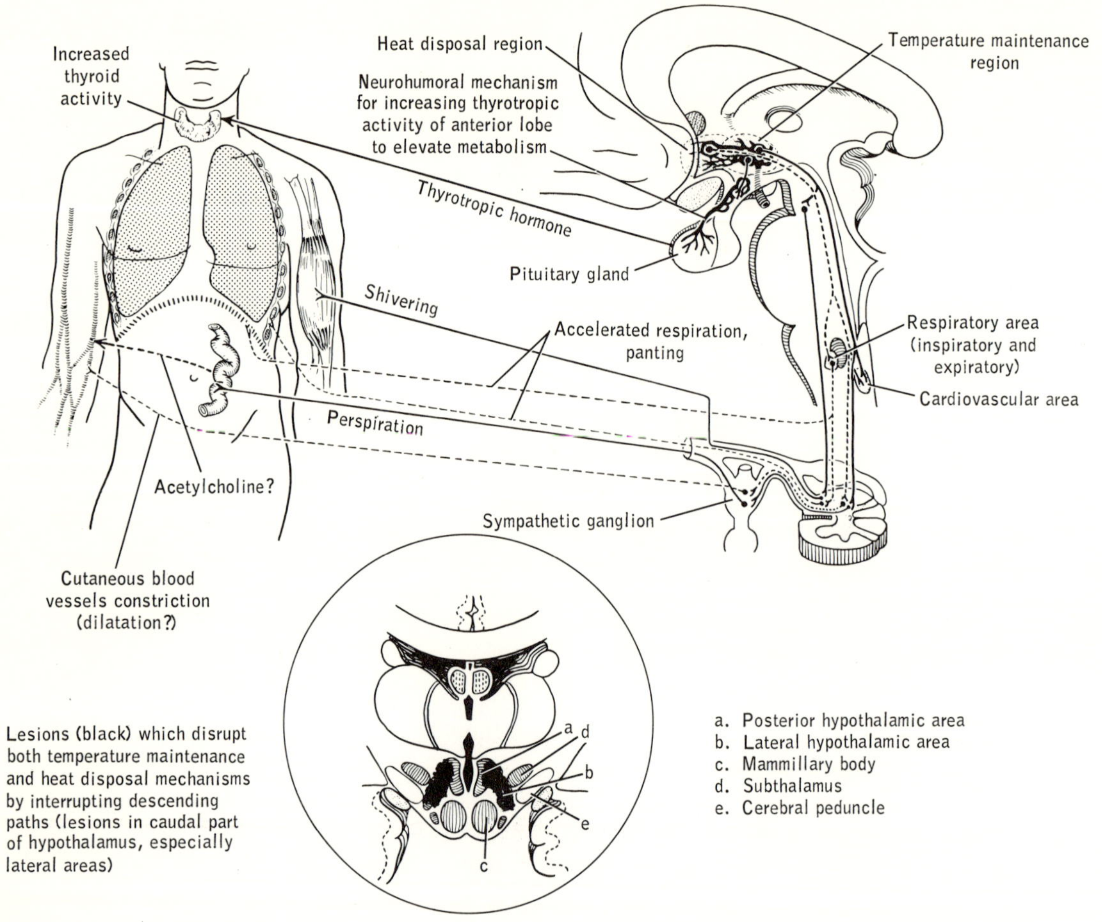

Fig. 21-14. Temperature regulation. (*After Netter Ciba Clinical Symposia.*)

one set is regarded as the *heat-loss* or *heat-dissipation center,* the other as the *heat-production* or *-conservation center.*

The heat-loss center is a relatively small area in the anterior hypothalamus, about 4 mm from the midsagittal line between the anterior commissure and the optic chiasma; it extends rostrally into the preoptic area. When the blood temperature rises, the cells of this center discharge over descending hypothalamic efferents to the respiratory and cardiovascular centers of the brain stem and spinal cord. These centers respond by initiating vasodilatation and perspiration.

The neurons which compose the heat-production center are located mainly in the caudal portion of the lateral hypothalamus. When the temperature of the blood declines, these neurons discharge caudally over the same descending pathways utilized by those of the heat-loss center. This results in vasoconstriction, piloerection, increased cardiac rate, and elevated basal metabolic rate. Shivering is definitely a part of this process, since the rapid, involuntary contraction of the somatic musculature produces heat.[4]

Blood Pressure Regulation (Fig. 21-15.)

The reflex control of blood pressure has already been discussed in the chapters on the GVA

[4] This is further proof that the somatic efferent columns of the cord can be activated through the descending hypothalamic fibers.

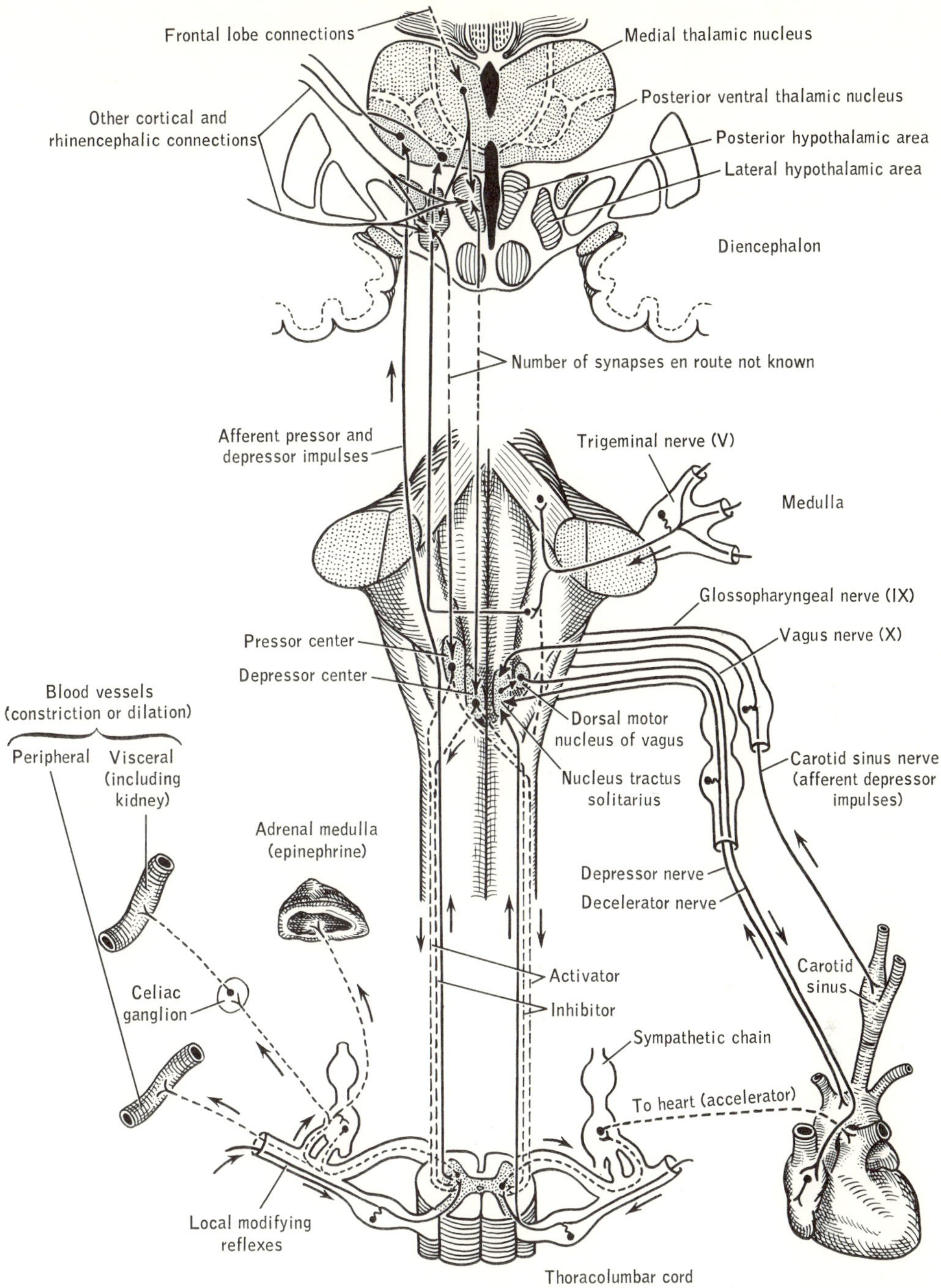

Fig. 21-15. Blood pressure regulation. (*After Netter Ciba Clinical Symposia.*)

and GVE systems. However, it should be indicated here that when generalized blood pressure changes are required, especially if the need is prolonged, the hypothalamus is activated and, through the same descending efferents, exerts influence upon the vasopressor and depressor centers of the reticular formation of the medulla. When the blood pressure change is initiated by psychic or emotional factors, it is certain that the hypothalamus is involved (Fig. 21-11). This is an important factor in the consideration of neurogenic or emotional hypertension in which the descending fibers from the hypothalamus activate the medullary vasopressor center. This, in turn, through the reticulospinal tract, accelerates the heart and produces mesenteric vasoconstriction directly through nerve fibers and indirectly through epinephrine secreted by the adrenal medulla under the activating influence of the thoracolumbar autonomic fibers.

Appetite Control (Fig. 21-16.)

There is good supportive evidence that the hypothalamus is important in regard to appetite and thus is directly involved in the problems of obesity and malnutrition. These subjects will be discussed further under Clinical Considerations.

Sleeping-waking Mechanism (Fig. 21-17.)

It has been shown that if a normal, nonfatigued person receives a certain amount of stimulation, from whatever source, he will remain

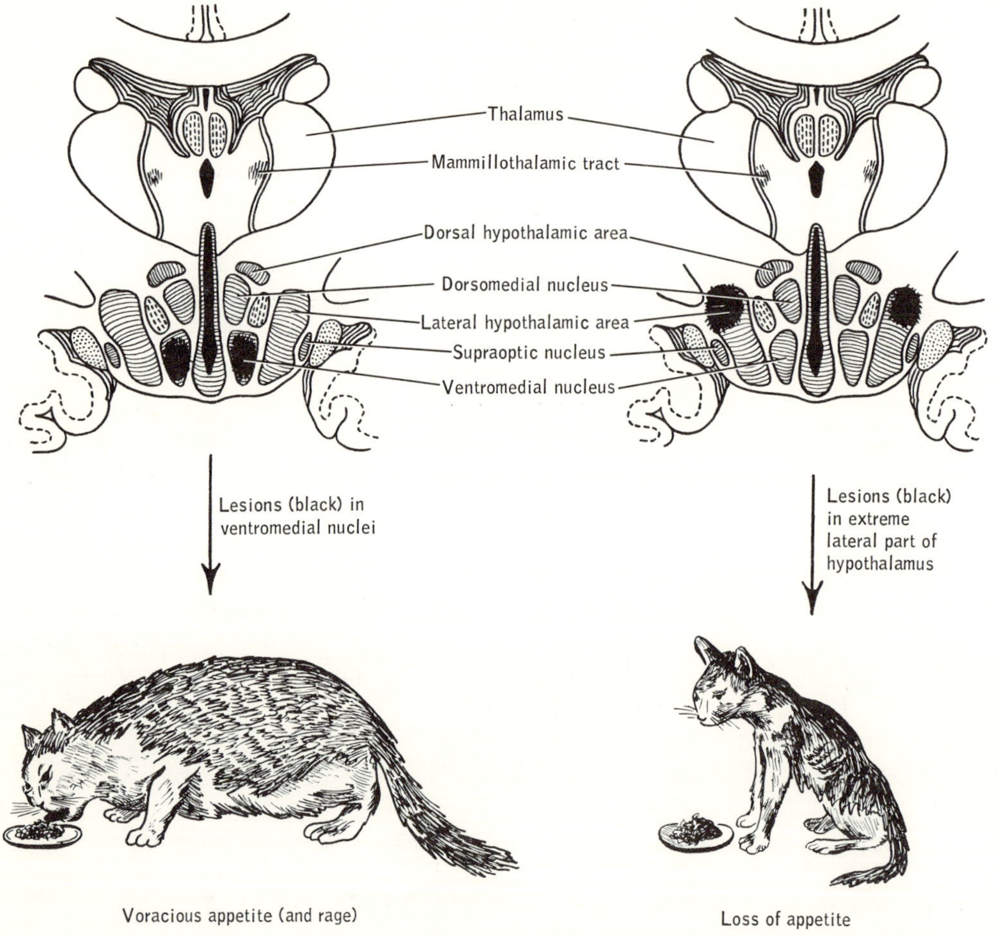

Fig. 21-16. Hypothalamic control of appetite. (*After Netter Ciba Clinical Symposia.*)

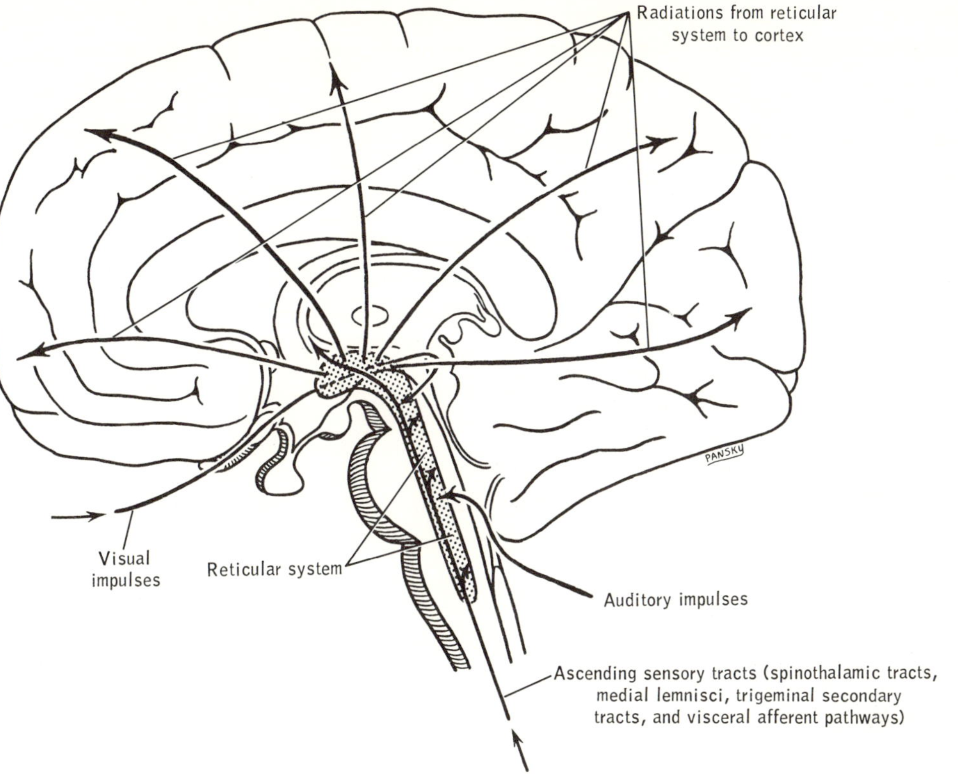

Fig. 21-17. Sleep-waking mechanism. (*After Netter Ciba Clinical Symposia.*)

awake and conscious of his surroundings. This means that when sufficient ascending impulses reach the cortex, it is activated. Normally the great sensory pathways, passing through thalamic nuclei to the cortex, are important in this connection. However, it has been shown experimentally that with these pathways intact, somnolence will occur with bilateral lesions placed in the posterior hypothalamus. It is apparent, therefore, that the reticular system of the brain stem, which receives collaterals from all the sensory systems and transmits their impulses into the hypothalamus, is of major importance in cerebral activation. The reticular system then passes through the thalamus to exert a generalized influence on the cortex.

It is difficult to understand the mechanism by which this reticular system is able to keep the proper number of cortical neurons active while the impulses traveling to the cortex directly by way of the afferent pathways are unable to do so. One explanation [5] may lie in the difference in distribution of the two systems. The primary sensory systems pass to relatively smaller areas of the cortex, while the reticular system is much more widespread. Another possibility is that since the reticular formation contains such enormous numbers of potential connections, one low-grade impulse entering it may fire off large numbers of others throughout the reticular formation. Thus, sleep may be looked upon as a condition resulting from a decreased flow of afferent impulses. This leads to an increase in the resistance at the synapses in the higher centers so that the few remaining afferent impulses cannot be integrated. This in its turn results in a loss of motor activity. There is some evidence for such a mechanism, since destruction of the reticular for-

[5] It is held by some that this system, like the cardiac pacemaker, is spontaneously active.

mation in the midbrain and the posterior end of the hypothalamus leads to a sleeplike condition.[6]

CLINICAL CONSIDERATIONS

Testing

There are no specific tests to be performed. However, certain symptoms commonly appear as a result of disease in this region. They include obesity, amenorrhea, diabetes insipidus, and disorders of sleep and of thermal regulation. In addition, emaciation, ulcerations of the alimentary tract, premature sexual development, and emotional disturbances are also attributable to hypothalamic disease. Frequently, certain of these symptoms appear together in a complex known as a hypothalamic syndrome; the diabetes insipidus and emaciation syndrome; the adiposogenital dystrophy complex; and a syndrome characterized by somnolence and disorders of temperature control.

Specific Pathology

The hypothalamus is subject to the same types of pathologic change found in other parts of the CNS. These changes may be precipitated by *trauma* resulting from surgery about the pituitary; from injury to the bones at the base of the skull; *degenerative processes* caused by disturbances of vascularity; *inflammatory lesions,* either primary within the nervous tissue, or in the meninges; and several types of *tumors,* arising in the posterolateral walls or floor of the third ventricle or in the hypophysis.

Hyperthermia

This condition is characterized by a very high temperature, sometimes terminating fatally. It has been encountered in man, particularly after surgery in or about the hypophysis, and is thought to be related to a destruction of the heat-loss center in the anterior hypothalamus. This may be coupled with a simultaneous irritation of the heat-production center located more posteriorly.

[6] It is possible that some cortical inhibitor center may later be found which will account for sleep.

Poikilothermia

Bilateral lesions in the posterior hypothalamus, behind the heat-production center, may cut off the temperature-control mechanism entirely from lower centers. This will leave body temperature completely at the mercy of the environment.

Diabetes Insipidus

This condition is characterized by great thirst with excessive water intake (polydypsia) and an unbelievably high urine production (polyuria). Although both these symptoms may be found in diabetes mellitus, the urine in diabetes insipidus is of low specific gravity and does not contain glucose. Lesions may occur in the supraoptic nucleus or in its projection through the infundibular stalk to the posterior pituitary. This cuts off the production of the antidiuretic hormone, leaving the diuretic substance[7] of the adenohypophysis unopposed.

Adiposogenital Dystrophy (Froehlich's Syndrome)

The two symptoms, adiposity and genital dystrophy, may occur together or separately. Most characteristically, fat tends to accumulate in the lower abdomen and around the hips, the so-called feminine type of distribution. The genitalia are underdeveloped, and there are changes in secondary sex characteristics. The exact site of the lesion in man is not known, but it appears from clinical experience that the anterior and lateral areas of the tuber cinereum and the ventromedial nucleus are involved. Recently, newer techniques have shown that lesions in the region of the ventromedial nucleus will cause marked increase in appetite, frequently associated with rage states. The aberration is so intense that an animal will eat heavily and wolfishly although it is already well fed. Since animals with destructive lesions in this region are somewhat less active than normal, they easily become obese. There is some feeling that the obesity is

[7] The production of the diuretic substance also appears to be in some way regulated by the hypothalamus; it has been noted that extensive hypothalamic lesions lead to oliguria (low urine production).

the result of changes in fat and carbohydrate metabolism resulting from the suppression of certain anterior lobe secretions. This theory is supported by the fact that in some experimental animals with lesions in this area, there is a tendency toward hypogonadism. In others, there seems to be a lack in the somatotropic hormone.

When lesions are placed in the lateral hypothalamic region, appetite is almost completely lost both in normal animals and in those with already existing ventromedial nuclei lesions.

There is further evidence that the hypothalamus exerts regulatory influences on the anterior lobe, chiefly through humoral substances in the hypothalamiconeurohypophyseal portal system of veins. These influences include lesions of the median eminence, causing loss of sexual activity and atrophy of the genitalia.

Hypertension (Fig. 21-18.)

Although hypertension usually subsides when the emotional episode passes, the periods of hypertension may be long in the so-called chronic worrier. When prolonged, the high pressure may permanently alter the kidney in such a way that it secretes abnormal amounts of renin (a renal vasopressor substance) which can lead to a continuous hypertension, even in the absence of stress. It is also felt that the same factors which overstimulate the hypothalamus in the manner just described may also cause it to secrete a substance into the blood stream (a neurosecretion) which is carried to the anterior pituitary. This, in turn, is stimulated to secrete adrenocorticotropic hormone. An oversecretion of the adrenal cortex may also be concerned with hypertension.

Amenorrhea, Impotence, and Sexual Infantilism

This symptom complex may arise as a result of disorders in either the hypothalamus or the hypophysis. With destruction of the anterior and tuberal portions of the hypothalamus, there is loss of the regulatory secretions which govern the production of gonadotropic hormones. The exact nature of the sexual disorders will depend upon the patient's sex and age when the lesion occurs. In children, development of sexual organs and the sexual functions are retarded. If the lesion occurs after puberty, there may be a regression of sexual function and a reversal of secondary sexual characteristics that is especially noticeable in males. An opposite effect is the so-called *pubertas precox,* the premature development of the genitalia and sexual function. In this condition the hypothalamic control mechanism is in some way blocked, permitting an unchecked secretion of gonadotropin. It is sometimes associated with internal hydrocephalus. More frequently, however, especially when the signs appear very early, it may be related to a hematoma. When the signs occur later, they are often caused by tumors, encephalitis, or meningitis.

Disorders of Sleep

These may occur as a result of encephalitis. They may consist of the occurrence of short periods of sleep during normal waking hours or of prolonged periods of sleep. The latter condition can result from destruction of the caudal hypothalamus or from damage in the transition zone between diencephalon and mesencephalon, perhaps as far down as the central tegmental area in the mesencephalon. Insomnia has also been described in cases of encephalitis. It may be due to an irritative phase of the disease. There may or may not be disturbances of temperature regulation.

Disorders of "Emotions"

Inflammations, vascular disturbances, and neoplasms in or about the hypothalamus have led to many aberrant activities. Sometimes these take the form of impaired memory or of maniacal outbursts with excitement and destructiveness. Sudden and unreasonable seizures of crying and laughing may also occur. Anxiety states or periods of apathy may be seen. Loss of inhibitions with indecent behavior is not uncommon. It should be pointed out that any of these conditions (or all of them) may also be symptomatic of diseases in other parts of the nervous system. They may result from the activities of these other parts following hypothalamus destruction.

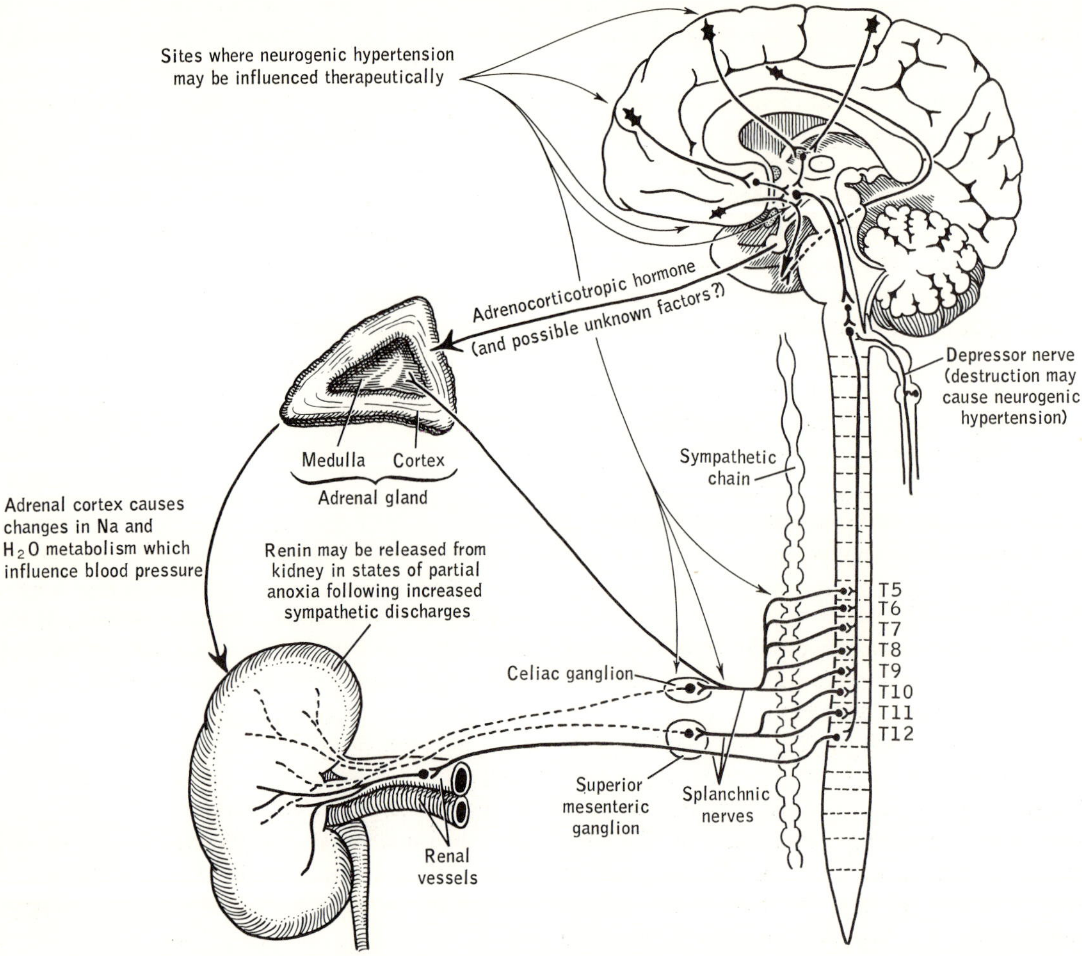

Fig. 21-18. Neurogenic and humoral hypertension. Emotional tension, anxiety states, and other mental stresses induce hypothalamic stimulation, which in turn influences peripheral circulation. (*After Netter Ciba Clinical Symposia.*)

Miscellaneous Effects

Through animal experimentation, it has also been shown that stimulation of the hypothalamus produces ovulation (in rabbits); lesions in the central area result in a fall of metabolic rate; stimulation and inhibition of certain regions speed up or slow down the production of thyrotropic hormones; hyperglycemia has resulted from stimulation of the hypothalamus and if prolonged in the tuberal region, will cause a decrease in sensitivity to insulin. Hypothalamic lesions have been shown in some animals to cause an increase in sensitivity to insulin. In pancreatectomized cats, this has led to a reduction in insulin requirements.

SUMMARY

I. Parts

A. Definite nuclei: preoptic, supraoptic, paraventricular, posterior, dorsomedial, ventromedial, tuberal, and mammillary

- *B*. Regional divisions: anterior, lateral, and dorsal

II. Afferent connections
- *A*. Fornix
  1. Origin—hippocampus and dentate gyrus
  2. Termination—mammillary nuclei
  3. Function—one of chief paths from cortex to hypothalamus; may be involved in emotions and memory
- *B*. Medial forebrain bundle
  1. Origin—septal nuclei (of olfactory brain)
  2. Termination—mammillary nuclei and lateral area
  3. Function—ascending fibers from midbrain tegmentum to hypothalamus; descending fibers to lateral hypothalamus and midbrain tegmentum; olfactovisceral and olfactovisceroso-matic correlation in hypothalamus and hemispheres
- *C*. Periventricular fibers
  1. Origin—dorsomedial and midline nuclei of thalamus
  2. Termination—anterior, tuberal and posterior areas
  3. Function—cerebral influence on visceral function
- *D*. Stria terminalis
  1. Origin—amygdaloid complex
  2. Termination—preoptic nucleus and anterior area
  3. Function—part of the olfactovisceral reflex relay system
- *E*. Mammillary peduncle
  1. Origin—tegmentum of mesencephalon
  2. Termination—mammillary nuclei
  3. Function—possible activation of hypothalamus through ascending reticular fibers; correlation of gustatory and visceral sense with the somatic afferents from mucous membranes of nose and mouth
- *F*. Strio—and pallidohypothalamic fibers
  1. Origin—putamen and globus pallidus (possible subthalamic nucleus and zona incerta)
  2. Termination—ventromedial, dorsomedial, paraventricular and mammillary nuclei
  3. Function—coordination of somatic and visceral motor function
- *G*. Corticohypothalamic fibers
  1. Origin—area 6, through septal area and thence through medial forebrain bundle
  2. Termination—posterior nucleus, mammillary nuclei, and lateral area
  3. Origin—posterior orbital cortex
  4. Termination—paraventricular and ventromedial nuclei
  5. Origin—frontal cortex
  6. Termination—supraoptic nucleus
  7. Origin—area 23 of gyrus cinguli through anterior nucleus of thalamus to descend in the mammillothalamic tract
  8. Termination—mammillary nuclei
  9. Function—mediation of conscious influence over visceral activity

III. Efferent connections
- *A*. Mammillothalamic tract (bundle of Vicq d'Azyr)
  1. Origin—medial mammillary nucleus
  2. Termination—anterior nucleus of thalamus (and via relays to gyrus cinguli)
  3. Function—part of hypothalamic activation of cortex by way of anterior thalamic nucleus; reciprocal circuit through gyrus cinguli; thalamocortical impulses from hypothalamus resulting from correlation of gustatory and olfactory impulses
- *B*. Mammillotegmental tract
  1. Origin—medial mammillary nucleus
  2. Termination—central reticular nucleus of the mesencephalic tegmentum
  3. Function—part of descending control mechanism of autonomic centers in brain stem and spinal cord

C. Periventricular fibers

1. Origin—posterior nuclei, tuberal nuclei, and supraoptic nuclei
2. Termination—dorsomedial and midline nuclei of the thalamus; tegmental nuclei of the mesencephalon; parasympathetic nuclei of the brain stem; the vital centers in the medullary reticular formation (i.e., cardiac and respiratory); the intermediolateral column of the cord—all of these through the dorsal longitudinal fasciculus (of Schütz) and through the reticulospinal tract
3. Function—probably supplemental, carrying hypothalamic control to brain stem parasympathetic nuclei and vital centers

D. Hypothalamohypophyseal fibers

1. Origin—supraoptic and paraventricular nuclei
2. Termination—neurohypophysis
3. Origin—tuberal nuclei
4. Termination—neurohypophysis
5. Function—activation of posterior lobe of pituitary with influence on secretion of adenohypophysis

22 THALAMIC RELAY AND CORRELATION CENTER TO THE CORTEX

STRUCTURE

Gross

The thalamus is the largest portion of the diencephalon. Its gross relationships to the mesencephalon, internal capsule, and basal nuclei of the telencephalon have already been described (Chap. 2).

Thalamic Nuclei (Figs. 22-1 to 22-5.)

The thalamus is divided into two parts by a sheet of myelinated fibers called the *internal medullary lamina*. This divides the thalamus into a medial and a lateral area. Each of these major areas is further subdivided into specific nuclear masses. The medial portion consists of the dorsomedial (Fig. 25-15) and anterior nuclei (Figs. 25-15 to 25-17); the latter is enclosed within the medullary lamina. The lateral portion is divided into a dorsal and ventral tier of nuclei. The caudal projection of the ventral tier is referred to as the *metathalamus*. Further subdivisions into still smaller areas become enormously complicated, since 30 or more nuclei are recognized. However, since some are of an uncertain functional status, the discussion here will be limited, in so far as possible, to those with more definite connections and significance. On this basis, the tertiary divisions are as follows: the *dorsomedial* area consists of the *dorsomedial, submedial,* and *habenulopeduncular tract nuclei;* the dorsal portion of the lateral nucleus is divided, from front to back, into the *dorsolateral* (Fig. 25-14), *posterolateral* (Fig. 25-14), and *pulvinar* (Fig. 25-13) nuclei; the ventral portion of the lateral thalamic mass consists of the *anterior ventral, lateral ventral* (Figs. 25-15, 25-16), and *posterior ventral nuclei.* The posterior ventral nucleus is usually described as consisting of the *posteromedial ventral* (*arcuate* or *semilunar*) *nucleus* (Fig. 25-14), adjacent to which a separate *accessory arcuate* or *semilunar nucleus* may be found; and the *posterolateral ventral nucleus*. The metathalamus also has two distinct nuclear masses, namely the *medial* (Fig. 25-13) and *lateral geniculate bodies* (or *nuclei*) (Fig. 25-14).

In addition to the above more obvious divisions, there are two other scattered sets of nuclei: (1) nuclei of the midline, which make up the lamina of gray substance lining the third ventral and which are particularly prominent in its dorsal half and also in the massa intermedia (when the latter is present); (2) nuclei scattered in the internal medullary lamina, the so-called *intralaminar nuclei,* which include the *paracentral, lateral central, centrum medianum* (Fig. 25-14), and *parafascicular*.[1]

[1] It is now quite common to group these four nuclei together with the three subdivisions of the medial thalamus (dorsomedial, submedial, and habenulopeduncular tract nuclei) in a unit referred to simply as the *medial nuclei*—probably a more logical arrangement when the nuclei are considered on a functional basis.

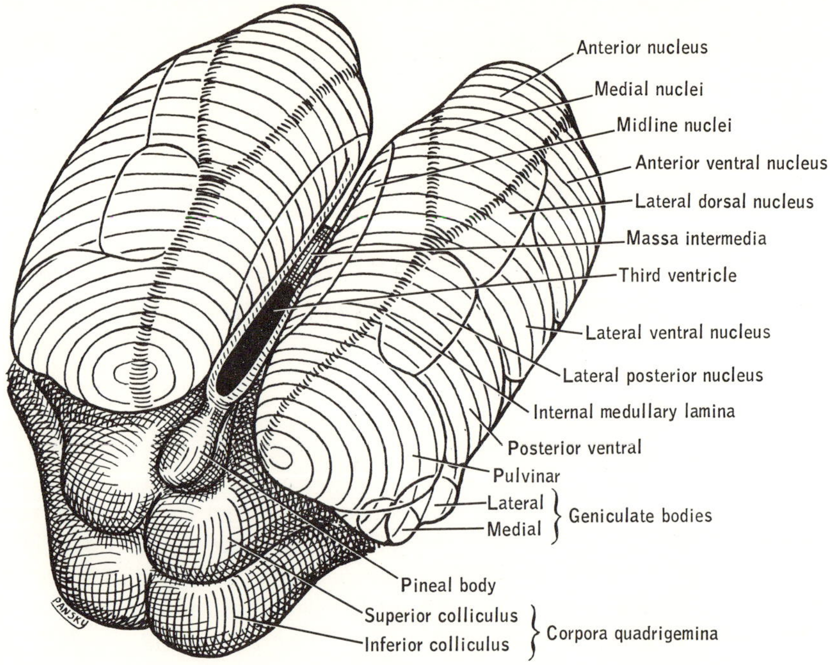

Fig. 22-1. Dorsal view of the thalamus showing the major divisions.

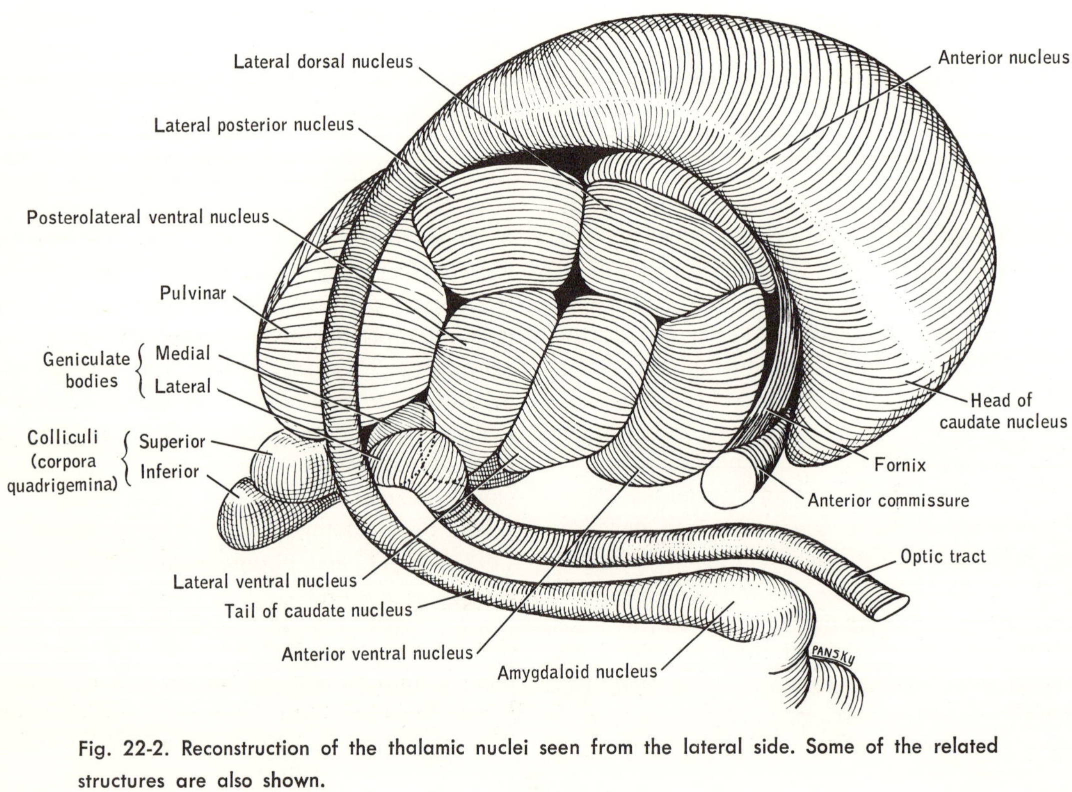

Fig. 22-2. Reconstruction of the thalamic nuclei seen from the lateral side. Some of the related structures are also shown.

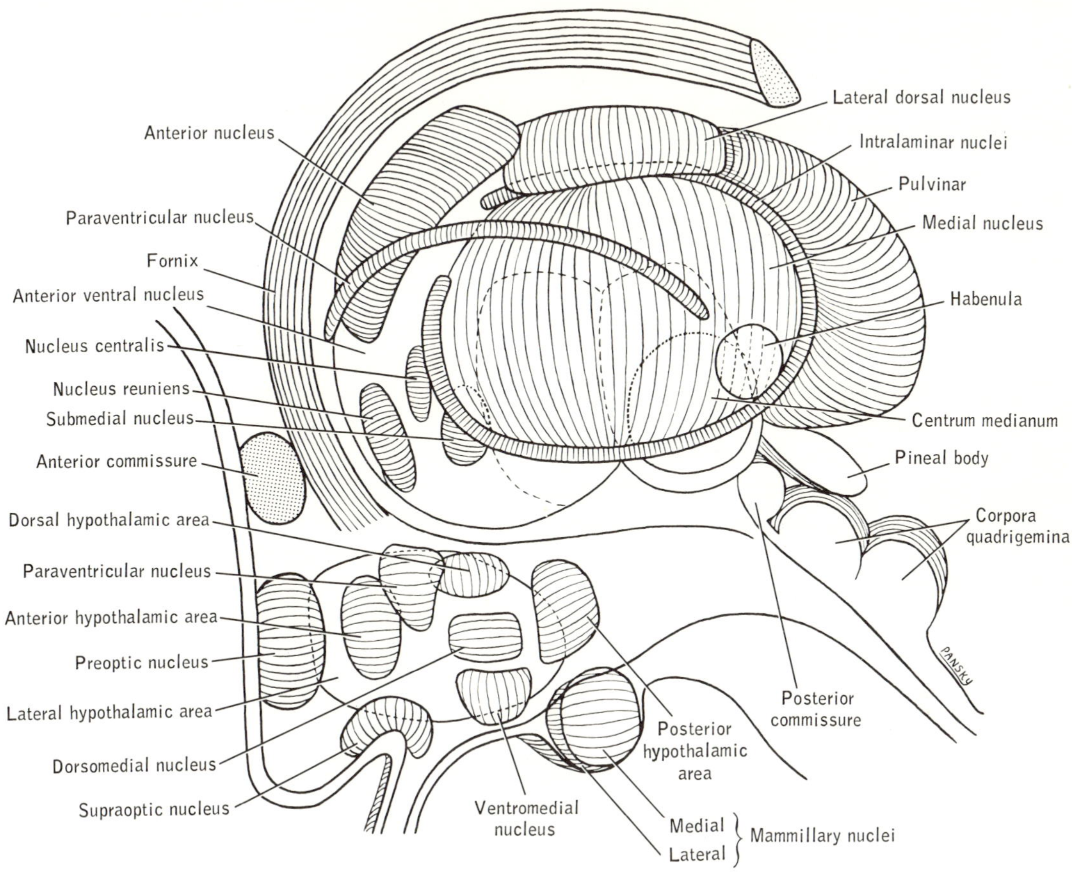

Fig. 22-3. Reconstruction of the major thalamic nuclei seen from the medial side.

FUNCTIONAL CLASSIFICATION OF THE THALAMIC NUCLEI

Three general nuclear groups are considered. The first, and probably oldest, sometimes classified as *nuclei of the thalamic reticular system,* are the *midline* and *intralaminar nuclei,* the fibers of which are primarily related to the rhinencephalon, the hypothalamus, and possibly the striatum, with no projections to the neocortex. The second group is made up of the nuclei in the ventral tier of the lateral thalamus, including the metathalamus. These nuclei are primarily *cortical relay* (extrinsic) in nature, receiving terminals from all the great ascending systems of the body and sending efferents to the neocortex. The third group is comprised of *association* (*intrinsic*) *nuclei.* They receive few, if any, ascending sensory fibers, their afferents being mainly from other parts of the brain while their efferents are distributed particularly to association areas of the cortex. The anterior and medial nuclei, together with the nuclei in the dorsal part of the lateral nucleus, make up this group.

CONNECTIONS OF THE NUCLEI

Nuclei of the Midline (Fig. 22-6.)

These nuclei receive terminals and many collaterals from the spinothalamic tracts, the trigeminothalamic tracts, and the medial lemniscus. It also appears that some of the fibers from the tectal region and certain thalamic nuclei also reach the midline complex. Some efferents descend into the hypothalamus and into the basal ganglia; others appear to reach portions in both the medial and lateral thalamic areas. It is said that these nuclei are important for impulses arising in the viscera, and it has been suggested that integration here permits some appreciation of pain.

Cortical Relay Nuclei

Sensory Systems

Posteromedial Ventral Nucleus. (Fig. 22-7.) This nucleus serves the GSA and GP systems. The afferents enter by way of the trigeminothalamic tract. The efferents pass through the posterior limb of the internal capsule to areas 1, 2, and 3 on the postcentral gyrus (Fig. 23-10).

Posterolateral Ventral Nucleus. (Fig. 22-7.) This area is also a relay center in the GSA and GP systems. The afferents are the lateral and ventral spinothalamic tracts and the medial lemniscus. The efferents pass through the posterior limb of the internal capsule to areas 1, 2, and 3 of the postcentral gyrus (Fig. 23-11).

Medial Geniculate Body (Nucleus). (Fig. 9-24.) This is an SSA relay area for hearing. The afferents travel from the cochlear nuclei via the lateral lemniscus and brachium of the inferior colliculus, plus possible relays from nuclei of the trapezoid body, lateral lemniscus, superior olive, and inferior colliculus. The efferents (auditory radiations) pass through the sublenticular part of the internal capsule as the geniculotemporal fibers to the transverse temporal gyrus. (Fig. 9-24.)

Lateral Geniculate Body (Nucleus). (Fig. 9-3.) This is a special somatic relay area for vision. The afferents enter through the optic tract and possibly relays from the nucleus of the su-

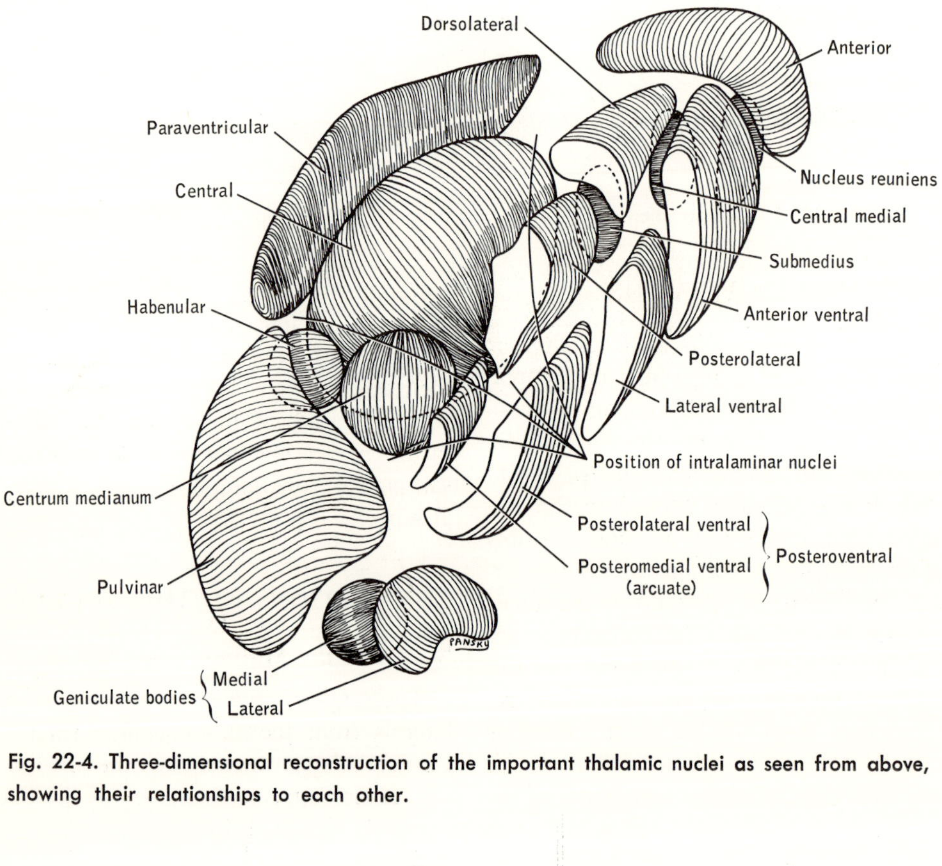

Fig. 22-4. Three-dimensional reconstruction of the important thalamic nuclei as seen from above, showing their relationships to each other.

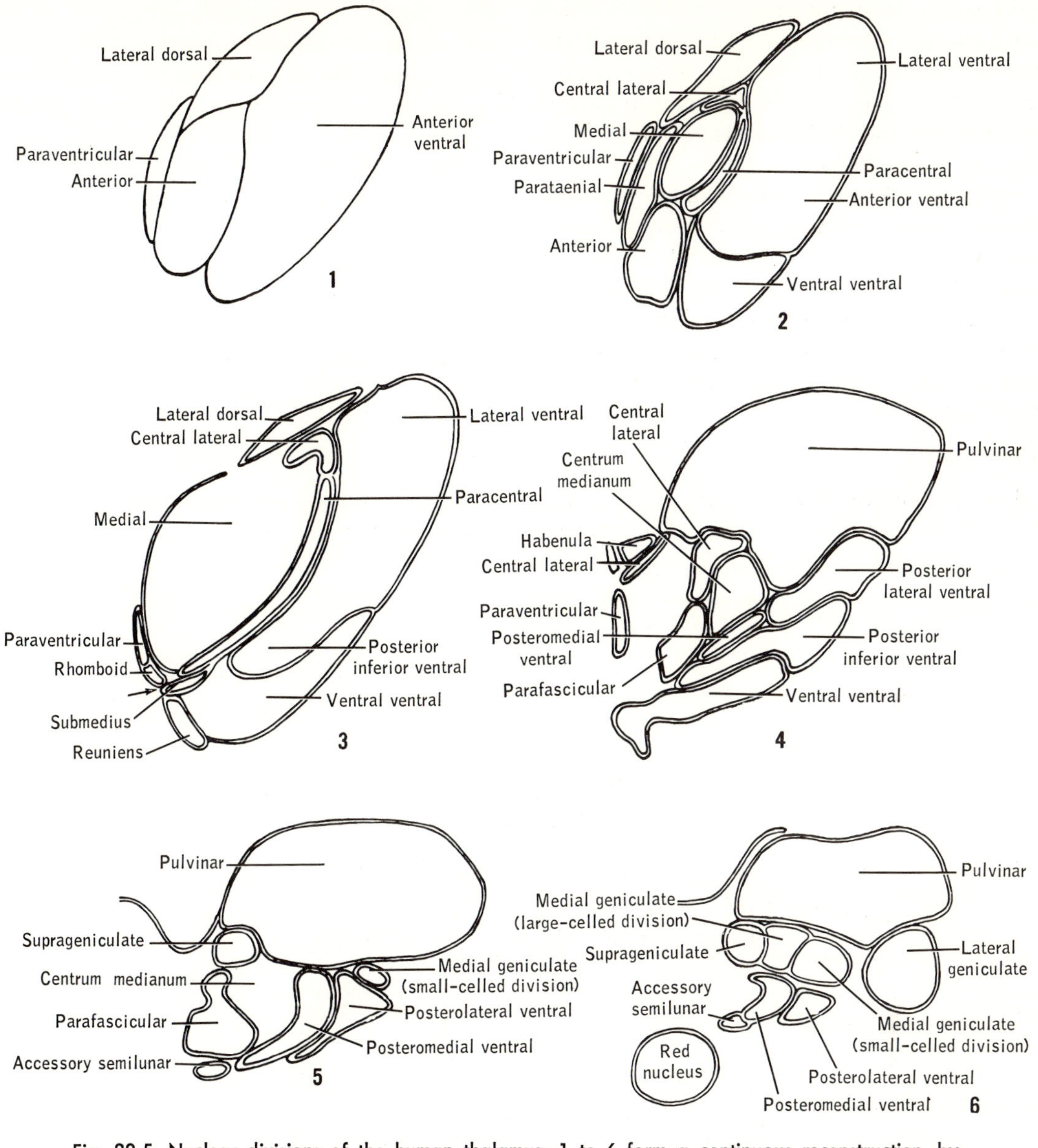

Fig. 22-5. Nuclear divisions of the human thalamus; 1 to 6 form a continuous reconstruction, by slices, of the outlines of the nuclei composing the human thalamus. They are cut in a plane perpendicular to the long axis of the brain stem. The central medial nucleus is not shown, but its location is indicated by an arrow in 3. (*Courtesy of Toncray and Krieg in Peele, The Neuroanatomical Basis for Clinical Neurology, McGraw-Hill Book Company, Inc., Blakiston Division, New York, 1954.*)

perior colliculus via the brachium of the superior colliculus. The efferents (optic radiations) travel through the retrolenticular part of the internal capsule as the geniculocalcarine tract to the cortex along the boundaries of the calcarine fissure (Figs. 9-5, 9-9, 23-10).

Accessory Arcuate (Semilunar) Nucleus. This is a relay center in the SVA system, for taste. The afferents are not definitely known but are possibly in the trigeminothalamic tracts. The efferents are believed to pass through the posterior limb of the internal capsule to reach the extreme ventral end of the postcentral gyrus. (Fig. 23-10.)

Motor System

Anterior Ventral Nucleus. (Fig. 22-8.) This is in the somatic motor system. The afferents arise from the globus pallidus via the fasciculus lenticularis and thalamic fasciculus. The efferents pass through the internal capsule to the frontal cortex.

Lateral Ventral Nucleus. (Fig. 22-9.) This is in the somatic motor system. The afferents are chiefly dentatothalamic fibers from the cerebellum by way of the superior cerebellar brachium. Others may also come from the red nucleus (rubrothalamic). The efferents travel through the posterior limb of the internal capsule to motor area 4 and to the premotor cortex, area 6.

Association Nuclei

Anterior Nucleus (Fig. 22-10.)

The afferents are chiefly fibers of the mammillothalamic tract. The efferent fibers have a wide

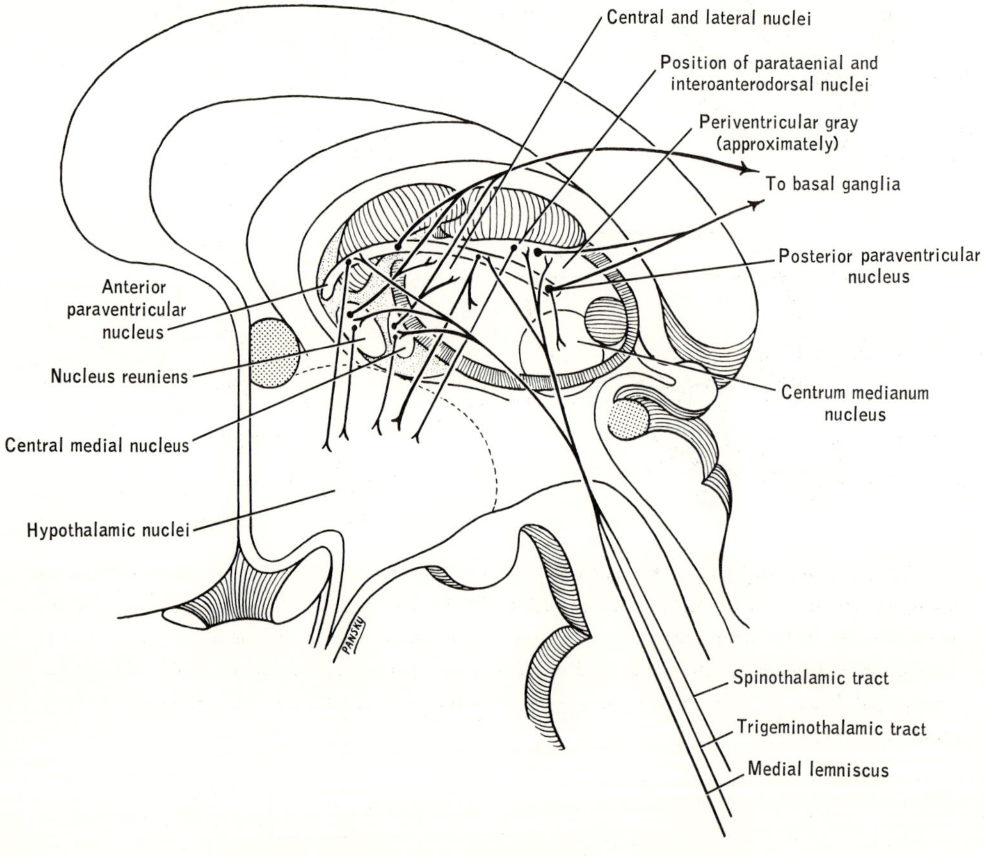

Fig. 22-6. Some of the connections of the midline nuclei.

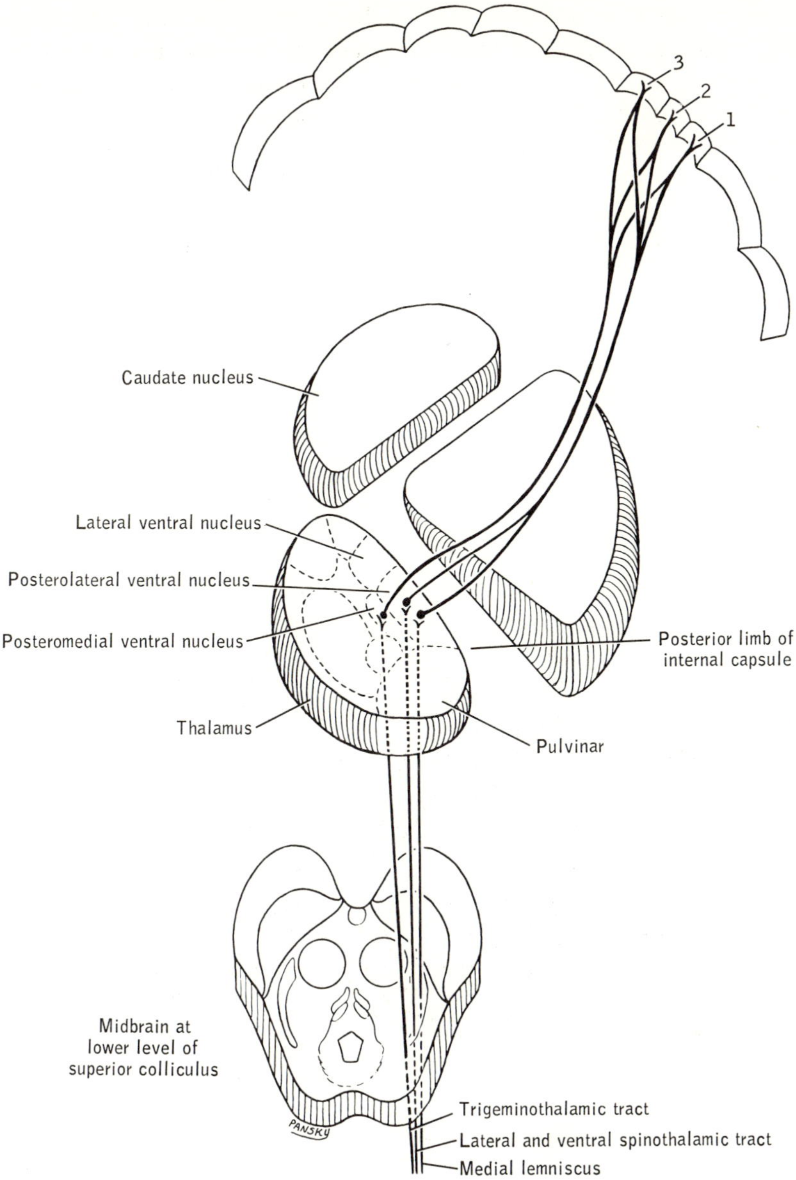

Fig. 22-7. Afferent and efferent fibers of the posterolateral ventral and posteromedial ventral nuclei of the thalamus.

distribution to the cortex of the inferior surface of the frontal pole, to the anterior part of the gyrus cinguli (area 32), to the intermediate part of that gyrus (areas 23 and 24), and to its retrosplenial part (area 29). (It was originally believed that this circuit was related to the olfactory system, but there is now some doubt about this relationship.)

Dorsomedial Nucleus (Fig. 22-10.)

The afferents come from a variety of sources, among them: the prefrontal cortex, hypothalamus, the midline, lateral and ventral posterior thalamic nuclei, putamen, centrum medianum, and pretectal region. Its efferents are also widespread, passing to the hypothalamus, pretectal zone, anterior nucleus of the thalamus, striatum, and frontal lobe of the cortex (areas 8, 9, 19, 11, 12, 45, 46, and 47; Fig. 23-8). Because of its variety of connections, this nucleus may be an integration center for somatic and visceral sensory impulses. Because of its connections to the striatum it may also influence the relationship between sensory and motor activity.

Submedial Nucleus (Fig. 22-10.)

Its afferents are probably similar to but less extensive than those of the dorsomedial nucleus,

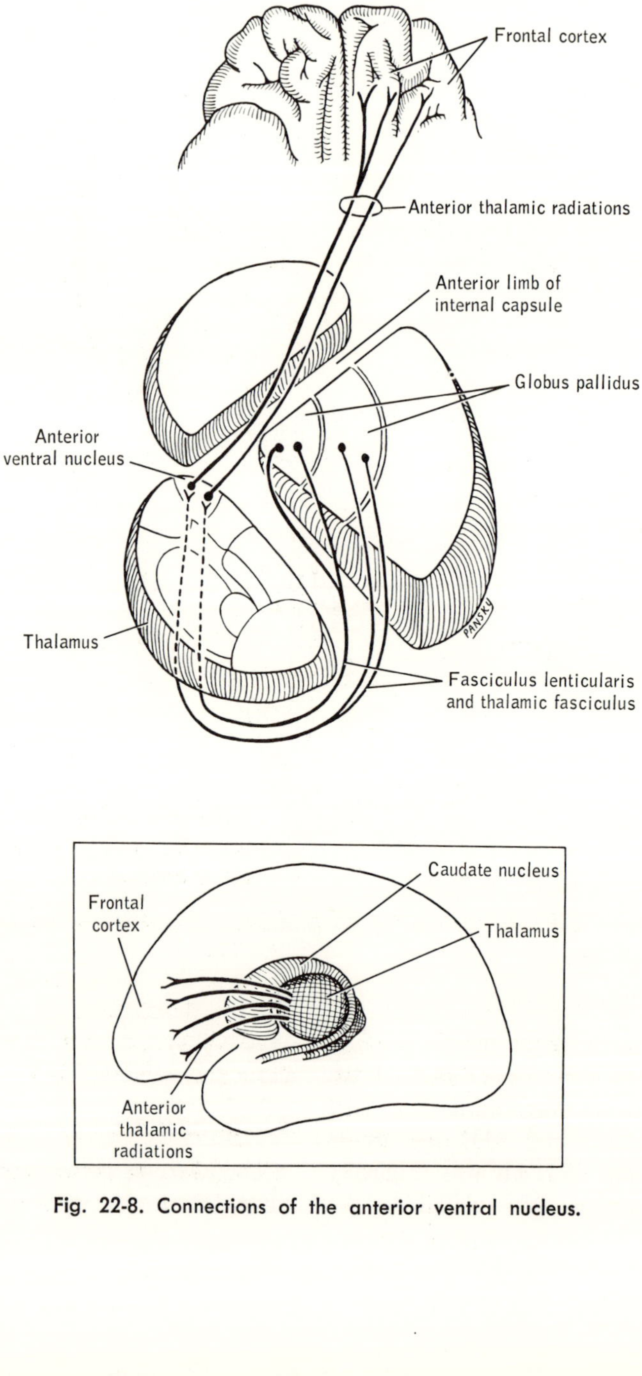

Fig. 22-8. Connections of the anterior ventral nucleus.

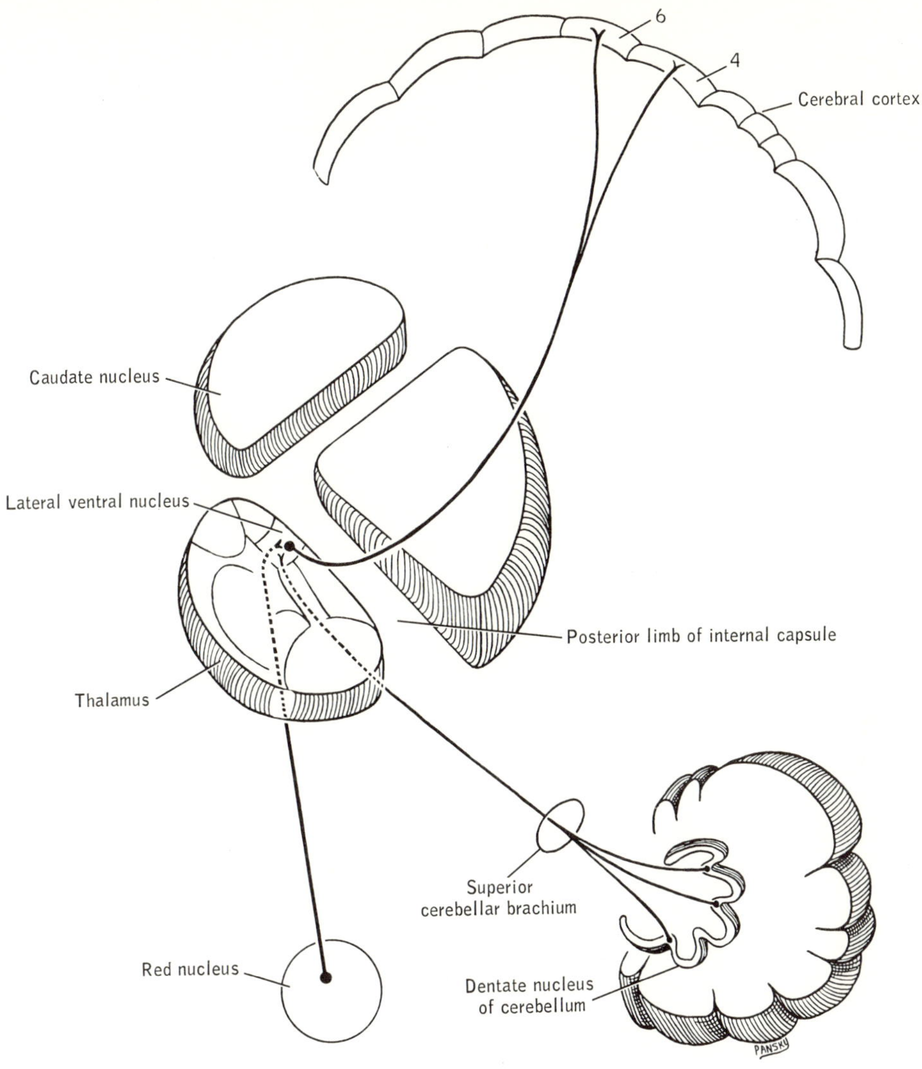

Fig. 22-9. Connections of the lateral ventral nucleus.

since the submedial nucleus is functionally grouped with the dorsomedial. Efferents from it are said to end in cortical areas 8 and 46.

Centrum Medianum Nucleus (Fig. 22-10.)

Although this rather large nucleus is actually one of the intralaminar nuclei, it is usually functionally grouped with the dorsomedial and submedial nuclei. The sources of its afferent fibers are uncertain, but it has been variously reported to receive sensory impulses from cranial nuclei V and X, from the medial geniculate body, the dentate nucleus, and the motor cortex. Its efferents are not clear either, but fibers are thought to go to the dorsomedial nucleus, caudate nucleus, and putamen.

Lateral Dorsal and Lateral Posterior Nuclei (Fig. 22-11.)

These two nuclei, forming the more rostral part of the dorsal tier of the lateral thalamic mass, are both considered association nuclei.

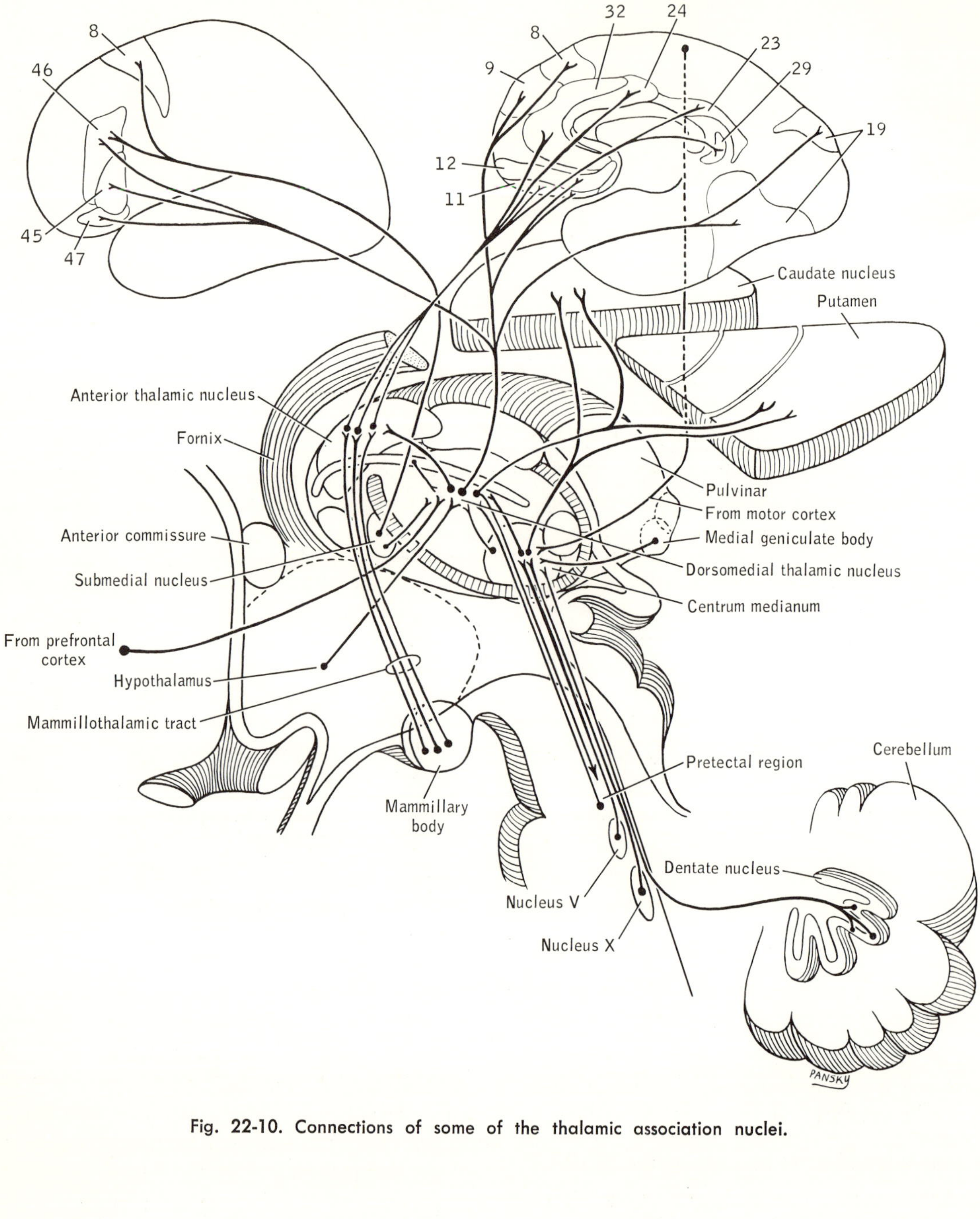

Fig. 22-10. Connections of some of the thalamic association nuclei.

Their afferents come from other thalamic nuclei, especially the ventral lateral and possibly some of the intralaminar nuclei. Their efferents are all thought to end in the parietal lobe, except for the postcentral gyrus.

Pulvinar Nucleus (Fig. 22-11.)

This nucleus is a large association area in the most posterior portion of the dorsal tier of the lateral thalamus. Its afferents arise in other parts of the thalamus, particularly in the nuclei in the ventral part of the lateral mass. It was once believed that both the geniculate nuclei sent fibers here, but this now seems doubtful. The amygdaloid nucleus and the inferior part of the temporal lobe also contribute fibers to this area. The efferents appear to terminate in the superior parietal lobe and in the angular and supramarginal areas. Some may even end in the occipital lobe. Because of the terminations of its efferents in cortical areas adjacent to the primary cortex for general and special somatic sense, it is thought to be intimately concerned with the association of the somatic senses.

Thalamic Reticular System

Up to this point, the thalamus has been considered as an integrating mechanism, both with and without cortical projections. When the latter are present, the cortical projection areas are specific. More recently, through electrical stimulation experiments, a far more extensive relationship between thalamus and cortex has been shown. The nuclei which exert this widespread influence belong to a "diffuse" thalamocortical mechanism, sometimes designated as the *thalamic reticular system*. This system is difficult to define anatomically, partially because many of its nuclei have been listed in other groups. Those nuclei, often classified as "midline," are considered "reticular." They are the *rhomboid, central medial,* and *reuniens*. To these are added four nuclei usually listed with medial group nuclei by most authors: the *centrum medianum, paracentral, central lateral,* and *parafascicular*. In addition, other authors place a portion of the anterior nucleus and the anterior ventral on the list of thalamic reticular nuclei. The *reticular nucleus proper,* often classified with the *lateral thalamic nuclei,* since it does, in part, separate the external medullary lamina from the internal capsule laterally, is also a member of this system. The evidence indicates that all these nuclei of the system are interconnected; the stimulation of one activates others.

It is not necessary to repeat afferent connections of this system since they have been given under the midline and medial group nuclei.

The efferents of this reticular mechanism may influence the cortex by way of other thalamic nuclei: the lateral dorsal, lateral posterior, and pulvinar, belonging to the dorsal tier of the lateral division; and the anterior thalamic nucleus, submedial nucleus, and possibly others of the medial group. (See Chap. 23.)

EVALUATION OF THALAMIC FUNCTION

In lower forms in which a cortex has not yet developed, the thalamus is the highest sensory correlation center. Here, there is an integration of visceral and somatic afferents, and appropriate motor responses are initiated through thalamic connections to the basal nuclei, for somatic activity, and to the hypothalamus for visceral activity. In man, the thalamus still maintains a measure of its original function in the correlation of motor and sensory activities, indicated by the fact that the lateral ventral and the anterior ventral nuclei lie in the neural stream between the cerebellum and cortex and the striatum and cortex, respectively. Nor are other functions, particularly in regard to visceral sense, pain, temperature, and simple touch, completely lost in man, even though the thalamus has been overshadowed by the evolution of the cerebral cortex. Since the cortex is the supreme sensory integration center, afferent impulses, originally fed into the thalamus, must be passed on to the cortex. Thus, the thalamus is now a relay center to the cerebrum, the posterior ventral nuclei and the metathalamus being important in this regard, all projecting to specific primary cortical areas: the gyri bounding the central fissure, including

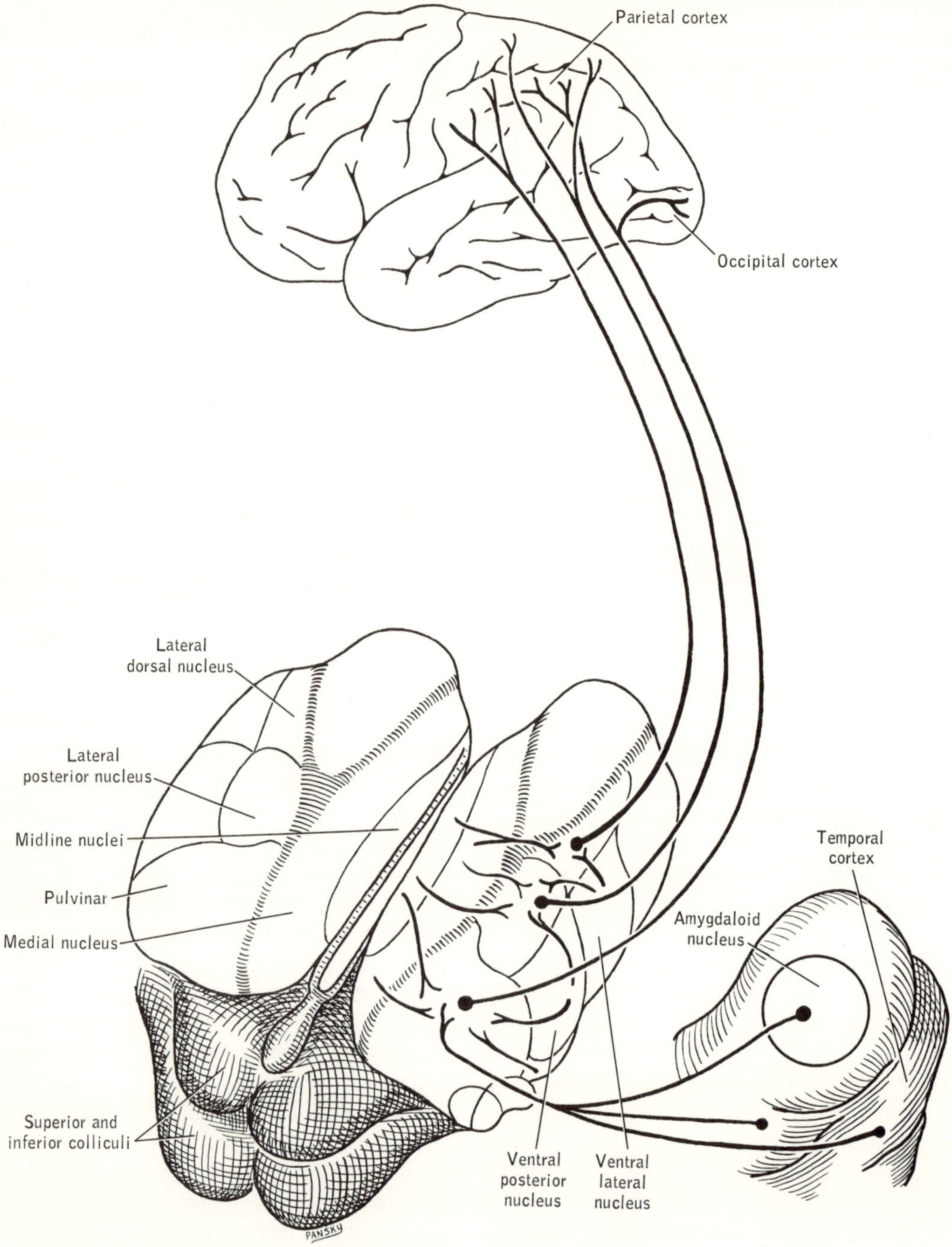

Fig. 22-11. Connections of the lateral dorsal nucleus, the lateral posterior nucleus, and the pulvinar.

areas 1, 2, and 3 (the somatosensory zones); the occipital pole region, area 17 (for vision); and the superior temporal gyrus, areas 41 and 42 (for hearing). These cortical areas, therefore, depend, for their activation, on sensory material already processed by the integration mechanism of the thalamus (Fig. 23-10).

The facilitation of thalamic integration is doubtless the underlying reason why the relay nuclei give rise to many efferent fibers destined for the associative (elaborative) nuclei of the thalamus: the lateral dorsal, lateral posterior, dorsomedial, and pulvinar. These nuclei likewise emit thalamocortical fibers directed not toward the primary sensory areas but to the so-called association cortex. Thus, general somatic impulses are carried to portions anterior and posterior to the pre- and postcentral gyri, the prefrontal and posterior parietal cortex, respectively. The more complex visual impulses reach the cortex rostral to the occipital pole in areas 18 and 19, while the more integrated auditory impulses reach area 22, which adjoins the primary auditory cortex in the temporal lobe (Fig. 23-11).

Intimately related to thalamic function are the two other aspects of sensation: affective and discriminative. On the one hand, *affective* sensation, which pertains to a feeling of mental strain, forms the basis of general bodily well-being or malaise. Included in this category are pain, temperature, agreeableness, disagreeableness, and some tactile sensations. The evidence seems clear that the thalamus itself is related to consciousness and simple recognition of touch, pain, temperature, and pleasant or unpleasant "affect" qualities. Thus, the reactions mediated through thalamic efferents to the hypothalamus or corpus striatum are primarily affective, the resulting reactions being immediate, excessive, and accompanied by general secretory, vasomotor, or other visceral changes.

The second aspect of sensation is *discriminative,* permitting stimuli to be compared as to intensity, locality, and relationships in time or space. On these discriminations the perception of form, size, and texture is based. Movements are also compared as to extent, direction, and sequence. However, although impulses carrying the information necessary for such discernment reach the thalamus and are relayed through and integrated by the thalamus, the cortex is essential in all matters of discrimination. This is amply borne out by the fact that in widespread cortical lesions, discrimination, including sense of position, is lost, while simple recognition of pain or touch, without localization, is retained. So, in contrast to affective sensation, discriminative sensations are precise, not excessive, and often delayed.

It is believed that the dorsomedial nucleus, which receives impulses from the lateral ventral thalamic areas, is the site for appreciation of the "affect" qualities of somatic sensation. Furthermore, the latter are integrated with visceral sensation, the resulting synthesis then being transmitted to the cortex. Hence, the cortex receives a blending of the somatic impulses which underlie cortical discrimination together with the so-called "feeling tone" produced through visceral activities. Therefore, the prefrontal cortex, the recipient of this thalamic discharge, is thought to be the area where discriminative cortical activities reach their greatest refinement.

Another aspect of thalamic function involves the thalamic reticular system. It is possible that this diffuse system may govern both local and general states of cortical response to incoming sensory stimuli. It has been suggested that specific thalamic relay nuclei permit the almost limitless diversified and intricate neural patterns which form the foundation for memory, thought, or complex behavior, while the force and the stimulus necessary to activate and sustain these cerebral circuits may be provided by the thalamic reticular system.

A functional evaluation of the thalamus would be incomplete without some consideration of the corticothalamic fibers. It has been established that any thalamic nucleus that sends its efferents to the cerebral cortex, receives, in turn, fibers coming down from the same cortical area. There are at least two possible reasons for this: (1) the cortex exerts a kind of inhibition influence on the thalamus, and (2) the cortex is a mechanism to make the thalamus more susceptible at certain times to afferent impulses of a particular sort, which in its turn will better influence this same cortical area. It has been suggested that this may be a mechanism for sensory attention. It is also obvious that the connection of the thalamus to the cortex and of the cortex to the thalamus forms a typical reverberating circuit, a mechanism which helps to maintain and amplify stimuli to ensure proper response.

CLINICAL CONSIDERATIONS

Testing

Little specific testing can be done. Because of the nature of the thalamus, with all the sensory and motor fibers passing through it, testing involves examination of the various sensory components over the body, including the special senses; observation of motor activity; and inquiry about the "feeling tone" of the patient.

Types of Pathologic Change

The position of the thalamus more or less protects it from trauma. However, like other portions of the nervous system, its function may be destroyed by tumor, inflammatory disease, or degenerative changes as a sequel to a primary vascular condition (thrombosis, embolism, or hemorrhage).

Specific Pathology

Clinically, there is described a symptom complex known as the *thalamic syndrome,* almost invariably due to thrombosis, in either the posterior cerebral artery or its thalamogeniculate branch. This syndrome is characterized by several findings. First, there is usually a contralateral hemiparesis, often associated with a transitory blockade, resulting from edema of the corticospinal tracts as they descend in the posterior limb of the internal capsule. Second, at the onset there is complete contralateral hemianesthesia and hemianalgesia. Gradually some of the superficial sensibility, such as that to pain, temperature, and gross touch, returns. However, the loss of position sense and stereognosis is usually permanent. There may or may not be sensory disturbances in the face, since the posteromedial ventral nucleus may be far enough medial to escape damage. The lateral geniculate body or its connecting fibers may also be involved in this lesion, which leads to a homonymous hemianopsia. A third and not uncommon finding is hyperaffectivity to superficial stimuli—the sensation of a pin, the movement of a brush, tickling, or touching being very unpleasant or even painful. In some instances there is severe contralateral intractable pain, either spontaneous or related to an ordinarily innocuous superficial cutaneous stimulus such as a movement or an emotional state. Another frequent occurrence is ataxia, characterized by the loss of deep sensibility and the appreciation of movement. In addition, certain involuntary movements may be encountered. The first of these is intention tremor, usually related to damage of the lateral ventral nucleus or its afferents (the dentatothalamic fibers from the cerebellum). When choreoathetoid movements are also seen, it is believed that the pallidothalamic fibers are involved in the lesion. Lastly, sometimes encountered in diseases of this region is the "thalamic hand," found on the contralateral side. In this condition, the fingers are flexed at the metacarpophalangeal joints, while the distal phalanges are extended. The wrist is flexed and pronated. However, in these cases, the muscle tone is actually reduced and the position of the extremity usually can be altered quite easily. Many neurologists feel that "thalamic hand" is due not to damage in the thalamus but rather to lesions in adjacent, nonthalamic structures.

DIVISIONS AND MAJOR NUCLEAR GROUPS OF THE THALAMUS

- Thalamus
  - Medial
    - Anterior nucleus
    - Dorsomedian nucleus
      - Dorsomedial nucleus
      - Submedial nucleus
      - Habenulopeduncular tract nuclei

INTERNAL MEDULLARY LAMINA

  - Lateral
    - Dorsal tier
      - Dorsolateral nucleus
      - Posterolateral nucleus
      - Pulvinar
    - Ventral tier
      - Anterior ventral nucleus
      - Lateral ventral nucleus
      - Posterior ventral nucleus
        - Posteromedial ventral nucleus (arcuate)
        - Accessory arcuate nucleus
        - Posterolateral ventral nucleus
      - Metathalamus
        - Medial geniculate body
        - Lateral geniculate body

MINOR THALAMIC NUCLEI AND FUNCTIONAL REGROUPING

- Nuclei of the midline
  - Rhomboid nucleus
  - Central medial nucleus
  - Nucleus reuniens
- Thalamic reticular nucleus
- Intralaminar nuclei
  - Paracentral nucleus
  - Lateral central nucleus
  - Parafascicular nucleus
  - Centrum medianum

→ Thalamic reticular system (nuclei of the midline, thalamic reticular nucleus, intralaminar nuclei)

- Intralaminar nuclei (as above)
- Nuclei of medial thalmus (see above)
  - Dorsomedial nucleus
  - Lateral central nucleus
  - Habenulopeduncular tract nucleus

→ Medial nuclei (intralaminar nuclei, nuclei of medial thalmus)

SUMMARY

- I. Functional classification
  - *A*. Nuclei of the thalamic reticular system, consisting of reticular nucleus proper plus nuclei of midline and the intralaminar nuclei. Primarily related to the rhinencephalon, hypothalamus, and corpus striatum with no projections to the neocortex.
  - *B*. Cortical relay nuclei (extrinsic), consisting of the nuclei in the ventral tier of the lateral division of the thalamus, including the metathalamus. These receive terminals of all great afferent systems, except the olfactory, and send projection fibers to the neocortex.
  - *C*. Association nuclei (intrinsic), consisting of the anterior nucleus, the medial nuclei, and the nuclei of the dorsal tier of the lateral division of the thalamus, including the pulvinar. These receive terminals from other parts of the brain and send efferents to association areas of the cortex.
- II. Connections
  - *A*. Nuclei of midline, taken as a nonspecific group
    1. Afferents from: spinothalamics; trigeminothalamics; medial lemniscus; visceral systems; corpora quadrigemina; and other thalamic nuclei
    2. Efferents to: hypothalamus; basal ganglia; and other parts of thalamus
    3. Function—cortical activation; hypothalamic stimulation; appreciation of pain(?)
  - *B*. Cortical relay nuclei
    1. Sensory systems
       - *a*. Posteromedial ventral nucleus
         - (1) Afferents from: the trigeminothalamic tracts serving the GSA and GP systems of the head
         - (2) Efferents to: specific primary sensory cortex of the postcentral gyrus (areas 1, 2, and 3)
         - (3) Function—relay general somatic (and proprioceptive) impulses from head to areas 3, 1, 2 on postcentral gyrus
       - *b*. Posterolateral ventral nucleus
         - (1) Afferents from: the lateral and ventral spinothalamic tracts and the medial lemniscus serving the GSA and GP systems of the trunk and extremities
         - (2) Efferents to: specific primary sensory cortex of the postcentral gyrus (areas 1, 2, and 3)
         - (3) Function—relay general somatic (and proprioceptive impulses from limbs and trunk to cortical areas 3, 1, 2 on postcentral gyrus
       - *c*. Medial geniculate body
         - (1) Afferents from: the lateral lemniscus and brachium of the inferior colliculus, serving the SSA system for hearing
         - (2) Efferents to: specific primary sensory cortex of the superior temporal gyrus (areas 41 and 42)
         - (3) Function—relay auditory (special somatic) impulses to cortical areas 41 and 42 on superior temporal gyrus
       - *d*. Lateral geniculate body
         - (1) Afferents from: the optic tract (and perhaps brachium of superior colliculus) serving the SSA system for vision
         - (2) Efferents to: specific primary sensory cortex along the calcarine fissure and at the occipital pole (area 17)
         - (3) Function—relay optic (special somatic) impulses to cortical area 17 along calcarine fissure of occipital lobe
       - *e*. Accessory arcuate
         - (1) Afferents from: probably the

trigeminothalamics serving the SVA system for taste

(2) Efferents to: specific primary cortex at extreme ventral end of postcentral gyrus (area 43)

(3) Function—relay gustatory (special visceral) impulses to cortical area 43 at lower end of postcentral gyrus

2. Motor systems

a. Anterior ventral nucleus

(1) Afferents from: globus pallidus via fasciculus lenticularis and thalamic fasciculus

(2) Efferents to: frontal motor areas

(3) Function—relay of influence of globus pallidus on cortical area 6 and perhaps others for stabilization of voluntary and automatic action

b. Lateral ventral nucleus

(1) Afferents from: dentate nucleus of the cerebellum, via the brachium conjunctivum (some direct, others relayed through red nucleus)

(2) Efferents to: motor and premotor cortex (areas 4 and 6)

(3) Function—relay cerebellar influence directly to motor cortex, area 4 on precentral gyrus; stabilization of voluntary action

C. Association nuclei

1. Anterior nucleus

a. Afferents from: mammillary nuclei via mammillothalamic tract

b. Efferents to: gyrus cinguli (areas 23, 24, 29, and 32)

c. Function—relay impulses from hypothalamus to gyrus cinguli; part of "emotion circuit"

2. Dorsomedial nucleus

a. Afferents from: prefrontal cortex; hypothalamus; pretectal zone; other thalamic nuclei, such as midline, lateral ventral, posterior ventral, and centrum medianum

b. Efferents to: hypothalamus; pretectal zone; anterior nucleus of the thalamus; corpus striatum; and frontal lobe cortex (areas 8, 9, 11, 12, 19, 45, 46, and 47)

c. Function—integration of somatic and visceral function and the motor activity in response to these functions; influences hypothalamic activity

3. Submedial nucleus

a. Afferents from: similar to dorsomedial nucleus

b. Efferents to: cortex (areas 8 and 46)

c. Function—probably similar to 2. above

4. Centrum medianum nucleus

a. Afferents from: uncertain, but it is said that sensory impulses arising in nerves V and X reach this nucleus; medial geniculate body; dentate nucleus; and motor cortex

b. Efferents to: caudate nucleus; putamen; dorsomedial nucleus of the thalamus

c. Function—relay in the reticular activating system; activation of globus pallidus through diffuse afferent system

5. Lateral dorsal and lateral posterior nuclei

a. Afferents from: other thalamic nuclei (i.e., lateral ventral, intralaminar)

b. Efferents to: all parietal cortex, except postcentral gyrus

c. Function—relay from other thalamic nuclei to associative areas of cortex

6. Pulvinar nucleus

a. Afferents from: amygdaloid complex; inferior temporal cortex; other thalamic nuclei, i.e., those in ventral tier of lateral division *b*. Efferents to: cortex of superior parietal lobe; the supramarginal area; the angular gyrus; occipital lobe

c. Function—relay acoustico-visual integration to associative areas of cortex in parietal and occipital lobes

D. Thalamic reticular system

1. Afferents from: see nuclei given above
2. Efferents to: other thalamic nuclei, i.e., lateral dorsal; lateral posterior; pulvinar; anterior; submedial (other medial nuclei?). In this way it influences the cortex.
3. Function—relay in the reticular activating system

23 THE CEREBRUM AS THE HIGHEST CENTER OF THE CENTRAL NERVOUS SYSTEM

STRUCTURE

Gross

The position and relations of the principal sulci and gyri, together with the divisions into lobes, have already been discussed (Chap. 2).

Microscopic

Cortex (Gray Matter)

Cell Types. (Fig. 23-1.) *Pyramidal Cells.* These are the most characteristic cells found in the cortex and are one of the two most numerous. As the name implies, they have the shape of pyramids, the apices of which are directed toward the brain surface as apical dendrites. Other, finer dendrites may sprout from any part of the surface of the cell. The latter usually extend horizontally with branching in the vicinity of the parent cell. The single axon, springing from the base of the cell, is directed internally toward the white matter. In some cases, the axons actually enter the white substance; in others, they terminate in deeper layers of the cortex. Each cell has a large, round, vesicular nucleus and contains distinct Nissl bodies. The size of the cells varies considerably. They are classified as small when their height is 10 to 12 micra; medium, from 20 to 30 micra; large, from 45 to 50 micra; and giant, when the height exceeds 100 micra. These last are the pyramidal cells of Betz.

Stellate Cells (Granule Cells). These are small polygonal or triangular cells with a dark nucleus and a small amount of cytoplasm. They measure 4 to 8 micra at their widest point. Each cell has numerous small dendrites coursing in all directions and a short axon which branches in the vicinity of the cell body. Some of the larger of these cells resemble the pyramidal cells although they are not so large. Their apical dendrites also extend toward the surface while the single axon may enter the white matter.

Fusiform Cells (Spindle). In these, the long axis of the spindle-shaped cell is perpendicular to the surface. A dendrite is attached to each end of the cell. The deeper one ramifies within the same cortical layer containing the cell body, the superficial one, running toward the surface, often reaches the most external layer. The axon springs from the middle or lower part of the cell and runs into the white matter.

Horizontal Cells (of Cajal). These are small spindle- or pear-shaped cells with their axons extending horizontally, parallel to the surface, and remaining, throughout their length, within the cortical layer containing the cell body. The dendrites are short and also remain in this same layer.

Ascending Axon Cells (of Martinotti). These cells are small and polygonal in shape, with short dendrites arborizing in the vicinity of the cell body. Their axons are directed toward the surface, each giving off collaterals to all cortical layers through which they pass.

Intracortical Fibers. (Fig. 23-2.) These may be classified according to their direction as either *radial* or *tangential.* The former run in fine bundles at right angles to the brain surface and include the axons of the pyramidal, fusiform, large stellate and Martinotti cells as well as ascending afferent and association fibers which terminate in the cortex. The tangential fibers run horizontally, parallel to the surface, and often are found in distinct bands. They are of several types: the terminal branches of afferent projection or association fibers, the axons of which usually reach a certain cortical depth and then bifurcate into horizontal branches; the axons of horizontal and granule cells; and the collaterals of the pyramidal and fusiform cells.

Layers. (Fig. 23-3.) The six basic cortical layers usually described are indicated below, starting with the most external.

Molecular or Plexiform (*I*). This layer contains few cells, those present being the small stellate and horizontal types. There is a fairly dense layer of tangential fibers composed of axons of these cells; the dendrites of deeper-lying pyramidal and fusiform cells; and the axon terminals of Martinotti cells.

Outer Granular Layer (*II*). This layer is made up of many closely packed, small pyramidal cells. Their apical dendrites all enter the molecular layer. Their axons pass deep, many ending within the cortex, others entering the white substance. Terminating within this layer are some axons from the deeper Martinotti cells. Dendrites from fusiform cells and still deeper-lying pyramidal

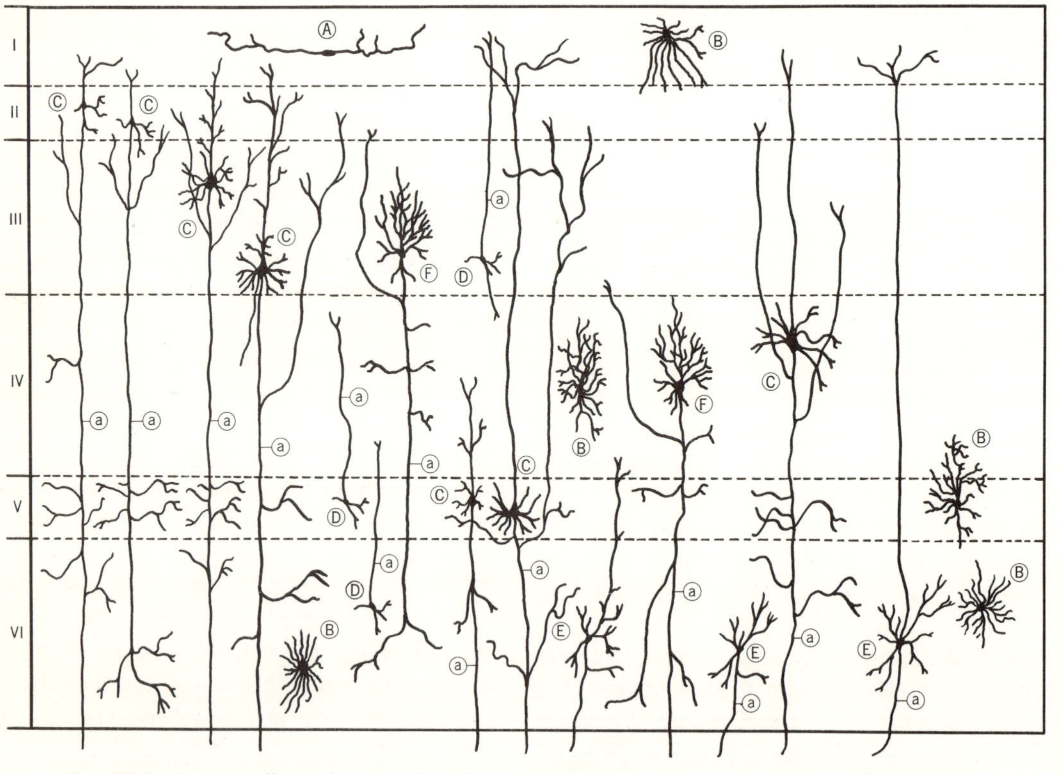

Fig. 23-1. Nerve cells and neuroglia of the cerebral cortex. *A*, horizontal cells of Cajal; *B*, neuroglia; *C*, pyramidal cells, medium and large; *D*, cell of Martinotti; *E*, fusiform cell (spindle cell); *F*, stellate cell (granule cell). Cells are placed according to the layer of the cortex in which they are usually found. Axons are indicated by (*a*).

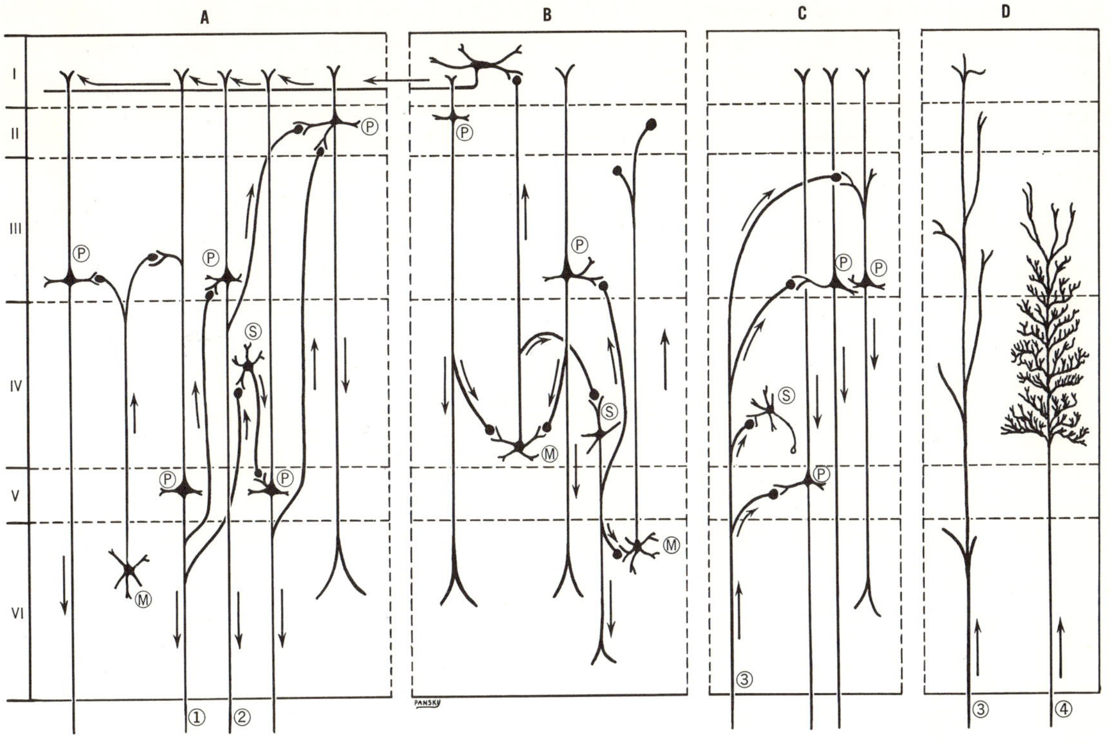

Fig. 23-2. Diagram illustrating cortical fibers. (*Based on data by de No', in Peele, The Neuroanatomical Basis for Clinical Neurology, McGraw-Hill Book Company, Inc., Blakiston Division, New York, 1954.*) The black spheres represent points of synapse. *A*, connections of efferent cortical neurons; *B*, connections of intracortical neurons; *C*, connections of afferent (thalamocortical) neurons; *D*, mode of termination of afferent cortical fibers. *P*, pyramidal cell; *M*, Martinotti cell; *S*, spindle cell. (1) projection efferent; (2) association efferent; (3) specific afferent; (4) association afferent.

cells pass through this layer to reach the molecular layer.

Outer Pyramidal Layer (III). This is made up of pyramidal cells, among which are scattered stellate and Martinotti cells. Sometimes this layer is subdivided into an outer zone, in which lie medium pyramidal cells; and an inner zone, composed of large pyramidal cells. The apical dendrites of both sizes run superficially to reach the molecular layer. Most of the axons run internally, leave the cortex, and enter the white substance. Some, however, remain in the cortex. A band of horizontal fibers, the band of Kaes-Bechterew, may also be seen in the outer portion of this layer.

Inner Granular Layer (IV). The majority of cells are of the small stellate variety. They are numerous and closely packed. The axons of many are short and remain within this layer. Some of the larger cells have axons running to deeper cortical layers. The entire layer contains a large number of horizontal fibers, the so-called *external band of Baillarger*. These are mainly the terminal ramifications of the thalamocortical radiations, since this is the receiving layer for most impulses arising in subcortical levels.

Inner Pyramidal Layer (V). This layer is composed chiefly of medium and large pyramidal cells, among which are also scattered stellate and Martinotti cells. The apical dendrites of the large cells penetrate all the way to the outermost layer of the cortex, those of the small ones apparently ramifying mainly in layer IV. All axons of these cells enter the white substance. In the deeper part of this layer is a considerable band of horizontal fibers, the *internal band of Baillarger.*

Fusiform Layer (VI). The predominant cell type here is the fusiform cell, the long axis of which is perpendicular to the surface. Interspersed among the fusiform cells are cells of Martinotti, stellate cells, and small pyramidal cells. The dendrites of the larger fusiform cells reach the outer plexiform layer, but those of the smaller ones reach layer IV only, while a few may even remain in layer VI. The axons of the fusiform cells enter the white substance. The sixth layer is sometimes further subdivided into an outer portion, containing closely packed, large cells, and an inner portion, containing smaller, more loosely arranged cells.

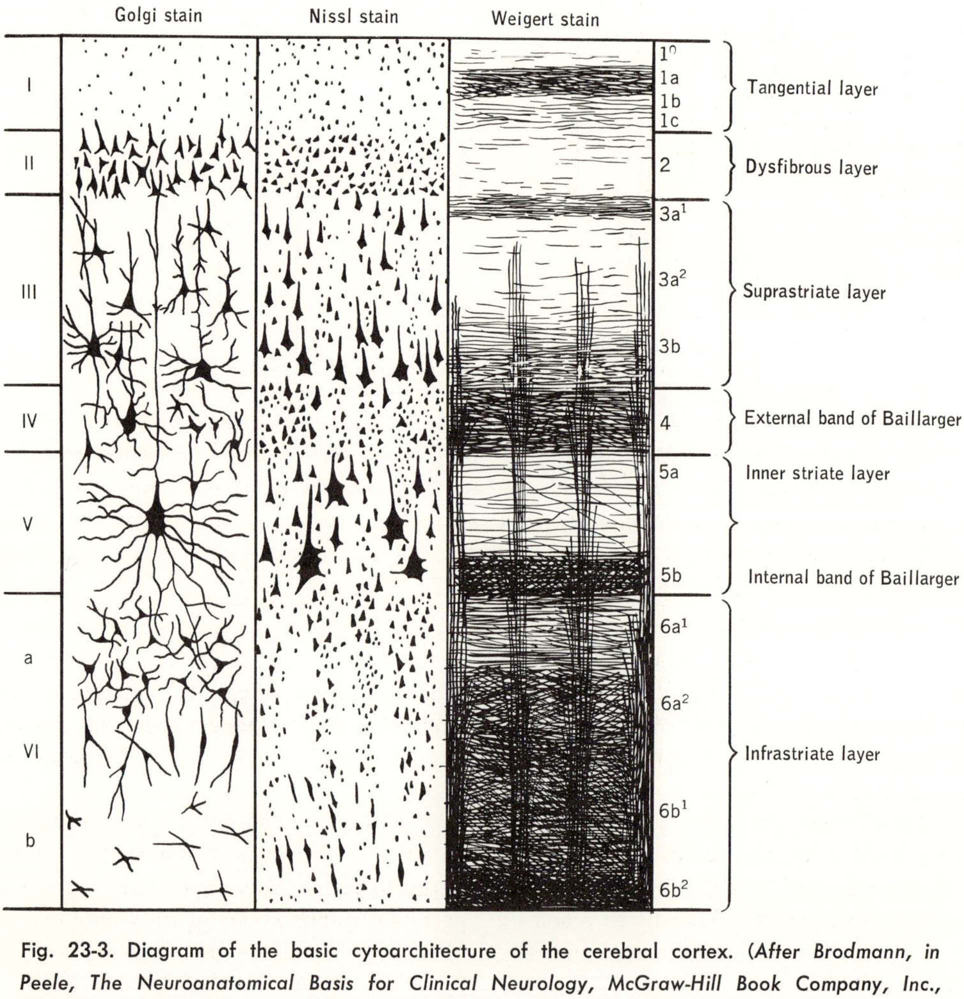

Fig. 23-3. Diagram of the basic cytoarchitecture of the cerebral cortex. (*After Brodmann, in Peele, The Neuroanatomical Basis for Clinical Neurology, McGraw-Hill Book Company, Inc., Blakiston Division, New York,* 1954.) (I) molecular layer; (II) outer granular layer; (III) outer pyramidal layer; (IV) inner granular layer; (V) inner pyramidal layer; (VI) fusiform layer. Certain subdivisions are also indicated: (3a′) band of Bechterew; (4) external band of Baillarger; (5b) internal band of Baillarger.

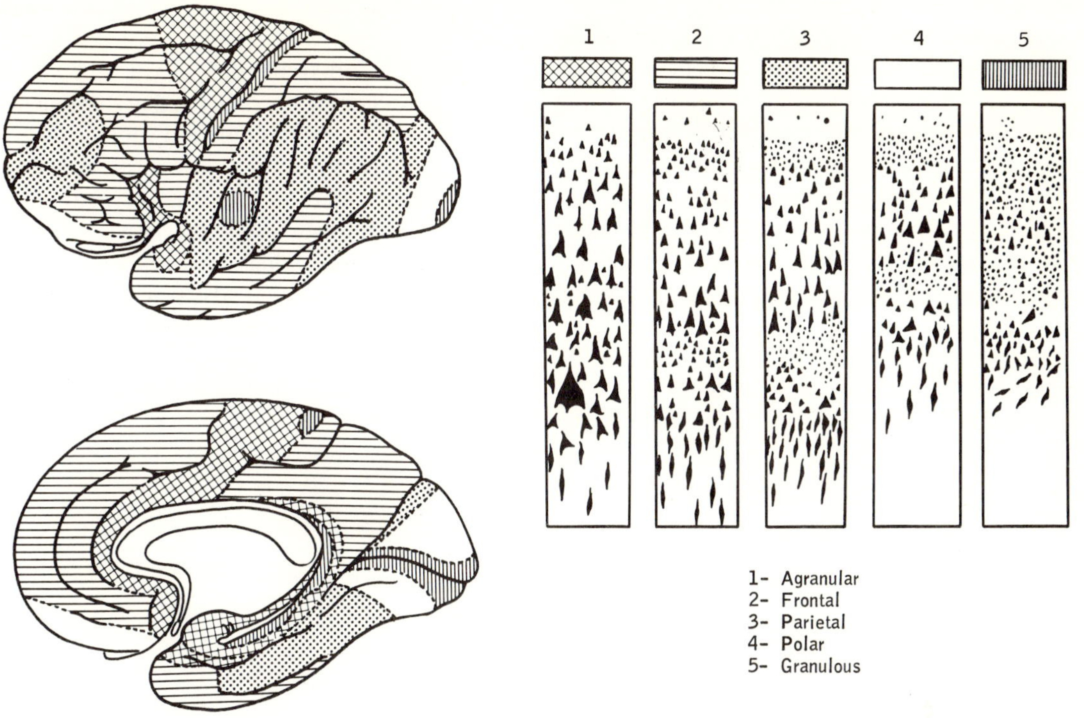

Fig. 23-4. The five fundamental types of cortex. (*After Economo, in Peele, The Neuroanatomical Basis for Clinical Neurology, McGraw-Hill Book Company, Inc., Blakiston Division, New York, 1954.*)

Types of Cortex. (Fig. 23-4.) There is considerable variation in thickness and cellular development in the cortical layers. In addition, there are differences in the total thickness of the cortex, the number of afferent and efferent fibers, and in the number, distinctness, and position of the horizontal bands (band of Kaes-Bechterew; internal and external bands of Baillarger). On the basis of these variations, several types of cortex have been described. For this classification, the reader is referred to the work of von Economo.

FIBERS OF THE CORTEX

Afferent Fibers (Corticipetal)

In any area of the cortex, two types of afferent fibers are recognized; specific and nonspecific.

Specific

These fibers arise in nuclei outside the hemispheres and belong chiefly to the somesthetic, optic, and auditory systems. They terminate in the primary sensory areas.[1]

Somesthetic. (Chap. 8.) These fibers arise in the posteromedial ventral and posterolateral ventral nuclei of the thalamus, relaying sensation of pain, temperature, and light touch upward from the trunk and head. This group of thalamocortical projections is found in the posterior part of the lenticulothalamic portion of the internal capsule (Figs. 2-16, 23-5). *General proprioception* from the same body areas probably follows this same course.

Optic. (Chap. 9.) All the optic radiations arise in the lateral geniculate nucleus. Those arising

[1] Most of them end in cortical layer IV, although some may continue into layer III.

more dorsally in this nucleus, destined to terminate in that part of the occipital lobe above the calcarine fissure, travel in the retrolenticular part of the internal capsule. The remainder of the optic fibers, arising in the lateral and ventral portions of the lateral geniculate body, which terminate in the occipital lobe, caudal to the calcarine fissure, first pass horizontally in the sublenticular part of the posterior limb of the internal capsule before turning posteriorly toward the visual cortex.

Auditory. (Chap. 9.) These fibers arise in the medial geniculate body and, in their course to the superior temporal gyrus, pass horizontally in the sublenticular part of the internal capsule.

Vestibular and General Visceral. (Chaps. 13 and 10.) Ascending fibers belonging to these systems (special proprioception and general visceral afferent, respectively) are known to exist. Even though vague, there is conscious recognition of position and balance and there is an awareness of the viscera. From what is known of the cortical areas which receive these fibers, it seems certain that they must travel in the lenticulothalamic part of the internal capsule. *The special visceral afferent* fibers for taste probably follow this same course.

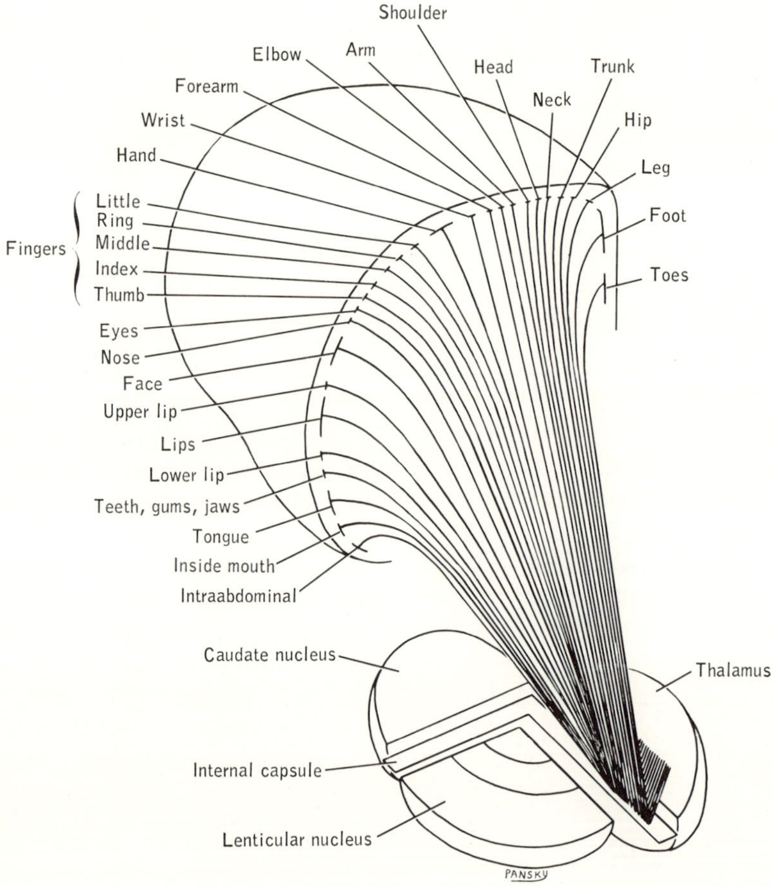

Fig. 23-5. Sensory sequence in the postcentral cortex and internal capsule. (*Adapted from Penfield and Jasper, Epilepsy and the Functional Anatomy of the Human Brain, Little, Brown & Company, Boston, 1954.*)

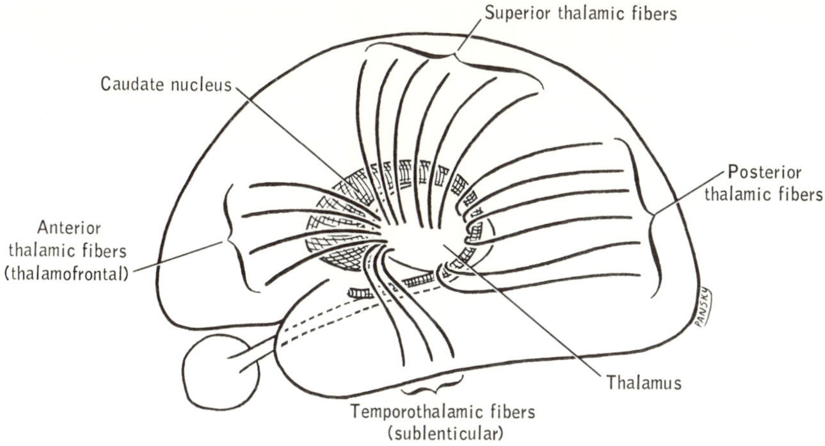

Fig. 23-6. Thalamocortical radiations.

Nonspecific

These are the thalamocortical radiations arising in the elaborative or associational thalamic nuclei (Fig. 23-6). They end in cortical[2] areas adjacent to the primary sensory cortex.

From the dorsomedial nucleus, definitely, and perhaps from some of the lateral nuclei, fibers destined for the frontal lobe ascend through the anterior limb of the internal capsule.

The lateral ventral thalamic nucleus sends its fibers into the rostral part of the lenticulothalamic part of the internal capsule for distribution to the frontal lobe.[3]

The lateral and posterior nuclei project mainly to the parietal and occipital lobes through the retrolenticular part of the internal capsule.

The anterior thalamic nucleus appears to project through the anterior limb of the internal capsule.

Association Fibers

These fibers arise in one cortical area to terminate in other cortical areas of the same side. They give off branches to several cortical layers.[4] Association fibers may be short, running from one gyrus to its next nearest neighbor (arcuate fibers), or they may be long, extending from the most remote portions of the hemisphere. These bundles have been indicated and the specific ipsilateral cortical connections have already been discussed (Chap. 2).

[2] They terminate chiefly in layer IV and possibly in layer III.

[3] Distribution is mainly in areas 4 and 6.

[4] The chief arborization is in layers II and III, but there are some branches in layers V and VI.

Commissural Fibers

These neurons arise in the cortex of one hemisphere, cross the midline, and are distributed to similar cortical areas of the opposite hemisphere. Their endings are comparable to those of the association fibers.

There are three major pathways by which the two halves of the cerebrum are united across the midline. Two of these, the anterior and hippocampal, interconnect parts of the archipallium. The third, the corpus callosum, by far the largest, unites the two neopallial hemispheres. (Chap. 2.)

Anterior Commissure

The position of this bundle has been noted elsewhere (Chap. 2; Fig. 25-19). It crosses through the lamina terminalis. After crossing, the fibers are found to be arranged in two groups. The rostral group is smaller and consists of fibers uniting the two olfactory bulbs. The caudal group interconnects the pyriform and amygdaloid regions.[5]

Hippocampal Commissure

Its position and relations have been indicated in the sections on gross anatomy (Chap. 2) and the special visceral afferent (olfactory) system (Chap. 11). The fibers unite the two hippocampi and the dentate gyri. At first, these commissural fibers accompany those of the fornix, going through its fimbria and posterior pillars. As the latter converge beneath the splenium of the corpus callosum, the commissural fibers diverge medially, cross the midline,[6] and penetrate the fornix of the opposite side to reach the hippocampus and dentate gyrus.

Corpus Callosum

Its position and important relations have already been indicated in the gross (Chap. 2; Figs. 25-13 to 25-20). With the possible exception of a few fibers from the middle and inferior temporal gyri which may cross in the anterior commissure, all the other neocortical areas are connected through this commissure.

Those fibers from the prefrontal cortexes traverse the most anterior part of the corpus and arch rostrally as soon as the crossing occurs. In the posterior part of the corpus, the fibers interconnecting the occipital lobes bend posteriorly immediately after crossing the midline. The fibers in the middle part run transversely, but after crossing, they sweep superiorly and inferiorly within the hemisphere to reach the appropriate regions of the opposite cortex. The superior fibers, in particular, intermingle with the fibers of the internal capsule in a region known as the *corona radiata*. It should be recalled that the occipital radiations of the corpus callosum form the roof and lateral wall of the posterior horn of the lateral ventricle. The term *tapetum* is often applied to the callosal fibers in this position.

[5] Some investigators now feel that parts of the middle and inferior temporal gyri, which are neocortical, are also united by fibers in the posterior part of the anterior commissure.

[6] The area between the pillars of the fornix where the commissural fibers cross is called the *psalterium*.

Although the complete distribution of all the fibers in the corpus callosum of man is not known, there is evidence for some very specific interconnections. For the sake of completeness, these are given in the footnote below.[7]

Intracortical Fibers (Fig. 23-2.)

The cortex contains many neurons the axons of which remain entirely within the cortical layers. These are chiefly small cells with ascending, horizontal, or short axons. Even the pyramidal, fusiform, and large stellate cells with axons leaving the cortex contribute to the intracortical mechanism by giving collaterals to other cortical layers.[8] This arrangement makes possible a direct synaptic relation between the cells of layer VI and the great afferent systems terminating in layer IV. The pyramidal, fusiform, and large stellate cells in the deeper layers of the cortex

[7] The precentral gyrus is believed to receive fibers from areas 4, 6, 1, 5, and 7 of the other side (area 4 from the opposite 4, 5, and 6, while area 6 receives from the contralateral 6 only). Area 4s transmits to the opposite area 32, and area 6 sends callosal fibers to contralateral 6, 4, 1, 5, and 39. Areas 1, 5, and 39 of the parietal lobe receive fibers from the frontal lobe areas 4 and 6. The parietal cortex appears to transmit callosal fibers from areas 1 and 2 to areas 1, 2, 3, and 4; from area 5 to opposite 5, 3, 2, 1, and 4; from area 7 to the contralateral 7, 5, 2, and 1. In addition, there is some evidence for fibers from the region of the superior parietal lobule reaching the contralateral area 4γ, and for others, originating in the region of the interparietal sulcus, to run to the frontal pole area of the other side. The chief known interconnections between the occipital lobes run through the occipital radiations of the corpus callosum, uniting areas 18 and 19, the visual association areas, on either side. The chief commissural fibers of the temporal lobe, which pass by way of the corpus callosum, unite areas 41 and 42, the auditory receptive zone.

[8] The pyramidal cells found in layers II, III, and IV have some dendrites in their respective layers of origin, but their apical dendrites extend outward to the molecular layer (I). As their axons descend, they give off some recurrent collaterals to their own layer, but mainly horizontal collaterals are distributed to layers V and VI. Furthermore, most of the pyramidal cells in layer V extend their apical dendrites into layer I. However, some of the pyramidal cells in layer V have shorter apical dendrites which reach only to layer IV, while the short, basal dendrites ramify in layer V. The fusiform cells in layer VI show a similar distribution: the superficial dendrites reach layers I through IV; the deep dendrite ramifies within layer VI.

send their axons out of the cortex but have the horizontal type of collateral that runs at right angles to the stem axon into any layer. In addition, recurrent collaterals ascend and ramify in more superficial layers.[9] In this way, any activating impulse reaching a neuron in the efferent layers can spread laterally through this layer or be returned to the superficial layers in the same territory, setting up short, reverberating circuits.

It is obvious that the stellate cells with short axons, the horizontal cells, and the cells with ascending axons (Martinotti) make possible almost limitless intracortical connections: locally, within the same layer; from layer to layer, vertically; and horizontally, from one region to another. Because of this arrangement, it has been suggested that a given vertical strip of cortex is a basic, physiologic unit—a complete intracortical arc, composed of afferent, associational, and efferent connections. Within each strip, afferent impulses are constantly being shifted from superficial to deeper layers and back again to the superficial, finally leaving the cortex through efferent channels. Since all the vertical chains are interconnected horizontally, a cortical excitation induced at a specific point, by the incidence of an afferent impulse, may spread to adjoining units.

Efferent Fibers (Corticifugal)

These are of three sorts: projection, to subcortical centers; association, to other parts of the same hemisphere; and commissural, to the cortex of the contralateral hemisphere.

Projection Fibers

These are axons of pyramidal cells lying mainly in layer V (possibly in other layers). Axons of fusiform cells, especially in layer VI, also contribute to the mass of projection fibers. Among the fibers belonging to this group are corticothalamic, corticospinal, corticobulbar, corticorubral, corticostriate, and corticopontine. The *corticothalamic fibers* will not be described specifically. In general, the same areas of the cortex receiving projection fibers from a particular thalamic nucleus will give rise to descending fibers, which follow the same course to terminate in that nucleus. *Corticospinal fibers* occupy an intermediate position in the rostral region of the lenticulothalamic part of the internal capsule. The fibers are arranged so that those destined for the cervical region lie nearest to the genu while those for the foot are farther posterior (Figs. 2-16, 23-7). The *corticobulbar fibers* descend, from the motor areas of the cortex, in the genu and extreme rostral edge of the lenticulothalamic portion of the internal capsule (Fig. 2-16). *Corticorubral fibers,* arising in the frontal lobe, descend in the lenticulothalamic part of the internal capsule, close to the corticospinal group but lie perhaps slightly farther laterally. *Corticostriate* and *corticonigral fibers* arise from the posterior part of the frontal lobe and the parietal lobe. It seems likely that they lie in the lenticulothalamic part of the capsule, accompanying corticospinal and corticorubral fibers. The corticopontine fibers are usually designated according to their lobe of origin. *Frontopontine* fibers arise in the frontal lobe and descend in the anterior limb of the internal capsule. *Temporopontine* and *occipitopontine* fibers apparently traverse the sublenticular portion of the internal capsule.

At the rostral border of the midbrain, the corticospinal, corticobulbar, and corticopontine fibers from the internal capsule converge into massive bundles called the *cerebral peduncles* (Figs. 2-37, 2-38). Although widely separated just below the diencephalon, the peduncles converge and lie close together at the rostral border of the pons. The fibers running through the basis pedunculi are somewhat segregated, depending on their origin and destination. For convenience, the peduncle can be divided into fifths. In the most medial fifth lie the frontopontine fibers, while the temporopontine fibers lie at the other extreme in the lateral fifth. Between these two, and occupying the intermediate three-fifths, are the corticospinal fibers. In the medial portion of the latter zone are many corticobulbar fibers des-

[9] Most of these manifestations are in layers II and III, but some may even reach layer I.

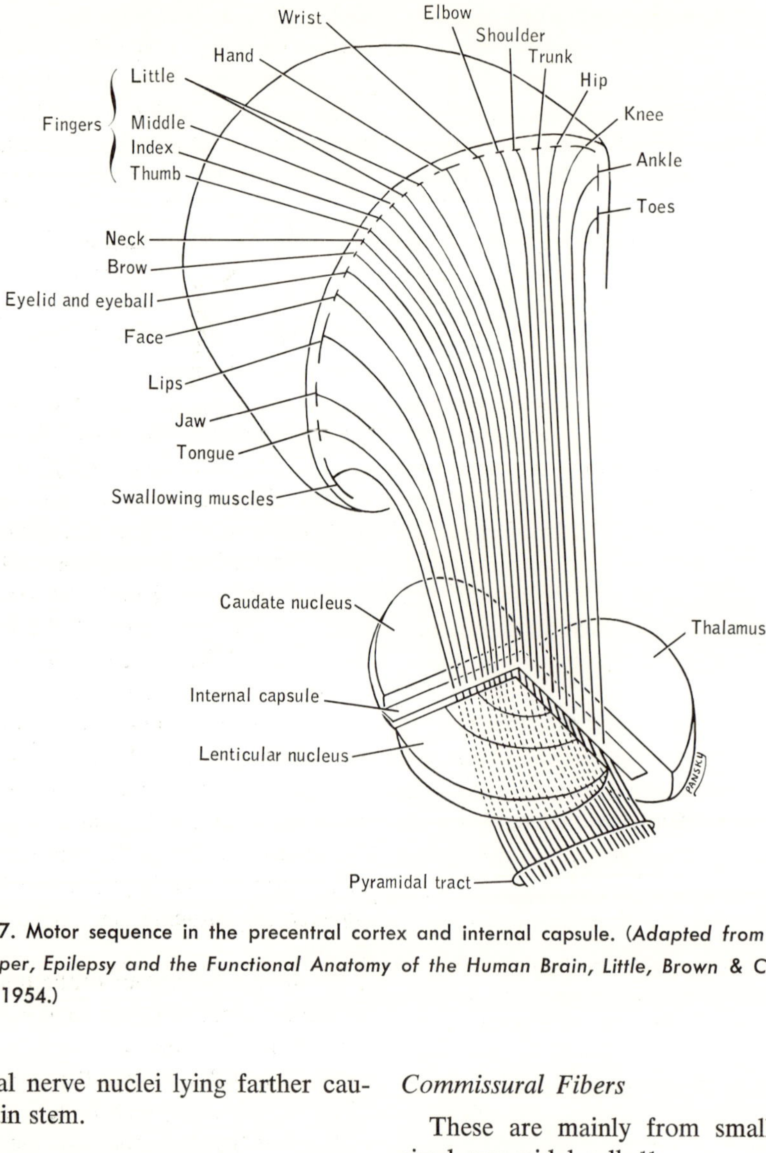

Fig. 23-7. Motor sequence in the precentral cortex and internal capsule. *(Adapted from Penfield and Jasper, Epilepsy and the Functional Anatomy of the Human Brain, Little, Brown & Company, Boston, 1954.)*

tined for cranial nerve nuclei lying farther caudally in the brain stem.

Association Fibers

These arise chiefly from the small or medium-sized pyramidal cells.[10] The fusiform cells of the deepest layer, VI, also contribute association fibers. The large, stellate cells of this same layer may give rise to the very short association fibers, the arcuate, running from one gyrus to the next, by curving beneath the intervening sulci.

[10] Particularly from those cells in layers II and III and to a lesser degree from layer V.

Commissural Fibers

These are mainly from small and medium-sized pyramidal cells.[11]

CORTICAL AREAS

Over the past 50 years, several investigators have mapped the cortex according to variations in structural characteristics. Although the original maps indicated some 20 areas, more recent work has subdivided many of these into a grand total of 200 or more zones. Experimental and

[11] Mainly in layers III and V.

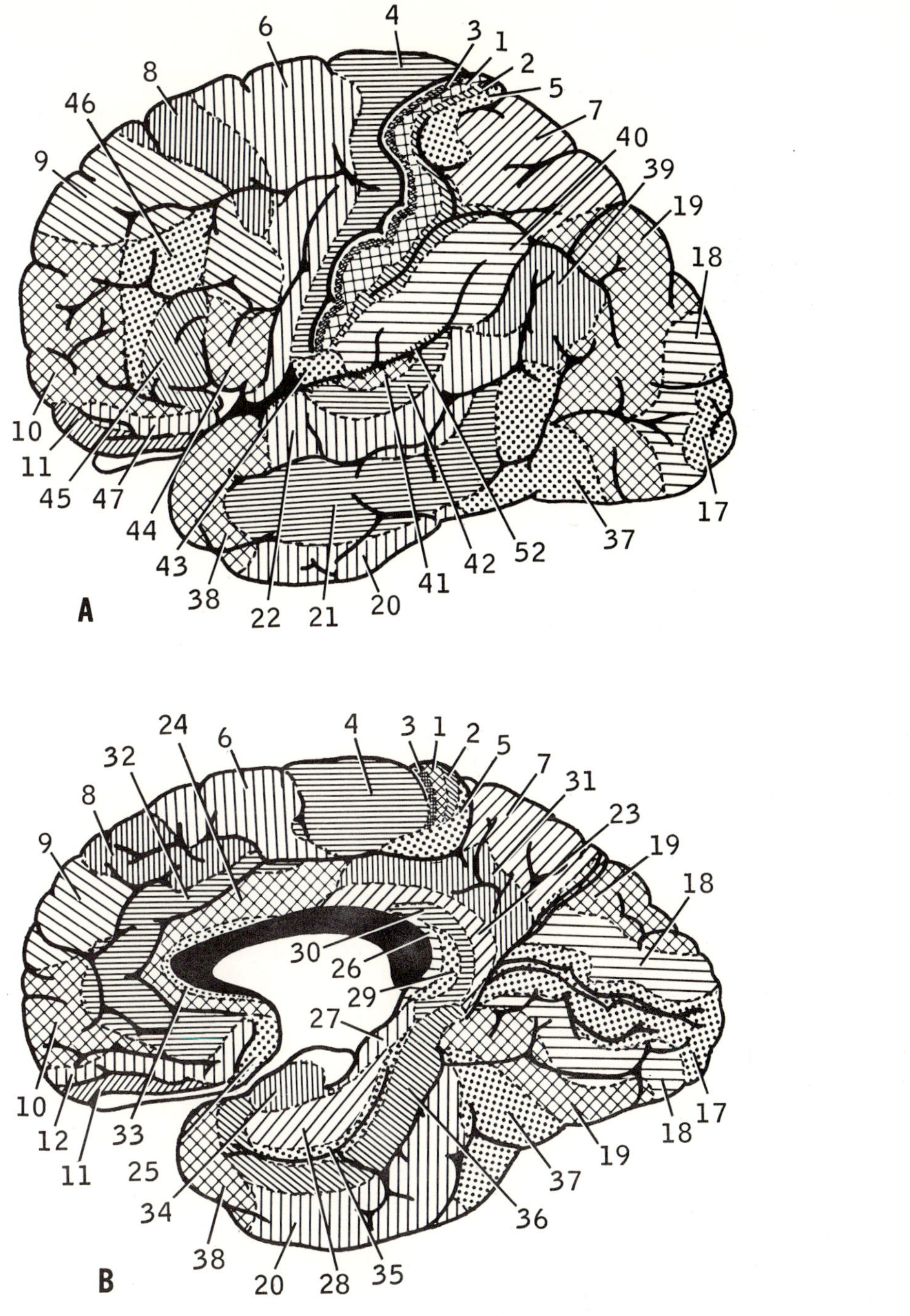

Fig. 23-8. Cytoarchitectural maps of the human cerebral cortex. (*Adapted from Brodmann, in Peele, The Neuroanatomical Basis for Clinical Neurology, McGraw-Hill Book Company, Inc., Blakiston Division, New York,* 1954.) *A.* Lateral surface. *B.* Medial surface.

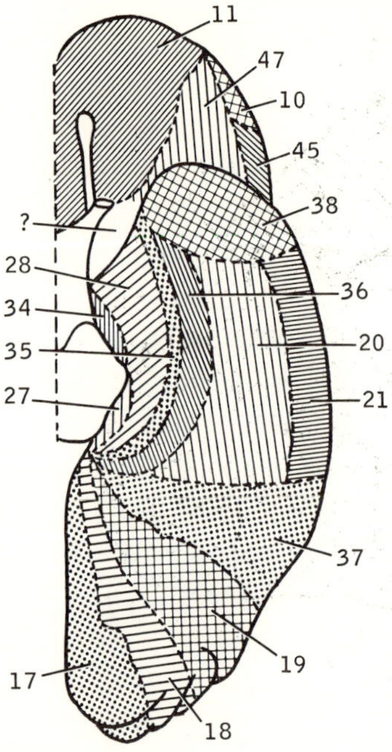

Fig. 23-9. Cytoarchitectural maps of the human cerebral cortex as seen on the basal surface. *(Adapted from Brodmann, in Peele, The Neuroanatomical Basis for Clinical Neurology, McGraw-Hill Book Company, Inc., Blakiston Division, New York, 1954.)*

pathologic research has demonstrated specific functional differences among a large number of these zones. Since many of these functional areas will be frequently referred to, the cortical maps, based upon the investigation of Brodmann[12] (Figs. 23-8, 23-9), have been included.

Primary Sensory Areas (Fig. 23-10.)

Somesthetic

This is the region of the postcentral gyrus, including its medial extension into the paracentral lobule. It receives fibers from both the posteromedial and posterolateral ventral nuclei of the thalamus, which, in turn, act as relays for fibers of the spinothalamic tracts, the medial lemniscus, and the trigeminothalamic bundles. Thus, this cortical zone subserves all general somatic sensibility, both superficial and deep. Each small part on the opposite side of the body has a point-for-point representation on the cortex. According to the cortical maps, the primary somesthetic region includes areas 3, 1, and 2. It should be emphasized that this sensory cortex is not primarily concerned with the recognition of sensory modalities, which is a thalamic function, but is important in discrimination, particularly in the recognition of spatial relations, the appreciation of similarities or differences between objects, and the recognition of stimuli of different intensities.

Visual

This zone, located chiefly on the medial side of the hemisphere, in the walls of the calcarine fissure, includes portions of the cuneus and the lingual gyrus. A variable amount (usually small) of visual cortex extends over onto the lateral aspect of the occipital lobe. This entire visual region is indicated on the maps as area 17. It receives its fibers from the lateral geniculate nucleus via the retrolenticular part of the internal capsule, as the geniculocalcarine tract. The macular portion of the retina is represented on the caudal third of the area. The paracentral retina is represented in the middle portion, while the peripheral retina is represented on the most rostral portion of this area. The upper retina projects to the cuneate portion of area 17, while the lower retina projects to the part belonging to the lingual gyrus. In area 17, the separate impulses from the two retinae are blended into a single image. There are several other prime functions for this area. Among them are the perception of color; the localization of objects in space, related to the optic axis; the recognition of shape; and the discrimination of shape. The final recognition of objects seen, however, depends upon integration in other regions of the hemisphere.

Auditory

This region lies on the upper surface of the superior temporal gyrus, most of it facing the

[12] Although there might be some justification for using other maps, with different designations, Brodmann's work seems to be more generally used.

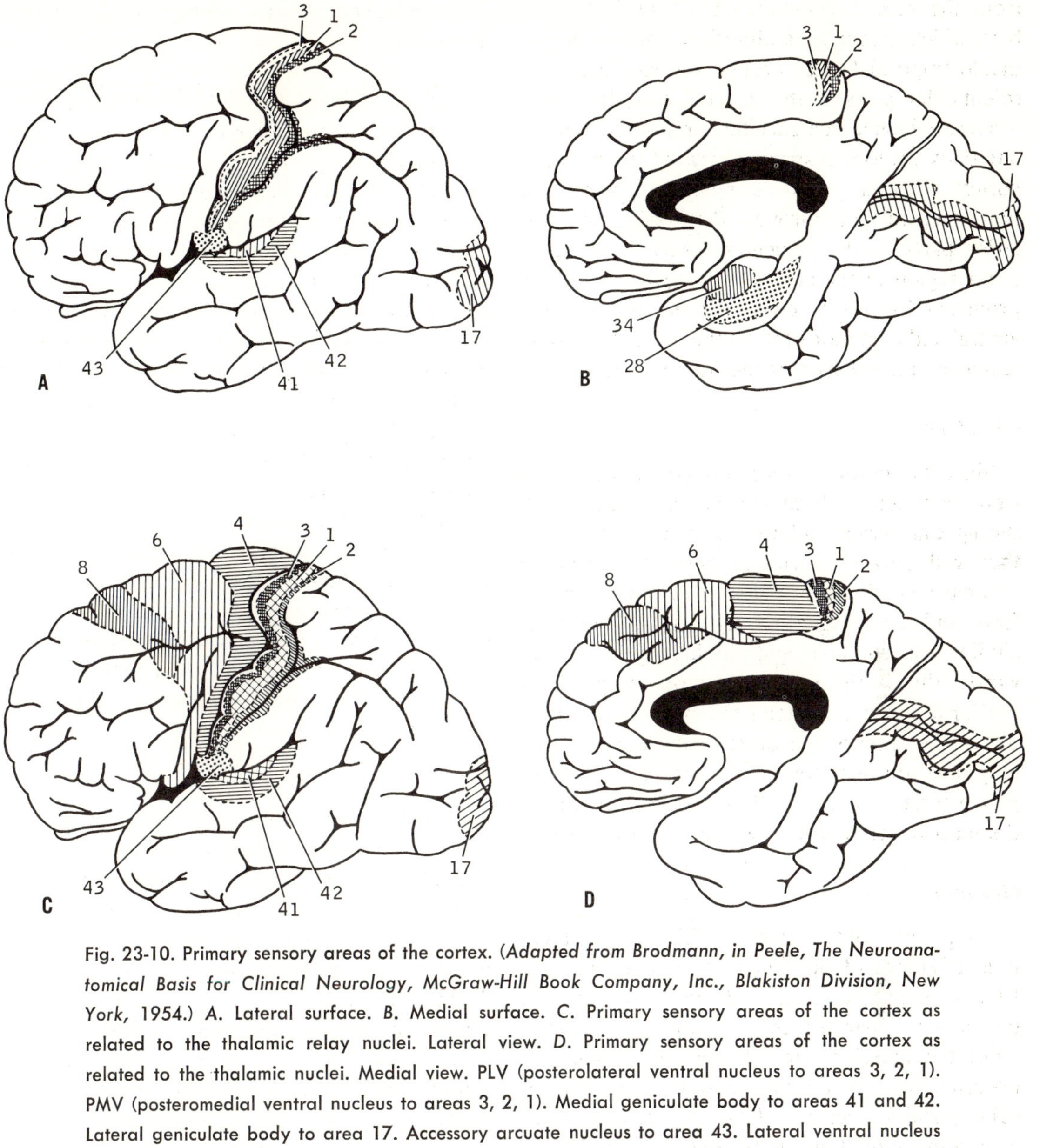

Fig. 23-10. Primary sensory areas of the cortex. (*Adapted from Brodmann, in Peele, The Neuroanatomical Basis for Clinical Neurology, McGraw-Hill Book Company, Inc., Blakiston Division, New York, 1954.*) *A.* Lateral surface. *B.* Medial surface. *C.* Primary sensory areas of the cortex as related to the thalamic relay nuclei. Lateral view. *D.* Primary sensory areas of the cortex as related to the thalamic nuclei. Medial view. PLV (posterolateral ventral nucleus to areas 3, 2, 1). PMV (posteromedial ventral nucleus to areas 3, 2, 1). Medial geniculate body to areas 41 and 42. Lateral geniculate body to area 17. Accessory arcuate nucleus to area 43. Lateral ventral nucleus to areas 4, 6, and 8.

lateral (sylvian) fissure. Here are one or two small gyri, known as the *transverse gyri* (of Heschl), which run transversely across the main gyrus. The more rostral of these is believed to be the primary auditory receptive area, designated on the map as area 41. Immediately surrounding the latter, except for its medial side, is a narrow strip of cortex numbered area 42, which, according to some investigators, should be included as a part of the primary receptive zone. Others consider area 42 to be associative in nature. The auditory receptive cortex receives from the medial geniculate body projection fibers which travel as auditory radiations or geniculotemporal fibers through the sub- and retrolenticular parts of the internal capsule. There is some evidence that specific parts of the geniculate body project to specific parts of the auditory cortex so that impulses resulting from high tones are relayed through the dorsal and anterior parts of the geniculate body to the posterior region of the cortical area; while impulses produced by lower tones, passing through the ventral and posterior parts of the geniculate body, reach the rostral part of the auditory cortex.

Olfactory

Since the cortical areas concerned with smell were completely discussed in connection with the special visceral afferent system (Chap. 11), they will only be reviewed here. The primary cortical receptive zones seem to be the prepyriform and periamygdaloid regions, the latter including the semilunar and ambient gyri. In other words, this is the lateral olfactory gyrus (prepyriform) as it lies along the rostrolateral border of the anterior perforated substance and the gray mass that has covered the amygdaloid complex (periamygdaloid). Both of these represent the most rostral portions of the pyriform lobe.

Gustatory

As pointed out elsewhere (Chap. 11), there is a difference of opinion as to where this area lies. Among the suggested locations are the uncus, or a part of the neighboring temporal lobe; the anterior part of the insula; and the opercular part of the postcentral gyrus. The insular position seems to have the least support. The intimate relationship between taste and smell gives some logic to the uncus, since it is so close to the primary olfactory cortex. More recent evidence indicates that the opercular region, at the foot of the postcentral gyrus, in the region adjacent to the insula, is the primary gustatory cortex, designated as area 43 on the map. In this position, the primary taste cortex lies close to the somatic representation of the tongue and to the motor centers controlling jaw and tongue movements.

Secondary Sensory Areas (Fig. 23-11.)

Heretofore, this discussion has dealt with only a relatively small portion of the cortex and in the light of a specific function, i.e., as the center of sensory reception. Each area of the cortex receives specific sensory impulses from peripheral receptors. On reaching the cortex, these impulses produce sharply defined sensations (vision, touch, etc.). Sensations of position and movements are also accurate. However, although awareness of sensation has now been brought to its highest level, the perceptive level required for the recognition of an object has not yet been attained. This requires the association of the primary stimuli into progressively more complex sensory combinations, which, naturally, necessitates a spreading over a somewhat wider field. Thus, there are regions closely adjoining the primary receptive centers, sometimes called *parasensory areas* or *sensory psychic areas,* which serve to elaborate primary sensory impulses into unisensory perception.

Somesthetic Perception

The secondary cortex for this system has been described as lying around the inferior end of the central fissure, area 43, and a part of the rostral area 40. In addition to its obvious connections to the associative cortex, the primary sensory cortex is strongly connected to other cortical zones.[13] The underlying reasons for the connections of the sensory areas with the motor cortex are obvious, for it is through such interrelations that sensory recognition may initiate voluntary action. However, it may not be clear why there are connections to the more posterior portions of the parietal lobe. This may be explained by the fact that although the primary, together with its adjacent secondary, cortex is capable of integrat-

[13] Thus, area 1 receives fibers from areas 4, 6, 39, 40, 5, and 7, while at the same time it gives efferents to 4, 5, 7, and 39. Although afferents to area 2 have not been proved, efferents from area 2 appear to reach areas 31 and 32. Because of its location, the interconnections of area 3 have not been established.

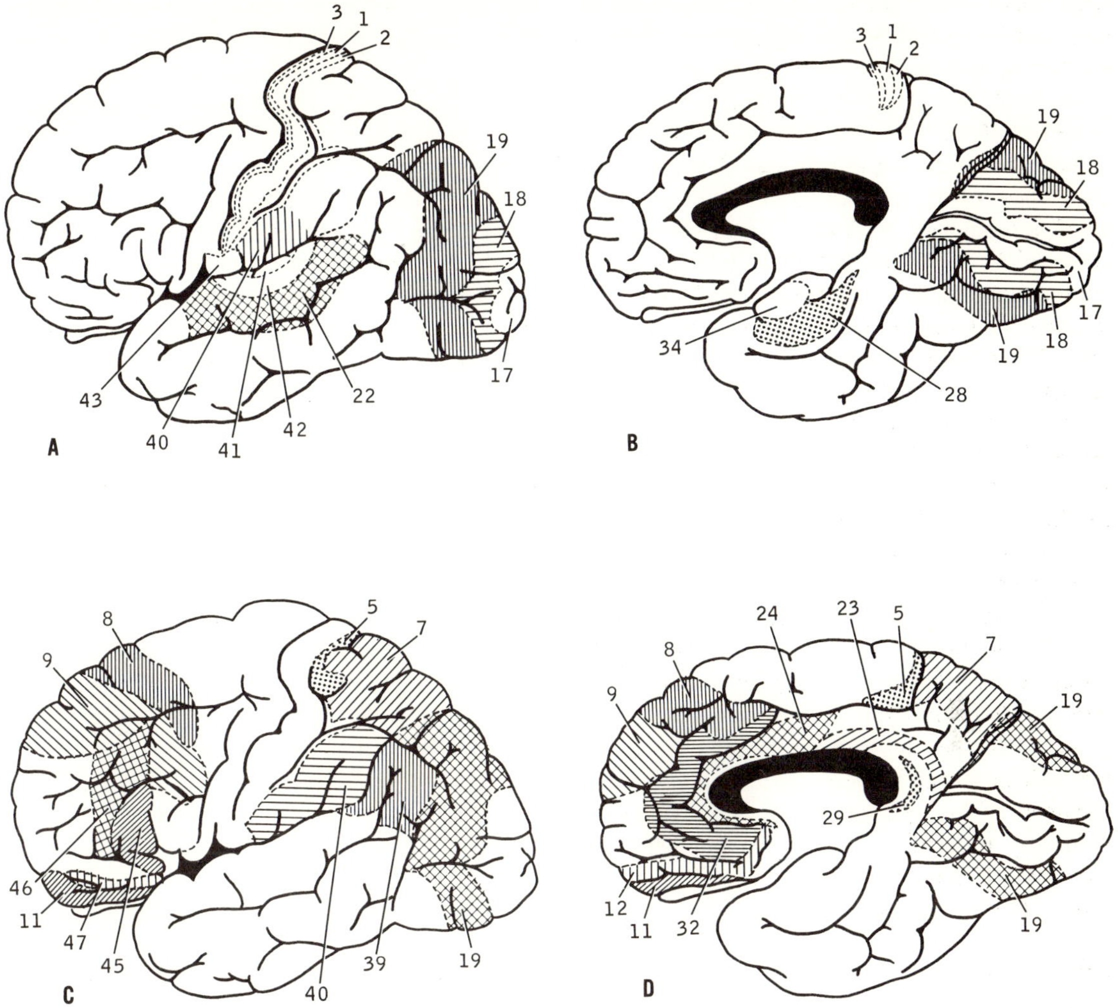

Fig. 23-11. Secondary sensory areas of the cortex. (*Adapted from Brodmann, in Peele, The Neuroanatomical Basis for Clinical Neurology, McGraw-Hill Book Company, Inc., Blakiston Division, New York, 1954.*) A. Lateral surface. *B.* Medial surface. C. Cortex related to associative thalamic nuclei. Lateral view. *D.* Cortex related to associative thalamic nuclei. Medial view. Anterior nucleus to areas 23, 24, 29, and 32. Dorsal medial nucleus to areas 8, 9, 11, 12, 19, 45, 46, 47. Submedial nucleus to areas 8 and 46. Lateral dorsal and lateral posterior nuclei to areas 5, 7, 19, 39, and 40. Pulvinar to areas 5, 7, 19, 39, and 40.

ing, localizing, and comparing afferent impulses of the GSA and GP systems, in order to gain the concept of form, size, or texture, it is necessary to blend tactile, proprioceptive and pressure impulses. This requires further integration, which occurs in the posterior parietal lobe, probably with the assistance of the nonspecific thalamic nuclei and their projections.

Visual Perception

On the maps, the visual perceptive areas are indicated as 18 and 19. It has been shown that the primary visual cortex, area 17, has short association fibers leading into area 18 and, through the latter, to area 19. Both areas 18 and 19 send fibers back into 17, thus forming reverberating circuits.[14] Area 18 is of particular importance, at least as far as the purely visual impulses are concerned. The interpretation of the printed word is thought to be a function of this cortical zone, in the region of the left angular gyrus, including parts of the rostral portion of the occipital lobe and the posterior part of the parietal lobe. The positive spatial localization of an object in relation to self also seems to be a function of this same general region. The visual cortical areas also give rise to various projection fibers, some going to the pons (corticopontine), some to the tectum of the mesencephalon (corticotectal), and still others to the tegmentum (corticotegmental), including the oculomotor complex and possibly the parabducens and abducens nuclei. It is through such circuits as these to the lower centers that the involuntary or automatic movements of the eyes are initiated. Fixation on objects, whether moving or stationary, can be maintained through these cortical connections. Included in this mechanism, too, are the accommodation reflexes involving the pupillary and ciliary muscles in the adjustment to near and far vision. (Chaps. 9 and 14.)

Auditory Perception

The larger part of the superior temporal gyrus surrounding areas 41 and 42 is definitely auditory associative cortex. It is given number 22 on the map and is, of course, strongly interconnected with both areas 41 and 42.[15] The primary auditory cortex perceives simple auditory impulses. However, the integrative mechanism of the associative cortex is required for the appreciation of intricate sounds. The blending of auditory impulses necessary for the interpretation of sounds, such as speech, occurs in this same general region, especially in the dominant hemisphere (the left, for right-handed individuals). There are few projection fibers to lower centers. Corticogeniculate (to the medial geniculate body) and corticotectal fibers (to the roof of the mesencephalon) have been described. Such projection fibers are probably important in the conscious effort to "listen," which involves tension changes on the part of the tensor tympani and stapedius muscles. Also the turning of the head and eyes to follow the source of sound, during conscious and attentive states, uses such cortical circuits originating in areas 41 and 42. That the auditory cortex is in corticocortical relationship to the motor speech area should not be surprising. The connections posteriorly to the visual association areas are logical, when one considers the relationship between sight and sound.

Olfactory Perception

The chief associative olfactory region seems to be the entorhinal area, which includes most of the rostral portion of the hippocampal gyrus and is designated on the map as area 28. This area shows many associative connections to the neocortex of the temporal lobe, for the most part through the perirhinal cortex, area 35 (in the rhinal fissure), and perhaps through the caudally located retrosubicular area 48, which lies behind area 35.[16] These olfactory centers are important in associating smell with both visceral and somatic activities. The connections with the neocortical regions bring smell into a position to initiate voluntary action and bring it also into association with other afferent systems, relating it to the learning and memory complex.

[14] In addition, areas 18 and 19 are interconnected to area 37 and appear to receive fibers from auditory areas 41, 42, and 22.

[15] In addition to these connections, fibers leave the primary auditory cortex to reach area 8 (the eye field); areas 18 and 19; areas 6, 44, 43, and 1 of the frontal and parietal lobes, respectively; and areas 21 and 37, mainly in the inferior and posterior parts of the temporal lobe. The auditory associative cortex also has connections to areas 45 and 10, in the frontal and parietal opercular zones.

[16] It may also be connected with the hippocampal formation around the hippocampal fissure and with the transitional cortex, the presubiculum, and subiculum.

Motor Areas (Fig. 23-12.)

Pyramidal

Impulses which initiate muscular activity may arise in the cortex. The zone chiefly responsible for movements requiring skill lies on the precentral gyrus in area 4.[17] The axons from this area pass by way of the corticospinal and corticobulbar tracts to terminate about cranial or spinal motor cells (Chap. 20). It was once believed that all the so-called pyramidal fibers arose from the giant pyramidal cells (of Betz), in the posterior part of area 4. However, it has been proved that only a very small percentage of fibers in the medullary pyramids, for example, have such an origin and that smaller pyramidal cells in area 4 also contribute to this bundle. Perhaps even more surprising is the revelation that other cortical areas also send fibers into this system.[18] It also appears that motor areas 6 and 8 send out "pyramidal" fibers. The muscles in a specific body region have a definite point-for-point relationship to portions of the precentral gyrus (Fig. 23-7). It is obvious that the areas involving movements of the hand, jaw, tongue, and lips seem disproportionately extensive when compared with those for other, larger parts of the body. This is essential, since greater skill is required in the use of the hand and in speaking than for other types of movement.

The numerous corticocortical interconnections of area 4 are given in the footnote below.[19]

Since further experimentation has been done using various sorts of electrical stimuli applied directly to the cortex, some of the cortical areas shown above have been further subdivided. These divisions are well demonstrated on the maps of Foerster (Fig. 23-13). The type of movement elicited by such stimulation varies. Some movements are characterized by contractions of small muscle groups or even of individual muscles. Such responses are referred to as "isolated" or "discrete." When the muscular contractions are more widespread, they are called

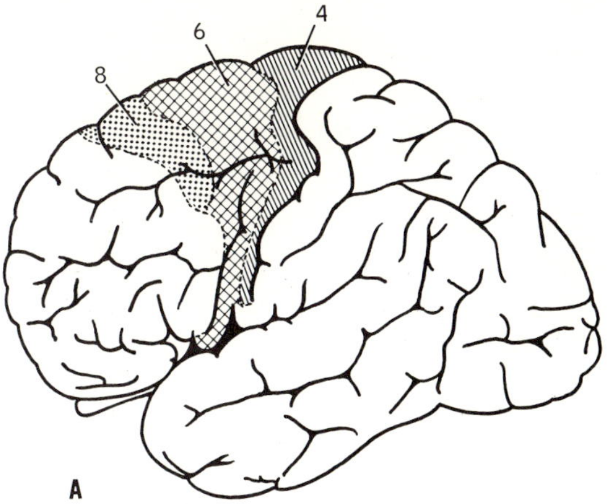

A

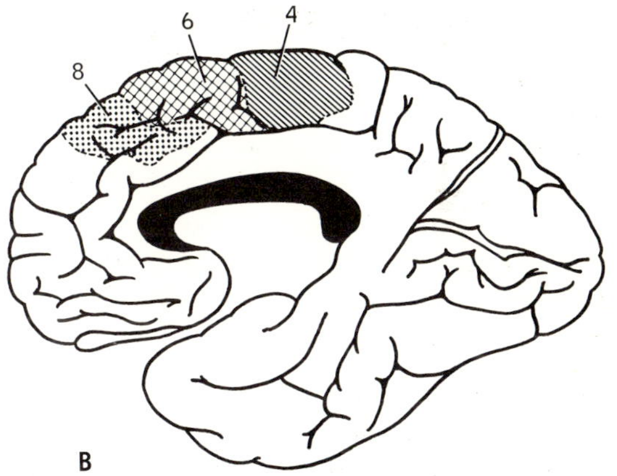

B

Fig. 23-12. Motor areas of the cortex. (*Adapted from Brodmann, in Peele, The Neuroanatomical Basis for Clinical Neurology, McGraw-Hill Book Company, Inc., Blakiston Division, New York, 1954.*) A. Lateral, B. medial surface.

[17] It should be noted that there are also fibers arising in area 4 which are said to belong to the extrapyramidal system.

[18] Areas 3, 1, 2, 5, and 7 give rise to pyramidal fibers in lower animals.

[19] It receives fibers from areas 6, 8, 9, and 10 of the frontal lobe; from areas 3, 1, 2, 5, and 7 (possibly 39 and 40) of the parietal lobe; and areas 21 and 22 of the temporal lobe. From the opposite hemisphere, it receives fibers from areas 4, 6, 1, 5, and 7. Area 4 sends efferent association fibers to areas 1, 5, 6, 7, and 39 (area 4s also sends fibers to area 32). It should also be recalled that both areas 4 and 6 receive thalamocortical fibers from the anterior and lateral ventral nuclei of the thalamus.

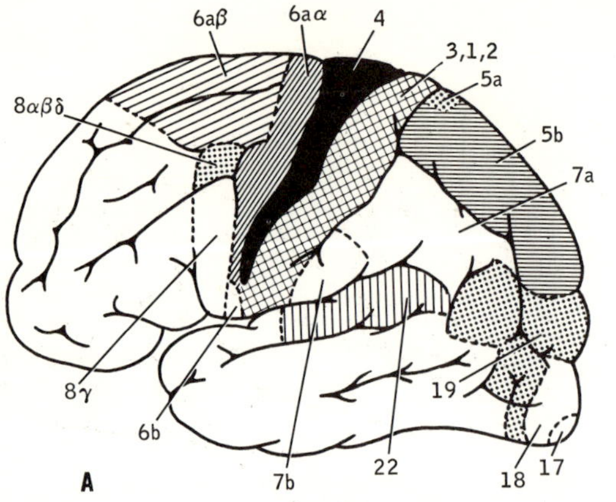

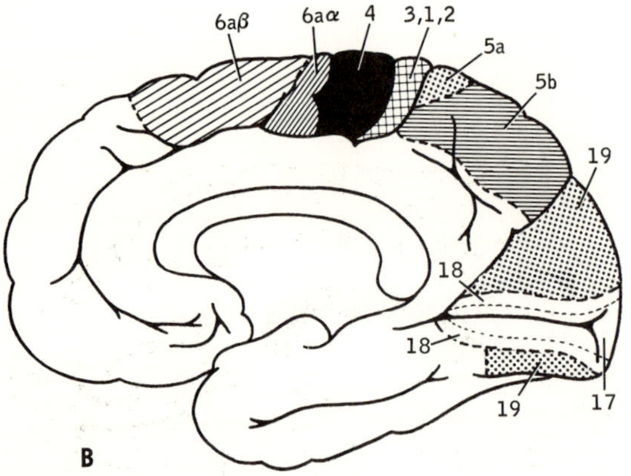

Fig. 23-13. Human cerebral hemispheres showing areas of excitable cortex. (*Adapted from Foerster, in Peele, The Neuroanatomical Basis for Clinical Neurology, McGraw-Hill Book Company, Inc., Blakiston Division, New York, 1954*). *A.* Lateral, *B.* medial surface.

"mass movements," which are further classified as either *adversive,* involving turning of the head, eyes, or limbs to one side; or *synergic,* involving flexion or extension. When area 4 is stimulated, isolated movements occur. When areas 6aα, 3, 1, and 2 are excited, isolated movements also occur, provided area 4 is intact; when area 4 is ablated, stimulation of these regions results in mass movements. If the stimulus is applied to areas 6aβ, 5a, 5b, and 22, head, eyes, and trunk rotate to the opposite side (adversion), together with synergic flexion or extension of the contralateral extremities. The presence or absence of area 4 does not affect this activity. Stimulation of areas 8α, 8β, and 19 results in turning of the head and eyes to the opposite side. The stimulus applied to 6aβ produces rhythmic coordinated movements by muscles controlled by cranial nerves V, VII, IX, X, and XII. The most common flexor synergy pattern is the flexion and abduction of the arm and flexion of the forearm, with the hand pronated and the fist either open or closed. Extension is less commonly seen but is also associated with the pronated hand. With this action in the upper extremity, there is a corresponding flexion pattern in the lower extremity which involves a flexion at the hip and knee with dorsal flexion of the foot and toes. When the extensor pattern occurs, all these movements are exactly opposite in the corresponding joint. As a result of these experiments and other considerations, it was concluded that only that part of the cortex through which isolated movements could be elicited should be considered pyramidal. All the other areas, stimulation of which produces mass movements, are to be considered extrapyramidal.

In concluding the study of this portion of the motor apparatus, the function of the pyramidal system may now be summarized. (1) It is the only initiator of isolated voluntary movements. (2) It facilitates the mechanisms fundamental to the maintenance of muscle tone. (3) It maintains the deep reflexes at low threshold.

Extrapyramidal (Fig. 23-14.)

Any performance which requires precision or dexterity involves the activity of large numbers of muscles. Generally, those muscles located toward the distal ends of the extremities may be considered the "prime movers" in the act. As they contract, regardless of what the action is, the muscles opposing them must either undergo complete inhibition or must at least be relaxed to a certain degree. However, if the finger muscles are to have a solid base against which to work, the wrist must be fixed. This requires the correct amount of tension exerted by the muscles acting on the wrist, in this case called the *synergists.* Other synergists necessarily must act upon the elbow and shoulder, fixing them or permitting the proper amount of movement. For some feats of skill, the muscles of the trunk, both lower extremities, and the opposite upper limb may be involved. This often calls for rapid changes in posture and alterations in the degree of contraction of all the muscles performing the act. The pyramidal system makes possible the selection for use of an individual muscle and coordinates its contraction with the activity of the opposing muscles (antagonists) and the synergists. An entire series of these prime movers can rapidly be thrown into action, and just as rapidly, the necessary alterations are made in antagonists and synergists. The extrapyramidal system makes possible the essential postural adjustments for the activity of the active limbs and maintains the proper tone, so important for easy muscular action.

There appear to be many areas of the cortex which send fibers into the extrapyramidal system. It is believed that the major portion of such fibers arises in areas 4, 4s, and 6. In addition, areas 8, 9, 19, 24, 3, 1, 2, and 7 also contribute to the group. It should now be recalled that these same areas, in various combinations,[20] discharge to the caudate nucleus, putamen, globus pallidus, substantia nigra, subthalamus, red nucleus, midbrain tegmental nuclei, and the reticular nuclei of the lower brain stem.

Belonging to this system are also fibers which end in pontine nuclei as a part of the corticopontocerebellar circuit. The frontopontocerebellar fibers arise in areas 6, 4, and 10. They enter the anterior limb of the internal capsule, traverse the cerebral peduncle in its medial one-fifth, and terminate in the homolateral pontine nuclei. From here fibers arise which cross the midline and ascend in the contralateral brachium pontis

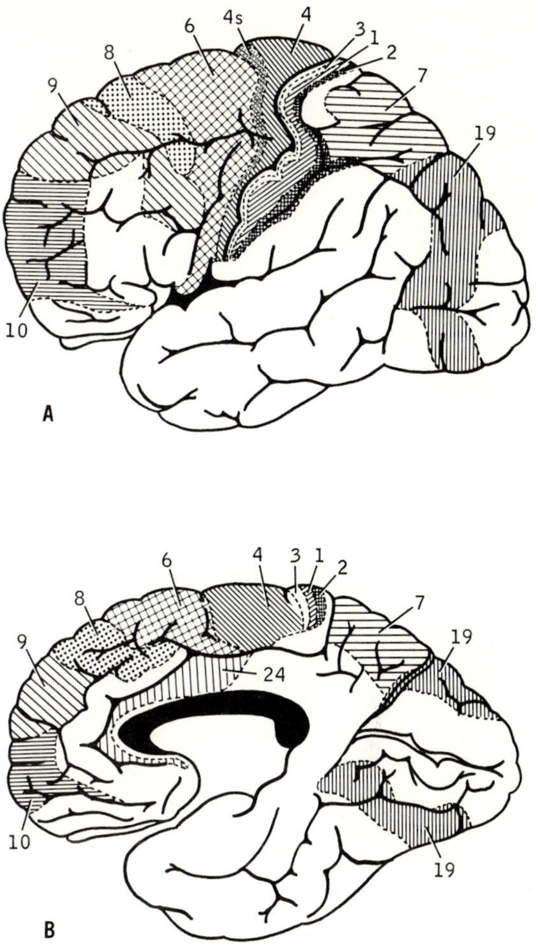

Fig. 23-14. Extrapyramidal area of the cerebral cortex. *A.* Lateral, *B.* medial surface.

to the cerebellum. Temporopontocerebellar fibers arise from the caudal parts of the middle and inferior temporal gyri, enter the posterior limb of the internal capsule through the sublenticular portion, and descend in the lateral one-fifth of the cerebral peduncle. On entering the pons, the disposition is the same as that of the frontopontine group.[21] It is the corticopontocerebellar circuit that brings the influence of the cerebellum to bear upon voluntary action.

[20] Areas 4s, 8, 9, 24, 2, and 19 discharge to the caudate nucleus; area 6 and part of 4 project to the putamen; area 6 sends fibers to the globus pallidus; areas 4, 4s, and 6 project to the substantia nigra, subthalamus, and tegmental nuclei of the midbrain; areas 4 and 6 are also believed to be connected to the red nucleus; area 19 discharges to the putamen; and areas 4s, 8, 24, 2, and 19 have efferents leading to the medullary reticular nuclei, especially to the inhibitor center.

[21] There are also believed to be occipitopontocerebellar fibers arising in area 19 which accompany the temporopontine fibers and parietopontocerebellar fibers arising in the superior parietal lobule.

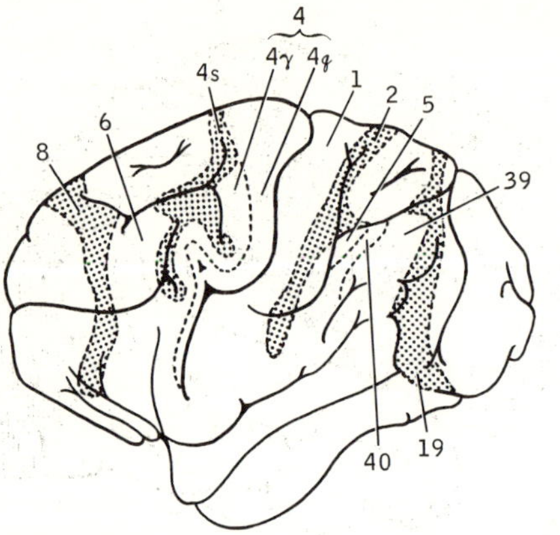

Fig. 23-15. Diagram of the suppressor strips of the brain of the chimpanzee. (*Adapted from Bucy, in Ranson and Clark, Anatomy of the Nervous System, 10th ed., W. B. Saunders Company, Philadelphia, 1959.*)

It has been shown by some investigators that electrical stimulation of certain cortical areas in the absence of large portions of the pyramidal system will produce mass movements. Such areas are 6aα, 6aβ, 3, 1, 2, 5, 8, 19, and 22. However, stimulation of certain other portions of the cortex has quite the opposite effect. Among the first of these zones, called inhibitor strips, to be located was 4s. Stimulation of strip 4s abolishes resistance to passive movement and suppresses movements resulting from the stimulation of area 4γ.[22, 23] Later, several other strips ("s" areas) were found; namely, 8s, 2s, 19s (Fig. 23-15) and 24s. It is claimed that stimulation applied to any of these areas can inhibit or suppress motor responses elicited by activation of area 4γ and relax any existing muscular tension. In fact, it now seems possible that stimulation of any of these suppressor zones can suppress the cortical electrical activity of any part of the cortex. One group of investigators reported that all the "s" zones have corticocortical connections with area 32; and that area 24s may be the most powerful of the suppressor strips, since stimulation here not only inhibits muscular action induced by the activation of area 4γ, prevents afterdischarge, and abolishes deep reflexes, but also, in unanesthetized cats, suppresses normal walking. It is possible, however, that this zone (24s) acts back upon all cortical areas as a regulator of cortical activity, perhaps working in relation to the thalamic and brain stem reticular systems.

In general, then, one might summarize the extrapyramidal system as one which activates large muscle groups and simultaneously suppresses the activity of others in the production of stereotyped movement patterns; suppresses mechanisms underlying tone; and elevates the threshold of deep reflexes. Its function, however, is adapted to the performance of the pyramidal system, for it should be understood that any complex movement involving skill depends upon the proper cooperation between these two portions of the motor apparatus.

CORTICAL ASSOCIATION

Just as the afferent and efferent systems at the lowest levels of the CNS are related through association neurons, so they are related in the cerebrum. It seems likely that the vast majority of the estimated 14 billion cortical neurons is of the association type. The ever-increasing number of these neurons, keeping pace with the evolutionary changes, has increased the possibilities of reaction enormously by opening many more pathways between the sensory and motor areas.

In general, the sensory areas lie posterior to the central fissure. However, it should be obvious that the conscious recognition of many things is far more involved than the possibilities encompassed within the boundaries of unisensory per-

[22] In monkeys, stimulation of 4s leads to the depression of the extensor tone, while stimulation of 4s and 6 together leads to a relaxation of flexor tone. In animals with fully functional pyramidal systems but under light anesthesia, stimulation applied to any part of area 4 inhibited tonus, and this inhibition could be selectively produced by stimulating specific points. This topical inhibition, which these experiments indicated was carried through the pyramidal system, may be important in reciprocal innervation.

[23] More recently, experiments with implanted electrodes in unanesthetized animals failed to indicate suppressor strips.

ception. Thus, it is necessary for associations to be made linking the various parasensory areas into complex neural patterns by which their impulses are blended into multisensory perceptions. For example, tactile and kinesthetic stimuli are combined into perceptions of form, size, and texture. However, the final recognition of an object may require visual or auditory impressions, as well. For these final intricate associations the logical location is the large cortical territory lying among the unisensory perceptive zones.[24]

Even as this receptive-perceptive mechanism is described, it is necessary to consider another large and perhaps most important function of the cortex, *associative memory*. The ability to recall past sensory experiences and to correlate them with traces of former reactions is the basis of learning. The exact mechanism underlying memory is open to speculation. One theory is based upon the knowledge that external influences can modify the structure of various tissues; it is also known that such processes occur in other parts of the nervous system below the cortex. Thus, it is possible that neurons of the cortex represent the ultimate in modifiability. Hence, changes in the cortex, because of its tremendous capacity for modification by the receipt of external stimuli, alter the action of stimuli reaching the cortex at a later time and furnish the basis of conscious and unconscious memory. Others prefer to explain memory on more structural considerations, based upon cerebral architecture. Thus, memory depends upon the setting up by nerve impulses, resulting from externally applied stimuli, of perpetually reverberating circuits through neural side chains.[25] Then, when some facilitating impulse, which may take any form, lowers the threshold of the side chain, a memory circuit is allowed to enter consciousness. Such circuits as these occur in the large associative areas of the cortex and quite probably within some of the other regions, the specific functions of which are not definitely established. That such might be the case has been demonstrated in man, in whom the stimulation of certain regions on the temporal lobe brought out a definite re-creation of past events, or the memory of persons long gone, or the recollection of words of a poem or song. Actually, these memories were complete, would persist as long as the stimulus was applied, and could be repeated if the same stimulus were applied to the same spot. Interestingly enough, the same emotional pattern which was associated with the original event accompanied the recollection, particularly if the emotion were fear. As a matter of fact, cortical stimulation sometimes elicited the emotion alone and not the complete memory picture.

It now should be clear that any object, regardless of its nature, is ultimately represented by a fabric of memories woven together, in a set pattern, from the fibers of the sensory systems which once had been activated by stimuli. Then, at a later time, an impulse, initiated by something seen, heard, or felt, "pulls upon the proper string" and releases the pattern from the intricate maze within the fabric. At this point, the object is recognized or remembered as having been seen or felt or heard before.

Although this discussion has mentioned somesthetic, visual, or auditory perceptions, it should be clear that there are many times when olfactory impulses are also woven into the pattern.

It now becomes necessary to consider another aspect of cortical function. Heretofore, the receptive-perceptive (appreciative) portions have been described. The extensive areas lying rostral to the central fissure must now be discussed.

Within the frontal lobe, primary motor centers have been demonstrated. Thus, in area 4, there are points the activity of which leads to the contraction of individual muscles or small groups of muscles required for special movements of the limbs or face. Superimposed on the primary motor centers are intricate association zones related to the action phase of cortical function.

[24] This includes all the cortex bounded superiorly and rostrally by areas 5 and 7 (the somesthetic psychic area), posteriorly by area 18 (the visual psychic zone), and caudally by area 22 (the auditory psychic area).

[25] This is a dynamic way of "storing" sensory information.

These are the premotor (paramotor) areas essential for complicated activities such as locomotion, mastication, swallowing, and, perhaps most complex of all, speaking.[26]

The responses appropriate for meeting the over-all situation in which the individual finds himself are initiated, it is true, in the cerebral cortex. They probably begin in specific primary sensory areas of the cortex, passing via internuncial neurons into association areas adjoining the primary centers, and finally, after traversing a myriad of association fibers involving widespread regions of the cortex, terminate about the cells in area 4. The latter, then, far from being the center of origin for voluntary action, serves merely as a tool by which the whole cortex exerts its influence over lower motor neurons. In this way, the manner of response to various combinations of stimuli is immeasurably influenced by sensory impressions built up and stored in association regions over an entire lifetime.

Many reactions which pass as voluntary are actually in the nature of cortical reflexes, completely automatic, and apparently occurring without thought as to how they arose. In other words, motor responses follow a regular pattern created by innumerable repetitions of a given stimulus. For example, the driver of a car stops suddenly when a traffic light changes or a pedestrian suddenly appears in the road ahead. In these instances, stimuli applied to the retina initiate impulses which traverse the optic pathway to its primary center in the calcarine cortex. From here, through association fibers, other impulses pass to adjoining areas of the occipital lobe (parasensory) and continue forward through portions of the parietal cortex to end, finally, among the neurons of the frontal motor areas. From here fibers descend to the lumbosacral cord, causing the lower limb to apply the brake. The same sort of reaction can be initiated through the auditory system. Thus, it should be obvious that much of motor activity is initially reflex in character and that its patterns are established through repeated sensory associations (practice) in the cortex.

The olfactory system is also capable of initiating and reinforcing motor activity through cortical connections. It is held by some that the hippocampus is an associative and integrative area for this system. It is likewise possible that it is the principal effector zone. Axons from cells in the hippocampus form the alveus which curves medially over the hippocampus, just below the floor of the inferior horn of the lateral ventricle. These fibers extend medially to form the fimbria of the fornix (the fimbria is comprised of the fibers of origin of the fornix). The majority of fibers in the fornix terminate in the mammillary bodies. Thus, through the fornix, the influence of the hippocampus is brought to bear upon other cortical areas in the following way. Fibers arising in the mammillary bodies pass by way of the mammillothalamic tract to terminate in the anterior nucleus of the thalamus. From the anterior nucleus, some fibers ascend to the frontal lobe (possibly including area 4) and to several areas of the gyrus cinguli.[27] Fibers arising in parts of the gyrus cinguli, especially area 24, terminate in the caudate nucleus, the bulbar inhibitory center, and other areas of the cortex itself, to affect motor activity.

Thus, it can be seen that the cortex influences action in several ways which set it apart from the purely associational systems of the reflex mechanism from which it evolved. Among these ways are the following: it allows for a delay in response to external influences, permits a variety of possible responses, and aids in the integration of responses.

Lying rostral to the premotor area is an extensive region of cortex known as the prefrontal; it is especially highly developed in man. It is known that this region receives strong thalamic projections from the dorsomedial thalamic nucleus, which, likewise, is at its developmental peak in man. Here, the cortex is related to autonomic centers through the hypothalamus and,

[26] The term *praxis* is applied to the performance of these essentially cortical acts, and this performance is based upon the recollection of similar acts executed sometime in the past.

[27] They ascend especially to areas 23, 24, 29, and 32.

via the uncinate fasciculus and cingulum, to the rostral portions of the temporal lobe, to which has been ascribed the function of storage of specific memory. There are also direct and indirect connections with the parietal and occipital association areas. Thus, any or all of the complex and intricate memory patterns developed in other portions of the brain can be assembled here in even more complex pictures. It is these patterns which make possible the higher mental faculties, namely, abstract thinking, judgment, development of ethical standards, and the control of emotional behavior. Thus, on a purely speculative basis, one might consider the possibility that the prefrontal cortex is concerned not primarily with memory or general intelligence but with foresight. Inherent here is the ability not only to recognize a problem as a current incident but to relate it to the past and to anticipate its future possibilities. It is said that the prefrontal regions are responsible for giving direction to, and initiative for, mental processes. Here, too, lies the capacity to make personal adjustments. The influence of this part of the cortex on the control of emotional reactions is probably exerted, together with that of the limbic lobe, by way of the hypothalamus and the autonomic nervous system.

The authors do not wish to leave the impression that there are distinctly functional divisions of the cortex—one, receptive-perceptive, another, expressive, etc. What must be constantly kept in mind is that the divisions represent highly integrated phases of a constant, uninterrupted process and that every action which grows out of it depends upon the working together of all portions of the brain. A destruction of any part of this total mechanism will cause defects in function of the whole cortex, and the severity of the defects will be proportional to the extent of the destruction. However, because of this functional and anatomic division, the symptoms will be more a reflection of defects in *understanding,* when the lesions are in the caudal half of the hemisphere; they will reflect defects in *doing,* when the lesions lie in the rostral half of the cortex.

Limbic System [28]

The term *limbic system* is often used and certainly warrants discussion but it was felt that this should be postponed until the anatomy and physiology of its components had been studied.

There is not complete agreement concerning its constituent parts. However, the following arrangement has found fairly wide acceptance. First, there is a cortical component, the limbic lobe which consists of the subcallosal gyrus, the gyrus cinguli, the hippocampal gyrus together with the hippocampal formation and dentate gyrus. Second, is the subcortical component made up of the amygdaloid complex, the septal nuclei, the hypothalamus, epithalamus and anterior thalamic nucleus. From the foregoing, it should now be obvious that many of these areas play important roles both in the olfactory system (special visceral afferent) and in the control mechanism of the autonomic system (general visceral efferent). Due to these relationships the term *visceral brain* is also applied to this system.

Because of its location, this system is in a position both to receive and associate oral, visceral, sexual and basic sensory impulses and to discharge them through its numerous connections with the hypothalamus. Furthermore, all of the adjacent regions of the hemisphere subserving auditory, visual, gustatory and general somatic functions relay impressions to the hippocampal gyrus through intercortical association fibers. It should also be pointed out that this ancient system, whose cortical components are both archi- and paleopallial, is also anatomically related to the neocortex by way of thalamo and hypothalamocortical connections. Thus, the old and new are able to work together. It has been said that what a person feels is mediated by the visceral brain but what he knows belongs to the neocortex. The limbic system gives the emotional background for intellectual functions.

As just implied, this system is related to emotion. By definition, emotion is a strong feeling

[28] Part of the discussion of both the Limbic and Reticular Activating Systems has been adapted from the *Visceral Brain* and *Reticular Activating System* through the courtesy of the Schering Corporation.

toward an object which usually results in some definite physical expression. It is individually felt or experienced and is outwardly manifested by behavioral patterns which express private feelings on the subject. There are also internal expressions of emotion which are affected by the visceral brain through the autonomic nervous system.

Predominantly emotionally determined, the activities associated with the limbic system are concerned with the preservation of the species and the preservation of self.

This system has been implicated clinically with peptic ulcer and hypertension. It also appears that the secretion of ACTH and the sex hormones are influenced by it.

CONSCIOUSNESS

Without responsiveness to impressions made by the senses, without awareness of one's own thoughts and actions, none of what has been said of cortical function would have significance. From time to time, the site of consciousness has been variously placed. It is difficult to localize it sharply, but there seems little doubt that it is chiefly the result of cortical activity. However, the diencephalon seems to be a prime prerequisite if consciousness is to exist. Destruction at that level often leads to somnolence, while stimulation of the thalamic reticular formation or the reticular formation of the brain stem, transmitted through the thalamus, alters cortical electrical activity. Therefore, no discussion of consciousness would be complete without mention of the reticular activating system (RAS).[28] The parts of this system have already been enumerated (see Chap. 22).

It has been shown that arousal to a waking state can be accomplished in the absence of the specific ascending sensory fiber tracts. In other words, there is an extralemniscal system which receives impulses from all sensory systems and carries them upward through a series of relays to influence widespread cortical areas in an alerting reaction. It extends the length of the CNS from spinal cord through the medulla, pons, midbrain, subthalamus, hypothalamus and the ventromedial thalamus. Direct stimulation of the reticular formation in the brain stem produces changes in the EEG which are identical to those seen in awaking from sleep.

Functions ascribed to the reticular system are: general arousal, the transition from sleep to waking; and general alerting or attentiveness. The relation of the RAS to consciousness is difficult to establish. Consciousness has been defined as an "awareness of environment and of self." It is perhaps alertness that characterizes the waking state, the level of consciousness which is affected over-all by the RAS.

Some investigators have gone so far as to state that the RAS integrates corticofugal impulses into memory patterns and thus is related to the learning process.

It has also been postulated that there are descending corticoreticular pathways from specific cortical areas. Through such pathways the degree of consciousness may be controlled by the cortex, thus setting up a selective mechanism for conscious responsiveness.

Because of its direct relationship to the hypothalamus and also through the influence of the latter on the pituitary gland, the RAS is also implicated in emotions.

CLINICAL CONSIDERATIONS

Testing

Since the cortex represents the ultimate receptive center for the afferent systems and the highest level of control for the voluntary motor apparatus, and since the internal capsule is the great fiber pathway connecting the cortex with lower levels, tests already described for the integrity of each of the systems help in localizing lesions. However, because of the nature of cortical function, most of the tests for cerebral disease must necessarily be designed to show defects in association or integration. Thus, one must determine several facts about the receptive-appreciative areas. Recognition (*gnosis*) should be tested, the patient being asked to identify various common objects by handling them without actually seeing them. Tests for recognition of objects by sight should also be included. The ability to understand common words, both spoken and written, should be investigated. Simple memory tests and tests for normal associations should be given.

The expressive side of cortical function is also examined. Tasks requiring the use of the extremities, particularly the fingers and, to a lesser degree, the toes, should be given the patient. The examiner should listen to the patient's speech, giving attention not only to sound formation, but to the words and to the order in which they are spoken. The ability to write must also be ascertained. The presence or absence of muscle paralysis and its nature and location are determined. The examiner inquires about the possible occurrence of seizures which may involve voluntary muscles, and whether such involuntary contractions are seen over a wide area of the body. If this is the case, it is helpful to find out which sets of muscles contract first. Emotional reactions should be observed, and information concerning social behavior should be sought. It also is logical to investigate the state of activity of the autonomic nervous system.

Several other tools available to the physician are helpful in localizing cortical lesions. The first is the x-ray, particularly the ventriculogram and pneumoencephalogram (Chap. 4), through which the ventricular system and subarachnoid space are visualized. Angiography has also become an important aid in the diagnosis and localization of intracranial lesions. A radiopaque substance, such as Diodrast, is injected into the internal carotid artery just above its origin, outlining the cerebral arteries. Films taken a few seconds later show the venous system (venogram). A second diagnostic tool is the electroencephalogram (EEG), a valuable addition to the neurologist's armamentarium (Fig. 23-16). The basis of electroencephalography is that the human brain generates electrical potentials which can be measured, amplified, and recorded by placing electrodes on the scalp. Changes in amplitude and frequency of the brain waves occur in various disease processes. The EEG is especially valuable in the diagnosis of the convulsive disorders and in the localization of various intracranial lesions such as neoplasms, trauma, abscesses, hematomas, etc. It has likewise been shown that various conditions, actions, and substances, such as drowsiness, sleep, age, hypoxia, acapnia, hypoglycemia, opening and closing of the eye, attention drugs, etc., may alter the "brain wave" pattern. The EGG has its limitations, however, and normal-appearing records may be obtained in spite of clinical evidence of severe organic brain disease.

Another means of detecting the presence of tumors in the cerebrum is the ECHOGRAM (Fig. 23-17). In this procedure, a series of ultrasonic waves is beamed across the head and the echo is recorded. A shift in the midline peak toward the left, for example, would indicate a lesion in the right hemisphere.

Manifestation of Cortical Lesions

Paralysis

In this section, this term is used to apply only to loss or impairment of motor function.

Flaccid. This type of paralysis, together with muscular atrophy, has been discussed in another chapter (Chap. 14).

Spastic. As the name implies, there is an increase in muscle tone, as well as an exaggeration of deep tendon reflexes. It is probably more clinically sound, in dealing with this symptom as related to cortical lesions, to include it as a manifestation encompassed within the complex upper motor neuron syndrome. It seems pointless to become involved in an academic discussion of the effects of lesions purely within the pyramidal or extrapyramidal parts, for even under ideal experimental conditions, it is virtually impossible to separate the two. There is little doubt that most lesions seen in clinical practice involve both parts of the upper motor apparatus. In summary, damage to the pyramidal portion is responsible for lack of voluntary motor response. Hypertonia, hyperreflexia, and clonus are due to loss of the extrapyramidal part. The former is a sign of deficit of the initiating forces normally sup-

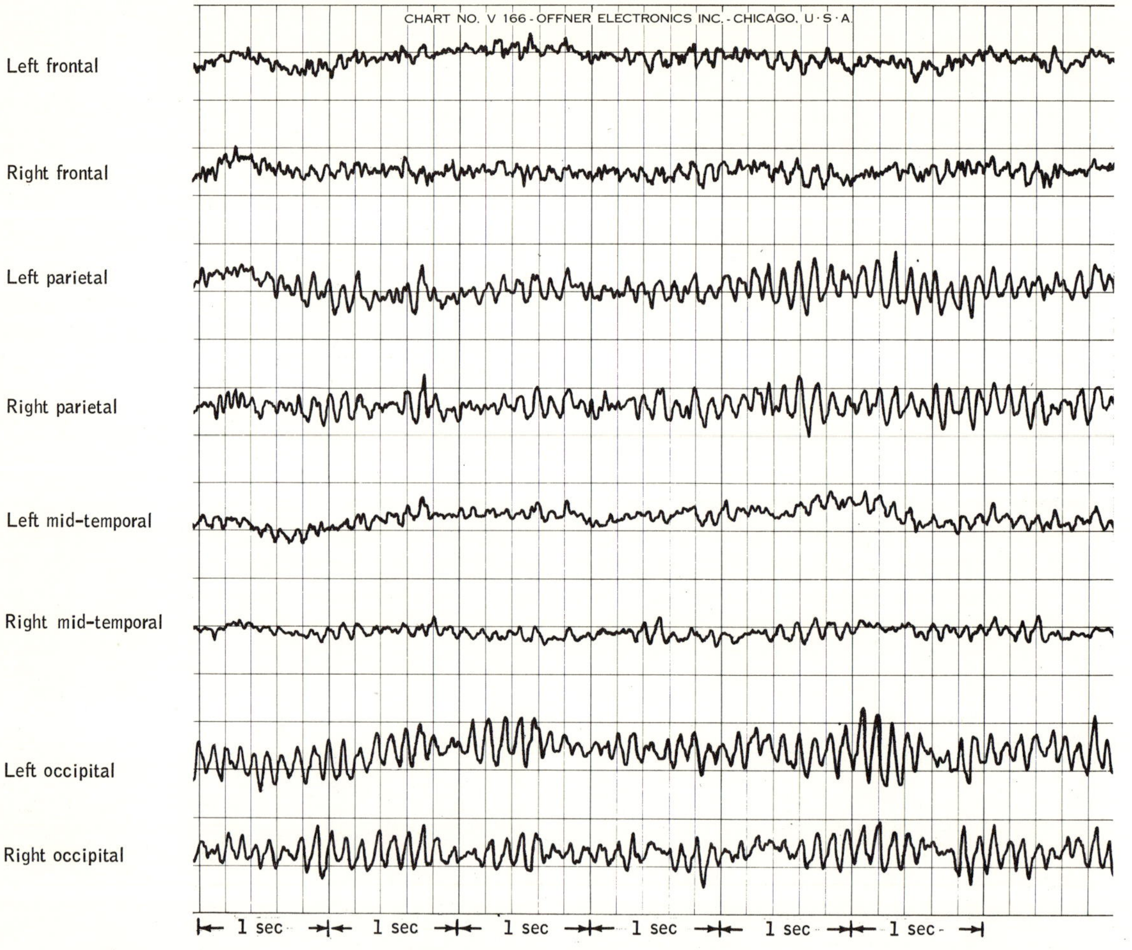

Fig. 23-16. Normal electroencephalogram showing typical patterns from the frontal, parietal, temporal, and occipital areas of both hemispheres.

plied by the pyramidal apparatus; the latter is a sign of release from the normal control exerted over lower centers by the extrapyramidal connections.

Apraxia

In a general way, this is a condition in which there is loss of ability to perform purposeful movements although there is no paralysis. Three varieties have been described; ideational, motor, and ideomotor. *Ideational* apraxia is believed to be due to loss of the ideational concept of the act and is often manifested in diffuse brain disorders such as cerebral arteriosclerosis. *Motor* apraxia is thought to represent a loss of the kinesthetic memory of an act. The purpose of the intended act is usually apparent but the execution remains defective. It is usually associated with lesions on or near the precentral gyrus. *Ideomotor* apraxia refers to a state in which the patient cannot perform an act correctly although old habitual motor acts can be accomplished spontaneously or regularly and often with perseveration. It is associated with lesions of the dominant cerebral hemisphere, frequently involving the supramarginal gyrus.

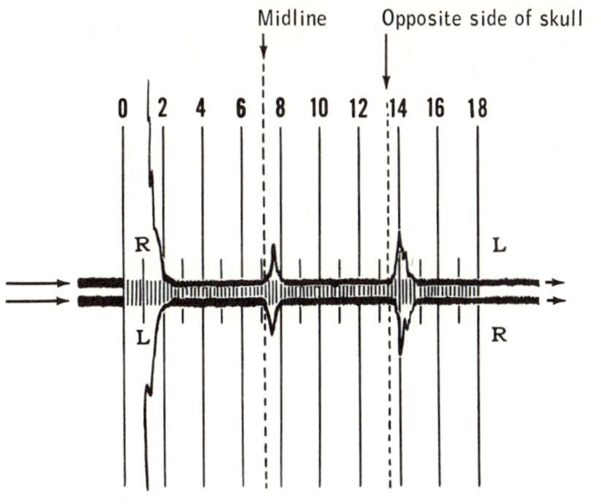

Fig. 23-17. Normal echogram. A tumor would result in a shift in the midline peak toward one side or the other.

Agnosia

This term means the loss of ability to recognize the import of sensory stimuli. In an extensive cortical lesion, the individual may not recognize an object by using all the great afferent routes because of the damage to the major association regions. However, it is not uncommon for only one of the sensory systems to be involved, in which case the term applied to this condition is referable to that particular aspect. For example, *asterognosis* is the inability to recognize the form and nature of objects by touch, while *visual agnosia* is the loss of ability to recognize that which is seen. When used in this specific sense, the lesion is usually located in the association area of that system.

Autotopagnosia (Body Image Agnosia)

This deals with the inability to localize or orient correctly the different parts of the body. Lesions in the posterior portion of the parietal lobe, especially in the dominant hemisphere, may lead to this condition.

Aphasia (Fig. 23-18.)

In general, this may be defined as the loss of power of expression by speech or writing, or it may be a loss of the powers of comprehending spoken or written words. Hence, there are two major types of aphasia, one concerned with the receptive mechanism, *receptive aphasia,* and the other with the expressive part of cortical function, *expressive aphasia.* Actually, most aphasias are not pure but are mixtures of both types (*mixed aphasia*).

Receptive. In this class are usually included two subdivisions, although the term *sensory aphasia* is often used to cover both. In order to distinguish between the two, the term sensory aphasia will be used in the sense of *word deafness.* In such conditions, spoken words are not understood although hearing is normal. Lesions are usually in the superior or posterior part of

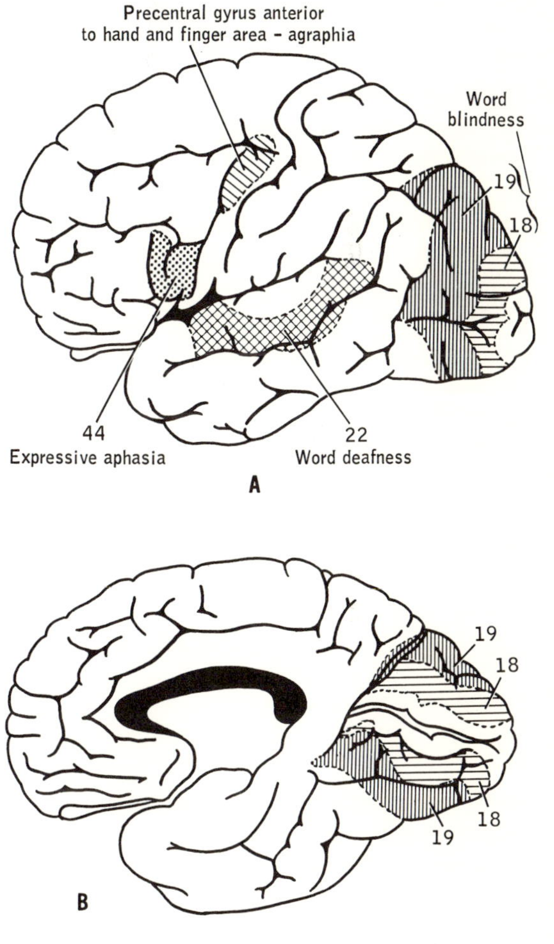

Fig. 23-18. Cortical areas involved in aphasias. A. Lateral, B. medial surface.

the superior temporal gyrus of the dominant hemisphere. The other type of receptive aphasia is *alexia,* or *word blindness*. In these cases, the patient cannot interpret the written word although vision is normal. The lesion is usually in the transition area between the occipital and parietal lobes, in areas 18 and 19. The angular gyrus is often mentioned in this connection.

Expressive (Ataxic Aphasia). Within this class, two motor complexes are involved also. One, usually called simply *motor aphasia,* denotes the loss of ability to carry out the coordinated movements of lips, tongue, palate, and larynx necessary for speaking although there is no paralysis of any of the muscles in the parts mentioned. Lesions causing this condition are found in Broca's speech area 44, which includes the triangular and opercular portions of the inferior frontal gyrus. The term *agraphia* is usually applied to the instances in which the patient cannot write although there is no paralysis of the muscles of the fingers, forearm, or arm. The lesion is probably located in the frontal lobe, just rostral to the hand and finger areas of the precentral gyrus.

Two other aphasias are often mentioned: (1) *amnestic* (*nominal*) *aphasia,* the defective use of words, the inability to name objects, colors, etc., often coupled with a loss of memory for words; (2) *semantic aphasia,* the inability to understand words and phrases or the significance and relations of things in the environment. The latter, in particular, occurs with extensive lesions in the inferior parietal lobule and parts adjacent to it.

Anesthesia

This has been discussed under the GSA system. In cortical lesions, particularly involving areas 3, 1, and 2, there is loss of localization of peripheral stimuli although awareness, especially of pain, and, to a lesser degree, of temperature, is possible at the thalamic level.

Anopsia

In the sense used here, it means a lack of vision due to a cortical lesion in area 17 of the occipital lobe.

Anosmia

In this defect, in which there is a loss of smell, a lesion occurs in such a way as to interrupt the olfactory tracts or to involve the semilunar or ambient gyri or the rostral end of the hippocampal gyrus. In complete anosmia, both sides are affected.

Ageusia

This is inability to taste. A central lesion leading to such a deficit would undoubtedly lie in the parietal opercular region. To be complete, it would have to be bilateral.

Anesthesia, Anopsia, Spastic Paralysis

Because of the representation of nearly all the systems, a lesion in the posterior limb of the internal capsule can produce symptoms referable to the somesthetic senses, vision, hearing to a lesser degree, as well as the voluntary motor system. Nowhere else in the central nervous system could a relatively small lesion produce such widespread effects in so many systems. This is the outstanding characteristic of capsular lesions.

Types of Pathology

The same types of pathologic change noted elsewhere in the nervous system may be encountered here, viz., tumors, congenital malformations, inflammatory disease, degenerative or vascular disease, or trauma.

Symptoms of Specific Pathology

Jacksonian Epilepsy

The signs seen in this condition are motor. It usually begins with clonic convulsive movements of a small muscle or a small group of muscles. These movements, then, may spread, eventually involving most of the muscles on one side of the body. At least in the beginning, the lesion is irritative in nature. It may be due to a tumor, a scar, or gummas of various sorts located within or encroaching upon the precentral gyrus. However, this condition can also be found in the absence of apparent pathologic alterations. Since surgery may be of value in the treatment of this condition, it is important to notice which sets of muscles are first to contract during the seizure, because this usually indicates the focal point of the lesion. Since each of the muscle groups has a constant representation on the precentral gyrus, this observation helps the surgeon determine the site for exploration.

Hemiplegia

Spastic paralysis of muscles of the opposite side of the body, due to an upper motor neuron lesion, has been discussed elsewhere (Chap. 20). In connection with the cortex, a lesion would have to involve a major portion of the precentral gyrus to produce this condition.

Severe Anxiety States or Depression

Thus far, in considering clinical cases, the concern in this book has been primarily with organic disease which has led to a destruction of, or encroachment upon, nuclei or fiber pathways. In a book of this kind, it is not possible even to speculate upon the innumerable functional states which lie in the field of psychiatry or psychology. However, certain surgical procedures, sometimes lumped under the heading of prefrontal lobotomy, deserve some attention. They affect the connections between the frontal lobe and the thalamus. In general, they are most successful in dealing with severe obsessive-compulsive and paranoid states, anxiety and agitated states, schizophrenic psychoses, and intractable pain. In frontal leukotomy or lobotomy, the cortical-subcortical connections in the frontal lobe (usually about the level of the anterior part of the lateral ventricle) are severed. Topectomy refers to the bilateral removal of cortical areas, usually 9 and 10, of the brain. In cortical undercutting operations, performed relatively less frequently, the connections are interrupted at a level just below the cortex. In the operation of thalamotomy, a lesion is made in the dorsomedial nucleus of the thalamus by means of stereotaxic devices. Actually, bilateral leukotomy may transform the depressed patient into one who is almost too easygoing. He may be overcontented with the status quo and lack the drive to pursue a planned course. He may not be able to adapt well to unexpected events. However, although there may be difficulty in abstract thinking, there is no loss of general intelligence, nor is the ability to reason on concrete matters greatly impaired.

SUMMARY

I. Primary sensory—sensory receptive
   A. Somesthetic: postcentral gyrus; termination for GSA system; areas 1, 2, and 3
   B. Visual: on both sides of the calcarine fissure, on medial side of occipital lobe, and at the occipital pole, area 17
   C. Auditory: upper part of the superior temporal gyrus, areas 41 and 42
   D. Olfactory: the prepyriform and periamygdaloid cortex, areas 34 and anterior 28
   E. Gustatory: most ventral end of postcentral gyrus, area 43

II. Secondary sensory—sensory perceptive
   A. Somesthetic: area 40 (and 43?)
   B. Visual: areas 18 and 19
   C. Auditory: area 22
   D. Olfactory: posterior 28 (and 35?)
   E. Gustatory: ?

III. Motor
   A. Pyramidal: predominantly area 4, but also areas 6 and 8. Sends fibers by way of corticobulbar and corticospinal tracts to terminate about lower motor neurons
   B. Extrapyramidal: areas 2, 4γ, 4s, 6, 8, 9, 19, and 24. Sends fibers from
      1. 4s, 8, 9, 19, and 24 to caudate nucleus
      2. 4 and 6 to putamen
      3. 6 to globus pallidus
      4. 4γ, 4s, and 6 to substantia nigra and tegmental nuclei
      5. 4 and 6 to red nucleus (?)
      6. 4s, 8, 19, and 24 to medullary reticular nuclei (?)
   C. Corticopontile circuit
      1. Areas 4 and 6 (and 10?) to pontile nuclei as part of the frontopontine

fibers in the corticopontocerebellar pathway

2. Parts of the middle and inferior temporal gyri as a part of the temporopontine fibers in the corticopontocerebellar pathway

IV. Suppressor strips: cortical areas designated as 2s, 4s, 8s, 19s, and 24s

V. Fibers

A. Afferents

1. Specific

a. Somesthetic: from the posteromedial ventral and posterolateral ventral nuclei of the thalamus through the posterior limb of the internal capsule to primary cortical areas on the postcentral gyrus (areas 1, 2, and 3); for pain, temperature, and touch from the head, neck, trunk, and extremities

b. Proprioceptive: essentially the same as under Somesthetic

c. Visual: from the lateral geniculate body of the thalamus via geniculocalcarine fibers in the sub- and retrolenticular parts of the internal capsule to the primary visual cortex (area 17)

d. Auditory: from the medial geniculate body of the thalamus via geniculotemporal fibers in the sublenticular part of the internal capsule to the primary auditory cortex (areas 41, 42)

e. Olfactory: from the olfactory bulb or anterior or lateral olfactory nuclei through lateral olfactory striae to the prepyriform, periamygdaloid, and ambient gyrus cortex (areas 34 and 28)

f. Gustatory: from the accessory arcuate nucleus of the thalamus through the posterior limb of the internal capsule to the most ventral end of the postcentral gyrus (area 43)

2. Nonspecific

a. From the dorsomedial nucleus, and perhaps some of the lateral nuclei, through the anterior limb of the internal capsule to the frontal lobe (areas 8, 9, 11, 12, 19, 45, 46, and 47)

From the anterior nucleus, through the anterior limb of the internal capsule to the gyrus cinguli (areas 23, 24, 29, and 32)

b. From the submedial nucleus to the frontal cortex (areas 8 and 46)

c. From the lateral dorsal and lateral posterior nuclei, through the posterior limb of the internal capsule to all parietal cortex, except the postcentral gyrus; and to the occipital lobe

B. Association fibers: see Chap. 2

C. Commissural fibers

1. Anterior commissure

a. Rostral part: unites the olfactory bulbs

b. Caudal part: joins the pyriform and amygdaloid regions as well as the middle and inferior temporal gyri of the two hemispheres

2. Hippocampal: unites the two hippocampi and dentate gyri

3. Corpus callosum: unites all areas of the neocortex in the two hemispheres except the middle and inferior temporal gyri

D. Efferents (descending projection)

1. Corticothalamic: to same thalamic areas that contribute thalamocortical fibers (afferents) to the cortex
2. Corticobulbar
3. Corticospinal
4. Corticostriate
5. Corticorubral
6. Corticonigral
7. Corticotegmental
8. Corticopontile

24 CLINICAL CASES

Case 1

A woman, aged 38, came to her doctor complaining that for the past several months she had noticed an increasing weakness, first in her right hand, and later in her left. When questioned, she revealed that actually, before she had noticed the onset of the weakness, she had injured her right hand, on two occasions, separated by several weeks. Once she had burned herself with the iron, the other time she had cut herself with a knife, but in neither case did she suffer pain. Even superficial examination indicated that the metacarpal bones of both hands stood out clearly, suggesting atrophy of the intrinsic muscles of the hand. When asked to abduct or adduct the fingers, adduct the thumb, or oppose the fifth digit, she could not do so. It was also discovered that there was a bilateral analgesia over the medial side of the hand, extending about to midpalm, including the ring finger and part of the middle finger. The area of analgesia extended up the forearm, involving the medial half of the volar surface and nearly half of the dorsal side. Up the arm, on the anterior surface, the region involved was the medial two-thirds of that surface to near the level of the axilla. The entire medial aspect of the arm was also insensitive to pain. On the dorsal side, less than the medial half was affected. There was a slight drooping of the eyelids, particularly marked on the right, with pupillary constriction also noticeable on this side. The right eyeball appeared to be more deeply set in the orbit. There was some weakness in both flexion and extension of the wrist, with a slight amount of atrophy of the muscles of the forearm.

Diagnosis. (Fig. 24-1.) This is a case of *syringomyelia.* The pathologic process soon breaks the commissures carrying fibers from the dorsal gray columns to the lateral spinothalamic tracts. Since these fibers cross almost immediately, there is a bilateral loss of pain and temperature sense corresponding roughly to the area of the lesion but not extending elsewhere, since the spinothalamic tracts themselves are undamaged. As the cavity enlarges, it encroaches on the ventral gray columns and destroys them in an area corresponding to the maximum area of the lesion. This is the reason for the flaccid paralysis with atrophy. The dermatomes involved in the analgesia indicate that the pathologic change lies at levels C8 and T1. This is further confirmed by the atrophy of the intrinsic muscles of the hand. There is also indication, from the position of the spread of analgesia, that C7 is becoming involved. The appearance of ptosis, miosis, and enophthalmos, all signs of Horner's syndrome, indicates that the intermediolateral cell column, giving rise to white rami of the thoracolumbar autonomic nerves, has been destroyed, at least to the level of T2 on the right side. Apparently, the cavity had not pushed so far toward the left.

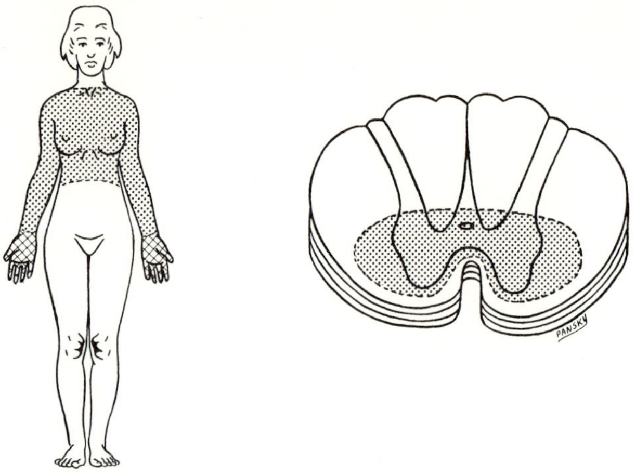

Fig. 24-1. Case 1.

Case 2

A 21-year-old male construction worker complained that he was somewhat indisposed and inclined to feel chilly. He also complained of headache and of a slight stiffness of the neck. He became worse during the following day and his temperature rose to 100.2°F. He passed a restless night and the following morning showed signs of weakness in both upper extremities; the weakness was more marked on the right. During the day, there was a progressive increase in the paralysis, and toward night there seemed to be a speech defect. That evening a physician was called, and the following was disclosed: there was no impairment in function of cranial motor nerves III, IV, V, VI, VII, or XII; pupillary reflexes were normal; there was a noticeable speech defect; respiration was shallow; the patient yawned continuously and complained that the room was stuffy; except for a slight movement of the hand, the right upper extremity was completely paralyzed, the left was very weak; stiffness in the neck was marked, particularly in flexion and extension; there were no abnormalities in muscular action or reflexes in the lower extremities. The respiratory difficulty became rapidly worse, and complete failure occurred early the following morning. There were no signs of circulatory involvement.

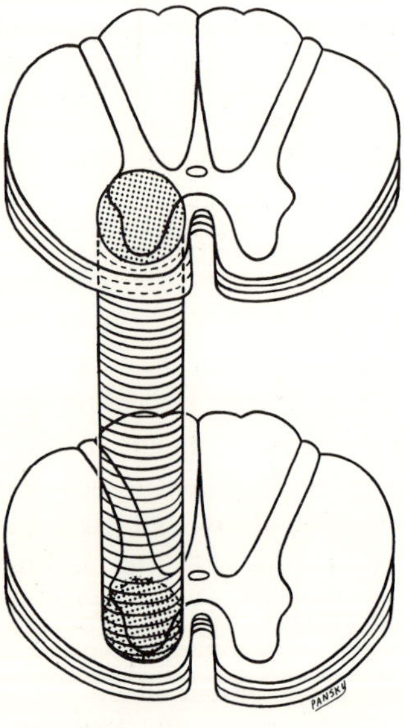

Fig. 24-2. Case 2.

Diagnosis. (Fig. 24-2.) This is a case of *poliomyelitis* involving the cervical cord, extending at least as far caudally as C7. The disease process encompassed the origin of the phrenic nerve as well as the nerves to the accessory respiratory muscles. The motor cells in the ventral gray columns at all these levels were destroyed.

Case 3

A man, aged 45, reported to his physician that for the past 4 years, he had experienced sharp pains in his lower extremities and, to a lesser extent, around the axilla. The episodes of pain became more frequent and sometimes were so severe that sedation was required. Within the past year he had begun to experience difficulty in walking. Examination revealed that his gait was unsteady and broad-based, with a flinging or flapping of legs and feet. A positive Romberg sign was present. Cranial nerves were intact except that pupils were unequal, irregular, and miotic and did not react to light but constricted on accommodation convergence (typical *Argyll Robertson pupils*). Motor power was intact. Deep tendon reflexes were absent in both lower extremities. Position and vibratory sensations were absent in both lower extremities and slightly impaired in the upper extremities.

Diagnosis. (Fig. 24-3.) All the symptoms indicate *tabes dorsalis*. The patient later admitted to exposure to syphilis but showed no external manifestations. The disease process first attacked the dorsal roots of the lower spinal nerves. This irritation was the cause of the pain experienced earlier. Later, most of the medial divisions of the dorsal roots were destroyed and, of course, the dorsal funiculus from these levels degenerated. It was the loss of these fibers that accounted for the loss of reflexes and the appearance of the Romberg sign. The Argyll Robertson pupil indicated that the disease had destroyed the pretectal zone, which is essential in the light reflex but is not involved in accommodation.

Case 4

A 40-year-old man gave the following history when admitted to the neurologic service. About a year previously, he had noted definite diminution of strength in his right hand. Three or four months later, shrinkage of the muscles in that hand became apparent. About the same time, the onset of the same symptoms was noted in the left hand. Approximately 1 year after his difficulties began, he found some trouble in walking, his legs seemed weak, and there was evidence of wasting of the musculature of the lower extremities, more noticeable on the right than on the left. Recently he had been forced to remain in bed as he could no longer get about. Examination revealed weakness of both upper extremities (especially distally in both hands) and of both lower extremities, which were also spastic. Atrophy and fasciculations of the musculature of both upper extremities and of the right lower extremity were present. Deep tendon reflexes were absent in both upper extremities and hyperactive in both lower extremities. Abdominal reflexes were absent bilaterally, and there were bilateral Babinski reflexes.

Diagnosis. (Fig. 24-4.) The loss of volitional movement, plus hyperreflexia, abnormal reflexes, and spasticity in certain areas, is indicative of an upper motor lesion. The loss of deep reflexes, with atrophy and degeneration, is typical of a

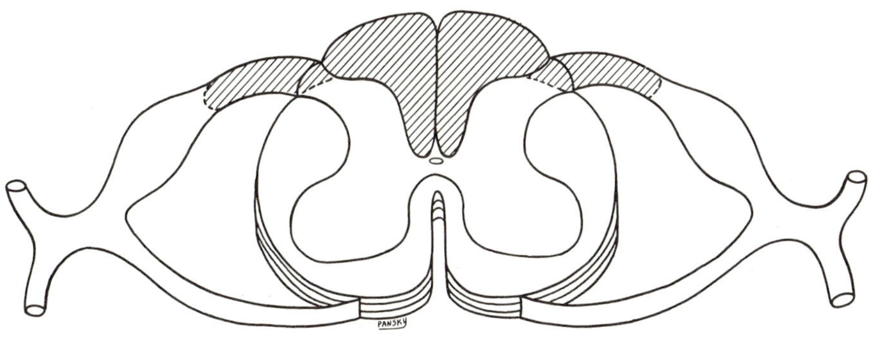

Fig. 24-3. Case 3.

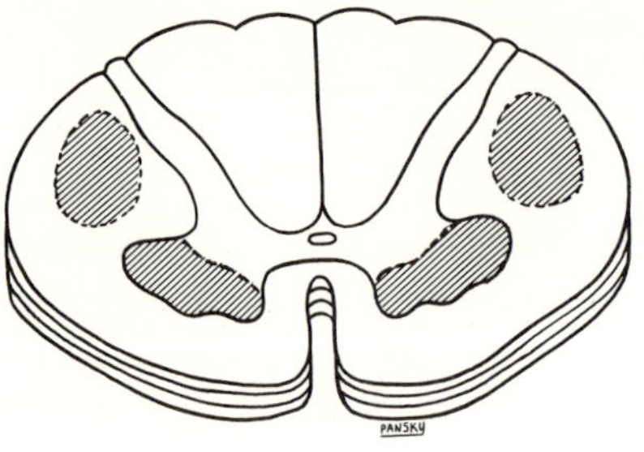

Fig. 24-4. Case 4.

lower motor neuron defect. This condition, called *amyotrophic lateral sclerosis,* selectively attacks the motor system, causing degeneration not only of the corticospinal tracts but also of the ventral gray columns.

Case 5

A 40-year-old woman was first seen by the neurological service 2 years after an accident concerning which she gave the following information: she had fallen backward down the stairs; on recovering consciousness some 30 minutes later, she was completely paralyzed in all extremities and had no feeling in her arms; she was hospitalized, and surgery was suggested. This she refused and shortly thereafter she was sent home, with her condition essentially unchanged. Gradually, she regained use of her upper limbs, but her legs were still paralyzed. Within a few weeks, sensation returned to both upper extremities. Later, the paralysis began to disappear from the left lower limb but it still felt "numb." Examination revealed the following: all the cranial motor nerves responded normally; light and accommodation reflexes were normal; voluntary movement and reflexes were normal in both upper extremities; there was no voluntary movement in the right lower extremity, but the knee jerk was exaggerated and there was slight rigidity; position sense was also lost in this limb; sensations of pain and temperature were normal on the right side; the left lower extremity showed normal voluntary movement, reflexes, and position sense; the loss of pain and temperature sense was complete over the entire left lower limb, and this condition extended onto the trunk to just above the inguinal ligament. A later follow-up proved that the conditions enumerated above persisted for the remainder of her life.

Diagnosis. (Fig. 20-5.) The loss of voluntary movement in the right lower limb, with spasticity and hyperreflexia, indicates an upper motor neuron lesion on the right side, somewhere between the brachial and lumbosacral plexuses. This is further supported by loss of position sense on the same side caused by damage to the posterior funiculus of that side. The loss of pain and temperature sensation on the left also points to a lesion on the right side, since these modalities cross to the opposite lateral spinothalamic tract within two segments of the level of entry into the cord. This fact helps to localize the damaged area to about the tenth thoracic level, on the right. This is the typical *Brown-Séquard syndrome,* due to a degeneration caused by a permanent vascular insufficiency resulting from trauma to the vessels in this area.[1]

Case 6

A 65-year-old man suddenly lapsed into unconsciousness for several hours. When he regained consciousness, he found that he could neither speak nor move his right arm or leg. In a few days, he was able to talk, although he still was unable to use his tongue properly. A few weeks later he was examined by a physician who made the following observations: there was a definite spastic paralysis of the right upper and lower extremities, with increased reflexes, absent abdominal reflexes, and a positive Babinski reflex; no atrophy was noted; the protruded tongue deviated to the left and definite atrophy was observed on the left side of the tongue; no paralysis could be detected in larynx, pharynx, or palate, nor were the jaws, face, or eyes involved; pain and temperature reception were normal over the entire trunk and head; there

[1] In the case here presented, the symptoms resulted primarily from vascular damage to one side of the cord. This syndrome is more commonly encountered when the cord is actually cut by bone fragments, bullets, knives, etc.

was almost complete loss of position and vibratory sense and of two-point discrimination over the right half of the body, exclusive of the face.

Diagnosis. (Chap. 20.) The left-sided deviation of the tongue with atrophy indicated a lesion involving the nucleus or fibers of the left hypoglossal nerve. Since both extremities on the right showed spastic paralysis, typical of an upper motor neuron lesion, the pyramidal tract on the left, above the decussation, was involved. In this case, *hemiplegia alternata hypoglossi,* there was also loss of position and vibratory sense and tactile discrimination on the right. Since the medial lemniscus lies just dorsal to the pyramid, it was included in the lesion and, since it is rostral to the sensory decussation, caused symptoms referred to the right side of the body.

Case 7

A 55-year-old woman complained of dizziness and fell down before help could reach her. She did not lose consciousness. It was noted at the time that both eyes turned toward the right and that her speech was not normal. However, she was not given a complete examination for over 2 months. At this time, it was found that both muscle tone and reflexes were normal and equal in all four extremities. However, there was some incoordination in both the right limbs. There was no detectable paralysis of the jaws, facial muscles, or tongue, but an inspection of the pharynx showed that the uvula was directed toward the left, indicating a right-sided paralysis of the palate. Laryngoscopic investigation also suggested paralysis of the right vocal cord. When standing with her feet together and eyes closed, the patient tended to fall to the right. There was loss of pain and temperature sensations on the right side of the face and left side of the entire trunk. Tactile sensation was normal.

Diagnosis. (Fig. 24-5, Chap. 16.) The initial dizziness and conjugate deviation to the right indicate a disturbance of an irritative nature involving the right vestibular nuclei. With time, degeneration involving some of the right vestibular nerve fibers had occurred, as indicated by the patient's tendency to fall to the right. Loss of

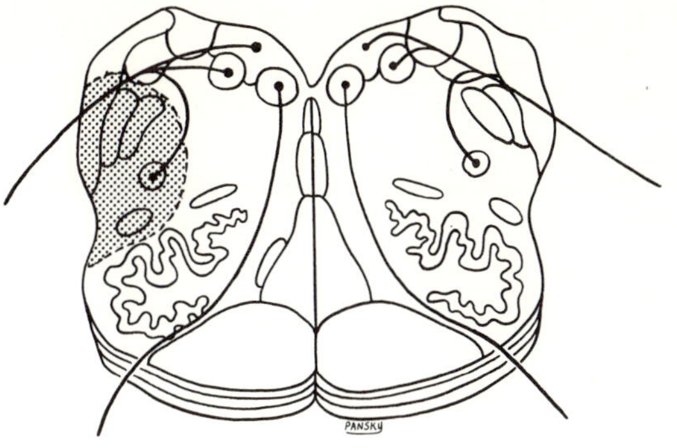

Fig. 24-5. Case 7.

pain and temperature sensation on the left side of the body is conclusive proof of interruption of the lateral spinothalamic tract on the right; loss of these senses on the right side of the face suggests involvement of the spinal V tract and its nucleus. The paralysis of the palate and vocal cord on the right indicates damage to the nucleus ambiguus and emerging vagal fibers on the right. The slight incoordination is suggestive of some involvement of the cerebellum or its connections. In this case, a *thrombus* had developed in the *posterior inferior cerebellar artery,* which led to the destruction of the dorsolateral portion of the right side of the medulla, including the inferior portion of the restiform body containing the dorsal spinocerebellar tract; the ventral spinocerebellar tract; the lateral spinothalamic tract; the spinal V tract and its nucleus; part of the nucleus ambiguus; emerging fibers of the vagus; and the caudal group of vestibular nuclei.

Case 8

A young boy, aged 8, was admitted to the neurological service. There was no history of birth injury, nor had there been any unusual childhood diseases. His growth and development were normal. About 6 months previously, however, he had screamed with severe pain in the back of his neck and had vomited, these events occurring when he first got out of bed in the morning. Similar attacks of pain and vomiting recurred at varying intervals. His mother also noted that he carried his head tilted to the right and walked unsteadily. Recently, these episodes had become very frequent and the boy was unable to play. Examination in the clinic indicated the following: on percussion, the head gave a "cracked-pot" sound; the head was tilted to the right; there was a slight stiffness of the neck; both optic disks were swollen but the visual fields were normal; there was a course nystagmus on looking to the left, with a quicker, finer nystagmus on looking to the right; the pupils were equal and the light reflexes were normal; the eye movements were normal; the remainder of the cranial nerves were intact; the extremities, especially on the left, were hypotonic; there was bilateral heel-to-knee and finger-to-nose ataxia and intention tremor, again more marked on the left; gait was wide-based and unsteady with a tendency to reel toward the left; there were no sensory or reflex changes and no pathologic reflexes.

Diagnosis. The boy was taken to surgery, where it was found that a large growth had developed in the *left cerebellar hemisphere.* It was removed and was found to be an *astrocytoma* of the hemisphere. Convalescence was uneventful.

Case 9

A young girl, aged 14, was admitted to the hospital for diagnosis. According to the history, her birth had been normal and uncomplicated. There had been no unusual illness or accidents during her childhood and her growth and development were normal. About a year before this admission, the girl began to complain of "ringing or buzzing" in her right ear, a condition which had persisted since. Shortly thereafter, the school physician reported that the girl was "hard of hearing" in the right ear. As time went on, there was some dizziness and she complained of difficulty in seeing. Later, weakness and awkwardness of the right upper extremity appeared. Although her appetite was good, she was experiencing difficulty in swallowing solid foods. Examination revealed the following: nystagmus to the left; the patient was unable to follow the examiner's finger when moved to her right and, when this was tried with both eyes open, she complained of double vision; at rest, the right eye tended to turn inward; the pupils were regular, equal, and responded normally to light; the visual fields were normal, but there was some papilledema bilaterally; the right side of her face, including the muscles above the eye, showed evidence of paralysis; an inspection of the pharynx showed that the uvula was directed toward the left and the right side of the palate drooped; tests revealed that there was almost 100 per cent loss of hearing in the right ear, in both air-conducted and bone-conducted sound; the caloric tests in the right ear produced no eye responses, while on the left, nearly normal responses were induced; there were weakness and an intention tremor of the right upper extremity.

Diagnosis. The findings given above suggested a tumor of the posterior fossa on the right side, and surgery was recommended. At operation, a tumor was found in the *right cerebellopontine angle,* involving the following cranial nerves: VI, VII, VIII, IX, and X. There was also some pressure on the inferior part of the cerebellum. This is a typical *acoustic neurinoma.*

Case 10

A woman, aged 44, told the examining physician that beginning several months before, she had experienced rather severe headaches in the frontal region, which she had attributed to sinusitis. Somewhat later, she noticed weakness in her right upper extremity and clumsiness of the fingers of that hand. There was also weakness of the right lower extremity. With the onset of the muscular weakness, speech difficulties appeared, and there was trouble with vision. Questions about the ocular disturbance showed it to be double vision (diplopia). Examination revealed that the left pupil was larger than the right, and that when seen from in front, the left eye turned outward and somewhat downward. There was no convergence in this eye, nor could light or accommodation reflexes be elicited. There was ptosis of the left lid. There was no voluntary action in either extremity on the right. The Achilles and patellar reflexes were both exaggerated, and a positive Babinski reflex was found, all on the right side. There was paralysis of the facial muscles below the eye on the right, and the tongue, when protruded, deviated to the right, but there was no sign of atrophy.

Diagnosis. (Chap. 20.) The eye signs, characterized by a dilated pupil, with no response to light or accommodation; a petosis of the lid; lack of convergence with a lateral downward deviation, owing to the unopposed action of the lateral rectus and superior oblique muscles, all point to the destruction of the third nerve or nucleus, including the autonomic component for pupillary constriction. The spastic paralysis, with hyperreflexia on the opposite side of the body, suggests an upper motor lesion including the corticobulbar fibers to the muscles of the face and tongue. The only place where the third nerve on one side lies close to the upper motor neurons for the other side is in the midbrain, where the emerging fibers of the oculomotor nerve are next to the medial side of the basis pedunculi. Thus, a tumor here would account for all the signs, including the headache. This is a case of *hemiplegia alternata oculomotoria,* or *Weber's syndrome.*

Case 11

A young girl, aged 13, was admitted to the medical clinic for observation. The family history was negative. Her birth was normal and uncomplicated. There was no record of serious illness during infancy or early childhood. During her first years of life, growth and development had been normal. Recently, there had been little growth and she remained slender and underweight. Her mental development was normal. When she was about 8 years old, she had developed a persistent polyuria, accompanied by polydipsia. At that time she was given Pitressin, with striking results. Examination revealed that she was undersized, underweight, and undernourished with no evidence of pigmentation or cutaneous tumors; her genitalia were infantile; her optic nerve heads showed slight pallor; her vision was normal, but there was complete bitemporal hemianopsia; her blood sugar level was low.

Diagnosis. The findings suggested a tumor in or near the anterior hypothalamus, and surgery was recommended. At operation, a *growth* was discovered which had disrupted the *optic chiasma* and encroached upon the hypothalamus in the region of the *infundibulum* and *tuber cinereum.*

Case 12

A man, aged 62, fainted while attending a hotly contested ball game. He was unconscious for nearly 48 hours. When he regained consciousness, he was paralyzed in both extremities on the right. Seven weeks later he was given a thorough examination. At this time, there was hyperreflexia and spasticity in both the right upper and lower extremities. When protruded, the tongue deviated toward the right but there was no atrophy. Paralysis of the facial muscles, on the right side, below the eye, was noted. There was impairment of all modalities of sensation over the entire right side of the body and face, but the various sensory modalities were affected to different degrees. The sensations of position, vibration, and two-point touch were lost completely. There was some loss of temperature sense, but pain appeared little affected in the same area. The pupils responded normally to light, but it was found that the patient suffered from right homonymous hemianopsia.

Diagnosis. The spastic paralysis on the right indicated an upper motor neuron lesion. Since there was paralysis of the tongue, without atrophy, and since only the facial muscles below the eye were involved, proof for destruction of both corticospinal and corticobulbar fibers was complete. The sensory disturbances were of major importance. Position and vibratory sense and tactile discrimination require cortical connections. There was impairment of thermal sense, but pain was recognized. This would indicate that the lesion is high, above thalamic levels, since the thalamus may be the conscious center

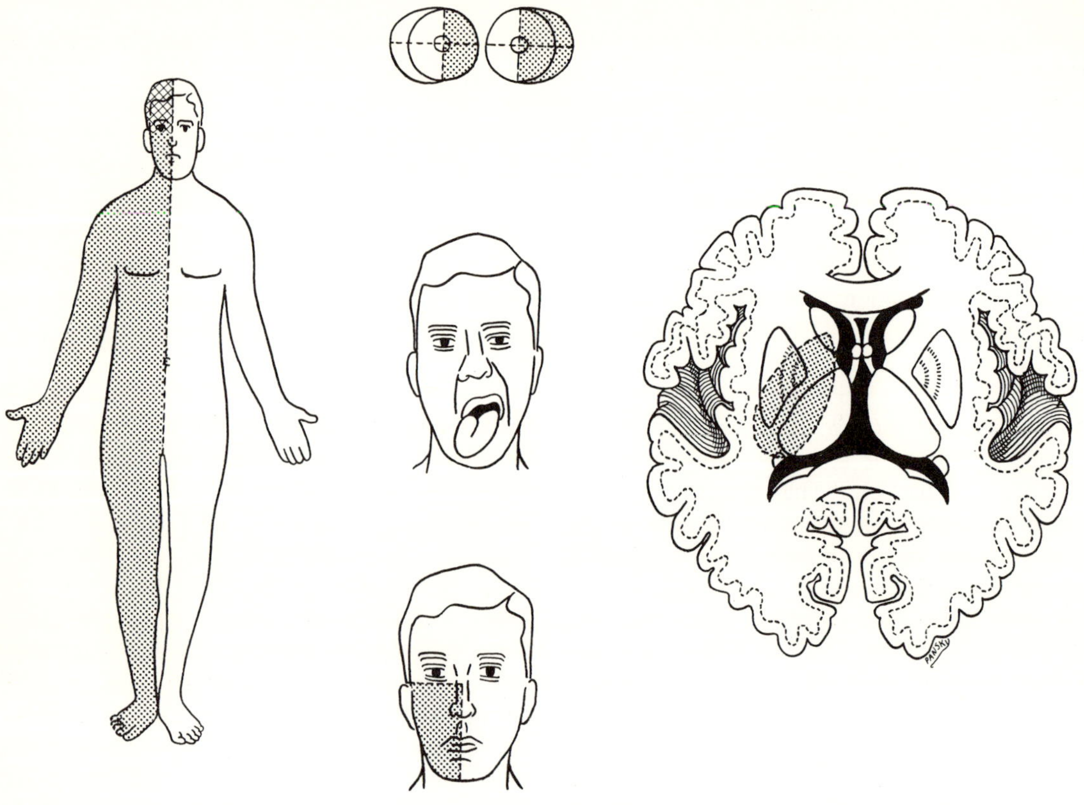

Fig. 24-6. Case 12.

for pain. The visual defect is characteristic of lesions in either the optic or geniculocalcarine tracts. A single lesion which involves the upper motor neurons and, at the same time, encompasses the general and special somatic systems, together with proprioception, would have to lie in the *posterior limb of the internal capsule*. The manner of onset of the symptoms suggested a *hemorrhage* in that region of the capsule. (Fig. 24-6.)

Case 13

A young man, aged 20, was referred to a neurologist with the following history. At the age of 18 he had suffered an attack of subacute bacterial endocarditis, which had been treated with heavy doses of penicillin over a period of 6 weeks. One day, about 8 months previous to the present visit, he had suddenly fainted and had been unconscious for several hours. Although consciousness returned, his mind was "hazy" for 5 or 6 days and he was not able to speak. Examination revealed spasticity in the right upper extremity, with loss of voluntary movement but no atrophy. There were no disturbances in the right lower or in either of the left extremities. The protruded tongue deviated to the right, but there was no atrophy. The facial muscles, below the eye, on the right were paralyzed. There were no visual defects nor somesthetic disturbances.

Diagnosis. Spastic paralysis in the right upper extremity means upper motor neuron involvement. The paralysis of the facial muscles below the eye also indicates upper motor rather than lower motor neuron lesions. The paralysis of the tongue, without atrophy, also supports this view. Because of the inclusion of the cranial motor defects, the lesion could lie in the cortex, subcortical white matter, internal capsule, or basis pedunculi. However, in the latter two locations, a lesion would almost certainly cause a paralysis in the lower extremity as well. A capsular lesion would also show severe sensory disturbances. By elimination, the cortex remains. This location is confirmed by the presence of motor aphasia, the loss of speech resulting from an involvement of Broca's area in the frontal opercular area of the dominant hemisphere. Since this is a right-handed individual, the lesion is on the *left side,* including *the lower part of the precentral gyrus* and the *frontal operculum.* This is doubtless the result of an *embolism* in the branch of the *middle cerebral artery* supplying this region. The medical history contributes the evidence of endocarditis, in which emboli are not uncommon. (Fig. 24-7.)

Case 14

A man, aged 52, came to the clinic complaining of pains and weakness in his legs. Over the past few weeks the pain had become more severe; his legs were so sensitive that even the touch of a bed sheet was almost intolerable and it was now very difficult for him to walk. His family history was negative and there was no report of any recent severe illness or injury. He did say, however, that he had been a consistently heavy drinker for years and in the past few months, his alcohol consumption had increased. Examination revealed that the patient was undernourished, to the point of emaciation. There was a bilateral loss of the deep reflexes at both knee and ankle. The muscles were atonic and flaccid and there was indication of some atrophy. Although the patient could walk, he showed the peculiar "stepping gait" (need to raise feet to keep from tripping) characteristic of bilateral foot drop. Sensory impairment of the "stocking" variety was observed on both extremities. In this case, all forms of sensation, especially touch and position sense, were greatly impaired, but there was hypersensitivity to a pin prick. The skin of the lower extremities was

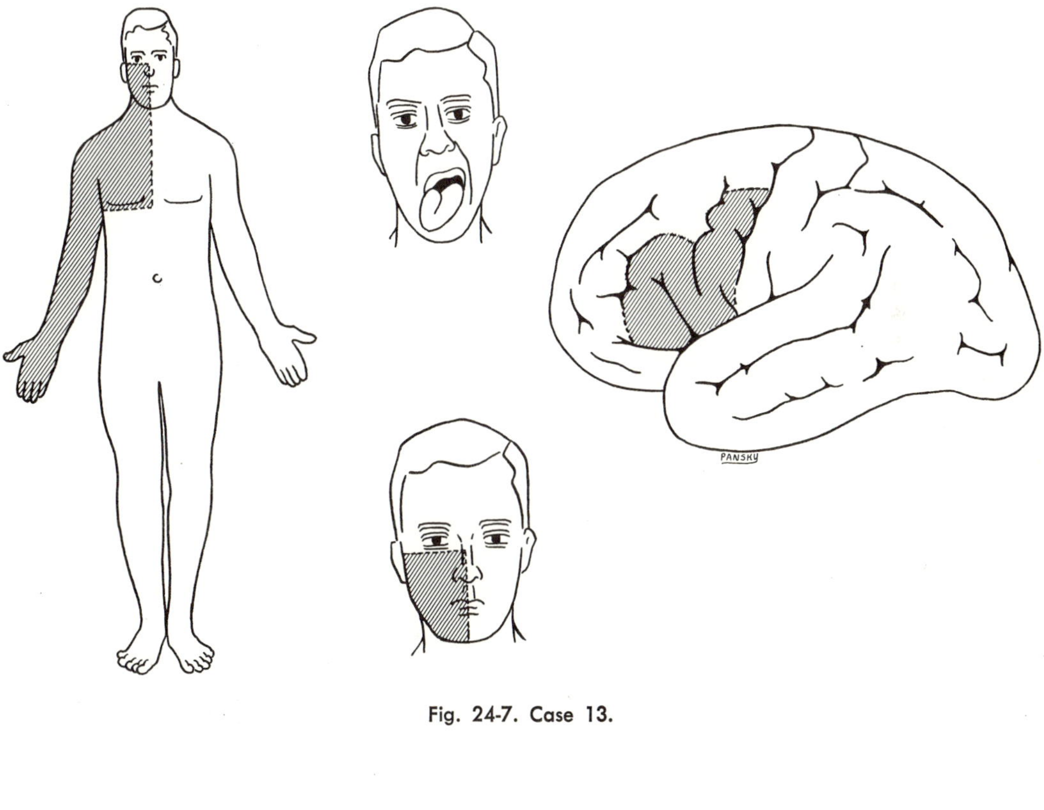

Fig. 24-7. Case 13.

somewhat reddened and there was edema. Except for a tremor in the upper limbs, no other signs were observed. The cranial nerves were normal.

Diagnosis. The severe and progressive symptoms, with flaccidity and atrophy, are characteristic of lower motor neuron lesions. The coloration of the skin and edema are suggestive of involvement of the autonomic fibers to the blood vessels of the lower extremity. The gradual loss of sensations of touch with an early hypersensitivity to pain are often indicative of an inflammatory process with progressive degeneration of peripheral nerves. These signs, together with the history of heavy drinking, lead to the diagnosis of a *peripheral neuritis* (*neuropathy*) due to alcohol (alcohol polyneuropathy).

Case 15

A man, aged 64, was admitted to the clinic. He said that perhaps 2 years previously he had been bothered by a shaking in his left arm, beginning in the fingers. Since that time the shaking had spread to his neck and right arm. At this time, a tentative diagnosis of paralysis agitans was made, and the case was followed for several years. During the next 2 years the condition spread to involve his lower limbs. When last examined, the following positive signs were seen: a fine-to-moderate rhythmic tremor was seen in his upper extremities; when standing, the head sagged forward and the shoulders were stooped with ventral flexion of the trunk; the arms were somewhat extended and adducted and flexed except for the distal phalanges, which were extended; the gait was slow and deliberate and there was no associated swinging of the arms while walking; there had been a definite increase in muscular rigidity since the previous examination; the face was masklike and without change of expression. On the negative side, no true paralysis was found although voluntary motor action was slowed; the deep reflexes were intact; the abdominal reflexes were present and somewhat hyperactive; there was no Babinski sign; there were no abnormalities in pupillary reaction; there were no sensory disturbances over the trunk, and both motor and sensory cranial components were normal.

Diagnosis. (Fig. 19-16.) A diagnosis of *paralysis agitans* (*Parkinson's disease*) could be based on several outstanding features. Among these, the most important are lack of associated movements; marked changes in posture; expressionless face; increased muscular tonus and tremor. These signs, linked with the absence of evidence for pyramidal tract lesions, cranial nerve palsies, or sensory disturbances, make the diagnosis conclusive.

Case 16

A young man, aged 22, was referred to a neurologist by a physician representing the state athletic commission. The following history was obtained. The patient was a professional boxer. One night, several weeks previously, he had been knocked out in the last round of a preliminary event. He was unconscious for about 10 minutes. On regaining consciousness, he got up, and although still a bit hazy, he dressed, with some help, and was taken home by one of his handlers. On arrival, he appeared to have recovered completely. The following day he took it easy and there were no signs of any trouble. The second day, he began to feel dizzy and to experience a dull headache, which became progressively worse during the following several days. The dizziness was more severe, and there was occasional vomiting. However, all these signs disappeared by the end of a week, and for the next month or so he was free of symptoms. About 5 weeks after the initial knockout, he began training again. Two days later the headache, dizziness, and vomiting returned, accompanied by slight paralysis and weakness on the left side. His manager immediately took him to the commission doctor, who made the referral. On examination it was found that the pupil of the right eye was wider than the left, with a slight ptosis of the lid on the right; the optic disks were choked; there was a left-sided hemiplegia (spastic paralysis) especially marked in the upper extremity, with a considerable loss of voluntary movement in the fingers on that side; both Rinné's and Weber's tests indicated impairment of hearing of the central type, in both ears; there was some degree of mental confusion. At the same time, it was found that the temperature was normal but the pulse was slow. The cerebrospinal fluid pressure was elevated but was otherwise normal and showed no traces of blood.

Diagnosis. The history of trauma, followed by an asymptomatic (lucid) interval, which, in turn, was followed by headache, vertigo, and unilateral muscular weakness with signs of increased intracranial pressure, all point toward a *chronic* type of *subdural hemorrhage* (hematoma) resulting from trauma. The dilation of the right pupil, ptosis of the right lid, and spastic paralysis on the left indicated that the hematoma was on the right side. The greater severity of the paralysis in the upper extremity, plus the auditory defects, suggests that the hematoma lies over the lower part of the frontal and parietal lobes and the upper temporal lobe, centered close to the central sulcus.

Case 17

A young girl, aged 13, was brought to a neurologist at the suggestion of her family physician. She had a history of frequent sore throat. Three years previously, during an attack of sore throat, she had complained of soreness in her joints. At that time, her family was told that she had rheumatic fever. Early in the present year she had an especially severe attack of tonsillitis. During the girl's recuperation from this illness, her mother first noticed involuntary, sudden, abrupt, and jerking movements in her daughter's right arm. Sometimes the movements involved the shoulder, sometimes the forearm and hand. More recently, involuntary tossing of the head had begun. The mother stated that these movements became exaggerated when the girl was excited, were less noticeable when she was resting quietly, and that she had never observed them at all while the girl was sleeping. The examination confirmed the mother's observations. A hypotonia was noted but the reflexes were quite normal. Although the patient at first appeared to be suffering from muscular weakness, as evidenced by dropping objects held in the hand, this was found to be because of the involuntary movements. There was some incoordination and awkwardness, especially when reaching for objects. With the arms outstretched, the hands were flexed at the wrist with overextension at the metacarpophalangeal joints. When the arms were stretched over the head, the palm, particularly of the right hand, turned outward with overpronation at the elbow. The face was more or less serene, the expression rather blank. There was evidence of irritability and emotional instability. There were no abnormal disturbances of sensation.

Diagnosis. The history of rheumatic fever, the recent sore throats, the choreiform movements, the "choreic hand" and "pronator sign" in a female of this age all contribute to the diagnosis of *Sydenham's chorea* (*St. Vitus' dance*).

Case 18

A woman, aged 65, consulted her physician because of persistent headache of several weeks' duration on the right side of the face, especially around the eye. She also complained of occasional double vision. At this time she was treated for sinusitis and was sent home. Several weeks later she returned, complaining that the pain was growing steadily worse. On examination it was found that the sinuses were clear and that there were no marked visual defects, either in acuity or fields. Test results for glaucoma were also negative. However, it was noted that there was exophthalmos, with pulsation, in the right eye; with both eyes open, the patient complained of double vision when the examiner's finger was moved toward the patient's right, and with the left eye covered, the right eye did not follow a moving object to the right; although other movements of the right eye were possible, they were definitely weaker and more difficult than on the left; all movements of the left eye were normal. Ophthalmoscopic examination indicated a right

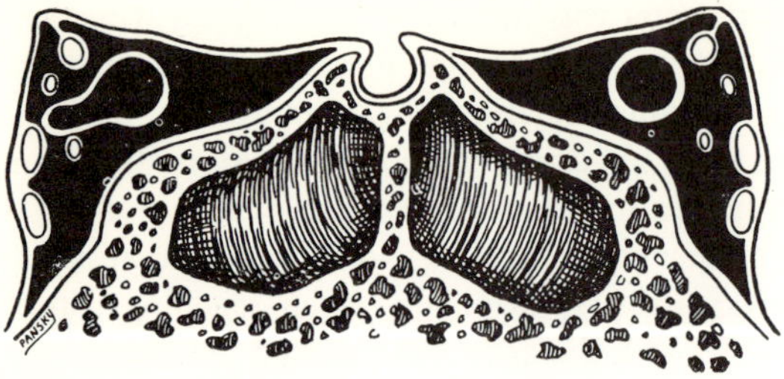

Fig. 24-8. Case 18.

papilledema. When pressure was applied to the right carotid in the neck, the pulsations in the right eye disappeared. Spinal fluid pressure and contents were normal. All other test results were negative.

Diagnosis. (Fig. 24-8.) The head pain, localized in the area of distribution of the ophthalmic division of the trigeminal nerve, in the absence of disease of the sinuses or primary disease of the eye, suggests an irritation along the course of the nerve. Paralysis of the lateral rectus muscle indicates a definite involvement of the abducens nerve, while weakness of the other extrinsic ocular muscles on the right suggests a progressive involvement of both the oculomotor and trochlear nerves. The disk sign and exophthalmos in the right eye indicate increased retro-ocular pressure, while the pulsations give evidence of an arterial involvement on that side. This was confirmed when the carotid artery in the neck was momentarily closed by pressure. Localization was made somewhat more exact by the fact that there is a place where an arterial enlargement could affect not only the sensory nerves but also the motor nerves to the extrinsic ocular muscles. The diagnosis was of an *aneurysm of the internal carotid artery* in the middle-to-anterior portion of the right cavernous sinus.

Case 19

A young boy, aged 5, was brought into the hospital during a summer hot spell complaining of a generalized intense headache. His parents indicated that he had vomited, had complained of a stiff neck, and seemed to be delirious, apathetic, and almost in a stupor. When asked whether the boy had had any fever, the parents said that there had been a very slight fever and that there might even have been some chills. Upon examination, the headache still persisted and neck stiffness was evident, with the neck muscles being sore to the touch, and an almost absolute inability to flex the neck muscles. On attempting to flex the head, there was flexion of the legs at the knees (Brudzinski sign) and from a flexed thigh, it was exceedingly difficult to extend the leg completely due to pain in the back (Kernig's sign). There was some mental confusion and the boy's temperature was 103°F.

Diagnosis. The history of headache, fever, mental confusion, and the obvious meningeal signs of neck stiffness, Brudzinski sign, and Kernig sign all indicate a diagnosis of *meningitis.* In meningococcic, pneumococcic, and streptococcic or staphylococcic infections the temperature is usually over 102°F. In TB meningitis, the temperature is usually between 100 and 101°F and in syphilitic meningitis, the temperature is usually normal. There may be associated chills, rapid pulse, and rapid respiration. Meningitis is most typically found in males, in children under 6, and occurs most frequently in the summer.

Case 20

A young man, aged 25, was referred to a neurologist by his family physician for diagnostic verification. The history concerned predominantly a condition of lower back pain which was first initiated when the patient bent over, several months earlier, in an attempt to lift a very heavy object. He said he felt a "snap in the back" and could hardly straighten out. Since then, there have been recurring episodes of back pain localized in the lower portion which at times have been brief, but now the pain has persisted for almost a week. The pain apparently is relieved somewhat by standing or lying down and is aggravated by bending, standing straight up, or even by coughing and sneezing. Recently, too, there has been leg pain in the left leg which seems to radiate along the back and side of the thigh. The leg pain is severe and it, too, seems to be aggravated by posture, coughing, sneezing, bowel movements, walking, and exertion in general. On examination, the neurologist found some loss of lumbar lordosis and spasm of the paravertebral muscles; manipulation of the leg was painful, lumbar spine movement was limited, extension of spine was painful, and lateral flexion of the spine was restricted. Walking was painful and the patient seemed to favor his left leg by limping slightly. Lasègués test was positive and there was a decrease in the Achilles reflex.

Diagnosis. The recurrent history, lower back pain following an attempt to lift a heavy object, limited lumbar spine movements, painful extension of the spine, pain relief and exaggeration by position change, pain on the straight leg-raising test, positive Lasègués test, and leg pain following the sciatic nerve distribution all point to a diagnosis of a *herniated disk* in the lumbar region impinging on the left sciatic nerve.

Case 21

A young man, aged 35, was brought to a neurologist on the advice of his family physician. Although the onset of the symptoms was a bit uncertain since they apparently began gradually and slowly, these were the facts as presented to the neurologist. There had been a gradual, slowly developing stiffness in the patient's back, which also involved his shoulder and hip joints. The stiffness of the "spine" had developed over many months. Initially there had been no pain, but soon pain occurred in the thorax, neck and lower back, and on both sides. On examination, the neurologist noted that there was no kyphosis, some muscular atrophy, a stiff, rigid, "poker" spine, the head was thrust forward and the trunk held rigid in walking, the spine muscles were in spasm, and there was hyperesthesia in pain zones. X-ray examination revealed some decalcification of the joints, blurring of joint faces, and a narrowing and obliteration of affective intervertebral disks.

Diagnosis. The diagnosis is based on the stiff spine, back pain, root pain, involvement of the hip and shoulder, no kyphosis, and atrophy of spine muscles with no cord involvement. The disease is referred to as *Spondylarthritis ankylopoietica* or *Marie-Strümpell's disease* or even *Spondylitis deformans*. The cause is unknown and the process is probably an infectious disease of the vertebral column and adjacent structures. Involvement of the hip and shoulder classifies this as Marie-Strümpell's disease.

Case 22

A woman, aged 45, was admitted to the hospital by her physician. Following fever and malaise, there had developed an acute inflammatory skin lesion, unilaterally in a girdle-like location in the middle of her right chest and back. There had also been a unilateral girdle-like eruption of vesicles on a red inflamed base with severe pain. The vesicles were distributed along an area innervated by spinal roots 8 to 10. There was also an accompanying paresthesia. The pain was sharp, knifelike, and there later developed a decreased sensitivity to touch. Following the patient's brief stay in the hospital, the eruption and the pain disappeared within 7 to 10 days.

Diagnosis. The unilateral involvement following distribution in the areas of spinal roots with anatomic precision, the typically radicular pain and vesicles all indicate a diagnosis of *Herpes zoster* (posterior poliomyelitis), an infectious disease of the dorsal spinal root, spinal root ganglion, and posterior horn of the spinal cord.

Case 23

A man, aged 50, noticed that his voice was suddenly getting hoarse and that he was having difficulty in swallowing. His physician referred him to a neurologist. The patient further developed dysarthria (a structural defect of speech; stuttering) and it was noticed that his shoulder and neck muscle, the trapezius, as well as the sternocleidomastoid, were paralyzed on the right side. On closer examination, there was found to be an ipsilateral paralysis of the right palate, an ipsilateral paralysis of the larynx on the right side, and an ipsilateral paralysis of the right tongue.

Diagnosis. This is a syndrome known as *Jackson's syndrome,* in which there is an ipsilateral paralysis of the palate, larynx, tongue, sternocleidomastoid and trapezius muscles due to a lesion which causes softening of the XIIth nucleus (hypoglossal), nucleus ambiguus and the XIth nucleus (accessory). Such a lesion is obviously located in the lower medulla.

Case 24

A 35-year-old woman developed hemiplegia of her left side (paralysis of one side of the body) and was admitted to the hospital where she was seen by a neurologist. On physical examination it was noted that besides the hemiplegia there was diplopia and internal strabismus of the right eye. There was also a loss of power to rotate the right eyeball outward. The external rectus muscle of the right eye was found to be paralyzed. There was no other cranial nerve involvement.

Diagnosis. The condition is diagnosed by the right external rectus muscle paralysis and the left hemiplegia (contralateral). This syndrome is known as the *Millard-Gubler syndrome* or *pontile syndrome* and involves a vascular lesion or tumor located in the pons (in this case in the right pons) where it can effectively destroy the VIth nerve and the pyramidal tract prior to its decussation, thus giving an ipsilateral cranial nerve involvement and a contralateral hemiplegia.

25 ATLAS OF SECTIONS OF THE BRAIN

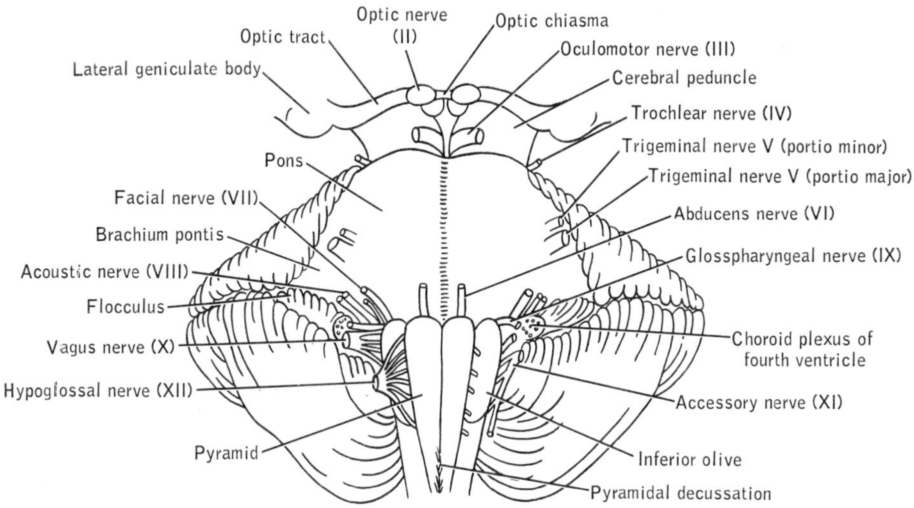

Outline of the brain stem showing level of sections illustrated in Figs. 25-1 to 25-12.

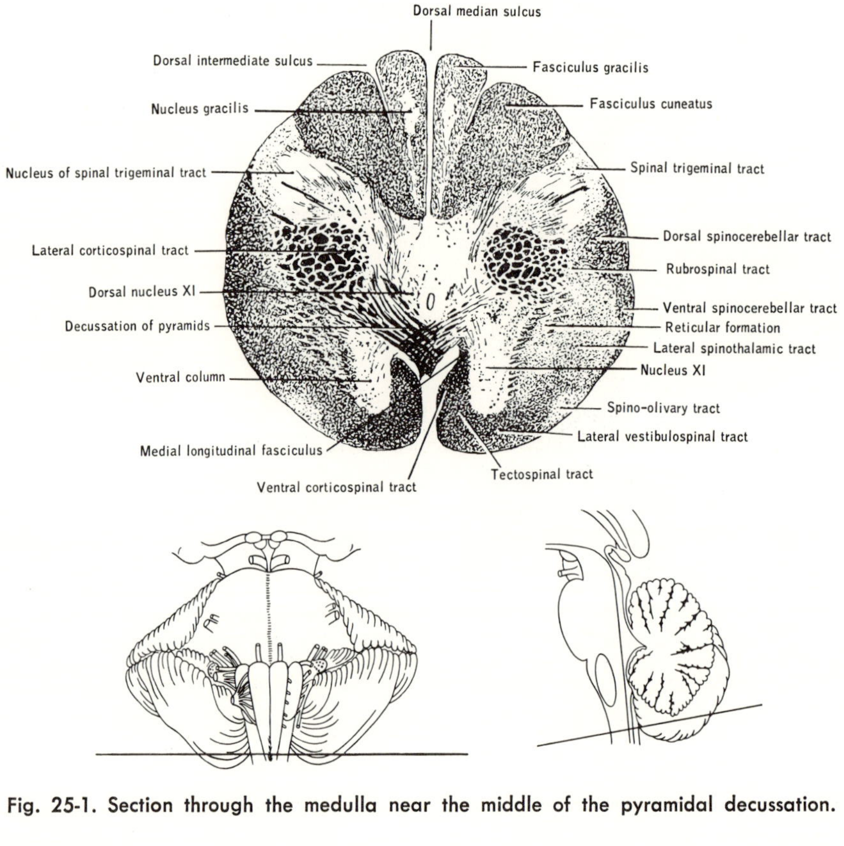

Fig. 25-1. Section through the medulla near the middle of the pyramidal decussation.

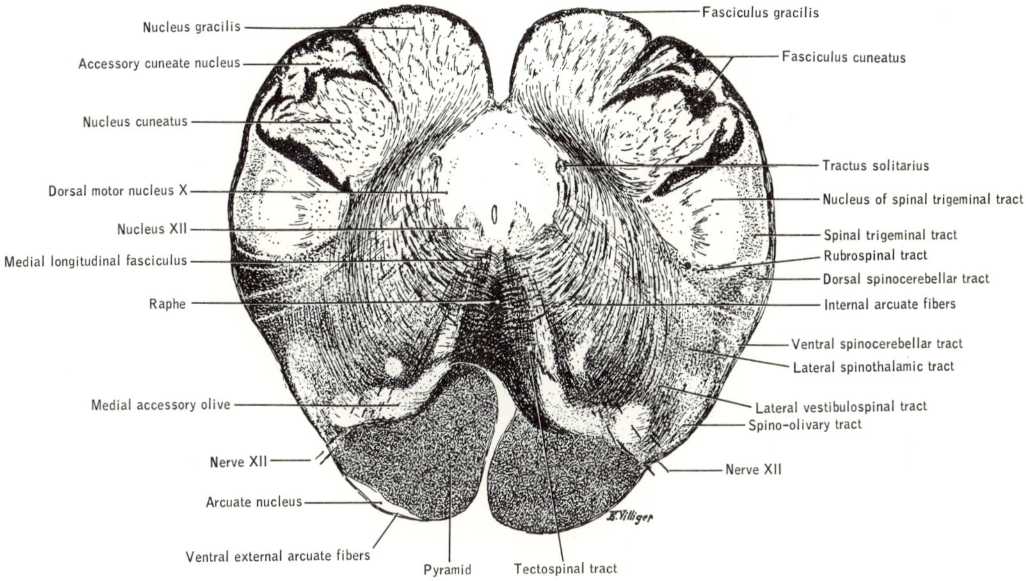

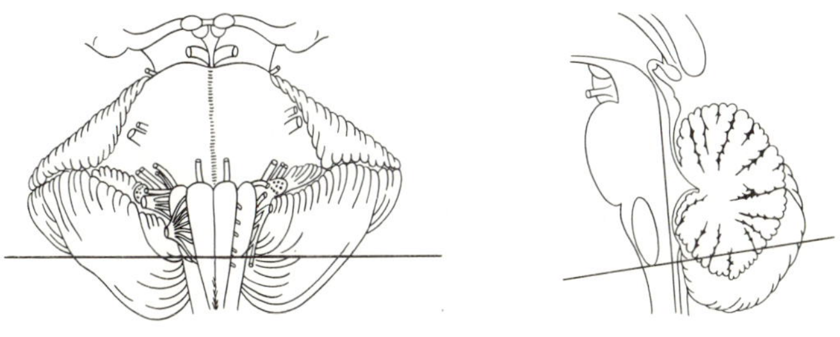

Fig. 25-2. Section through the medulla at the rostral end of the pyramidal decussation showing the internal arcuate fibers at the caudal level of the sensory decussation.

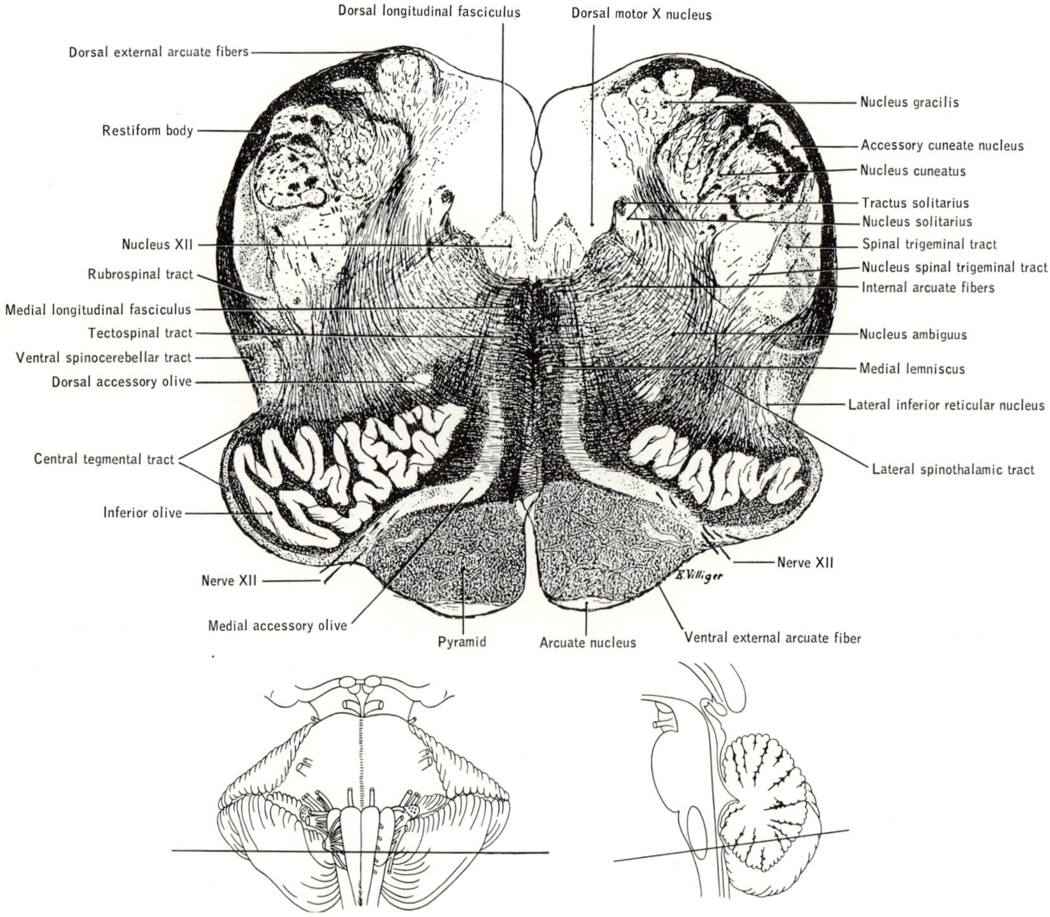

Fig. 25-3. Section of the medulla through the caudal portion of the inferior olive.

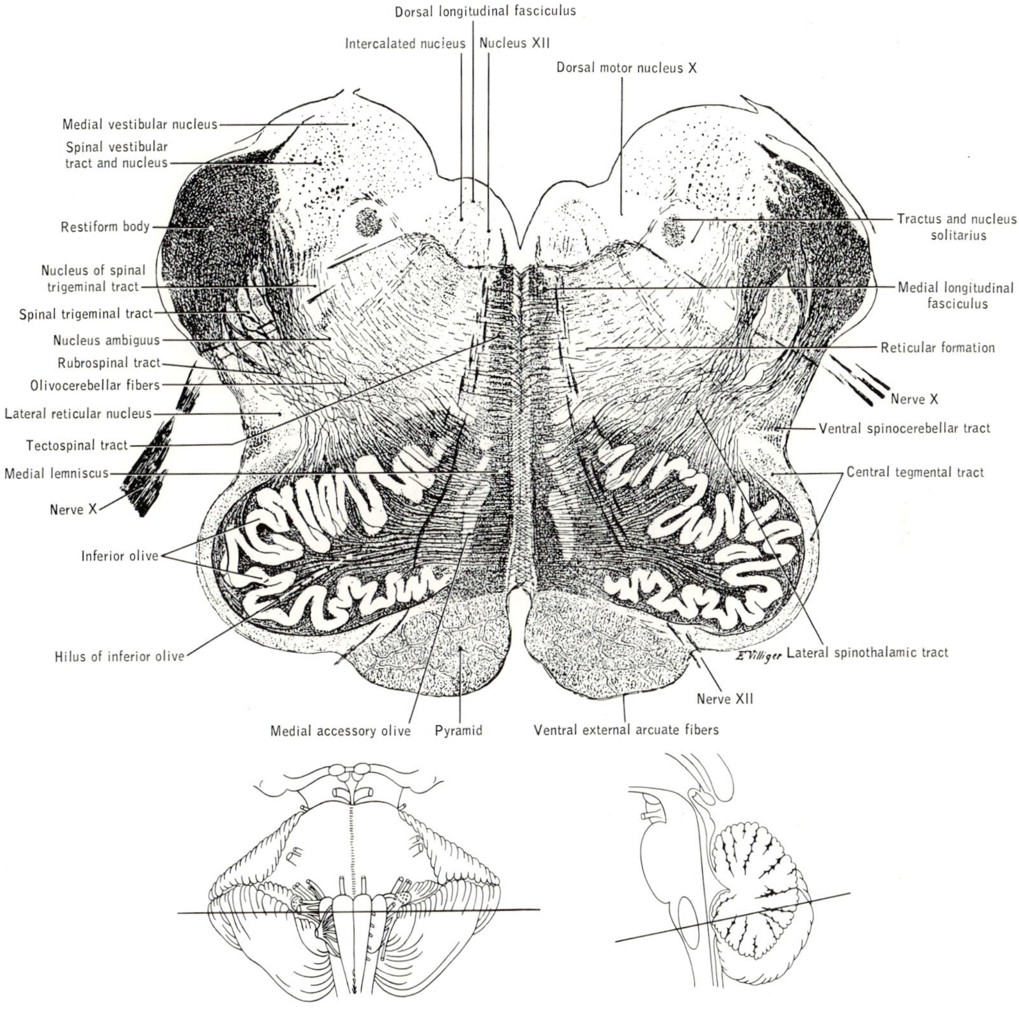

Fig. 25-4. Section of the medulla at the level of the emerging fibers of the vagus nerve (X).

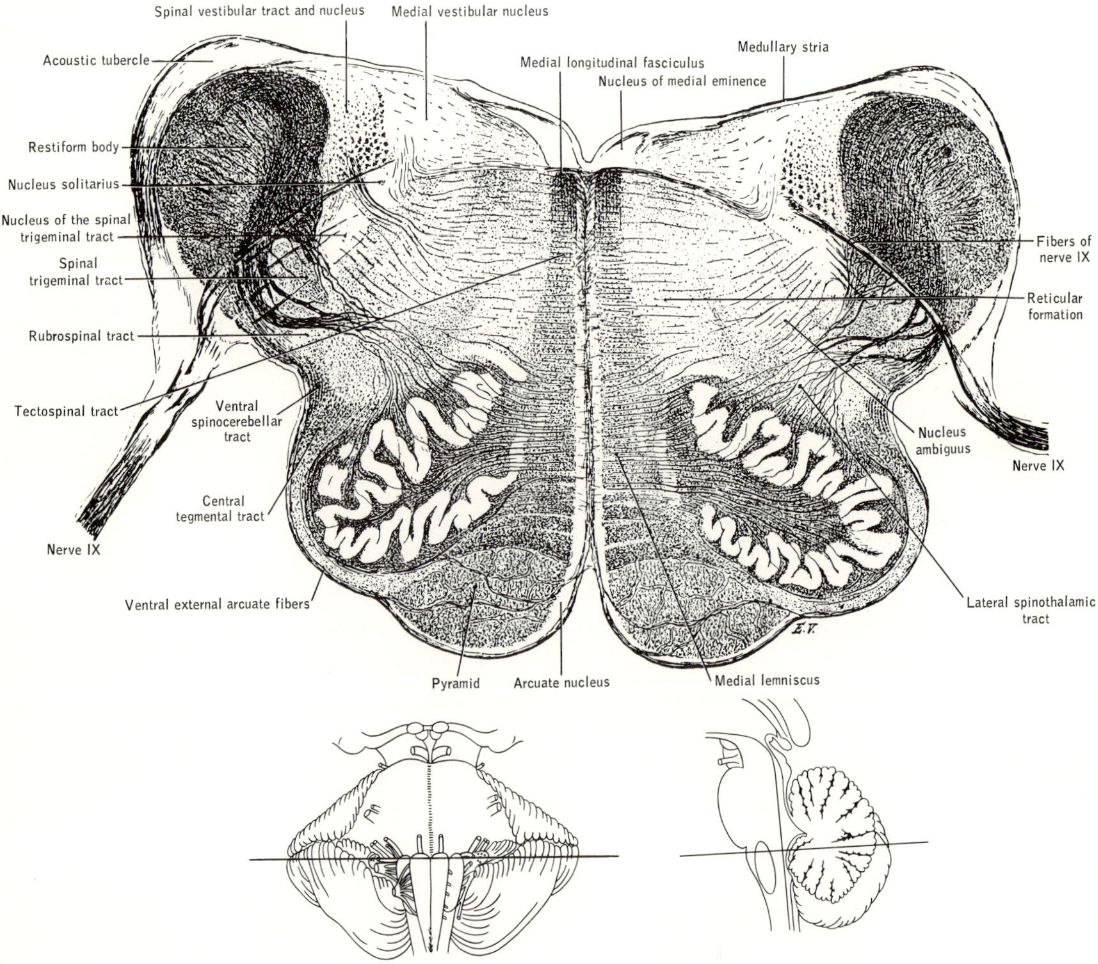

Fig. 25-5. Section of the medulla at the level of the glossopharyngeal nerve (IX).

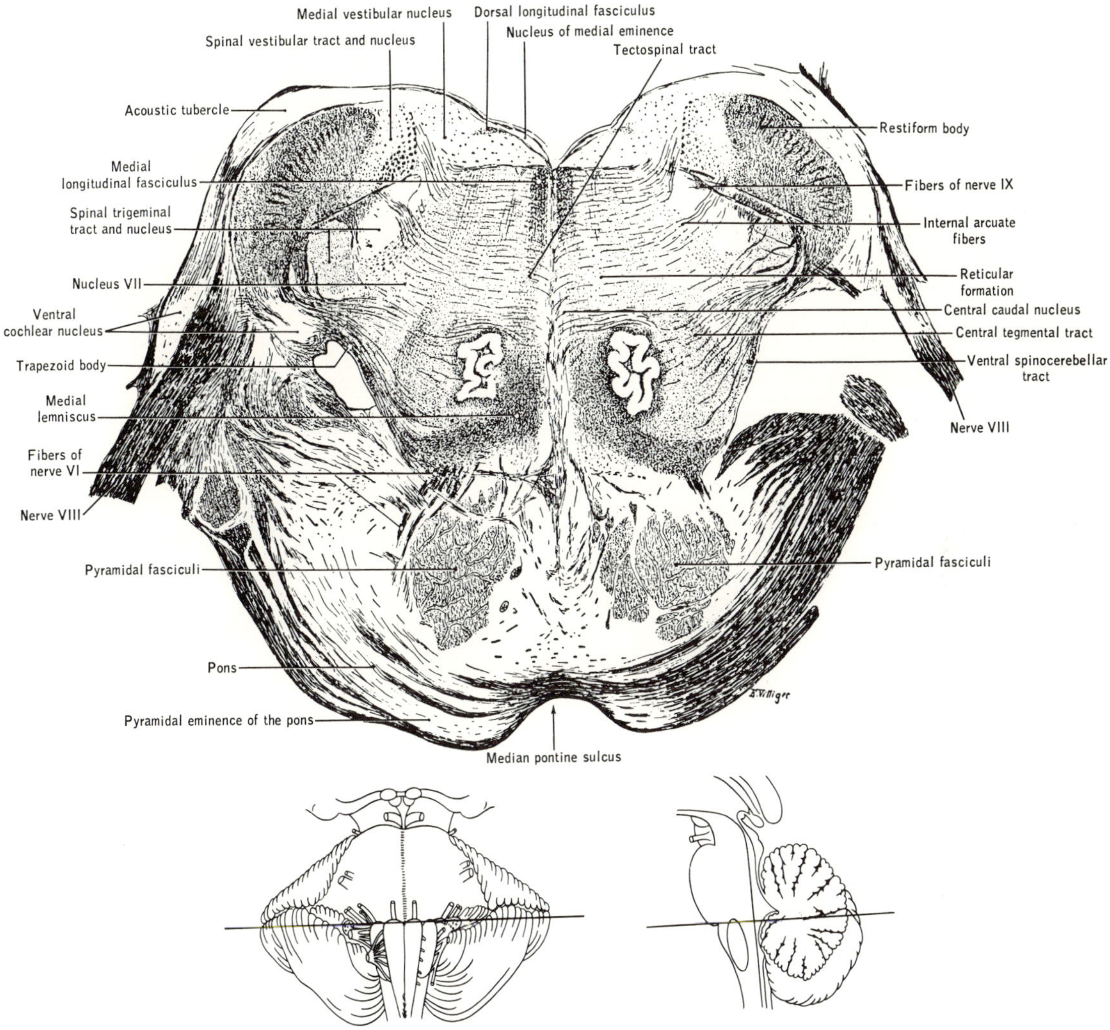

Fig. 25-6. Section of the lower portion of the pons through the superficial attachment of the acoustic nerve (VIII).

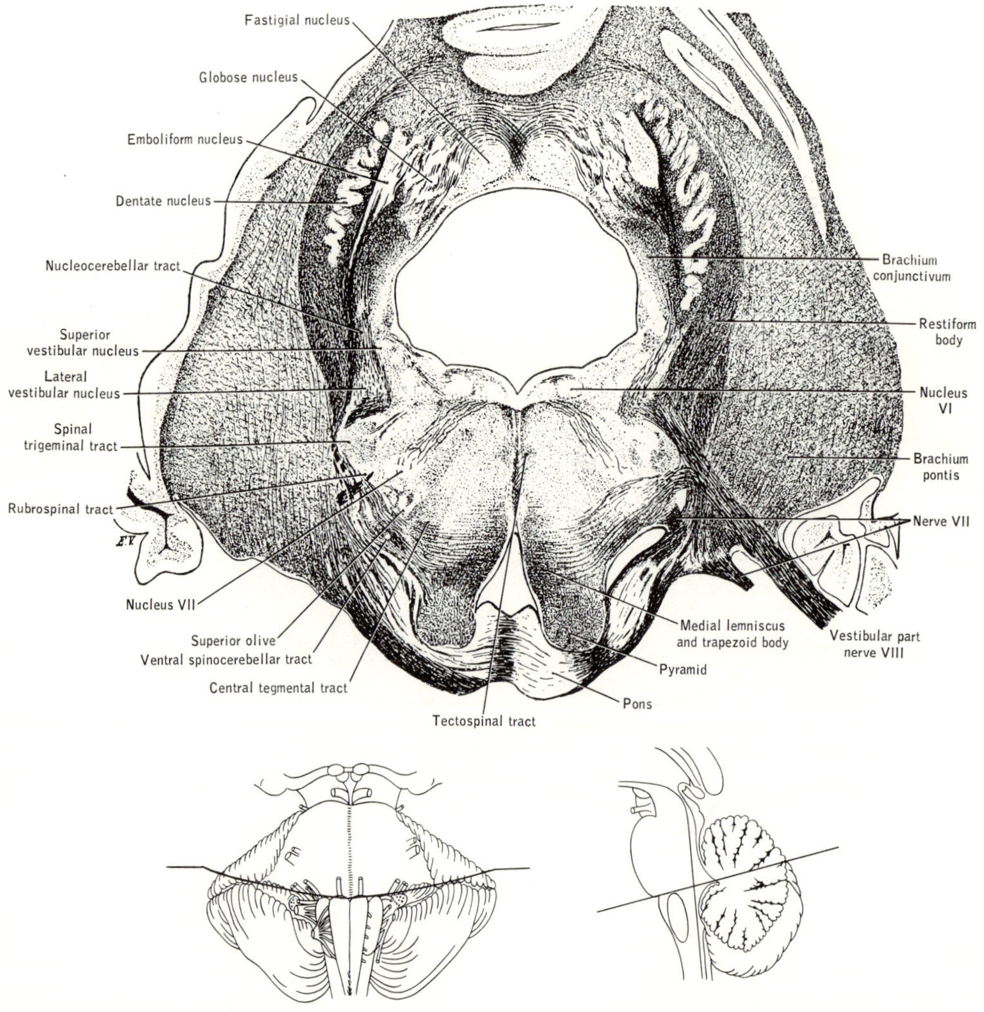

Fig. 25-7. Section of the pons at the level of the superficial attachment of nerve VIII and the nucleus of the facial nerve (VII).

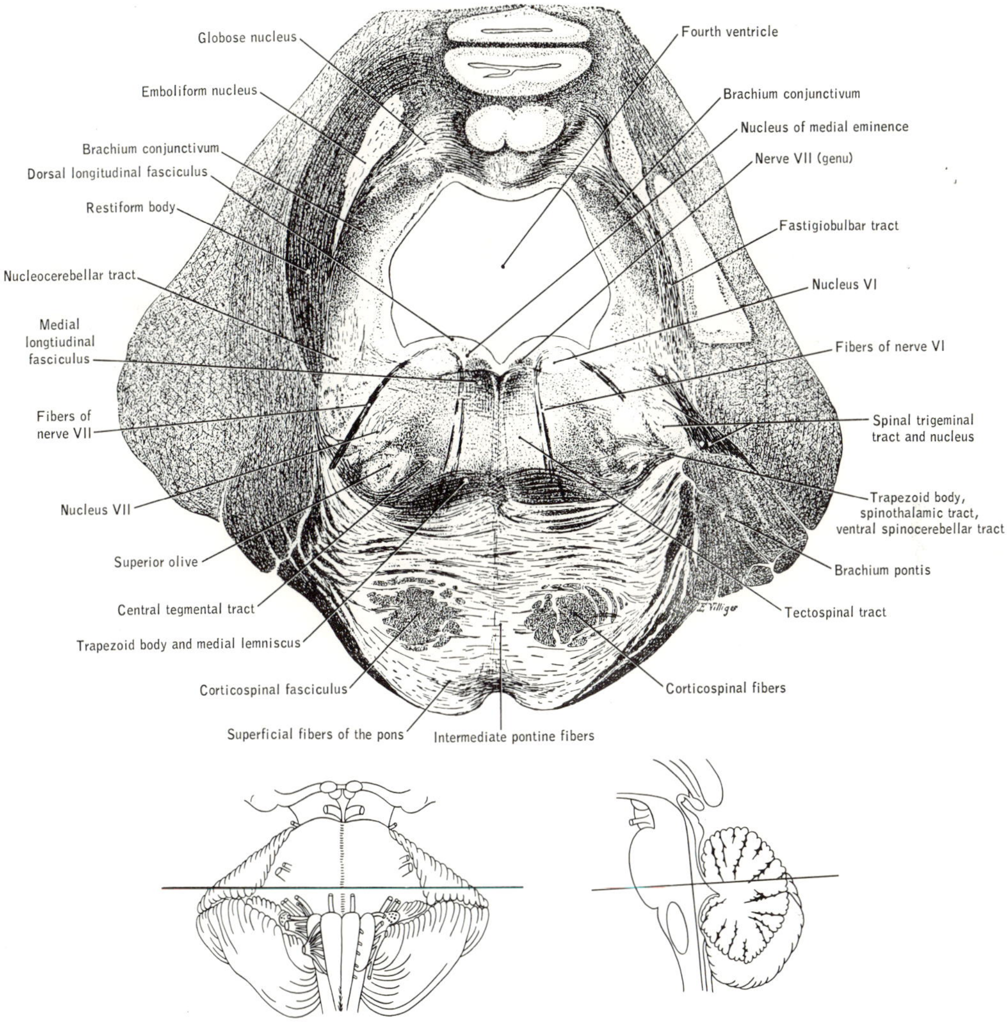

Fig. 25-8. Section of the pons through the level of the internal genu of nerve VII and the nucleus of the abducens nerve (VI).

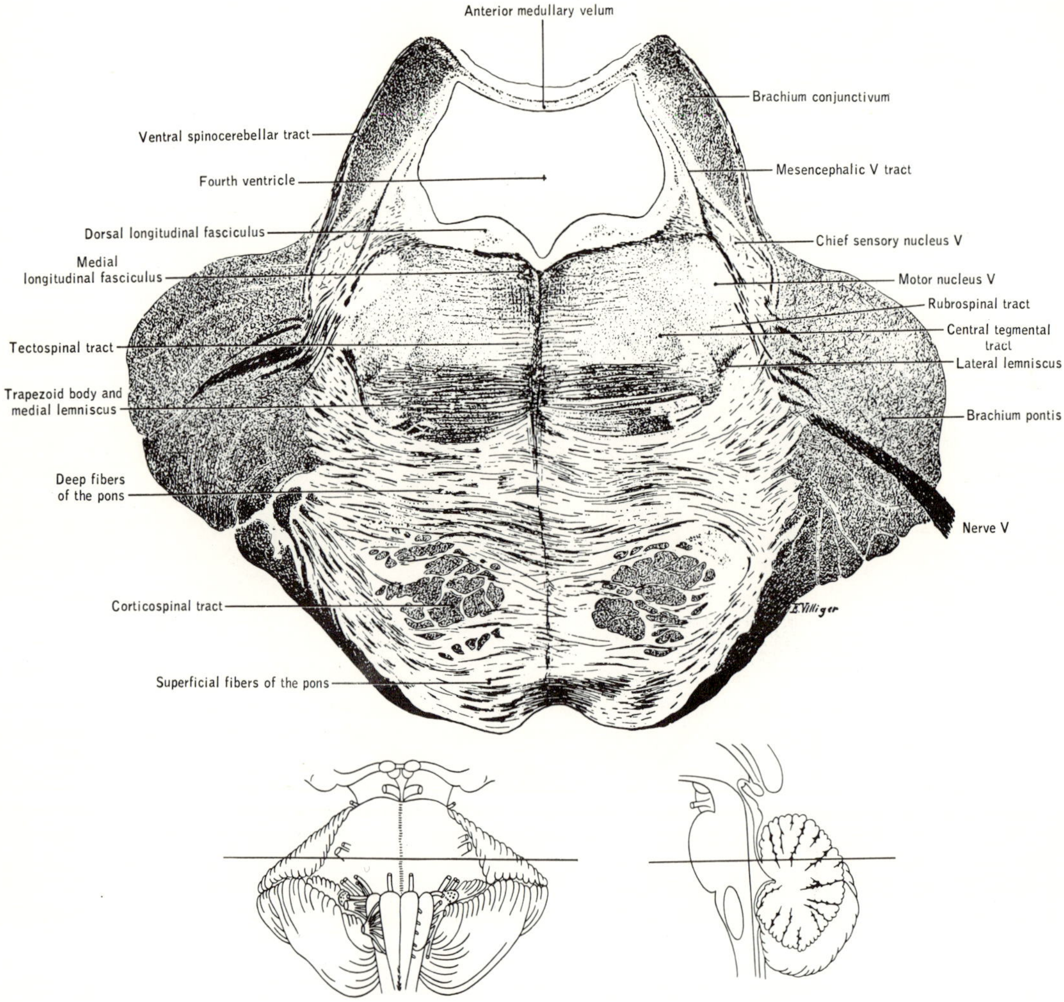

Fig. 25-9. Section of the pons at the level of the superficial attachment of the trigeminal nerve (V) together with the chief sensory and motor nuclei of nerve V.

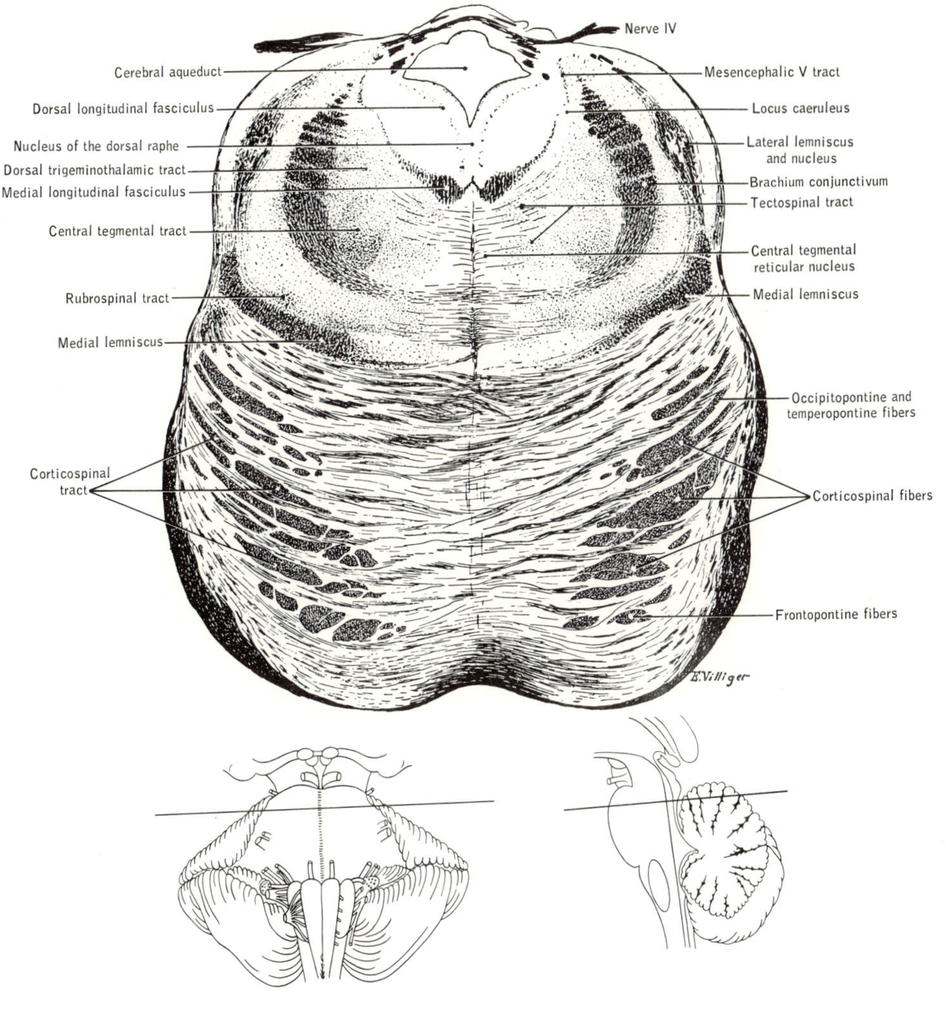

Fig. 25-10. Section through the mesencephalon at the caudal end of the cerebral aqueduct, showing the emerging fibers of the trochlear nerve (IV).

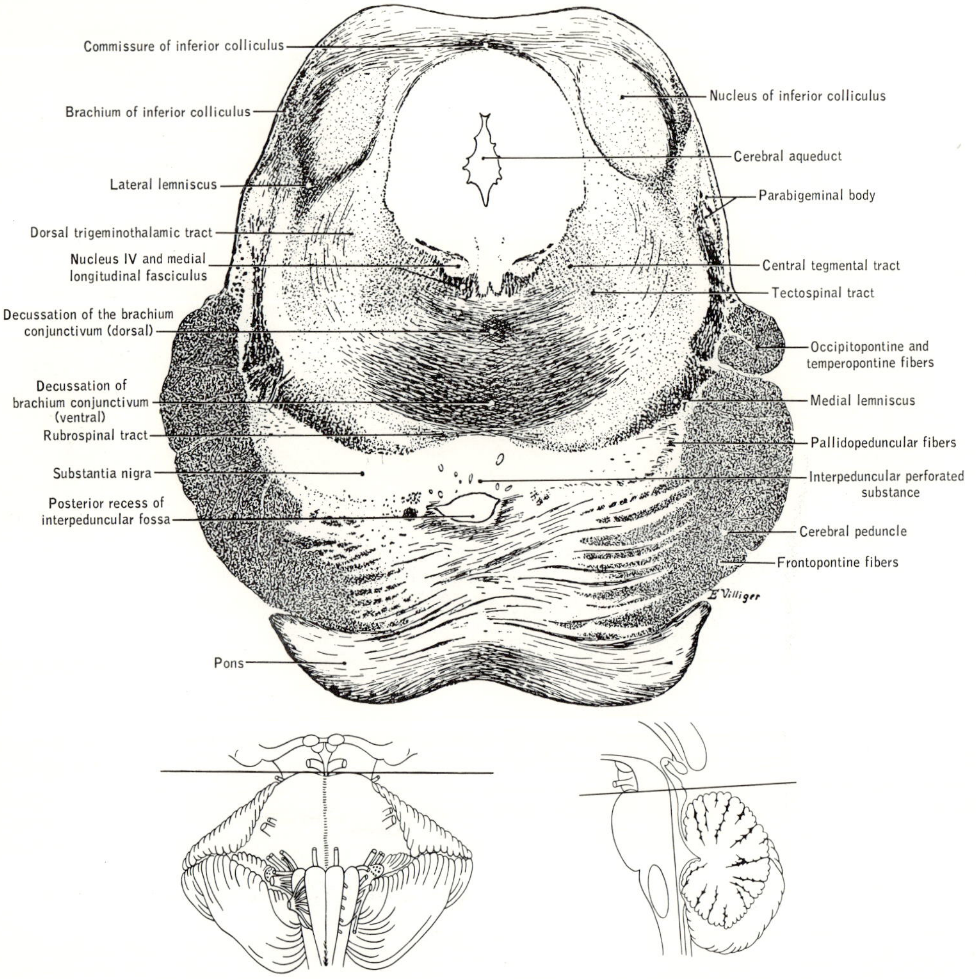

Fig. 25-11. Section of the mesencephalon at the level of the inferior colliculus, showing the nucleus of nerve IV.

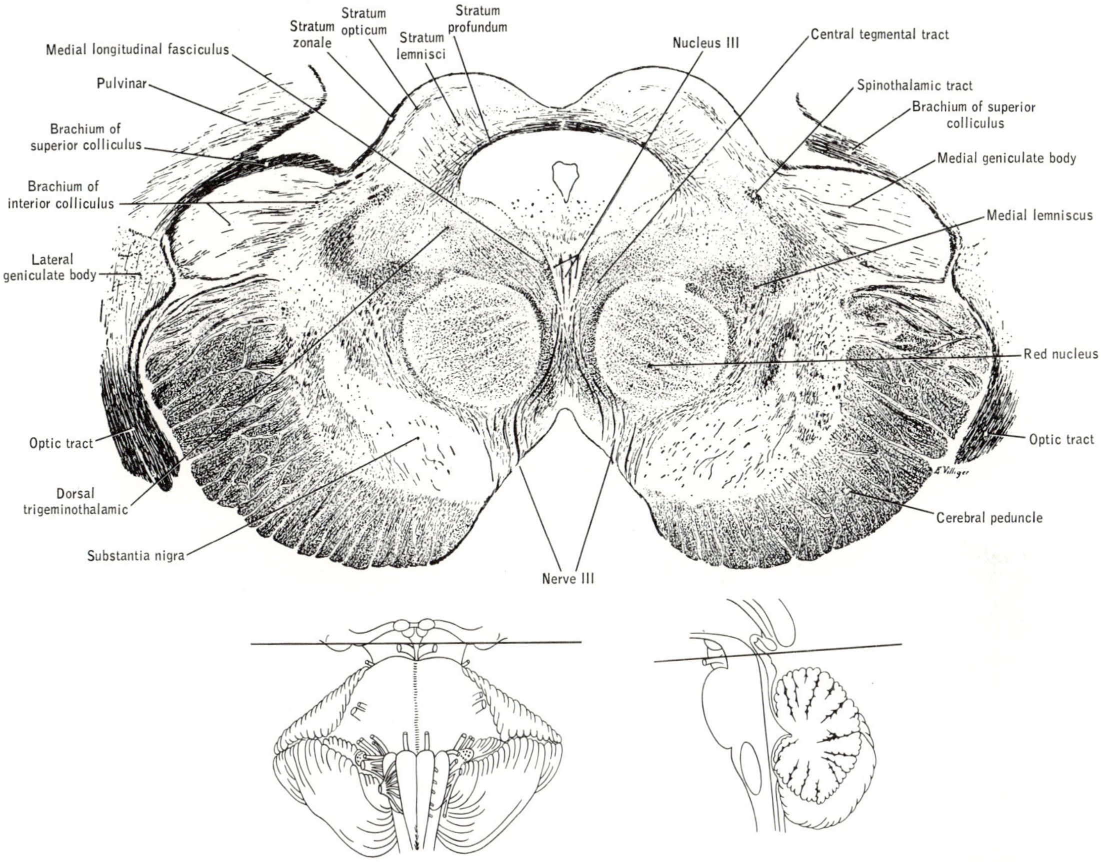

Fig. 25-12. Section of the mesencephalon showing the superficial attachment of nerve III as well as the caudal projection of the thalamus.

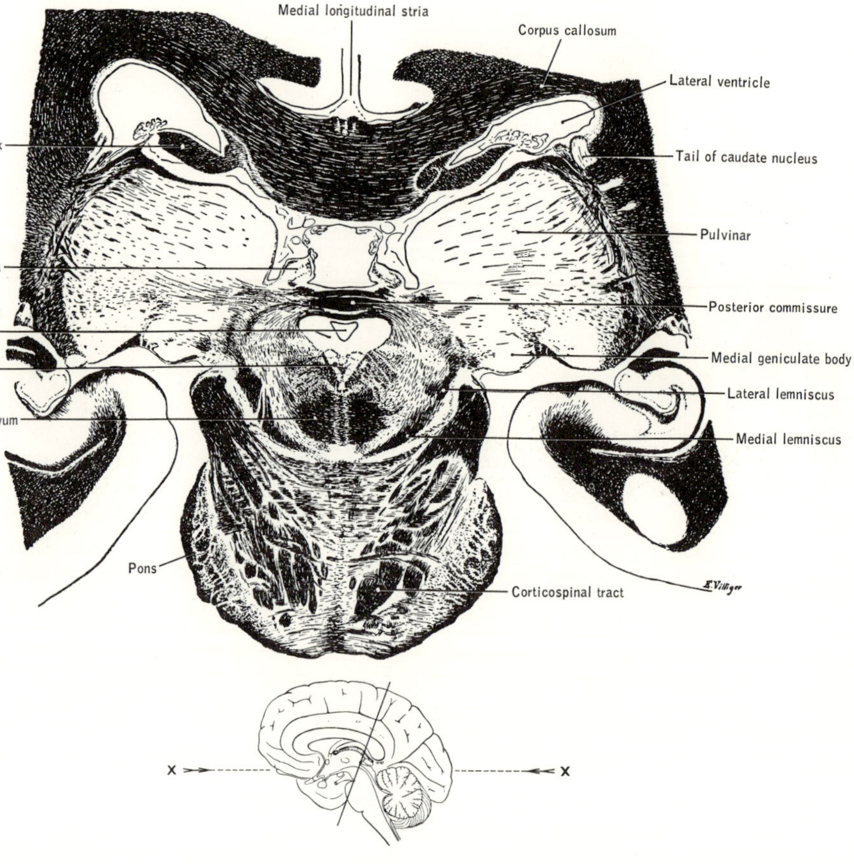

Fig. 25-13. Oblique section of the brain showing the pons, mesencephalon, and posterior commissure.

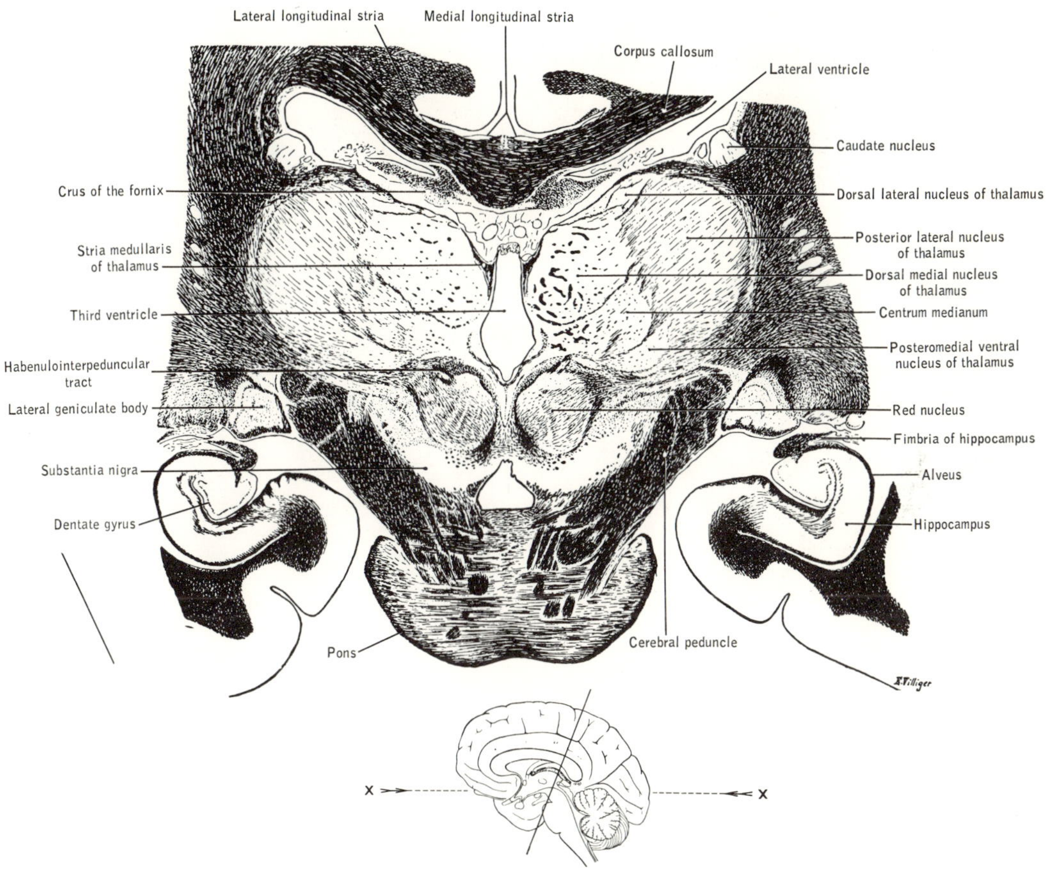

Fig. 25-14. Section of the brain showing some subdivisions of the thalamus.

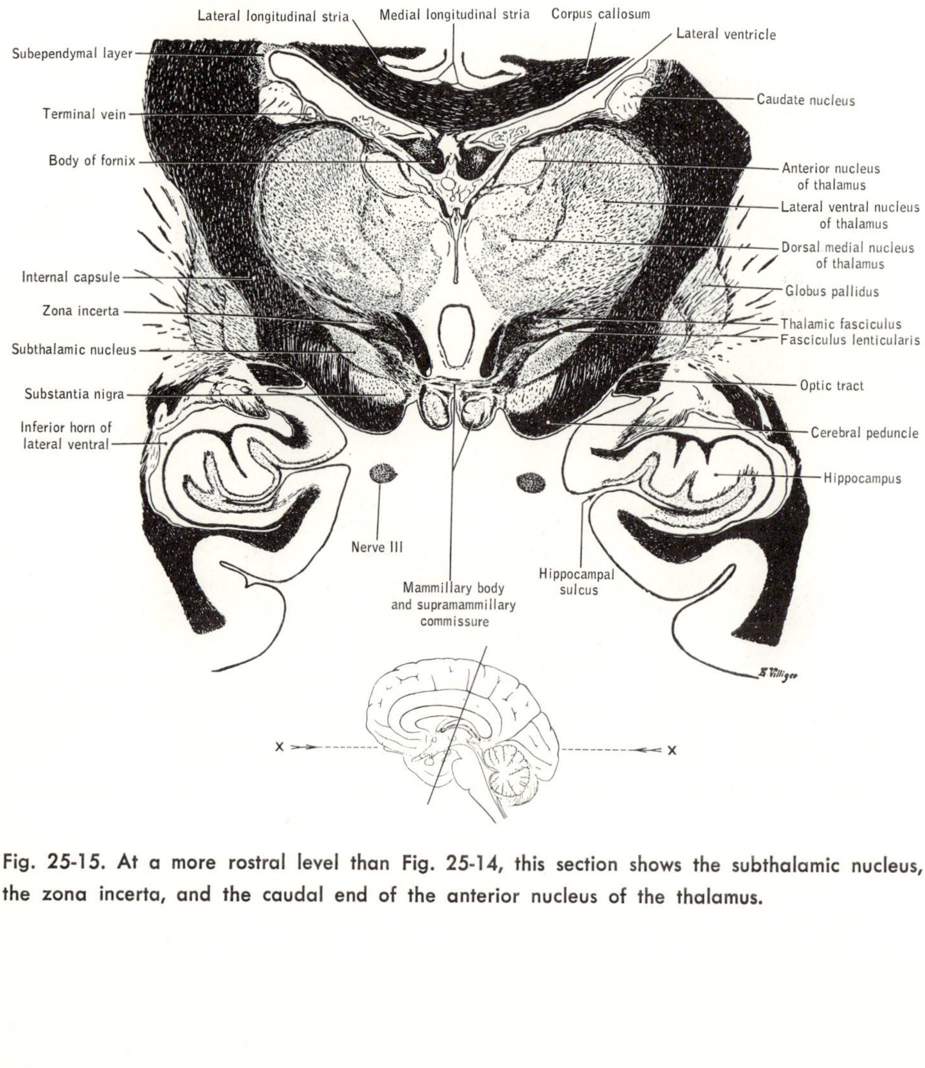

Fig. 25-15. At a more rostral level than Fig. 25-14, this section shows the subthalamic nucleus, the zona incerta, and the caudal end of the anterior nucleus of the thalamus.

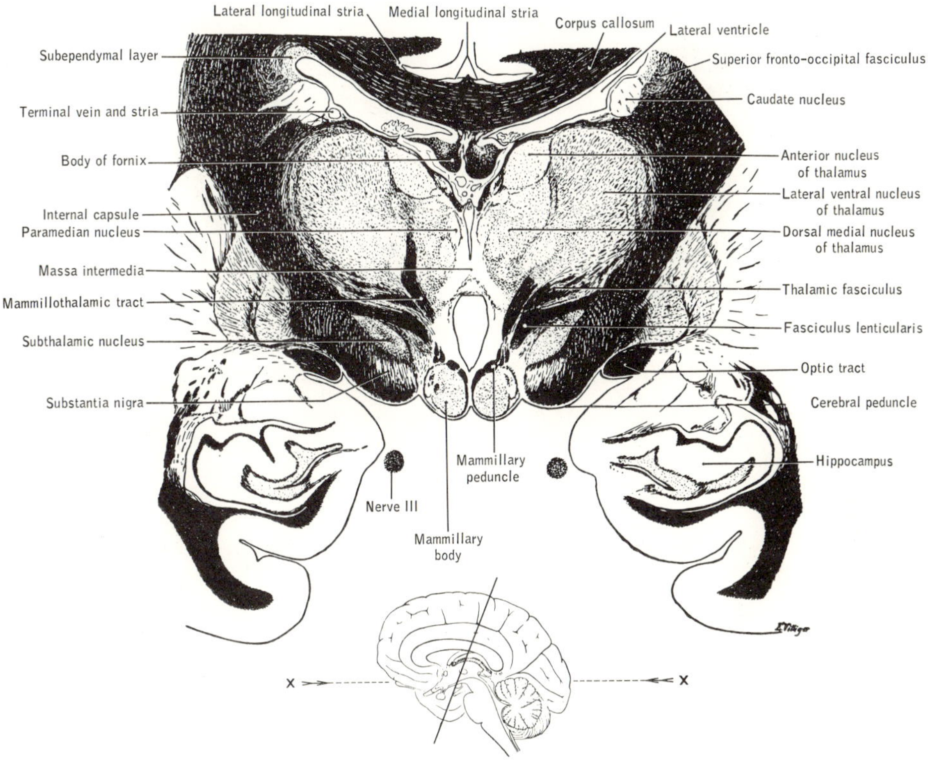

Fig. 25-16. This section is still farther rostral than that in Fig. 25-15, cutting the hypothalamus at the level of the lower portion of the mammillary bodies and the thalamus at the level of its anterior nucleus.

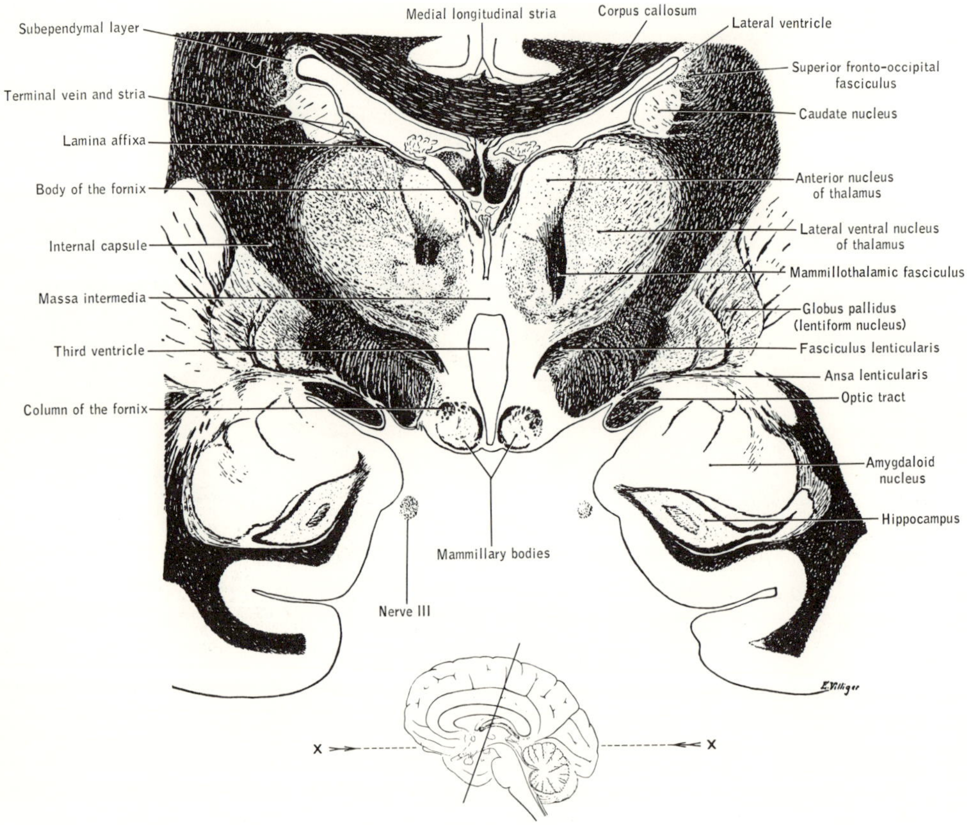

Fig. 25-17. This section passes through the rostral end of the mammillary bodies.

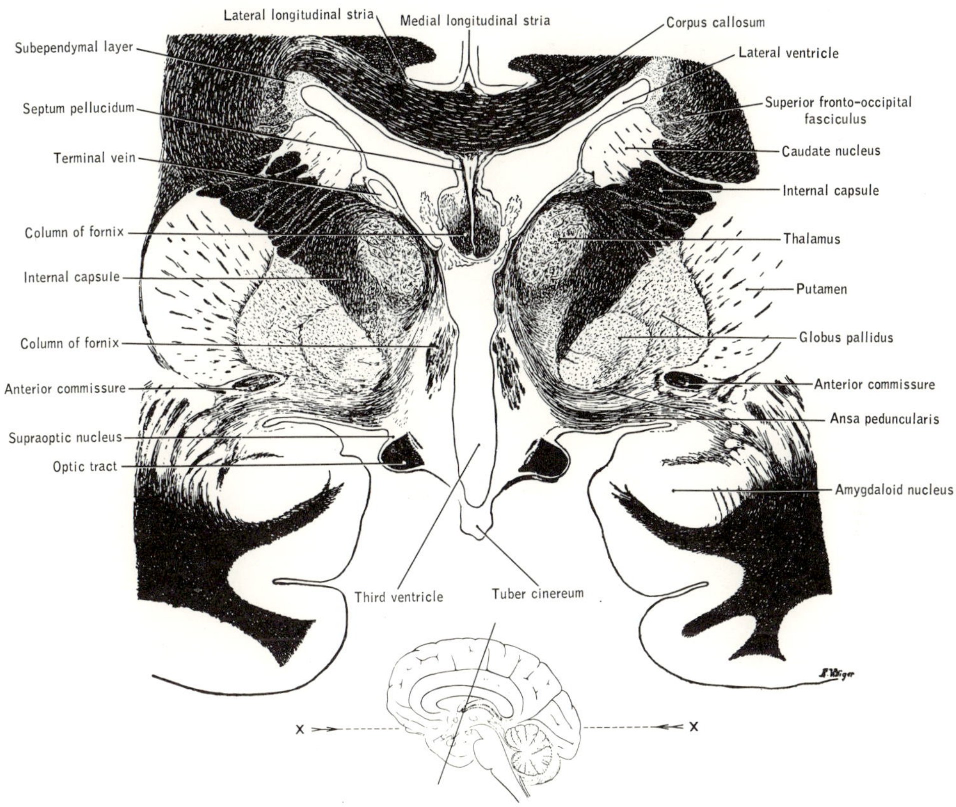

Fig. 25-18. This section passes through the extreme rostral end of the thalamus.

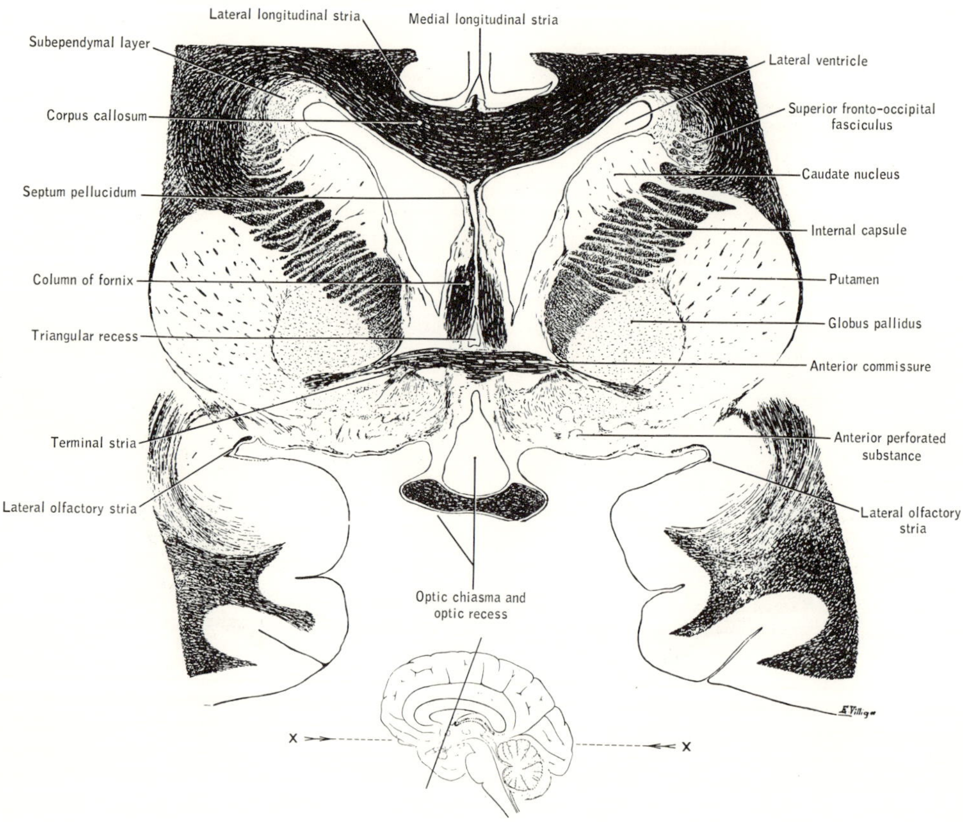

Fig. 25-19. Section of the brain at the level of the optic chiasma and the central portion of the anterior commissure.

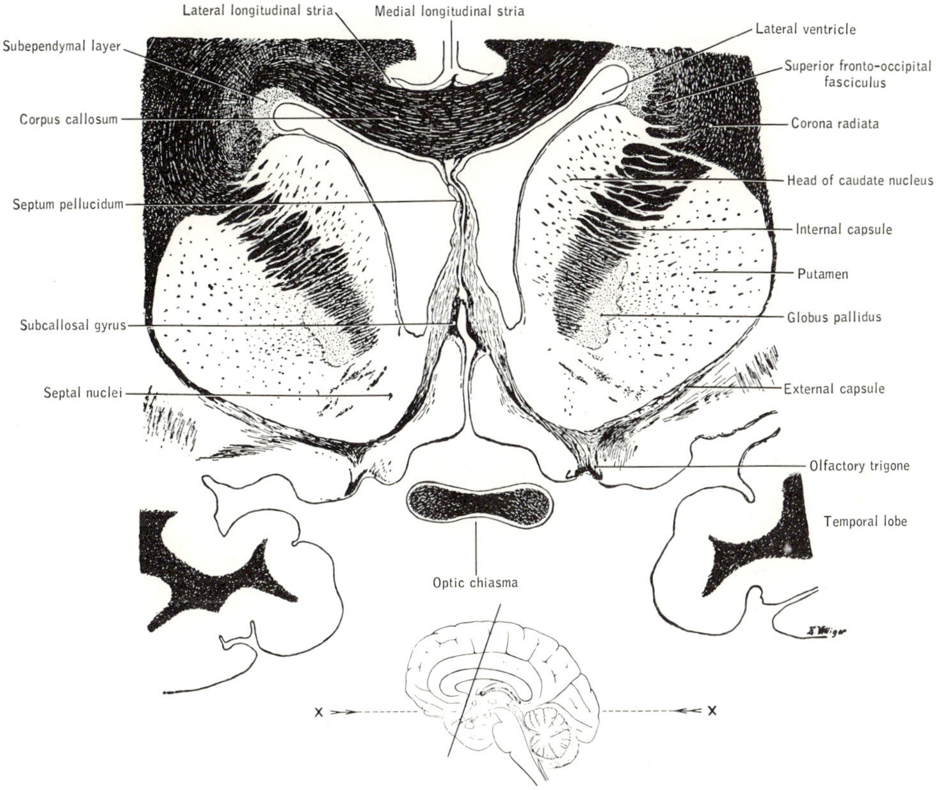

Fig. 25-20. Section through the rostral portion of the optic chiasma showing the union of the head of the caudate nucleus with the lenticular nucleus.

APPENDIX I EXAMINATION OF THE NERVOUS SYSTEM

The examination of the nervous system depends largely on inspection and palpation, occasionally upon percussion, and if vascular lesions are suspected, auscultation may be of value. The *history* is of great importance and the actual neurological examination is the observation of the patient's neurophysiology under a series of tests. The major testing categories are presented below.

A. Mental state
Consider the patient's state of awareness and degree of cooperation and, if there is any abnormality, evaluate the condition in terms of a toxic confusional state, a psychosis, dementia, or a word or thought disorder secondary to a cerebral disease.

B. Motor system
Determine whether all muscles are involved, or whether specific muscle groups are involved. Check the muscles for fatigability, tenderness, atrophy, degree of resistance to passive movement, strength of the muscles, and their ability to perform coordinated movements quickly. Tendon reflexes should be evaluated, keeping in mind the level of the central nervous system being tested. Some of the more common tests are:

1. Direct light reflex
   Light shined into eye causes pupil to constrict.
2. Consensual light reflex
   Light shined into one eye also causes opposite pupil to constrict.
3. Pupillary accommodation reflex
   On near vision eyes converge and pupils constrict; on distant vision pupils dilate. (In an Argyll-Robertson pupil there is light response but no accommodation.)
4. Corneal reflex
   Touch edge of cornea with cotton wisp and get closure of eyes.
5. Deep reflexes (actually stretching reflexes)
   a. Biceps M. (C5-C6)
   b. Brachioradialis M. (C5-C6)
   c. Scapulohumeral (C5-T1)
   d. Triceps M. (C7-C8)
   e. Upper abdominal Mm. (T8-T9)
   f. Middle abdominal Mm. (T9-T10)
   g. Lower abdominal Mm. (T11-T12)
   h. Quadriceps M. (L2-L4), knee jerk or patellar
   i. Adductor Mm. (L2-L4)
   j. Hamstring Mm. (L4-S2)
   k. Achilles (L5-S2) ankle jerk
6. Superficial reflexes (receptors in skin and not in muscle)
   a. Upper abdominal (T5-T8)
   b. Midabdominal (T9-T11)
   c. Lower abdominal (T11-T12)
   d. Cremasteric (L1-L2)

e. Plantar (L4-S2)
f. Superficial anal (L1-L2)

7. Abnormal reflexes in pyramidal tract disease
   a. Clonus (an abnormal response of the stretch reflex from release of central inhibition)
      (1). Ankle
      (2). Patellar
      (3). Wrist
   b. Babinski sign (hallucal dorsiflexion reflex)
   c. Oppenheim's sign (hallucal dorsiflexion reflex)
   d. Grasp reflex
   e. Hoffman's sign
   f. Mayer's reflex
   g. Palm-chin reflex (Radovici's sign)
8. Meningeal irritation
   a. Kernig's sign
   b. Brudzinski's sign
   c. Nuchal rigidity
   d. Spinal rigidity
9. Coordination
   a. Ataxia
   b. Romberg's sign
   c. Check stance in standing, walking, with eyes closed, and direction of falling
10. Testing diadochokinesia (ability to arrest one motor system and substitute another)
    a. Test with alternating movements
    b. Stewart-Holmes rebound sign
11. Test for dyssynergia
    a. Finger-to-nose test
    b. Heel-to-knee test
12. The gait
    a. Ataxia (in cerebellar disease)
    b. Ataxia (in posterior column disease)
    c. Steppage gait: toe drop
    d. Spastic gait: hemiplegia
    e. Spastic gait: scissors gait (paraplegia)
    f. Propulsive gait: parkinsonian gait
    g. Clownish gait: Huntington's chorea
    h. Waddling gait: muscular dystrophy
    i. Bizarre gait: hysteria (use Hoover's sign)

C. Sensory system

Several types of sensation should be studied including pain (pin-prick), light touch, temperature, vibratory, and position sense.

1. Superficial pain
   Use pin-prick and compare symmetric zones with same degree of pressure.
2. Deep pain
   Can use pressure on eyeballs, testes, nerve trunks, and tendons.
3. Temperature
   Use both hot and cold, but not extremes.
4. Tactile sense
   Test with eyes closed.
5. Proprioceptive sense
   a. Position
   b. Pressure
   c. Vibratory
6. Testing higher integrative functions
   a. Stereognosis (ability to distinguish forms)
   b. Two-point discrimination
   c. Perception of figures on skin (graphesthesia)

D. Autonomic nervous system

1. Temperature regulation
2. Vasomotor disorders
   Vasospasm; vasodilatation; dermatographia.
3. Perspiration
   Localized areas of sweating may occur in syringomyelia, peripheral nerve disease, or neuropathy. Anhidrosis is a component of Horner's syndrome.
4. Trophic disturbances
5. Pilomotor reactions

E. Cranial Nerves

1. Olfactory
   Ask the patient to identify familiar odors such as tobacco, coffee, peppermint, etc.

2. Optic
   Use suitable tests for vision, depending on patient's acuity and ability to cooperate.
   Examine the fundi with an ophthalmoscope.
   Test visual fields by the confrontation method.
3. Oculomotor
   Check abnormalities of the eyelids.
   Check action of all eye muscles except the external rectus, superior oblique, and dilator muscles of pupil.
4. Trochlear
   Test the superior oblique muscle.
5. Trigeminal
   a. Motor division
      Look for tremor of the lips, involuntary chewing movements, and trismus (spasm of the masticatory muscles).
      Test the pairs of temporal and masseter muscles and compare muscle tension on both sides.
      Have patient open mouth and note any mandible deviation.
   b. Sensory division
      Test tactile perception of facial skin.
      Test sense of touch in oral mucosa.
      Test pain sensibility of skin and mucosa.
      Test corneal reflex.
6. Abducens
   Test the external rectus muscle.
7. Facial
   a. Motor
      Inspect the face in repose for flaccid paralysis.
      Check for upper or lower motor neuron lesion (UMN or LMN).
      UMN lesions do not affect the upper lid or forehead.
      (1). Face in repose
         Shallow nasolabial folds in both UMN and LMN.
         Palpebral fissure widened in LMN.
      (2). Elevation of eyebrow
         Elevation and wrinkling of forehead absent in LMN, present in UMN.
      (3). Frowning
         Lowering of eyebrows absent in LMN, present in UMN.
      (4). Tight eye closure
         Absent in LMN, lid closed normally in UMN.
      (5). Showing teeth
         The mouth does not elevate in either LMN or UMN.
      (6). Whistling
         Absent in both LMN and UMN.
      (7). Puffing cheeks
         Absent in both LMN and UMN.
      (8). Smiling
         The mouth does not elevate in LMN.
   b. Sensory (taste)
      Test anterior two-thirds of tongue with sugar, vinegar, quinine, and salt.
8. Acoustic
   a. Cochlear
      Rough quantitative test for hearing loss (whispered word, spoken word, ticking watch).
      Weber's test: Place tuning fork against forehead and note in which ear sound is heard best.
      Rinne's test: Tests both bone and air conduction.
   b. Vestibular
      Barany's test.
      Caloric test: Note nystagmus after applying hot and cold water in external ear.
      Pointing test.
      Labyrinthine tests for falling, positional nystagmus, past-pointing.

9. Glossopharyngeal
   Also has both motor and sensory fibers and is usually tested along with the vagus nerve.
   Test swallowing.
   Test for anesthesia of upper part of pharynx and soft palate.
   Test taste sensation of posterior third of tongue.
10. Vagus
    Have patient say "ah" and note uvula deviation.
    Note convergence of faucial pillars.
    Test gag reflex.
    Test areas of pharyngeal mucosa for areas of anesthesia.
    a. Larynx
       Watch laryngeal contours in neck to see if they elevate in swallowing.
       Note hoarseness, dyspnea, and inspiratory distress.
       Check vocal cords.
11. Accessory
    Palpate the upper borders of the trapezii while patient raises his shoulders against the resistance.
    Test the sternocleidomastoid muscle.
12. Hypoglossal
    When the tongue protrudes, look for tremors and other involuntary movements.
    Note any atrophy or tongue deviation.
    Test muscle strength by having patient push tongue against cheek while your hand resists from outside.
    Test lingual speech.

BIBLIOGRAPHY

Adelmann, H. B.: The problem of cyclopia, Quart. Rev. Biol., Part I, 2:161; Part II, 2:284, 1936.

Ades, H. W., and J. M. Brookhart: The central auditory pathway, J. Neurophysiol., 13:189, 1950.

Ades, H. W., and D. Raab: Recovery of motor function after two-stage extirpation of area 4 in monkeys, J. Neurophysiol., 9:55, 1946.

Adrian, E. D.: *The Basis of Sensation: The Action of Sense Organs,* W. W. Norton & Company, Inc., New York, 1928.

Adrian, E. D.: Afferent areas in the cerebellum connected with the limbs, Brain, 66:289, 1943.

Adrian, E. D., and B. H. C. Matthews: The Berger rhythm: potential changes from the occipital lobes in man, Brain, 57:355, 1934.

Alpers, B. J.: *Clinical Neurology,* F. A. Davis Company, Philadelphia, 1947.

Anson, B. J., and W. G. Maddock: *Callander's Surgical Anatomy,* 3d ed., W. B. Saunders Company, Philadelphia, 1952.

Anthony, C. P.: *Textbook of Anatomy and Physiology,* 4th ed., The C. V. Mosby Company, St. Louis, 1955.

Arey, L. B.: *Developmental Anatomy,* 6th ed., W. B. Saunders Company, Philadelphia, 1954.

Bach, L. M. N., and H. W. Magoun: The vestibular nuclei as an excitatory mechanism for the cord, J. Neurophysiol., 10:331, 1947.

Bailey, F. R.: *Textbook of Histology,* 14th ed., by W. M. Copenhaver and D. D. Johnson, The Williams & Wilkins Company, Baltimore, 1958.

Bailey, P.: *Intracranial Tumors,* Charles C Thomas, Springfield, Ill., 1948.

Bailey, P., and G. von Bonin: *The Isocortex of Man,* University of Illinois Press, Urbana, Ill., 1951.

Bailey, P., G. von Bonin, E. W. Davis, H. W. Garol, and W. S. McCulloch: Further observations on associational pathways in the brain of *Macaca mulatta,* J. Neuropathol. Exptl. Neurol., 3:413, 1944.

Bailey, P., H. W. Garol, and W. S. McCulloch: Cortical origin and distribution of corpus callosum and anterior commissure in the chimpanzee, J. Neurophysiol., 4:564, 1941.

Baker, A. B., H. A. Matzke, and J. R. Brown: Poliomyelitis. III. Bulbar poliomyelitis; a study of medullary function, A.M.A. Arch. Neurol. Psychiat., 63:257, 1950.

Barker, D.: The innervation of the muscle spindle, Quart. J. Micr. Sci., 89:143, 1948.

Barnes, S.: Degeneration in hemiplegia: with special reference to a ventrolateral pyramidal tract, the accessory fillet and Pick's bundle, Brain, 24:463, 1901.

Barnes, W. T., H. W. Magoun, and S. W. Ranson: The ascending auditory pathway in the brain stem of the monkey, J. Comp. Neurol., 79:129, 1943.

Beattie, J., G. R. Brow, and C. N. Long: Physiological and anatomical evidence for the existence of nerve tracts connecting the hypothalamus and spinal sympathetic centers, Proc. Roy. Soc., London, B., 106:253, 1930.

Beck, E.: The origin, course and termination of the prefrontopontine tract in the human brain, Brain, 73:368, 1950.

Benda, C. E., and S. Cobb: On the pathogenesis of paralysis agitans, Medicine, 21:95, 1942.

Berger, H.: Über das Elektrenkepathalogramm des Menschen, Arch. Psychiat. Nervenkrankh., 87:527, 1929.

Bing, R., and W. Haymaker: *Regional Diagnosis*

in Lesions of the Brain and Spinal Cord, 11th ed., The C. V. Mosby Company, St. Louis, 1940.

Bloom, W., and D. W. Fawcett: *A Textbook of Histology,* 8th ed., W. B. Saunders Co., Philadelphia, 1962.

Bonin, G., von: Architecture of the precentral motor cortex and some adjacent areas, in *The Precentral Motor Cortex,* 2d ed., by P. C. Bucy (ed.), University of Illinois Press, Urbana, Ill., 1949.

Bornstein, W. S.: Cortical representation of taste in man and monkey, Yale J. Biol. and Med., 12:719, 1940.

Bosma, J. F., and E. Gellhorn: Electromyographic studies of muscular coordination on stimulation of the motor cortex, J. Neurophysiol., 9:263, 1946.

Botterell, E. H., and J. F. Fulton: Functional localization in the cerebellum of primates, J. Comp. Neurol., 69:31, 1938.

Boynton, E. P., and M. Hines: On the question of threshold in stimulation of the motor cortex, Am. J. Physiol., 106:175, 1933.

Brock, S.: *Basis of Clinical Neurology,* The Williams & Wilkins Company, Baltimore, 1945.

Brodal, A.: Experimentelle Untersuchen über die olivo-cerebellare Lokalisation, Z. ges. Neurol. Psychiat., 169:1, 1940.

Brodal, A.: Central course of afferent fibers for pain in facial, glossopharyngeal and vagus nerves. Clinical observations, Arch. Neurol. Psychiat., 57:292, 1947.

Brodal, A.: The hippocampus and the sense of smell. A review, Brain, 70:179, 1947.

Brodal, A.: *Neurological Anatomy,* Oxford University Press, New York, 1948.

Brodmann, K.: Vergleichende Lokalisationslehre der Grosshirnrinde in ihren Prinzipien dargestellt auf Grund des Zellenbaues, Johann Ambrosius Barth, Munich, 1909.

Brodmann, K.: *Die allgemeine Chirurgie der Gehirnkrankheiten. Neue Deutsch Chirurgie,* Bd. 11, Ferd. Enke Verlag, Stuttgart, 1914.

Brouwer, B.: Projection of the retina on the cortex in man, Research Publs., Assoc. Nervous Mental Disease, 13:529, 1934.

Buchanan, A. R.: *Functional Neuroanatomy,* 3d ed., Lea & Febiger, Philadelphia, 1957.

Bucy, P. C.: Cortical extirpation in the treatment of involuntary movements, Research Publs., Assoc. Nervous Mental Disease, 21:551, 1942.

Bucy, P. C.: Effects of extirpation in man, in *The Precentral Motor Cortex,* 2d ed., by P. C. Bucy (ed.), University of Illinois Press, Urbana, Ill., 1949.

Bucy, P. C.: Relation to abnormal involuntary movements, in *The Precentral Motor Cortex,* 2d ed., by P. C. Bucy (ed.), University of Illinois Press, Urbana, Ill., 1949.

Bucy, P. C., and J. F. Fulton: Ipsilateral representation in the motor and premotor cortex in monkeys, Brain, 56:318, 1933

Bumke, O., and O. Foerster: *Handbuch der Neurologie,* Bd. 5, Springer-Verlag, Berlin, 1936.

Cameron, D. E., and M. D. Pradas: Bilateral frontal gyrectomy:psychiatric results, Research Publs., Assoc. Nervous Mental Disease, 27:534, 1948.

Campbell, A. W.: *Histological Studies on the Localization of Cerebral Function,* Cambridge University Press, New York, 1905.

Caton, R.: The electric current of the brain, Brit. Med. J., 2:278, 1875.

Chang, H.-T., T. R. Rugh, and A. A. Ward, Jr.: Topographical representation of muscles in motor cortex of monkeys, J. Neurophysiol., 10:39, 1947.

Clark, G.: The mode of representation in the motor cortex, Brain, 71:320, 1948.

Clark, G.: Suppression and facilitation—a review, Quart., Chicago Med. School, 10:14, 1949.

Clark, G., and J. W. Ward: Responses elicited from the cortex of monkeys by electrical stimulation through fixed electrodes, Brain, 71:332, 1948.

Clark, W. E. L.: The mammalian oculomotor nucleus, J. Anat., 60:426, 1926.

Clark, W. E. L.: The topography and homologies of the hypothalamic nuclei in man, J. Anat., 70:203, 1935.

Clark, W. E. L.: The visual centers of the brain and their connexions, Physiol. Revs., 22:205, 1942.

Clark, W. E. L.: The connexions of the frontal lobes in the brain, Lancet, 1:353, 1948.

Clark, W. E. L., J. Beattie, G. Riddogh, and N. M. Dott: *The Hypothalamus,* Oliver & Boyd, Ltd., Edinburgh, 1938.

Clark, W. E. L., and R. H. Boggan: On the connections of the anterior nucleus of the thalamus, J. Anat., 67:215, 1933.

Cobb, Stanley: *Foundations of Neuropsychiatry,* The Williams & Wilkins Company, Baltimore, 1941.

Cobb, Stanley: *Borderlands of Psychiatry,* Harvard University Press, Cambridge, Mass., 1943.

Cobb, Stanley: *Emotions and Clinical Medicine,* W. W. Norton & Co., New York, 1950.

Corning, H. K.: *Lehrbuch der topographischen Anatomie,* Auf. 14 u. 15, Verlag J. F. Bergman, Munich, 1923.

Corning, H. K.: *Lehrbuch der Entwicklungsge-*

schichte des Menschen, Auf. 14 u. 15, Verlag J. F. Bergman, Munich, 1925.

Courville, C. B.: *Pathology of the Central Nervous System,* Pacific Press Publishing Association, Mountain View, Calif., 1950.

Crosby, E. C., and J. W. Henderson: The mammalian midbrain and isthmus regions. II. Fiber connections of the superior colliculus, J. Comp. Neurol., 88:53, 1948.

Crosby, E. C., and T. Humphrey: Studies on the vertebrate telencephalon. II. The nuclear pattern of the anterior olfactory nucleus, tuberculum olfactorum and the amygdaloid complex in adult man, J. Comp. Neurol., 74:309, 1941.

Crosby, E. C., T. Humphrey and E. W. Lauer: *Correlative Anatomy of the Nervous System.* The Macmillan Co., New York, 1962.

Cunningham, D. J.: *Textbook of Anatomy,* 8th ed., by J. C. Brash and E. B. Jamieson (eds.), Oxford University Press, New York, 1947.

Curtis, H. J.: The intercortical connections of the corpus callosum as indicated by evoked potentials, J. Neurophysiol., 3:407, 1940.

Davis, H.: Physiology of hearing, in *Loose Leaf Medicine of the Ear,* by E. P. Fowler (ed.), Nelson, New York, 1939.

Davison, C.: The role of the globus pallidus and substantia nigra in the production of rigidity and tremor, Research Publs., Assoc. Nervous Mental Disease, 21:261, 1942.

DeJong, R. N.: *The Neurological Examination,* R. B. Hoeber, New York, 1950.

Denny-Brown, D., and E. H. Botterell: The motor functions of the agranular frontal cortex, Research Publs., Assoc. Nervous Mental Disease, 27:235, 1948.

Dow, R. S.: The evolution and anatomy of the cerebellum, Biol. Revs. Cambridge Phil. Soc., 17:179, 1942.

Dusser de Barenne, J. G.: Origin of the motor reactions produced by electrical stimulation of the cerebral cortex, Arch. Neurol. Psychiat., 31:1129, 1934.

Dusser de Barenne, J. G., H. W. Garol, and W. S. McCulloch: Physiological neuronography of the corticostriatal connections, Research Publs., Assoc. Nervous Mental Disease, 21:246, 1942.

Dusser de Barenne, J. G., and W. S. McCulloch: Sensorimotor cortex, nucleus caudatus and thalamus opticus, J. Neurophysiol., 1:364, 1938.

Dusser de Barenne, J. G., and W. S. McCulloch: Suppression of motor response obtained from area 4 by stimulation of area 4s, J. Neurophysiol., 4:311, 1941.

Eccles, J. C.: An electrical hypothesis of synaptic and neuromuscular transmission, Nature, 156: 680, 1945.

Eccles, J. C.: Acetylcholine and synaptic transmission in the spinal cord, J. Neurophysiol., 10:197, 1947.

Economo, C., von: *The Cytoarchitectonics of the Human Cerebral Cortex,* Oxford University Press, New York, 1929.

Economo, C., von, and G. Koskinas: Die Cytoarchitektonik der Hirnrinde der erwachsenen Menschen, Springer-Verlag, Vienna, 1925.

Elliott, H. C.: *Textbook of Neuroanatomy,* J. B. Lippincott Company, Philadelphia, 1963.

Elsberg, C. A., and E. D. Brewer: The sense of smell. X. A detailed description of the technique of two olfactory tests used for the localization of supratentorial tumors of the brain, Bull. Neurol. Inst., N. Y., 4:501, 1935.

Favill, J.: The relationship of eye muscles to semicircular canal currents in rotationally induced nystagmus, Research Publs., Assoc. Nervous Mental Disease, 6:530, 1929.

Fields, W. S., R. Guilleman, and C. A. Carton: Hypothalamic-hypophyseal interrelationships, Proceedings of the Houston Neurological Society, 3, 1955.

Foerster, O.: The cerebral cortex in man, Lancet, 2:309, 1931.

Foerster, O.: The dermatomes in man, Brain, 56:1, 1933.

Foerster, O.: Motorische Felder und Bahnen, in *Handbuch der Neurologie,* by O. Bumke and O. Foerster (eds.), Springer-Verlag, Berlin, 1936.

Foerster, O.: Sensible corticale Felder, in *Handbuch der Neurologie,* by O. Bumke and O. Foerster (eds.), Springer-Verlag, Berlin, 1936.

Ford, F. R.: *Diseases of the Nervous System in Infancy, Childhood and Adolescence,* Charles C Thomas, Publisher, Springfield, Ill., 1937.

Freeman, W., and J. W. Watts: Interpretation of function of frontal lobes based upon observations in 48 cases of prefrontal lobotomy, Yale J. Biol. and Med., 11:527, 1939.

Freeman, W., and J. W. Watts: Retrograde degeneration of the thalamus following prefrontal lobotomy, J. Comp. Neurol., 86:65, 1947.

Freeman, W., and J. W. Watts: Psychosurgery, in *The Treatment of Mental Disorders and Intractable Pain,* Charles C Thomas, Publisher, Springfield, Ill., 1950.

French, J. D., O. Sugar, and J. G. Chusid: Corticocortical connections of the superior bank of the sylvian fissure in the monkey, J. Neurophysiol., 11:185, 1948.

Fulton, J. F.: *Physiology of the Nervous System,*

2d ed., Oxford University Press, New York, 1943.

Fulton, J. F., and D. Sheehan: The uncrossed lateral pyramidal tract in higher primates, J. Anat., 69:181, 1935.

Galambos, R.: Suppression of auditory nerve activity by stimulation of efferent fibers to the cochlea, J. Neurophysiol., 19:424–437, 1956.

Gardner, E.: *Fundamentals of Neurology,* 3d ed., W. B. Saunders Company, Philadelphia, 1958.

Gardner, E., and H. M. Cuneo: Lateral spinothalamic tract and associated tracts in man, Arch. Neurol. Psychiat., 53:423, 1945.

Garol, H. W., and P. C. Bucy: Suppression of motor response in man, Arch. Neurol. Psychiat., 51:528, 1944.

Gellhorn, E.: The influence of alterations in posture of the limbs on cortically induced movements, Brain, 71:26, 1948.

Gellhorn, E., and L. Thompson: The influence of muscle pain on cortically induced movements, Am. J. Physiol., 142:231, 1944.

Gibbs, F. A., and E. L. Gibbs: *Atlas of Encephalography,* Addison-Wesley Publishing Company, Cambridge, Mass., 1950.

Gibbs, F. A., E. L. Gibbs, and W. G. Lennox: Cerebral dysrhythmias of epilepsy, Arch. Neurol. Psychiat., 39:298, 1938.

Gilbert, M. S.: Early development of the human diencephalon, J. Comp. Neurol., 62:81, 1935.

Givner, I.: Episcleral ganglion cells, Arch. Ophthalmol. Chicago, N.S., 22:82, 1939.

Glees, P.: The anatomical basis of corticostriate connexions, J. Anat., 78:47, 1944.

Glees, P., and P. D. Wall: Fiber connections of the subthalamic region and the centromedian nucleus of the thalamus, Brain, 69:195, 1946.

Globus, J. H.: *Practical Neuroanatomy,* William Wood & Company, Baltimore, 1937.

Grant, F. C., and L. M. Weinberger: Experiences with intramedullary tractotomy. I. Relief of facial pain and summary of operative results, Arch. Surg., 42:681, 1941.

Grant, J. C. B.: *An Atlas of Human Anatomy,* 3d ed., The Williams & Wilkins Company, Baltimore, 1951.

Gray, H.: *Anatomy of the Human Body,* 26th ed., by C. M. Goss (ed.), Lea & Febiger, Philadelphia, 1954.

Greep, R. (ed.): *Histology,* McGraw-Hill Book Company, Inc., Blakiston Division, New York, 1954.

Greischeimer, E. M.: *Physiology and Anatomy,* 7th ed., J. B. Lippincott Company, Philadelphia, 1955.

Grundfest, Harry, and B. Campbell: Origin, conduction and termination of the spino-cerebellar tract in cats, J. Neurophysiol., 5:275, 1942.

Ham, A. W.: *Histology,* 3d ed., J. B. Lippincott Company, Philadelphia, 1957.

Hamilton, W. J., J. B. Boyd, and H. W. Mossman: *Human Embryology,* 3d ed., The Williams & Wilkins Company, Baltimore, 1962.

Hammond, W. S., and C. L. Yntema: Depletion of the thoraco-lumbar sympathetic system following removal of neural crest in the chick, J. Comp. Neurol., 86:237, 1947.

Hardesty, I.: On the development and nature of neuroglia, Am. J. Anat., 3:229, 1904.

Hardesty, I.: On the occurrence of the sheath cells and nature of axon sheaths in the central nervous system, Am. J. Anat., 4:329, 1905.

Harris, G. W.: Neural control of the pituitary gland, Physiol. Revs., 28:139, 1948.

Harrison, F.: The hypothalamus and sleep, Research Publs. Assoc. Nervous Mental Disease, 20:635, 1940.

Hartridge, H.: The polychromatic theory, in *Recent Advances in the Physiology of Vision,* McGraw-Hill Book Company, Inc., Blakiston Division, New York, 1950.

Hausman, L.: Pure flaccid hemiplegia uncomplicated by sensory defect, Trans. Am. Neurol. Assoc., 65:217, 1939.

Haymaker, W.: *Bing's Local Diagnosis in Neurological Diseases,* 14th ed., The C. V. Mosby Company, St. Louis, 1956.

Haymaker, W. E., and M. B. Woodhall: *Peripheral Nerve Injuries; Principals of Diagnosis,* W. B. Saunders Co., Philadelphia, 1953.

Head, H.: *Studies in Neurology,* Oxford University Press, New York, 1920.

Hebb, D. O., and W. Penfield: Human behavior after extensive bilateral removal from the frontal lobes, Arch. Neurol. Psychiat., 44:421, 1940.

Herrick, C. J.: The functions of the olfactory parts of the cerebral cortex, Proc. Natl. Acad. Sci. U.S., 19:7, 1933.

Herter, C. A., and L. P. Clarke: *Diagnosis of Organic Nervous Diseases,* G. P. Putnam's Sons, New York, 1907.

Hertwig, R.: *A Manual of Zoology,* Henry Holt and Company, New York, 1905.

Hilton, J.: *On Rest and Pain, a Course of Lectures,* W. Wood & Co., New York, 1879.

Hines, M.: The anterior border of the monkey's motor cortex and the production of spasticity, Am. J. Physiol., 116:76, 1936.

Hines, M.: The motor cortex, Bull. Johns Hopkins Hosp., 60:313, 1937.

Hines, M.: Control of movements by the cerebral cortex in primates, Biol. Revs. Cambridge Phil. Soc., 18:1, 1943.

Hines, M.: Significance of the precentral motor cortex, in *The Precentral Motor Cortex,* 2d ed., by P. C. Bucy (ed.), University of Illinois Press, Urbana, Ill., 1949.

His, W., Jr.: Über die Entwickelung des Bauchsympathikus beim Hünchen und Menschen, Arch. Anat. u. Physiol. Anat. Ab., Suppl. S:137, 1897.

His, W., Jr.: *Die Entwickelung des menschlichen Gehirns wahrend der ersten Monate,* vol. 4, S. Hirzel Verlag, Leipzig, 1904, p. 176.

Hochstetter, F.: *Beitrage zur Entwickelungsgeschichte des menschlichen Gehirns,* Teil I, S.1, and Teil II, S.1, Deutiche, Vienna, 1929.

Holmes, G.: The cerebellum of man, Brain, 62:1, 1939.

Holmes, G.: The organization of the visual cortex in man, Proc. Roy. Soc., London, B., 132:348, 1944.

Holmes, G., and W. P. May: On the exact origin of the pyramidal tracts in man and other mammals, Brain, 32:1, 1909.

Huber, G. C.: The reptilian optic tectum, J. Comp. Neurol., 57:57–63, 1933.

Huber, G. C., E. C. Crosby, R. T. Woodburne, and L. A. Gillilan, J. O. Brown and B. Tamthai: The mammalian midbrain and isthmus region. Part I, The Nuclear pattern. J. Comp. Neurol., 78:129–534, 1943.

Ingram, W. R.: Nuclear organization and chief connections of the primate hypothalamus, Research Publs., Assoc. Nervous Mental Disease, 20:195, 1940.

Ingvar, S.: Studies in neurology. I. The phylogenetic continuity of the central nervous system. II. On cerebellar function, Bull. Johns Hopkins Hosp., 43:315, 1928.

Jacobsen, C. F.: Influence of motor and premotor area lesions upon the retention of skilled movements in monkeys and chimpanzees, Research Publs., Assoc. Nervous Mental Disease, 13:225, 1934.

Jasper, H. H.: Diffuse projection systems: the integrative action of the thalamic reticular system, Electroencephalog. and Clin. Neurophysiol., 1:405, 1949.

Jones, I. H.: Vestibular experiences, Laryngoscope, 59:354–368, 1949.

Jones, T., and W. C. Shepard: *A Manual of Surgical Anatomy,* W. B. Saunders Company, Philadelphia, 1945.

Jordan, H. E.: *A Textbook of Histology,* 9th ed., Appleton-Century-Crofts, Inc., New York, 1952.

Jordan, H. E., and J. E. Kindred: *Textbook of Embryology,* 5th ed., Appleton-Century-Crofts, Inc., New York, 1948.

Judovich, B. D., and W. Bates: *Segmental Neuralgia in Painful Syndromes,* F. A. Davis Co., Philadelphia, 1944.

Kappers, C. V. A., G. C. Huber, and E. C. Crosby: *The Comparative Anatomy of the Nervous System of Vertebrates,* The Macmillan Company, New York, 1936.

Keibel, F., and F. P. Mall: *Manual of Human Embryology,* J. B. Lippincott Company, Philadelphia, 1910.

Keiller, W.: *Nerve Tracts of the Brain Stem and Cord,* The Macmillan Co., New York, 1927.

Kimber, D. C., C. E. Gray, C. E. Stackpole, and L. C. Leavell: *Textbook of Anatomy and Physiology,* 13th ed., The Macmillan Company, New York, 1957.

Kingsbury, B. F.: The fundamental plan of the vertebrate brain, J. Comp. Neurol., 34:461, 1922.

Kodama, S.: Über die sogenannten Basalganglien, Schweiz. Arch. Neurol. Psychiat., 18:179, 1926.

Kremer, W. F.: Autonomic and somatic reactions induced by stimulation of the cingular gyrus in dogs, J. Neurophysiol., 10:371, 1947.

Krieg, W. J. S.: *Functional Neuroanatomy,* McGraw-Hill Book Company, Inc., Blakiston Division, New York, 1953.

Kreig, W. J. S.: Connections of the cerebral cortex of the monkey, Symp. Biol. Hung., 5:177–217, 1965.

Kuntz, A.: *The Neuroanatomic Basis of Surgery of the Autonomic Nervous System,* Charles C Thomas, Publisher, Springfield, Ill., 1949.

Kuntz, A.: *A Textbook of Neuroanatomy,* 5th ed., Lea & Febiger, Philadelphia, 1950.

Kurtz, S. M.: *Electron Microscopic Anatomy,* Academic Press, New York, 1964.

Langley, L. L., E. Cheraskin, and R. Sleeper: *Dynamic Anatomy and Physiology,* McGraw-Hill Book Company, Inc., New York, 1958.

Langworthy, O. R.: Development of behavior patterns and myelinization of the human fetus and infant, Carnegie Contrib. Embryol., 34, no. 228: 145, 1933.

Lanz, T., von, and W. Wachsmith: *Praktische Anatomie,* Springer-Verlag, Berlin, 1935.

Larsell, O.: The cerebellum: a review and interpretation, Arch. Neurol. Psychiat., 38:580, 1937.

Larsell, O.: *Anatomy of the Nervous System,* 2d ed., Appleton-Century-Crofts, Inc., New York, 1951.

Lassek, A. M.: The human pyramidal tract. II. A numerical investigation of the Betz cells of the motor area, Arch. Neurol. Psychiat., 44:718, 1940.

Lassek, A. M.: The pyramidal tract: basic considerations of corticospinal neurons, Research Publs. Assoc. Nervous Mental Disease, 27:106, 1947.

Levin, P. M.: Efferent fibers, in *The Premotor Cortex,* 2d ed., by P. C. Bucy (ed.), University of Illinois Press, Urbana, Ill., 1949.

Levin, P. M., and F. K. Bradford: The exact origin of the corticospinal tract in the monkey, J. Comp. Neurol., 68:411, 1938.

Lewis, D., and W. E. Dandy: The course of the nerve fibers transmitting the sensation of taste, Arch. Surg., 21:249, 1930.

Lewis, T.: *Pain,* The Macmillan Co., New York, 1942.

List, C. F.: Intraspinal epidermoids, dermoids and dermal sinuses, Surg. Gynecol. Obstet., 73:525, 1941.

Livingston, W. K.: *The Clinical Aspects of Visceral Neurology,* Charles C Thomas, Springfield, Ill., 1935.

Livingston, W. K.: *Pain Mechanisms,* The Macmillan Co., New York, 1943.

Lloyd, D. P. C.: Functional organization of the spinal cord, Physiol. Revs., 24:1, 1944.

Lloyd, D. P. C.: Facilitation and inhibition of spinal motor neurons, J. Neurophysiol., 9:421, 1946.

Lloyd, D. P. C., and H.-T. Chang: Afferent fibers in muscle nerves, J. Neurophysiol., 11:199, 1948.

Lorente de Nó, R.: Studies on the structure of the cerebral cortex. I. The area entorhinalis, J. Psychol. u. Neurol., 45:381, 1933.

Lorente de Nó, R.: Studies on the structure of the cerebral cortex. Continuation of study of ammonic system, J. Psychol. u. Neurol., 46:113, 1934.

Lorente de Nó, R.: Cerebral cortex: architecture, intracortical connections, motor projections, in *Physiology of the Nervous System,* 3d ed., by J. F. Fulton (ed.), Oxford University Press, New York, 1949.

McCulloch, W. S.: The functional organization of the cerebral cortex, Physiol. Revs., 24:390, 1944.

McCulloch, W. S.: Modes of functional organization of the cerebral cortex, Federation Proc., 6:448, 1947.

McCulloch, W. S.: Some connections of the frontal lobe established by physiological neuronography, Research Publs., Assoc. Nervous Mental Disease, 27:95, 1948.

McCulloch, W. S.: Cortico-cortical connections, in *The Precentral Motor Cortex,* 2d ed., by P. C. Bucy (ed.), University of Illinois Press, Urbana, Ill., 1949.

McCulloch, W. S., and H. W. Garol: Cortical origin and distribution of corpus callosum and anterior commissure in the monkey, J. Neurophysiol., 4:555, 1941.

McCulloch, W. S., C. Graf, and H. W. Magoun: A cortico-bulbo-reticular pathway from area 4s, J. Neurophysiol., 9:127, 1946.

McCulloch, W. S., and E. Henneman: The projection of area 19 to the reticular formation, Federation Proc., 7:79, 1948.

McLardy, T.: The thalamic projection to frontal cortex in man, J. Neurol. Neurosurg. Psychiat., N.S., 13:198, 1950.

MacLean, P. D.: Psychosomatic disease and the "visceral brain"; recent developments bearing on the Papez theory of emotion. Psychosom. Med., 11:338–353, 1949.

MacLean, P. D.: Limbic system and emotional behavior, A.M.A. Arch. Neurol. & Psychol., 73:130–134, 1955.

Magoun, H. W.: Descending connections from the hypothalamus, Research Publs., Assoc. Nervous Mental Disease, 20:270, 1940.

Magoun, H. W.: Bulbar inhibition and facilitation of motor activity, Science, 100:549, 1949.

Magoun, H. W., D. Atlas, W. K. Hare, and S. W. Ranson: The afferent path of the pupillary light reflex in the monkey, Brain, 59:234, 1936.

Magoun, H. W., and L. E. Beaton: The salivatory motor nucleus in the monkey, Am. J. Physiol., 136:720, 1942.

Magoun, H. W., and R. Rhines: An inhibitory mechanism in the bulbar reticular formation, J. Neurophysiol., 9:165, 1946.

Magoun, H. W., and R. Rhines: *Spasticity. The Stretch-reflex and Extrapyramidal Systems,* Charles C Thomas, Publisher, Springfield, Ill., 1947.

Marburg, O.: *Mikroskopisch-topographischer Atlas des menschlichen Zentralnervensystems,* Franz Deutiche, Leipzig, 1910.

Marburg, O.: Modern views regarding the anatomy and physiology of the vestibular tracts, Laryngoscope, 49:631–652, 1939.

Marburg, O.: The structure and fiber connections of the human habenula, J. Comp. Neurol., 80:211, 1944.

Maximow, A. A., and W. Bloom: *A Textbook of Histology,* 7th ed., W. B. Saunders Company, Philadelphia, 1957.

Mettler, F. A.: Relation between pyramidal and extrapyramidal function, Research Publs., Assoc. Nervous Mental Disease, 21:150, 1942.

Mettler, F. A.: Fiber connections of the corpus striatum of the monkey and baboon, J. Comp. Neurol., 82:169, 1945.

Mettler, F. A.: *Neuroanatomy,* 2d ed., The C. V. Mosby Company, St. Louis, 1948.

Mettler, F. A.: The nonpyramidal motor projections from the frontal cerebral cortex, Research Publs., Assoc. Nervous Mental Disease, 27:162, 1948.

Mettler, F. A., and C. C. Mettler: Role of the neostriatum, Am. J. Physiol., 133:594, 1941.

Meyer, A., E. Beck, and T. McLardy: Prefrontal leucotomy: a neuroanatomical report, Brain, 70:18, 1947.

Meyer, M.: Study of efferent connexions of the frontal lobe in the human brain after leucotomy, Brain, 72:265, 1949.

Meyers, R., D. B. Sweeney, and J. T. Schwidde: Hemiballismus: etiology and surgical treatment, J. Neurol., Neurosurg. Psychiat., N.S., 13:115, 1950.

Monakow, C., von: Biologisches und Morphogenetisches über die Mikrocephalia vera, Schweiz. Arch. Neurol. Psychiat., 18:191, 1926.

Monrad-Krohn, G. H.: *Clinical Examination of the Nervous System,* 7th ed., Paul B. Hoeber, Inc., New York, 1938.

Morris, H.: *Morris' Human Anatomy,* 11th ed., by J. P. Schaeffer (ed.), McGraw-Hill Book Company, Inc., Blakiston Division, New York, 1953.

Moruzzi, G., and H. W. Magoun: Brain stem reticular formation and activation of the EEG, Electroencephalog. and Clin. Neurophysiol., 1:455, 1949.

Murphy, J. P., and E. Gellhorn: The influence of hypothalamic stimulation on cortically induced movements and on action potentials of the cortex, J. Neurophysiol., 8:341, 1945.

Murphy, J. P., and E. Gellhorn: Further investigations on diencephalic-cortical relations and their significance for the problem of emotion, J. Neurophysiol., 8:431, 1945.

Nathan, P. W., and J. W. A. Turner: Efferent pathway for pupillary contraction, Brain, 65:343, 1942.

Neilson, J. M.: *Memory and Amnesia,* San Lucas Press, Los Angeles, Calif., 1958.

Netter, F. H.: *The Central Nervous System,* Ciba Pharmaceutical Products, Summit, N. J., 1950.

Newman, H. H.: *Vertebrate Zoology,* The Macmillan Company, New York, 1921.

Niemer, W. T., and H. W. Magoun: Reticulospinal tracts influencing motor activity, J. Comp. Neurol., 87:367, 1947.

Nulsen, F. E., S. P. W. Black, and C. G. Drake: Inhibition and facilitation of motor activity by the anterior cerebellum, Federation Proc., 7:86, 1948.

Papez, J. W.: Reticulospinal tracts in the cat. Marchi method, J. Comp. Neurol., 41:365, 1926.

Papez, J. W.: *Comparative Neurology,* Crowell-Collier Publishing Co., New York, 1929.

Papez, J. W.: A proposed mechanism of emotion, Arch. Neurol. Psychiat., 38:725, 1937.

Papez, J. W.: A summary of fiber connections of the basal ganglia with each other and with other portions of the brain, Research Publs., Assoc. Nervous Mental Disease, 21:21, 1942.

Papez, J. W., and W. A. Stotler: Connections of the red nucleus, Arch. Neurol. Psychiat., 44:776, 1940.

Parker, H. L.: *Clinical Studies in Neurology,* Charles C Thomas, Springfield, Ill., 1956.

Patten, B. M.: *Human Embryology,* 2d ed., McGraw-Hill Book Company, Inc., Blakiston Division, New York, 1953.

Patton, H. D., and T. C. Rugh: The relation of the foot of the pre- and postcentral gyrus to taste in the monkey and chimpanzee, Federation Proc., 5:79, 1946.

Peck, S. R.: *Atlas of Human Anatomy for the Artist,* Oxford University Press, New York, 1956.

Peele, T. L.: Cytoarchitecture of individual parietal areas in the monkey and the distribution of efferent fibers, J. Comp. Neurol., 77:693, 1942.

Peele, T. L.: *The Neuroanatomical Basis for Clinical Neurology,* McGraw-Hill Book Company, Inc., Blakiston Division, New York, 1954.

Penfield, W.: The cerebral cortex and consciousness, Harvey Lectures, 32:35, 1936.

Penfield, W.: Some observations on the cerebral cortex of man, Proc. Roy. Soc., London, B., 134:329, 1947.

Penfield, W.: Symposium on gyrectomy. Part I. Bilateral frontal gyrectomy and postoperative intelligence, Research Publs., Assoc. Nervous Mental Disease, 27:519, 1948.

Penfield, W., and E. Boldrey: Somatic motor and sensory representation in the cerebral cortex of man as studied by electrical stimulation, Brain, 60:389, 1937.

Penfield, W., and T. C. Erickson: *Epilepsy and Cerebral Localization. A study of the Mechanism, Treatment and Prevention of Epileptic Seizures,* Charles C Thomas, Publisher, Springfield, Ill., 1941.

Penfield, W., and J. P. Evans: Functional defects produced by cerebral lobectomies, Research

Publs., Assoc. Nervous Mental Disease, 13:352, 1934.

Penfield, W., and T. Rasmussen: Vocalization and arrest of speech, Arch. Neurol. Psychiat., 61:21, 1949.

Penfield, W., and T. Rasmussen: *The Cerebral Cortex of Man. A Clinical Study of Localization of Function,* The Macmillan Company, New York, 1950.

Petr, R., L. B. Holden, and J. Jirout: The efferent intercortical connections of the superficial cortex of the temporal lobe, J. Neuropathol. Exptl. Neurol., 8:100, 1949.

Pitts, R. F.: The respiratory center and its descending pathways, J. Comp. Neurol., 72:605, 1940.

Polyac, S. L.: *The Retina,* University of Chicago Press, Chicago, 1941.

Putnam, T. J.: Studies on the central visual system. IV. The details of the organization of the geniculostriate system in man, Arch. Neurol. Psychiat., 16:638, 1926.

Ranson, S. W.: Regulation of body temperature, Research Publs., Assoc. Nervous Mental Disease, 20:342, 1940.

Ranson, S. W., and P. R. Billingsley: Afferent spinal paths and the vasomotor reflexes. Studies in the vasomotor reflex arcs IV, Am. J. Physiol., 42:16, 1916.

Ranson, S. W., and S. L. Clark: *The Anatomy of the Nervous System,* 10th ed., W. B. Saunders Company, Philadelphia, 1959.

Ranson, S. W., and H. W. Magoun: The hypothalamus, Ergeb. Physiol., biol. Chem. u. exptl. Pharmakol., 41:56, 1939.

Ranson, S. W., and S. W. Ranson, Jr.: Efferent fibers of the corpus striatum, Research Publs., Assoc. Nervous Mental Disease, 21:69, 1942.

Rasmussen, A. T.: *The Principal Nervous Pathways,* 4th ed., The Macmillan Company, New York, 1952.

Rasmussen, A. T., and W. T. Peyton: The location of the lateral spinothalamic tract in the brain stem of man, Surgery, 10:699, 1941.

Rasmussen, A. T., and W. T. Peyton: The course and termination of the medial lemniscus in man, J. Comp. Neurol., 88:411, 1948.

Rasmussen, G. L.: The olivary peduncle and other projections of the superior olivary complex, J. Comp. Neurol., 84:141, 1946.

Rasmussen, G. L.: Further observations on the termination of the efferent cochlear bundle, Anat. Rec. 106:69–78, 1950.

Rasmussen, G. L.: Further observations of the efferent cochlear bundle, J. Comp. Neurol. 99: 61–74, 1953.

Ray, B. S., J. C. Hinsey, and W. A. Geohegan: Observations on the distribution of the sympathetic nerves to the pupil and upper extremity as determined by stimulation of anterior roots in man, Ann. Surg., 118:647, 1943.

Rhines, R., and H. W. Magoun: Brain stem facilitation of cortical motor response, J. Neurophysiol., 9:219, 1946.

Richardson, K. C.: The fine structure of the albino rabbit iris with special reference to the identification of adrenergic and cholinergic nerves and nerve endings in its intrinsic muscles, Am. J. Anat., 114:173–184, 1964.

Riley, H. A.: *An Atlas of the Basal Ganglia, Brain Stem and Spinal Cord,* The Williams & Wilkins Company, Baltimore, 1943.

Robinson, M. F., W. Freeman, and J. W. Watts: Personality changes after psychosurgery, Dig. Neurol. Psychiat., Inst. Living, 17:558, 1949.

Rose, J. E., and C. N. Woolsey: Organization of the mammalian thalamus and its relationship to the cerebral cortex, Electroencephalog. and Clin. Neurophysiol., 1:391, 1949.

Rouvière, H.: *Atlas aide-mémoire d'anatomie,* Masson et Cie, Paris, 1947.

Rylander, G.: Personality analysis before and after frontal lobotomy, Research Publs., Assoc. Nervous Mental Disease, 27:691, 1948.

Sachs, E., Jr., S. J. Brendler, and J. F. Fulton: The orbital gyri, Brain, 72:227, 1949.

Saunders, R. L. de C. H., W. H. Feindel, and V. R. Carvalho: X-ray microscopy of the blood vessels of the human brain, Part I, Medical and Biological Illustration, 15:108–122, 1965.

Saunders, R. L. de C. H., W. H. Feindel, and V. R. Carvalho: X-ray microscopy of the blood vessels of the human brain, Part II, Medical and Biological Illustration, 15:234–246, 1965.

Scarff, J. F.: Primary cortical centers for movements of upper and lower extremity in man; observations based on electrical stimulation, Arch. Neurol. Psychiat., 44:243, 1940.

Schreiner, L. H., D. B. Lindsey, and H. W. Magoun: Role of the brain stem facilitatory systems in the maintenance of spasticity, J. Neurophysiol., 12:207, 1949.

Schwartz, H. G., and G. Weddell: Observations on the pathways transmitting the sensation of taste, Brain, 61:99, 1938.

Seddon, H. J., P. B. Medawar, and H. Smith: Rate of regeneration of peripheral nerves in man, J. Physiol., 102:191, 1943.

Seletz, E.: *Surgery of Peripheral Nerves,* Charles C Thomas, Publisher, Springfield, Ill., 1951.

Shapiro, H. H.: *Maxillofacial Anatomy,* J. B. Lippincott Company, Philadelphia, 1954.

Sheehan, D.: The autonomic nervous system, Ann. Rev. Physiol., 3:399, 1941.

Sheps, J. G.: The nuclear configuration and cortical connections of the human thalamus, J. Comp. Neurol., 83:1, 1945.

Schaeffer, J. P. (ed.): *Morris' Human Anatomy,* 11th ed., McGraw-Hill Book Company, Inc., Blakiston Division, New York, 1953.

Sloan, N., and H. Jasper: Studies on the regulatory functions of the anterior limbic cortex, Electroencephalog. and Clin. Neurophysiol., 2:317, 1950.

Smith, W. K.: The functional significance of the rostral cingular cortex as revealed by its responses to electrical excitation, J. Neurophysiol., 8:241, 1945.

Smyth, G. E.: The systematization and central connections of the spinal tract and nucleus of the trigeminal nerve, Brain, 62:41, 1939.

Snider, R. S., W. S. McCulloch, and H. W. Magoun: A cerebello-bulboreticular pathway for suppression, J. Neurophysiol., 12:325, 1949.

Snider, R. S., H. W. Magoun, and W. S. McCulloch: A suppressor cerebello-bulbo-reticular pathway from the anterior lobe and paramedian lobules, Federation Proc., 6:207, 1947.

Spalteholz, W.: *Hand-atlas of Human Anatomy,* 7th ed., vol. 3, J. B. Lippincott Company, Philadelphia, 1955.

Spiegel, E. A.: Labyrinth and cortex. Electroencephalogram in stimulation of the labyrinth, Arch. Neurol. Psychiat., 31:469, 1934.

Spiegel, E. A., and I. Sommer: *Neurology of the Eye, Ear, Nose and Throat,* Grune & Stratton, New York, 1944.

Spofford, W. R.: *Neuroanatomy,* Oxford University Press, New York, 1942.

Starzl, T. E., and H. W. Magoun: Organization of the diffuse thalamic projection system, J. Neurophysiol., 14:133, 1951.

Streeter, G. L.: Factors involved in the formation of the filum terminale, Am. J. Anat., 25:1, 1919.

Strong, O. S., and A. Elwyn: *Human Neuroanatomy,* 5th ed., The Williams & Wilkins Company, Baltimore, 1964.

Sugar, O., L. V. Amador, and B. Griponissiotes: Corticocortical connections of the walls of the superior temporal sulcus in the monkey, J. Neuropathol. Exptl. Neurol., 9:179, 1950.

Sugar, O., J. D. French, and J. G. Chusid: Corticocortical connections of the superior surface of the temporal operculum in the monkey, J. Neurophysiol., 11:175, 1948.

Sugar, O., R. Petr, L. V. Amador, and B. Griponissiotes: Corticocortical connections of the cortex buried in intraparietal and principal sulci of monkey, J. Neuropathol. Exptl. Neurol., 9:430, 1950.

Sunderland, S.: The projection of the cerebral cortex on the pons and cerebellum in the macaque monkey, J. Anat., 74:201, 1940.

Taylor, E. W.: *Case Histories in Neurology,* W. M. Leonard, Boston, 1912.

Testut, L., and A. Latarjet: *Traité d'anatomie humaine,* vols. II & III, G. Doin & Cie, Paris, 1948, 1949.

Thorek, P.: *Anatomy in Surgery,* J. B. Lippincott Company, Philadelphia, 1956.

Tilney, F.: *The Brain, from Ape to Man,* Paul B. Hoeber, Inc., New York, 1928.

Tilney, F., and L. F. Warren: A contribution to the study of the epiphysis cerebri with an interpretation of the morphological, physiological and clinical evidence, Am. J. Anat. Memoirs. No. 9:7, 1919.

Toldt, C.: *An Atlas of Human Anatomy,* 2d ed., The Macmillan Company, New York, 1928.

Tongray, J. E., and W. J. S. Kreig: The nuclei of the human thalamus. A comparative approach, J. Comp. Neurol., 85:421, 1946.

Tower, S. S.: The pyramidal tract, in *The Precentral Motor Cortex,* 2d ed., by P. C. Bucy (ed.), University of Illinois Press, Urbana, Ill., 1949.

Villiger, E.: *Brain and Spinal Cord,* McGraw-Hill Book Company, Inc., Blakiston Division, New York, 1918.

Vonderahe, A. R.: Anatomic basis of emotion, Ohio State Med. J., 39:325, 1943.

Walker, A. E.: *The Primate Thalamus,* University of Chicago Press, Chicago, 1938.

Walker, A. E.: The spinothalamic tract in man, Arch. Neurol. Exptl. Psychiat., 43:284, 1940.

Walshe, F. M. R.: The giant cells of Betz, the motor cortex and the pyramidal tract: a critical review, Brain, 65:409, 1942.

Walzl, E. M., and V. Mountcastle: Projection of vestibular nerve to cerebral cortex of the cat, Am. J. Physiol., 159:595, 1949.

Ward, A. A., Jr.: The cingular gyrus: area 24, J. Neurophysiol., 11:13, 1948.

Ward, A. A., Jr.: The cingulate gyrus and personality, Research Publs., Assoc. Nervous Mental Disease, 27:438, 1948.

Ward, A. A., Jr., and W. S. McCulloch: The projection of the frontal lobe on the hypothalamus, J. Neurophysiol., 10:309, 1947.

Ward, A. A., Jr., J. K. Peden, and O. Sugar: Corticocortical connections in the monkey with special reference to area 6, J. Neurophysiol., 9:453, 1946.

Ward, J. W., and V. LeQuire: Responses elicited by electrical stimulation of the gyrus cinguli in unanaesthetized cats, Anat. Record, 106:91, 1950.

Wechsler, I. S.: *A Textbook of Clinical Neurology,* 6th ed., W. B. Saunders Company, Philadelphia, 1947.

Weddell, G., J. A. Harpman, D. G. Lambley, and L. Young: The innervation of the musculature of the tongue, J. Anat., 74:255, 1940.

White, J. C., R. H. Smithwick, and F. A. Simeone: *The Autonomic Nervous System,* 3d ed., The Macmillan Company, New York, 1952.

Whittier, J. R., and F. A. Mettler: Studies on the subthalamus of the Rhesus monkey. I. Anatomy and fiber connections of the subthalamic nucleus of Luys, J. Comp. Neurol., 90:281, 1949.

Whittier, J. R., and F. A. Mettler: Studies on the subthalamus of the Rhesus monkey. II. Hyperkinesia and other physiologic effects of subthalamic lesions, with special reference to the subthalamic nucleus of Luys, J. Comp. Neurol., 90:319, 1949.

Williams, J. F.: *A Textbook of Anatomy and Physiology,* 2d ed., W. B. Saunders Company, Philadelphia, 1928.

Woerdeman, M. W.: *Atlas of Human Anatomy,* McGraw-Hill Book Company, Inc., Blakiston Division, New York, 1950.

Wolff, H. G.: *Headache and Other Head Pain,* Oxford University Press, New York, 1948.

Woodburne, R. T., E. C. Crosby, and R. E. McCotter: The mammalian midbrain and isthmus regions. Part II. The fiber connections. A. The relations of the tegmentum of the midbrain with the basal ganglia in *Macaca mulatta,* J. Comp. Neurol., 85:67, 1946.

Yacorzynski, G. K., and L. Davis: An experimental study of the functions of the frontal lobes in man, Psychosomat. Med., 7:97, 1945.

INDEX